VOLUME EIGHTY-THREE

VITAMINS AND HORMONES

Pheromones

VOLUME EIGHTY-THREE

VITAMINS AND HORMONES

Pheromones

Editor-in-Chief

GERALD LITWACK

Chair, Department of Basic Sciences
The Commonwealth Medical College
Scranton, Pennsylvania

ELSEVIER

AMSTERDAM • BOSTON • HEIDELBERG • LONDON
NEW YORK • OXFORD • PARIS • SAN DIEGO
SAN FRANCISCO • SINGAPORE • SYDNEY • TOKYO
Academic Press is an imprint of Elsevier

Cover photo credit:
Pikielny, C.W. *Drosophila* CheB proteins involved in gustatory detection of pheromones are related to a human neurodegeneration factor. *Vitamins and Hormones* (2010) **83,** pp. 273–288.

Academic Press is an imprint of Elsevier
32 Jamestown Road, London, NW1 7BY, UK
Radarweg 29, PO Box 211, 1000 AE Amsterdam, The Netherlands
Linacre House, Jordan Hill, Oxford OX2 8DP, UK
30 Corporate Drive, Suite 400, Burlington, MA 01803, USA
525 B Street, Suite 1900, San Diego, CA 92101-4495, USA

First edition 2010

ISBN: 978-0-12-381516-3
ISSN: 0083-6729

For information on all Academic Press publications
visit our website at elsevierdirect.com

Printed and bound by CPI Group (UK) Ltd, Croydon, CR0 4YY

Transferred to digital print 2013

10 11 12 10 9 8 7 6 5 4 3 2 1

Contents

Contributors

C. Alaux
INRA, UMR 406 Abeilles et Environnement, Site Agroparc, Domaine Saint-Paul, Avignon, France

Julie Bakker
Neuroendocrinologie du Comportement, GIGA-Neurosciences, University of Liège, Belgium, and Netherlands Institute for Neuroscience, Amsterdam, The Netherlands, and Medical Center, Vrije Universiteit, Amsterdam, The Netherlands

Warrick J. Brewer
ORYGEN Youth Health Research Centre, Centre for Youth Mental Health, University of Melbourne, Victoria, Australia

Bruschini Claudia
Dipartimento di Biologia Evoluzionistica, Università degli Studi di Firenze, Firenze, Italy

Ana Maria Costa-Leonardo
Departamento de Biologia, Instituto de Biociências, Unesp—Univ Estadual Paulista, CEP 13506–900, Rio Claro—SP, Brasil

Sarah Y. Dewhirst
Biological Chemistry Department, Rothamsted Research, Harpenden, Herts, United Kingdom

Gabriela González-Mariscal
Centro de Investigación en Reproducción Animal, CINVESTAV-Universidad Autónoma de Tlaxcala, Tlaxcala, Tlax., México

David R. Grattan
Centre for Neuroendocrinology and Department of Anatomy and Structural Biology, University of Otago, Dunedin, New Zealand

Angel Guerrero
Department of Biological Chemistry and Molecular Modeling, Institute of Advanced Chemistry of Catalonia (CSIC), Barcelona, Spain

Nicolás Gutiérrez-Castellanos
Laboratori de Neurobiologia Funcional i Comparada, Departament de Biologia Cel·lular i Parasitologia, Facultat de Ciències Biològiques, Universitat de València, Dr. Moliner, 50, Burjassot, València, Spain

Ives Haifig
Departamento de Biologia, Instituto de Biociências, Unesp—Univ Estadual Paulista, CEP 13506–900, Rio Claro—SP, Brasil

John D. Harder
Department of Evolution, Ecology, and Organismal Biology, The Ohio State University, Columbus, Ohio

Jim Hardie
Department of Life Sciences, Imperial College London, Silwood Park campus, Ascot, Berkshire, United Kingdom

Eric Haubruge
Department of Functional and Evolutionary Entomology, Gembloux Agro-Bio Tech, Liege University, Gembloux, Belgium

Jan Havlicek
Department of Anthropology, Faculty of Humanities, Charles University, Prague, Czech Republic

J. Joe Hull
Molecular Entomology Laboratory, RIKEN Advanced Science Institute, Wako, Saitama, Japan, and USDA-ARS Arid Land Agricultural Research Center, 21881 N Cardon Lane, Maricopa, Arizona, USA

Leslie M. Jackson
Department of Evolution, Ecology, and Organismal Biology, The Ohio State University, Columbus, Ohio

Matthieu Keller
INRA, UMR 85 Physiologie de la Reproduction et des Comportements, Nouzilly, France, and CNRS, UMR 6175, Nouzilly, France, and Université François Rabelais de Tours, Tours, France

Kirill Kiselyov
Department of Biological Sciences, University of Pittsburgh, Pittsburgh, Pennsylvania, USA

Enrique Lanuza
Laboratori de Neurobiologia Funcional i Comparada, Departament de Biologia Cel·lular i Parasitologia, Facultat de Ciències Biològiques, Universitat de València, Dr. Moliner, 50, Burjassot, València, Spain

Caroline M. Larsen
Centre for Neuroendocrinology and Department of Anatomy and Structural Biology, University of Otago, Dunedin, New Zealand

Y. Le Conte
INRA, UMR 406 Abeilles et Environnement, Site Agroparc, Domaine Saint-Paul, Avignon, France

Luc Leblanc
Department of Plant Environmental Protection Science, University of Hawaii, Honolulu, Hawaii, USA

Jae Min Lee
Molecular Entomology Laboratory, RIKEN Advanced Science Institute, Wako, Saitama, Japan

Johan N. Lundström
Monell Chemical Senses Center, Philadelphia, Pennsylvania, USA, and Department of Psychology, University of Pennsylvania, Pennsylvania, USA, and Section of Psychology, Department of Clinical Neuroscience, Karolinska Institute, Stockholm, Sweden

A. Maisonnasse
INRA, UMR 406 Abeilles et Environnement, Site Agroparc, Domaine Saint-Paul, Avignon, France

Fernando Martínez-García
Laboratori de Neurobiologia Funcional i Comparada, Departament de Biologia Funcional i Antropologia Física, Facultat de Ciències Biològiques, Universitat de València, Dr. Moliner, 50, Burjassot, València, Spain

Alino Martínez-Marcos
Laboratorio de Neuroanatomía Humana, Departamento de Ciencias Médicas, Facultad de Medicina, Centro Regional de Investigaciones Biomédicas, Universidad de Castilla-La Mancha, Albacete, Spain, and Fac. Medicina Ciudad Real (UCLM). Avda. MOledores S/N. 13071 Ciudad Real

Shogo Matsumoto
Molecular Entomology Laboratory, RIKEN Advanced Science Institute, Wako, Saitama, Japan

Angel I. Melo
Centro de Investigación en Reproducción Animal, CINVESTAV-Universidad Autónoma de Tlaxcala, Tlaxcala, Tlax., México

Mark C. Mescher
Department of Entomology, Center for Chemical Ecology, The Pennsylvania State University, University Park, Pennsylvania, USA

Alice K. Murray
School of Biological Sciences, University of Liverpool, Liverpool, UK

Atsushi Ohnishi
Molecular Entomology Laboratory, RIKEN Advanced Science Institute, Wako, Saitama, Japan

Mats J. Olsson
Section of Psychology, Department of Clinical Neuroscience, Karolinska Institute, Stockholm, Sweden

Christos Pantelis
Melbourne Neuropsychiatry Centre, Department of Psychiatry, University of Melbourne, Victoria, Australia

Randen L. Patterson
Department of Biology, and Center for Computational Proteomics, The Pennsylvania State University, University Park, Pennsylvania, USA

Jaime C. Piñero
Department of Plant Environmental Protection Science, University of Hawaii, Honolulu, Hawaii, USA, and Cooperative Research and Extension, Lincoln University of Missouri, Jefferson City, Missouri, USA

John A. Pickett
Biological Chemistry Department, Rothamsted Research, Harpenden, Herts, United Kingdom

Claudio W. Pikielny
Department of Genetics and Neuroscience Center, Dartmouth Medical School, Hanover, New Hampshire, USA

Delphine Pillon
INRA, UMR 85 Physiologie de la Reproduction et des Comportements, Nouzilly, France, and CNRS, UMR 6175, Nouzilly, France, and Université François Rabelais de Tours, Tours, France

Gadi V. P. Reddy
Western Pacific Tropical Research Center, College of Natural and Applied Sciences, University of Guam, Mangilao, Guam, USA

Cervo Rita
Dipartimento di Biologia Evoluzionistica, Università degli Studi di Firenze, Firenze, Italy

S. Craig Roberts
School of Biological Sciences, University of Liverpool, Liverpool, UK

Liangyou Rui
Department of Molecular & Integrative Physiology, University of Michigan Medical School, Ann Arbor, Michigan, USA

Tamsin K. Saxton
Philosophy, Psychology and Language Sciences, University of Edinburgh, Edinburgh, UK

Benoist Schaal
Research Group in Developmental Ethology and Cognitive Psychology, Center for Taste and Smell Science, CNRS, Dijon, France

Mark J. T. Sergeant
Division of Psychology, Nottingham Trent University, Nottingham, United Kingdom

T. Seenivasagan
Defence Research & Development Establishment, Ministry of Defence, Government of India, Jhansi Road, Gwalior-474 002, MP, India

Todd E. Shelly
USDA-APHIS, Waimanalo, Hawaii, USA

Turillazzi Stefano
Dipartimento di Biologia Evoluzionistica, Università degli Studi di Firenze, Firenze, Italy, and Centro Interdipartimentale di Spettrometria di Massa (C.I.S.M.), Università degli Studi di Firenze, Firenze, Italy

Stefano Vaglio
Laboratory of Anthropology, Department of Evolutionary Biology "Leo Pardi," University of Florence, Florence, Italy

Damian B. van Rossum
Department of Biology, and Center for Computational Proteomics, The Pennsylvania State University, University Park, Pennsylvania, USA

Roger I. Vargas
U.S. Pacific Basin Agricultural Research Center, USDA, ARS, Hilo, Hawaii, USA

François J. Verheggen
Department of Functional and Evolutionary Entomology, Gembloux Agro-Bio Tech, Liege University, Gembloux, Belgium

R. Vijayaraghavan
Defence Research & Development Establishment, Ministry of Defence, Government of India, Jhansi Road, Gwalior-474 002, MP, India

Jing-Jiang Zhou
Centre for Sustainable Pest and Disease Management, Insect Molecular Biology Group, Biological Chemistry Division, Rothamsted Research, Harpenden, UK

Yingjiang Zhou
Department of Molecular & Integrative Physiology, University of Michigan Medical School, Ann Arbor, Michigan, USA

PREFACE

Pheromones are chemical substances generated by an individual that can affect another individual. The sensing individual may respond by some kind of specific response varying from alarm reactions to sexual behavior and to specific types of behavior in lower forms. The phenomenology of pheromones is particularly well documented for insects. Pheromone chemicals vary considerably from specie to specie. In this volume are reviewed many of the types of pheromones and their actions.

The volume opens with reviews of a more general nature and those that apply to humans in some cases. The first chapter deals with "Functional Neuronal Processing of Human Body Odors" by J. N. Lundstrom and M. J. Olsson. "Female Perception of Male Body Odor" is contributed by M. J. T. Sergeant. This is followed by "Current Issues in the Study of Androstenes in Human Chemosignalling" by J. Havlicek, A. K. Murray, T. K. Saxton, and S. C. Roberts. B. Schaal discusses "Mammary Odor Cues and Pheromones: Mammalian Infant-directed Communication about Maternal State, Mammae, and Milk." C. M. Larsen and D. R. Grattan describe "Exposure to Female Pheromones during Pregnancy causes Postpartum Anxiety in Mice." "Major Urinary Protein Regulation of Chemical Communication and Nutrient Metabolism" is reviewed by Y. Zhou and L. Rui. "Chemosensory Function of the Amygdala" is recorded by N. Gutierrez-Castellanos, A. Martinez-Marcos, F. Martinez-Garcia, and E. Lanuza. K. Kiselyov, D. B. van Rossum, and R. L. Patterson report on "TRPC Channels in Pheromone Sensing." "Alarm Pheromones: Chemical Signaling in Response to Danger" is the topic of F. J. Verheggen, E. Haubruge, and M. C. Mescher. Jiang-Jing Zhou describes "Odorant Binding Proteins in Insects" and C. W. Pikielny writes on "*Drosophila* CheB Proteins Involved in Gustatory Detection of Pheromones are Related to a Human Neurodegeneration Factor." S. Vaglio reports on "Volatile Signals During Pregnancy" and "Olfactory Sensitivity: Functioning in Schizophrenia and Implications for Understanding the Nature and Progression of Psychosis." This is followed by "Olfactory Systems in Mate Recognition and Sexual behavior" by M. Keller, D. Pillon, and J. Bakker. The last two chapters in this introductory section are those of A. I. Melo and G. Gonzalez-Mariscal on "Communication by Olfactory Signals in Rabbits: its Role in Reproduction" and "Chemical Communication and Reproduction in the Gray Short-tailed Opossum" (*Monodelphis domestica*) by J. D. Harder and L. M. Jackson.

A major topic in the discussion of pheromones is the information about lower forms, especially in the insect world. This is the area where a great deal of work has been done. To begin this topic, C. Alaux, A. Maisonnasse, and Y. Le Conte report on "Pheromones in a Superorganism: from Gene to Social Regulation." "Unraveling the Pheromone Biosynthesis activating Neuropeptide (PBAN) Signal Transduction Cascade that Regulates Sex Pheromone Production in Moths" is the subject of S. Matsumoto, A. Ohnishi, J. M. Lee, and J. J. Hull. C. Bruschini, R. Cervo, and S. Turillazzi elaborate on "The Pheromones in Social Wasps." G. V. P. Reddy and A. Guerrero introduce "New Pheromones and Insect Control Strategies." "Pheromones and Exocrine Glands in Isoptera" is reported by A. M. Costa-Leonardo and I. Haifig. W. S., Dewhirst, J. A. Pickett, and J. Hardie review "Aphid Pheromones." Then, R.I. Vargas, T. E. Shelly, L. Leblanc, and J. C. Pinero write about "Methyl Eugenol, Cue-Lure and Fruit Flies." T. Seenivasagan and R. Vijayaraghavan conclude this section with "Oviposition Pheromones in Haematophagous Insects."

Narmada Thangavelu of Elsevier helped in the process of completing this volume.

The scheme on the cover is reproduced from Figure 6 of the contribution by C. W. Pikielny entitled: "Drosophila CheB Proteins Involved in Gustatory Detection of Pheromones are Related to a Human Neurodegeneration Factor."

Gerald Litwack
April 13, 2010

CHAPTER ONE

Functional Neuronal Processing of Human Body Odors

Johan N. Lundström*,†,‡ and Mats J. Olsson‡

Contents

Abstract

Body odors carry informational cues of great importance for individuals across a wide range of species, and signals hidden within the body odor cocktail are known to regulate several key behaviors in animals. For a long time, the notion that humans may be among these species has been dismissed. We now know, however, that each human has a unique odor signature that carries information related to his or her genetic makeup, as well as information about personal environmental variables, such as diet and hygiene. Although a substantial number of studies have investigated the behavioral effects of body odors, only a handful have studied central processing. Recent studies have, however, demonstrated that the human brain responds to fear signals hidden within the body odor cocktail, is able to extract kin specific signals, and processes body odors differently than other perceptually similar odors. In this chapter, we provide an overview of the current knowledge of how the human brain processes body odors and the potential importance these signals have for us in everyday life.

* Monell Chemical Senses Center, Philadelphia, Pennsylvania, USA
† Department of Psychology, University of Pennsylvania, Pennsylvania, USA
‡ Section of Psychology, Department of Clinical Neuroscience, Karolinska Institute, Stockholm, Sweden

Vitamins and Hormones, Volume 83
ISSN 0083-6729, DOI: 10.1016/S0083-6729(10)83001-8

I. The Microsmatic Fallacy

Body odors carry information of great importance for individuals across a wide variety of species. That humans may be among these species has been, for a long time, dismissed outright. We now know, however, that each human has a unique odor signature that carries information related to his or her genetic makeup (Kwak *et al.*, 2010), as well as information about personal environmental variables, such as diet and hygiene (Havlicek and Lenochova, 2006; Penn and Potts, 1998b). Moreover, much like our fellow animals, humans seem to have the ability to extract biological and social cues from conspecific body odors (i.e., originating from the same species), and respond to those cues. Although the available literature on the central processing of human body odors (endogenous odors) has grown greatly of late, our understanding of this phenomenon is still dispersed and incomplete in many ways, and we recognize that, as a result of these knowledge gaps, some of the arguments we make in this overview are speculative. Nonetheless, it is our hope that this review identifies the important aspects of how the human brain processes body odors, and that this chapter will stimulate future discussions and research.

One long-standing view propagated in scientific and popular scientific literature and accepted by scientists and laymen alike is that the olfactory system plays a subordinate or unimportant role in human social lives. In reality, the US market alone spent more than $25 billion in 2001 on scented products in an effort to eliminate, hide, or enhance natural human body odors (Gilbert and Firestein, 2002). This directly contradicts the general view that the olfactory sense is in any way "residual" or subordinate to the other human sensory systems. The notion that humans do not use their sense of smell in everyday life can, arguably, be traced back (Schaal and Porter, 1991) to the writings of the French anatomist Pierre Paul Broca (1824–1880). Broca, best known for his discovery of the speech processing area subsequently named after him, labeled mammals as either microsmatic or macrosmatic entirely on the basis of the relative sizes of their olfactory systems and how important a role the olfactory system plays in their daily lives (Broca, 1888). Microsmatic animals, according to Broca's description, pay little attention to odors in their daily lives and possess an olfactory apparatus with little-to-no functional capacity. Humans were grouped with the microsmatic species on the basis of the small size of their olfactory system relative to those of other species. How Broca went about characterizing the size of the human olfactory system is not known, but we can likely assume that guessing played at least some part in his estimations. More recently, modern genetic techniques have demonstrated that mankind has more pseudo-olfactory genes than other comparative species, often taken as supportive evidence for Broca's notion (Glusman *et al.*, 2001; Rouquier *et al.*, 2000; Young *et al.*, 2002). However, comparative psychophysical studies of the olfactory function of humans and other species have demonstrated that olfactory performance is not directly correlated with the anatomical size of olfactory structures and the percentage of expressed olfactory genes (Laska and Freyer, 1997; Laska and Teubner, 1998; Laska *et al.*, 1999, 2005). Rather, olfactory performance appears to be dependent on the relevance of the message conveyed by a given odorant to an individual perceiving that odorant (Laska *et al.*, 2005). Together with recent advances in the scientific field of olfaction, these findings directly contradict Broca's influential but flawed notion of microsmatic humans and support the much different conclusion that odors exert a significant impact on a range of human behaviors.

II. Human Body Odor Perception and Production

The conscious percept, or mental impression, of a body odor often contains an emotional component that evokes polarized responses of strong like or dislike. For many of us, the two words "body odor" are sufficient to trigger an unpleasant percept related to heavy perspiration. Simple though that seems, the perception of body odor is multifaceted and more complex than a straightforward aversion to gym odor. Consider, for example, that the body odor of your lover may be a very pleasant percept, whereas the body odor of the person sitting next to you on the bus may be highly negative. Moreover, as we discuss in detail below, there is a clear distinction between the conscious and the nonconscious perception of body odors.

The importance of body odors has been demonstrated in the conscious selection of a potential partner in that the mere percept of body odors has a negative implication for women, but not for men (Herz and Cahill, 1997; Herz and Inzlicht, 2002). In addition, the impact that biological factors have on our percept of body odors has recently been indirectly demonstrated by several experiments. Our percept of body odors is dependent on the sexual orientations of both the donor and the perceiver (Martins *et al.*, 2005), and heterosexual women's percept of men's body odor varies over their menstrual cycle (Roberts *et al.*, 2004). Body odor is consciously perceived and its perception reflects a response to a small subset of the numerous chemical compounds (approximately 120) that comprise our body odor (Labows *et al.*, 1999). In contrast, we are typically not consciously aware of perceiving the specific compounds within our body odor that may serve as social signals.

Our body odors are primarily due to the elements from skin gland excretions and bacterial activity. The human skin contains three types of exocrine glands: eccrine, sebaceous, and apocrine glands. Eccrine glands populate the entire human body and represent the dominant type of sweat gland. The principal function of eccrine glands is to cool the body, and they respond mainly to thermal stimulation. The eccrine glands produce a clear and mostly nonodorous secretion comprised of more than 90% water (Sato, 1977). The sebaceous glands are found over much of the skin surface, with regional patches of higher density, and excrete sebum, a complex lipid mixture. What type of stimulation the sebaceous glands react to has not been well defined. The apocrine glands, nicknamed the "scent glands," differ from eccrine and sebaceous glands in structure and location. The ducts of apocrine glands exit through the shafts of hair follicles and are concentrated in areas of hair growth, such as the axillary area, the aureole of nipples, and the genitalia (Wysocki and Preti, 2000). Apocrine secretions contain most of the odorless precursors for the odorants that we commonly call "body odor." These secretions are small amounts of a milky lipid- and protein-rich fluid, the release of which is regulated mainly by psychological stimuli (Schaal and Porter, 1991). At the skin surface, bacteria metabolize this mixture of excretions and produce a plethora of volatile and nonvolatile substances (Gower and Ruparelia, 1993). The fact that body odors are formed by skin glands with distinct functions that respond to distinct exogenous stimuli is an important factor in our understanding of human body odors and the behavioral reactions they elicit. In short, not all body odors are created equal.

III. Central Processing of Body Odors

The mixture of chemical compounds causing our axillary body odor carries with it information that we are able to extract and utilize. Recent studies have demonstrated that humans produce individually unique body odors (Kwak *et al.*, 2010), which enable us to identify individuals (Lundstrom and Jones-Gotman, 2009; Olsson *et al.*, 2006; Russell, 1976; Wallace, 1977) and make accurate judgments about kinship based solely on body odor composition (Lundstrom *et al.*, 2009a; Porter, 1998; Porter and Moore, 1981; Weisfeld *et al.*, 2003).

Although a substantial number of studies have investigated the behavioral effects of body odors, only a handful have studied central processing. Bettina Pause was the first to explore how the human brain processes body odors. Using EEG, a method with very good temporal, but poor spatial resolution, Dr. Pause elegantly demonstrated that the human brain is able to discriminate between body odors despite an unawareness of this ability

(Pause *et al.*, 1999, 2006). Interestingly, the human brain appears to make a distinction between body odors originating from oneself and body odors originating from someone else, in this case, a stranger. Not only does the brain seem to process one's own body odors faster (Pause *et al.*, 1999), but it also allocates more neuronal processing to the resulting neuronal computations of one's own body odors than to the processing of body odors from an unrelated individual (Pause *et al.*, 2006). It has been repeatedly demonstrated that visual signals with high ecological importance are processed in a privileged way, often by neuronal networks residing outside of the main visual system (Dimberg and Ohman, 1983; Morris *et al.*, 1999; Schupp *et al.*, 2004). The complex mixtures we refer to as body odors, like the high-priority visual stimuli, convey large amounts of ecologically important information. The richness of information conveyed and the commonality among animal species indicate that the complex chemical mixture we refer to as body odors is a stimulus of ecological importance and as such, would receive preferential treatment by the brain. Indeed, a recent study from our lab seems to corroborate this notion (Lundstrom *et al.*, 2008).

In an effort to elucidate whether body odors are processed as common odors or whether they recruit a separate network, we measured how the brain responds to human body odors of varying origin as well as a mixture of common odors perceptually indistinguishable from human body odor (Lundstrom *et al.*, 2008). When we directly compared how the brain processes *body odors* with how it processes perceptually similar *fake body odor*, thus controlling for the effects caused by the conscious percept of the body odor, we found that body odors activate an elaborate network residing outside the main olfactory system. Body odors activate four main areas: the posterior cingulate cortex, the occipital gyrus, the angular gyrus, and the anterior cingulate cortex (see Fig. 1.1).

This particular combination of cortical areas forms an interesting network. The posterior cingulate cortex (PCC) is known to regulate emotional responses and actions (Cato *et al.*, 2004; Maddock, 1999), and the anterior cingulate cortex is primarily associated with attention processing (Botvinick, *et al.*, 1999). The occipital cortex activation was located within areas of the primary visual cortex, which suggests that the neuronal processing of body odors is similar to what has been previously demonstrated for emotional visual stimuli of high ecological importance, such as pictures of spiders or snakes. For these visual images, the PCC works in conjunction with the anterior cingulate cortex to determine and process the emotional stimuli (Fredrikson *et al.*, 1995). Although these two latter cortical areas (the PCC and anterior cingulate cortex) were predicted, we cannot assign a causal relationship between them within this dataset. It is possible, however, that body odors, in comparison with common odors, receive a more or less automatic heightened attention by virtue of their signal value. Seen from an evolutionary perspective, signals carrying important information

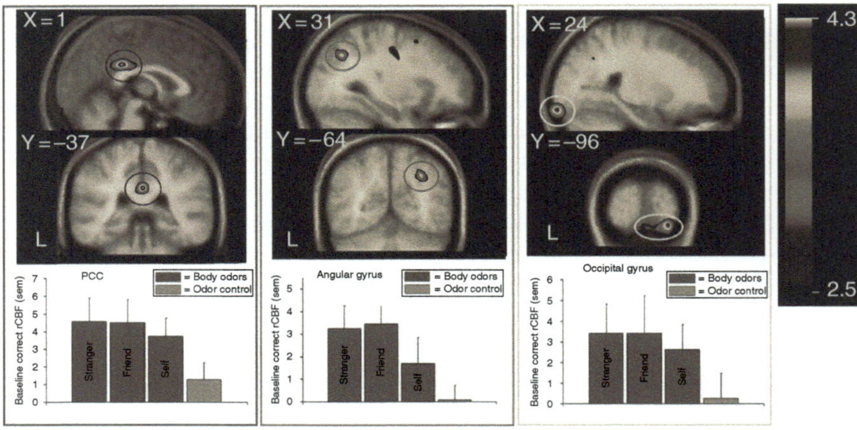

Figure 1.1 Statistical parametric maps (*t* statistics as represented by the color scale) of group averaged rCBF responses to processing of body odors superimposed on group averaged anatomical MRI. Blue circles mark increased rCBF in the posterior cingulate cortex (PCC), green circles mark increased rCBF response in the left angular gyrus, and yellow circles mark an increased rCBF response in the right occipital cortex. Coordinates denote center of activation and slice expressed according to the MNI world coordinates system. Left in upper row of pictures represents posterior and left in middle figures represents left side (L). Graphs under each statistical parametric map represent extracted baseline-corrected rCBF values within the activation peak, in each odor category. Error bars represent standard error of the mean (SEM). Reproduced with permission from Oxford University Press. (See Color Insert.)

or information related to recurrent survival threats might have been selected by evolutionary pressure to receive preferential processing, or, more specifically, direct access to areas of the brain regulating emotional and attentional processing. Such preferential processing would allow the information contained within human body odors to have a direct impact on human behavior by either affecting the saliency or directly heightening attention to specific stimuli.

Body odors also triggered a strong response in the occipital cortex, the so-called primary visual cortex. That there is a link between odor processing and visual processing has been demonstrated in a range of neuroimaging studies exploring neuronal processing of odors (Djordjevic *et al.*, 2005; Gottfried *et al.*, 2004; Royet *et al.*, 1999, 2001; Zatorre *et al.*, 2000) in the absence of visual stimulation. The combination of frequent olfactory stimulation-induced visual activations in olfactory neuroimaging studies, the absence of visual stimulation in this study, and the subjects' inability to distinguish human body odor from fake body odor stimuli suggests that visual activation is not a direct derivate of body odor processing. Moreover, a review of the aforementioned articles demonstrates no obvious common denominator that could explain the visual activation other than the presence of an olfactory stimulus. It could be speculated that the activation of the visual system is indicative of a preparedness mechanism. The presence of an odor arguably signals the imminent presence of an object, be it an individual with respect to body odors or a nice meal with respect to common odors, and the resulting cognitive mechanisms may prime or prepare the visual system for visual stimuli. Studies of the function of the angular gyrus, an area intimately connected to the creation of a visual body construct, support this theory. Disruption of the neuronal signals within this area is known to either abolish or alter how the human brain interprets the perception of its own and other individuals' bodies (Arzy *et al.*, 2006; Blanke *et al.*, 2002, 2004, 2005). Whether the angular gyrus serves as an important node in a modality-independent system for body representation remains to be demonstrated, however. The topic of cross-modal perceptual priming on a neuronal level is an emerging field where much is still to be learned, and with the emergence of high field strength MRI scanners, the future is ripe for interesting discoveries.

IV. Neuronal Processing of the Smell of Fear

Humans, like many other animals, seem to be able to identify the emotional state of a conspecific based solely on his or her body odor. A recent study collected body odor samples from individuals who watched either funny or scary movie sequences. Participants were later asked, in a forced-choice detection task, to identify the emotional state of the donors. Remarkably, participants were able to accurately identify both happy and fearful emotional odors at levels above chance value (Chen and Haviland-Jones, 2000), though they performed much better with body odor samples from fearful donors. A subsequent study replicated some of the findings reported by Chen and Haviland-Jones (2000) in that participants were able to identify a body odor as coming from a frightened individual (Ackerl *et al.*, 2002).

One can speculate that body odors originating from a fearful individual possess an inherently higher level of relevance to the perceiver, as they might signal danger in the surrounding environment (Ohman *et al.*, 2001b). In other words, given the high survival value, fearful stimuli might have been selected for, by evolution, to enjoy the benefit of an automatically higher level of attention and prioritized access to processing (Ohman and Mineka, 2001; Tooby and Cosmides, 1990). This might explain why participants seem to have an easier time identifying and discriminating the body odor sampled from a fearful individual. Interestingly, a recent study investigating the ability of body odors to modulate the acoustic startle reflex seems to support this notion (Prehn *et al.*, 2006). The acoustic startle reflex is an evoked preattentive reflex that is modulated by the affective valence and the extent to which the foreground stimulus merits attention and that is often used to investigate the emotional effect of stimuli (Dawson *et al.*, 1999; Koch, 1999). Prehn *et al.* (2006) demonstrated that body odors sampled during a state of anxiety were able to modulate the startle response, whereas body odors collected during a neutral emotional state were not. Body odors collected during a high anxiety state might thus modulate emotional processing of relevant stimuli in the surroundings (but see, Miltner *et al.*, 1994). Indeed, Chen *et al.* (2006) demonstrated that exposure to body odor samples collected during fearful stimuli rendered participants to process a fearful content in a word association task more slowly and more accurately. It might seem that the heightened accuracy in cognitive processing that fearful body odors produced is in congruence with the notion that these odors are preferentially processed or, as Chen *et al.* (2006) argue, that they modulate cognitive performance. One might, however, take the opposite stance. An instantaneous response to a fearful stimulus is at the core of fear-evoked responses (cf. Mineka and Ohman, 2002). The underlying evolution of cognition is not clear, but there is little evidence supporting the view that it emerged to enhance responses in fearful or stressful situations. Rather than carefully evaluate available options and their potential outcomes, an individual has a greater chance at survival if they are able to act instantly, with only minimal cognitive effort. Hence, the evolutionary pressure should have been on the promotion of false positive, rather than false negative errors in response to fear: the former is costly energy-wise, but the latter is potentially deadly. In other words, fearful stimuli should enhance reaction time at the cost of accuracy as previously demonstrated for fearful visual stimuli (Flykt, 2006; Ohman *et al.*, 2001a,b). Based on this, the assumption that fearful stimuli should increase accuracy and prolong the response time to lexical judgments requiring cognitive processing seems less plausible. However, in defense of the cognitive view are recent behavioral and imaging data that seem to indicate that body odor samples collected during a fearful or high emotional state are not processed in a manner similar to visual fearful stimuli, which provoke a fast and immediate response, but rather seem to modulate the cognitive evaluation or processing of relevant stimuli.

When asked to rate faces with an ambiguous emotional expression, women tend to rate them as being more fearful when exposed to body odors collected from men in a fearful state compared to body odor samples collected from men in a happy state (Zhou and Chen, 2009). Related results were obtained in a study by Mujica-Parodi *et al.* (2009), who collected body odor samples from volunteers performing a tandem parachute jump for the first time or while exercising. Exposure to the body odor samples collected during the parachute jump made the participants better at discriminating between the emotional faces presented to them. Unfortunately, neither of these two experiments reports data for response speed, thus making it impossible to infer anything about the trade-off between speed and accuracy. However, the aforementioned behavioral studies seem to indicate that body odors signaling fear or high levels of anxiety indeed modulate cognitive processing and increase accuracy of how certain salient stimuli in our surroundings are processed. This is contradictory to what is known for the processing of threatening visual stimuli, but in accordance with how the chemosensory system generally works. The speed of processing for chemosensory stimuli is significantly lower than that of visual or auditory stimuli (Wetter *et al.*, 2004). The estimated time difference between the onsets of the first perceptual and the first cognitive processing between the visual and olfactory system is as large as 200 and 400 ms, respectively (Olofsson *et al.*, 2008; Pause and Krauel, 2000). Relying on the olfactory system for early detection warning might therefore not be an optimal survival strategy for an individual, given how "slow" the brain is in processing chemosensory stimuli. However, since chemosensory stimuli are good at communicating messages over distance and remain reliable when the visual field is occluded, a good strategy would be to allow chemosensory stimuli to shape the slower and more deliberate processing rather than the initial and more rapid detection phase.

Two recent neuroimaging studies provide additional support for the notion that fear, or anxiety, can be communicated via our body odors (Mujica-Parodi *et al.*, 2009; Prehn-Kristensen *et al.*, 2009). Both studies sampled body odors from individuals undergoing a fear- or anxiety-inducing task as well as a physical exercise task as control. The aforementioned study by Mujica-Parodi *et al.* (2009) sampled body odors from individuals performing a tandem skydiving jump for their first time, whereas the study by Prehn-Kristensen *et al.* (2009) sampled body odors from individuals who were waiting for an important academic test. Although their design and analyses were quite similar, the studies produced different results. Mujica-Parodi and colleagues found that a central subcortical area, the amygdala (see Fig. 1.2), responded preferentially to the body odor sample collected during the skydiving jump when compared to the exercise sweat.

However, Prehn-Kristensen and colleagues found that a cortical network consisting of the fusiform gyrus, the insular cortex, PCC, and the precuneus responded preferentially to the anxiety sweat. Such large disparities between two studies so similar in design are, at first sight, hard to understand. However, this is an excellent example of how minor differences in the sampling of body odors have a large impact on the outcome. The body odor sampling by Mujica-Parodi *et al.* (2009), from volunteers performing a parachute tandem jump for the first time, who are presumably in a state of fear or at least very high anxiety, is quite different from the body

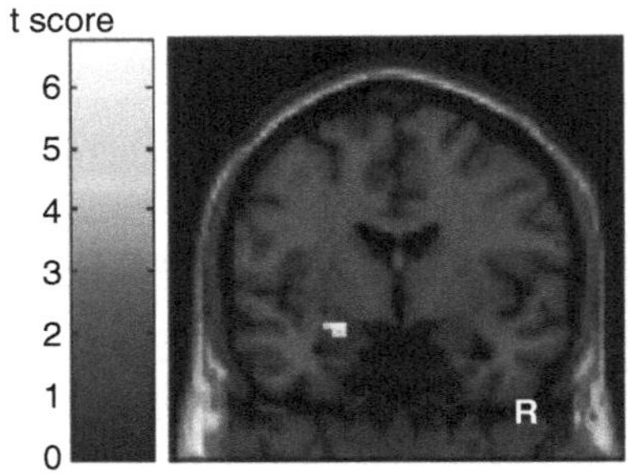

Figure 1.2 Statistical parametric maps (*t* statistics as represented by the color scale) of group averaged BOLD responses to the processing of fear-related body odors. Note the significant activation in the left amygdala. Reproduced with permission from the authors. (See Color Insert.)

odor sampled by Prehn-Kristensen *et al.* (2009), from students waiting to take an academic exam. It is probably safe to assume that jumping out of a plane would produce a more fearful state than waiting for an academic test, an act that is arguably more likely to induce high to moderately anxiety. Indeed, Mujica-Parodi and colleagues demonstrated by salivary cortisol measures that their subjects expressed at least very high levels of anxiety during the jump. The location of the main activity in the amygdala also supports the notion that it is indeed related to fear. The amygdala has repeatedly been linked to the processing of negative emotional stimuli (Morris *et al.*, 1999; Whalen *et al.*, 1998; Yamasaki *et al.*, 2002). Moreover, detection of threat-related stimuli and responses to them and other emotionally salient stimuli are mediated by the amygdala (LeDoux, 1992, 1996). However, although the amygdala is recognized as a major site of fear-plasticity (LeDoux, 2000), evidence suggests that it may not mediate feelings of fear *per se* (Dolan and Vuilleumier, 2003; LeDoux, 2000). Rather, the amygdala has been identified in all vertebrates studied to date as an important center in the identification of threats. In mice, the amygdala has been specifically identified as the main processing center of threat-related endogenous odors (Vyas *et al.*, 2007). One could postulate, therefore, that the amygdala should also be involved in the detection of threat-related olfactory stimuli in humans and not the processing of fear itself. The aforementioned study by Lundstrom *et al.* (2008) lends support to this notion. We demonstrated that smelling a stranger's body activated cerebral regions similar to those found to be active when viewing perceptually masked fearful faces (Morris *et al.*, 1998; Whalen *et al.*, 1998). Despite a low conscious recognition of the body odor's source, a marked response in the amygdala, insular, and precuneus cortex of all participating subjects was noted (see Fig. 1.3). In other words, the detection of a body odor signaling an unknown individual

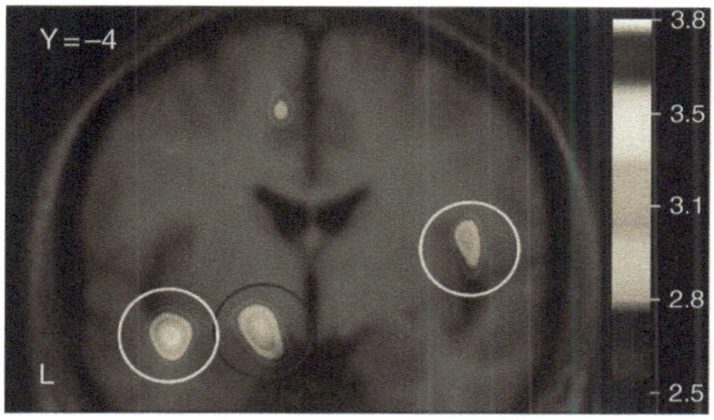

Figure 1.3 Group averaged rCBF response showed in statistical parametric map (*t* statistics as represented by the color scale) to the processing of the body odor of a stranger. Yellow circles mark bilateral increased rCBF in the insular cortex and red circles mark increased rCBF response in the amygdala. Left in figure represents left side (L). Reproduced with permission from Oxford University Press. (See Color Insert.)

(a stranger) in the near vicinity, or a body odor originating from an individual in a fearful state, could be hypothesized to act as a warning signal which would be processed by the amygdala.

Interestingly, the neuroimaging results obtained by Prehn-Kristensen and colleagues correspond to a great extent to the aforementioned results of body odor processing by Lundstrom *et al.* (2008). Activations were found in both studies within in the anterior and PCC as well as the insular and precuneus cortex. However, Prehn-Kristensen and colleagues' imaging design involved contrasting two natural body odors, whereas Lundstrom and colleagues contrasted natural body odors with a fake body odor consisting of natural odors. The control odor used in each study explains why these contrasts yield similar results.

As discussed above, body odors originate from various glandular sources and the mental and physical state of the individual has a large impact on which source is predominant at any given moment. In the samplings performed by Prehn-Kristensen and colleagues and Mujica-Parodi and colleagues, the emotional condition would have sampled predominantly from the apocrine glands and will be highly odorous while low in amount of sampled liquids. The exercise condition will sample predominantly from the eccrine glands and will have a weak odor but will also have a greater quantity of liquid. A contrast between these two conditions not only compares two emotional states, but also separates glandular excretions and two different amounts of stimulus. In the case of Prehn-Kristensen and colleagues' study, the contrast between anxiety sweat and exercise sweat would then result in cortical areas activated by sweat predominantly sampled from the apocrine glands when the perception of the body odor is controlled for, much like the design by Lundstrom *et al.* (2008). We would like to stress that this fact does not falsify or negate the obtained and published results. We are, however, arguing that the difference in the source of the body odors should be considered when interpreting the outcome. A more stringent control condition, although admittedly more cumbersome, would be to sample control body odor while participants perform a non-emotional task in the same physical state as during the experimental condition (see among others: Chen and Haviland-Jones, 1999; Chen *et al.*, 2006; Lundstrom *et al.*, 2008, 2009a). Nevertheless, the coherent message of these studies implies that humans, as do most other animals studied, have the ability to detect and process warning signals hidden within body odors. Moreover, it seems that these signals are able to modulate the cognitive processing of relevant stimuli in our surroundings. The natural human body odor consists of about 120 individual chemicals when sampled from a resting phase (Labows *et al.*, 1999). It would be of great interest to isolate which individual compound, or mixture of compounds, mediate these effects. Recent receptor studies in rodents imply that there is a single receptor transmitting these fear signals to the brain and that when it is rendered nonfunctional, the animal stops displaying fearful responses toward a natural threat odor (Kobayakawa *et al.*, 2007). It is not clear whether humans also express this receptor. If so, blocking the receptor or removing a component of the downstream pathway responsible for mitigating the warning signals might be a useful remedy in the treatment of social psychiatric disorders such as social phobia.

V. Are Body Odors Processed by the Main Olfactory System?

As discussed above, a network that is activated by body odor but unrelated to the conscious perception of a "body odor" is residing outside the main olfactory system has been identified (Lundstrom *et al.*, 2008; Prehn-Kristensen *et al.*, 2009). However, an important question left unanswered is whether body odors are processed within the common olfactory system. First, let us define what the human olfactory cortex entails. The olfactory sensory pathway starts with the receptor cells where odor molecules interact with receptors embedded in the olfactory mucosa situated on the roof of the nasal cavity. Their axons join in the olfactory nerve and project to the tufted and mitral cells of the olfactory bulb. The largest recipient of input from the olfactory bulb is the piriform cortex but only relatively recently was the greater neuronal olfactory network identified. Zatorre *et al.* (1992) were the first to outline the olfactory brain in humans. According to their findings, smelling odors result in brain activations in an area lying on the inferior junction of the frontal and temporal lobes, corresponding to the piriform cortex, and in another area in the right orbitofrontal cortex. Zatorre and colleagues proposed that these regions constitute the primary and secondary olfactory cortex, respectively. Later neuroimaging studies have verified Zatorre and colleagues' initial results. However, besides the piriform cortex, several other structures are involved in olfactory processing in various degrees. These structures include the olfactory tubercle, the periamygdaloid cortex, the anterior cortical nucleus, and the nucleus of the lateral olfactory tract of the amygdala (Carmichael *et al.*, 1994). From these set of anatomical structures receiving direct projections from the olfactory bulb, hence sometimes referred to as primary olfactory sensory areas, inputs are sent to another series of structures. These include the orbitofrontal cortex, the agranular insula, the hippocampus, the thalamus, medial and lateral hypothalamus, and ventral striatum and pallidum (Carmichael *et al.*, 1994). The region that receives the major cortico-cortical projections from the piriform cortex is the caudal orbitofrontal cortex (Carmichael *et al.*, 1994; Rolls *et al.*, 1996), and as such has traditionally been considered to constitute the secondary, or higher order, olfactory cortex. Interestingly, of the five published functional neuroimaging studies that have used intact body odor stimuli, none have reported activity within what is commonly referred to as olfactory cortex, namely the piriform cortex and the caudal orbitofrontal cortex (Lundstrom *et al.*, 2008, 2009a; Mujica-Parodi *et al.*, 2009; Prehn-Kristensen *et al.*, 2009; Zhou and Chen, 2008). In addition, if we view also minor projection areas from the olfactory bulb extending within the orbitofrontal cortex, the higher order olfactory cortex, there is only one study describing activation due to body odor perception. Zhou and Chen (2008) reports that body odors sampled while subjects were watching erotic videos activated the lateral orbitofrontal cortex. Although this area receives projections from the piriform cortex (Carmichael *et al.*, 1994), it is infrequently reported as active in olfactory neuroimaging studies. However, a recent study demonstrated that this area processes odor mixtures (Boyle *et al.*, 2008); the greater the disparity of odors within a mixture, the greater the signal within this area. Whether the results reported by Zhou and Chen (2008) are to some extent mediated by the disparity between the body odors and the single compound odor they used to contrast against, or whether the results are a result of body odor processing remains to be determined. Nevertheless, the basic fact remains that five neuroimaging studies, which have used a variety of methods and presented body odor stimuli reported as clearly perceived, have failed to activate the areas of the human brain that process common odors. One could argue that the conscious perception of body odors recruits areas outside the main olfactory system and that this mechanism is too transient to be detected by the olfactory cortices, areas with a demonstrated susceptibility to habitation effects (Poellinger *et al.*, 2001; Wilson, 2000).

Alternatively, one could argue that this is the result of the conscious trade-off made in neuroimaging analyses between risk of false positive and risk of false negative. Modern neuroimaging analyses correct only for false positive errors, whereas no correction exists for false negatives. In other words, lack of significant activity in a neuroimaging study can never be taken as evidence for the hypothesis that a specific area is not involved in the task at hand. However, the first argument can be rejected based on the clear activations in olfactory processing cortical areas for a nonendogenous control odor (fake body odor). In two studies, we presented a control odor consisting of nonendogenous components, which subjects identified as a natural body odor (Lundstrom *et al.*, 2008, 2009a). If the lack of activation in olfactory cortices is due to its cognitive processing, the same would hold for the nonendogenous control odor, which participants mistook for a natural body odor. Although statistically feasible, it is unlikely that five independent neuroimaging studies would produce five sets of similarly false negative results.

This lack of dependence on conscious awareness of the nature of the stimulus suggests that a biological model should be sought to explain the lack of noticeable processing in odor cortex. Tentative evidence for an early separation between the neuronal processing of endogenous odors and common odors can be found in the nonhuman animal literature. Two separate functional subsystems exist in the rodent olfactory system; one system is dedicated to the processing of common odors while another system produces innate responses to endogenous odors (Boehm *et al.*, 2005; Kobayakawa *et al.*, 2007). Whether body odors are processed mainly, or only, outside the main olfactory system in humans should be the focus of future studies.

As discussed above, several neuroimaging (Lundstrom *et al.*, 2008, 2009a; Prehn-Kristensen *et al.*, 2009) and behavioral results seem to be independent of conscious awareness of abilities. The ability to identify the body odors from either oneself (Lundstrom *et al.*, 2008) or one's sister (Lundstrom *et al.*, 2009a) is extremely high but participants express a very low conscious awareness. In most of the instances, although subjects are able to identify their own body odor and their sister's with 92% and 85% accuracy, respectively, subjects state that they are merely guessing. It is not clear where this disparity between the conscious estimate of one's ability to identify certain body odors and actual performance originates from. However, the anatomical organization of the olfactory pathway has one feature that is unique among our senses and might account for this discrepancy. The olfactory pathway lacks an early thalamic relay to transfer peripheral input into the brain. Whereas all the other senses project from the receptors to the brainstem and from there to the thalamus for further transfer to the primary sensory areas, the olfactory system projects directly from the receptors to the olfactory bulb and primary olfactory cortical areas (Carmichael *et al.*, 1994). The need of thalamic processing for conscious awareness was recently suggested (McAlonan *et al.*, 2008), implying that the late downstream contribution of the thalamus in olfactory processing might render it a mostly nonconscious process. The functional implications of this "negative" feature of the olfactory system remain, however, unknown (Plailly *et al.*, 2008).

VI. Kin Recognition via Body Odors

The ability to identify kin is ubiquitous among phyla and it is thought of as a vital evolutionary tool to promote one's genes by facilitating both nepotism and inbreeding avoidance (Lieberman *et al.*, 2007). It has long been known that we are able to make accurate judgments about kinship based solely on body odor composition (Lundstrom *et al.*, 2009a; Porter, 1998; Porter and Moore, 1981; Weisfeld *et al.*, 2003). The exact mediating mechanism behind kin recognition has yet to be elucidated, but it is believed that the signal within human body odors which facilitates this ability is determined by the human leukocyte antigen (HLA; in nonhuman animals, major histocompatibility complex, MHC), a highly polymorphic subset of the human genome involved in immunologic responses (Klein, 1986; Ober *et al.*, 1997; Penn *et al.*, 2002; Potts and Wakeland, 1993). The HLA is an immunologically important group of genes that regulates the discrimination of self/nonself within the immune system. The HLA has been demonstrated to be a good determinant of genetic similarity between two individuals due to being one of the most dimorphic gene complexes (Klein, 1986). Rodents have the ability to discriminate minute differences in MHC composition found in body odor, and discriminate kin and the degree of gene similarity (Beauchamp and Yamazaki, 2003; Eggert *et al.*, 1998; Hepper and Cleland, 1999; Mateo and Johnston, 2000, 2003; Yamazaki *et al.*, 2000). It is believed that the kin recognition mechanism is piggybacking on the more explored HLA/MHC-based mechanism.

The ability to discriminate very small differences in MHC composition is used in selection of mating partners where evidence suggests that the highest mating preference is for partners that are dissimilar in their genetic composition (Beauchamp and Yamazaki, 2003; Yamazaki *et al.*, 1993, 2000). Although the detailed genetic basis of this connection between MHC and mate preferences is not well understood, each individual's evolutionary drive to produce viable and fit offspring is believed to be the underlying cause (Apanius *et al.*, 1997; Penn and Potts, 1998a; Penn *et al.*, 2002). The evolutionary pressure to develop mechanisms for genetic similarity/dissimilarity judgments of potential mating partners could thus be hypothesized to be extremely high. Recent evidence promotes the idea that humans also have the ability to detect differences in HLA composition (Ober, 1999; Ober *et al.*, 1999; Sandro Carvalho Santos *et al.*, 2005; Wedekind and Furi, 1997; Weitkamp and Ober, 1999; Wedekind *et al.*, 1995).

The neuronal base for this ability was long unknown until Pause *et al.* (2006) demonstrated that the human brain is able to discriminate between minor differences in HLA composition based on EEG recordings also in the absence of a conscious awareness of this ability. However, although the likely mechanism mediating kin recognition is HLA identification, how the brain can perform this task is not known. In other animals, it has been suggested that this is done by the so-called self-recognition, or armpit mechanism (Mateo and Johnston, 2000, 2003). In other words, the animal identifies a kin by comparing the HLA/MHC composition with his or her own. Interestingly, the results from a recent neuroimaging study by Lundstrom *et al.* (2009a) support the notion that this mechanism is at play also in humans. When the cerebral activity was compared between when subjects identified the body odor of their siblings and that when they identified the body odor of a friend, that is, both were body odor stimuli but one was originating from a kin and the other from a nonkin, it was found that a neuronal network generally consistent with studies attempting to map the neuronal substrates of self-referential mental tasks was activated (Goldberg *et al.*, 2006; Gusnard *et al.*, 2001; Platek *et al.*, 2005). This suggests that kin recognition in human is based on the so-called self-referential mechanism, akin to other animals.

VII. The Stimulus Delivery Problem

The understanding of the neuronal processing of body odors is in its infancy and much remains unclear. Although there is now a substantial amount of behavioral studies investigating body odor processing, the first functional neuroimaging study of body odor processing was published as late as 2008. The reason for this scarcity is twofold. First, the field of olfactory perception, from which most researchers focusing on body odor processing originate from, is itself a small scientific field, especially in comparison with its larger siblings, the fields of visual and auditory perception. Second, the few studying body odor processing must contend with the incompatibility of chemosensory stimulus delivery and functional magnetic resonance imaging (fMRI). The technique of choice for most neuroimaging studies, fMRI boasts faster acquisition times and better resolution at a lower cost than the rival technique, positron emission tomography (PET). fMRI is based on the simple principle that the brain acts similar to any other muscle of the human body. When a muscle is working, it needs oxygen and nutrition, both of which are delivered through the bloodstream. fMRI assesses the minute differences in the degree of magnetism between oxygenized and deoxygenized hemoglobin by inducing a very strong and shifting magnetic field. Unfortunately, the high magnetic field strengths required to pick up these very weak signals make it impossible to have any ferrous metal inside the room where the scanner is located. This is not a significant problem for visual and auditory research since visual and auditory stimuli can be triggered from a distance, rapidly presented to a subject lying in the scanner, and just as rapidly removed. In contrast, chemosensory stimuli are chemical compounds whose size and density make rapid appearance and disappearance difficult. Despite this inherent difference between stimuli, olfactory stimuli must also be transported to the subject from outside the scanner and presented with a rapid onset and offset. The only way of accomplishing this is using an olfactometer (Kobal, 1981), a device capable of delivering odors in a controlled way without causing any thermal or tactile discomfort for the subject inside the scanner. Unfortunately, only a limited few are commercially available; all are limited to the presentation of liquid odorants and are therefore ill suited for the delivery of body odors. This means that the interested researcher needs to invest the time and money in building one himself or herself (Lorig *et al.*, 1999; Lundstrom *et al.*, 2009b), a task that can be daunting for many.

VIII. Conclusion

To conclude, behavioral studies using body odors as stimuli suggest that the complex mixture constituting human body odors is processed in a unique way due to the high behavioral relevance. Research suggest that endogenous chemical compounds within the body odors communicate various kinds of information that our sensory systems are able to extract and utilize. The mere fact that we are able to distinguish between individuals based solely on their body odors (Russell, 1976) and that our brains evoke differential responses to the stimulation of body odors originating from individuals with minute differences in their immunological composition demonstrates this capacity (Lundstrom and Jones-Gotman, 2009; Lundstrom *et al.*, 2009a; Pause *et al.*, 2006). What was once a divisive question in the scientific community, whether humans do use chemosignals in some form of social communication, can now be considered an undisputed statement (Beauchamp, 2000). What remains controversial is the chemical composition and appropriate label for the chemosignals themselves (cf. Beauchamp *et al.*, 1979; Doty, 2003). Specifically, whether or not humans communicate using so-called "pheromones" to communicate is still a matter of great debate. Body odor processing, however, is not an effect attributable to any specific compound, or "pheromone." A plethora of behavioral and neuroimaging data gathered from both human and nonhuman animal research strongly suggests that body odors contain signals detectable by and beneficial to conspecifics. Whether the effects of these signals are innate or learned, or whether they result from an interaction of both, is likely signal-dependant and remains to be elucidated.

ACKNOWLEDGMENTS

This work was supported by the National Institute on Deafness and other Communication Disorders—NIDCD (R03DC009869) and the Swedish Research Council—VR (2008-20712). We thank Amy R. Gordon for helpful comments and discussions.

REFERENCES

Ackerl, K., Atzmueller, M., and Grammer, K. (2002). The scent of fear. *Neuroendocrinol. Lett.* **23,** 79–84.

Apanius, V., Penn, D., Slev, P. R., Ruff, L. R., and Potts, W. K. (1997). The nature of selection on the major histocompatibility complex. *Crit. Rev. Immunol.* **17,** 179–224.

Arzy, S., Seeck, M., Ortigue, S., Spinelli, L., and Blanke, O. (2006). Induction of an illusory shadow person. *Nature* **443,** 287.

Beauchamp, G. K. (2000). *In* A perspective: Defining pheromones, The Monell Connection p. 2.

Beauchamp, G. K., and Yamazaki, K. (2003). Chemical signalling in mice. *Biochem. Soc. Trans.* **31,** 147–151.

Beauchamp, G. K., Doty, R. L., Moultan, D. G., and Mugford, R. A. (1979). Letter to the editor. *J. Chem. Ecol.* **5,** 301–305.

Blanke, O., Ortigue, S., Landis, T., and Seeck, M. (2002). Stimulating illusory own-body perceptions. *Nature* **419,** 269–270.

Blanke, O., Landis, T., Spinelli, L., and Seeck, M. (2004). Out-of-body experience and autoscopy of neurological origin. *Brain* **127,** 243–258.

Blanke, O., Mohr, C., Michel, C. M., Pascual-Leone, A., Brugger, P., Seeck, M., Landis, T., and Thut, G. (2005). Linking out-of-body experience and self processing to mental own-body imagery at the temporoparietal junction. *J. Neurosci.* **25,** 550–557.

Boehm, U., Zou, Z., and Buck, L. B. (2005). Feedback loops link odor and pheromone signaling with reproduction. *Cell* **123,** 683–695.

Botvinick, M., Nystrom, L. E., Fissell, K., Carter, C. S., and Cohen, J. D. (1999). Conflict monitoring versus selection-for-action in anterior cingulate cortex. *Nature* **402,** 179–181.

Boyle, J. A., Djordjevic, J., Olsson, M. J., Lundstrom, J. N., and Jones-Gotman, M. (2008). The human brain distinguishes between single odorants and binary mixtures. *Cereb. Cortex.* **19,** 66–71.

Broca, P. (1888). Mémoires d'Anthropologie. Reinwald, Paris.

Carmichael, S. T., Clugnet, M. C., and Price, J. L. (1994). Central olfactory connections in the macaque monkey. *J. Comp. Neurol.* **346,** 403–434.

Cato, M. A., Crosson, B., Gokcay, D., Soltysik, D., Wierenga, C., Gopinath, K., Himes, N., Belanger, H., Bauer, R. M., Fischler, I. S., Gonzalez-Rothi, L., and Briggs, R. W. (2004). Processing words with emotional connotation: An FMRI study of time course and laterality in rostral frontal and retrosplenial cortices. *J. Cogn. Neurosci.* **16,** 167–177.

Chen, D., and Haviland-Jones, J. (1999). Rapid mood change and human odors. *Physiol. Behav.* **68,** 241–250.

Chen, D., and Haviland-Jones, J. (2000). Human olfactory communication of emotion. *Percept. Mot. Skills* **91,** 771–781.

Chen, D., Katdare, A., and Lucas, N. (2006). Chemosignals of fear enhance cognitive performance in humans. *Chem. Senses* **31,** 415–423.

Dawson, M. E., Schell, A. M., and Bohmelt, A. H. (1999). Startle Modification: Implications for Neuroscience, Cognitive Science, and Clinical Science. Cambridge University Press, New York.

Dimberg, U., and Ohman, A. (1983). The effects of directional facial cues on electrodermal conditioning to facial stimuli. *Psychophysiology* **20,** 160–167.

Djordjevic, J., Zatorre, R. J., Petrides, M., Boyle, J. A., and Jones-Gotman, M. (2005). Functional neuroimaging of odor imagery. *Neuroimage* **24,** 791–801.

Dolan, R. J., and Vuilleumier, P. (2003). Amygdala automaticity in emotional processing. *Ann. NY Acad. Sci.* **985,** 348–355.

Doty, R. L. (2003). Mammalian Pheromones: Fact or Fantasy? *In* "Handbook of Olfaction and Gustation," (R. L. Doty, Ed.), 2nd edn., pp. 345–383. Marcel Dekker, New York.

Eggert, F., Muller-Ruchholtz, W., and Ferstl, R. (1998). Olfactory cues associated with the major histocompatibility complex. *Genetica* **104,** 191–197.

Flykt, A. (2005). Preparedness for action: Responding to the snake in the grass. *Am. J. Psychol.* **119,** 29–43.

Fredrikson, M., Wik, G., Fischer, H., and Andersson, J. (1995). Affective and attentive neural networks in humans: A PET study of Pavlovian conditioning. *NeuroReport* **7,** 97–101.

Gilbert, A. N., and Firestein, S. (2002). Dollars and scents: Commercial opportunities in olfaction and taste. *Nat. Neurosci.* **5,** 1043–1045.

Glusman, G., Yanai, I., Rubin, I., and Lancet, D. (2001). The complete human olfactory subgenome. *Genome Res.* **11,** 685–702.

Goldberg, I. I., Harel, M., and Malach, R. (2006). When the brain loses its self: Prefrontal inactivation during sensorimotor processing. *Neuron* **50,** 329–339.

Gottfried, J. A., Smith, A. P., Rugg, M. D., and Dolan, R. J. (2004). Remembrance of odors past: Human olfactory cortex in cross-modal recognition memory. *Neuron* **42,** 687–695.

Gower, D. B., and Ruparelia, B. A. (1993). Olfaction in humans with special reference to odorous 16-androstenes: Their occurrence, perception and possible social, psychological and sexual impact. *J. Endocrinol.* **137,** 167–187.

Gusnard, D. A. Akbudak, E., Shulman, G. L., and Raichle, M. E. (2001). Medial prefrontal cortex and self-referential mental activity: Relation to a default mode of brain function. *Proc. Natl. Acad. Sci. USA* **98,** 4259–4264.

Havlicek, J., and Lenochova, P. (2006). The effect of meat consumption on body odor attractiveness. *Chem. Senses* **31,** 747–752.

Hepper, P. G., and Cleland, J. (1999). Developmental aspects of kin recognition. *Genetica* **104,** 199–205.

Herz, R. S., and Cahill, E. D. (1997). Differential use of sensory information in sexual behavior as a function of gender. *Hum. Nat.* **8,** 275–286.

Herz, R. S., and Inzlicht, M. (2002). Sex differences in response to physical and social factors involved in human mate selection: The importance of smell for women. *Evol. Hum. Behav.* **23,** 359–364.

Klein, J. (1986). Natural History of the Major Histocompatibility Complex. John Wiley & Sons, New York.

Kobal, G. (1981). Electrophysiologische Untersuchungen des menschlichen Geruchssinns. Thieme Verlag, Stuttgart.

Kobayakawa, K., Kobayakawa, R., Matsumoto, H., Oka, Y., Imai, T., Ikawa, M., Okabe, M., Ikeda, T., Itohara, S., Kikusui, T., Mori, K., and Sakano, H. (2007). Innate versus learned odour processing in the mouse olfactory bulb. *Nature* **450,** 503–508.

Koch, M. (1999). The neurobiology of startle. *Prog. Neurobiol.* **59,** 107.

Kwak, J., Willse, A., Preti, G., Yamazaki, K., and Beauchamp, G. K. (2010). In search of the chemical basis for MHC odourtypes. *Proc. Biol. Sci.* (in press).
Labows, J. N., Reilly, J. T., Leyden, J. J., and Preti, G. (1999). Axillary Odor Determination, Formation and Control. *In* "Antiperspirants and Deodorants," (K. Laden, Ed.), 2nd edn.,2nd edn., Vol. 20, pp. 59–82. Marcel Dekker Inc., New York.
Laska, M., and Freyer, D. (1997). Olfactory discrimination ability for aliphatic esters in squirrel monkeys and humans. *Chem. Senses* **22,** 457–465.
Laska, M., and Teubner, P. (1998). Odor structure–activity relationships of carboxylic acids correspond between squirrel monkeys and humans. *Am. J. Physiol.* **274,** R1639–R1645.
Laska, M., Trolp, S., and Teubner, P. (1999). Odor structure–activity relationships compared in human and nonhuman primates. *Behav. Neurosci.* **113,** 998–1007.
Laska, M., Genzel, D., and Wieser, A. (2005). The number of functional olfactory receptor genes and the relative size of olfactory brain structures are poor predictors of olfactory discrimination performance with enantiomers. *Chem. Senses* **30,** 171–175.
LeDoux, J. E. (1992). Brain mechanisms of emotion and emotional learning. *Curr. Opin. Neurobiol.* **2,** 191–197.
LeDoux, J. E. (1996). The Emotional Brain: The Mysterious Underpinnings of Emotional Life. Simon & Shuster, New York.
LeDoux, J. E. (2000). Cognitive-emotional interactions: Listen to the brain. *In* "Cognitive Neuroscience of Emotion," (R. D. Lane and L. Nadel, Eds.), pp. 129–156. Oxford University Press, New York.
Lieberman, D., Tooby, J., and Cosmides, L. (2007). The Architecture of Human Kin Detection. *Nature* **445,** 727–731.
Lorig, T. S., Elmes, D. G., Zald, D. H., and Pardo, J. V. (1999). A computer-controlled olfactometer for fMRI and electrophysiological studies of olfaction. *Behav. Res. Meth. Instrum. Comput.* **31,** 370–375.
Lundstrom, J. N., and Jones-Gotman, M. (2009). Romantic love modulates women's identification of men's body odors. *Horm. Behav.* **55,** 280–284.
Lundstrom, J. N., Boyle, J. A., Zatorre, R. J., and Jones-Gotman, M. (2008). Functional neuronal processing of body odors differ from that of similar common odors. *Cereb. Cortex* **18,** 1466–1474.
Lundstrom, J. N., Boyle, J. A., Zatorre, R. J., and Jones-Gotman, M. (2009a). The neuronal substrates of human olfactory based kin recognition. *Hum. Brain Mapp.* **30,** 2571–2580.
Lundstrom, J. N., Gordon, A. R., Alden, E. C., Albrecht, J., and Boesveldt, S. (2009b). Methods for building an inexpensive computer-controlled olfactometer for temporally precise behavioral experiments. Submitted for publication. (under review).
Maddock, R. J. (1999). The retrosplenial cortex and emotion: New insights from functional neuroimaging of the human brain. *Trends Neurosci.* **22,** 310–316.
Martins, Y., Preti, G., Crabtree, C. R., Runyan, T., Vainius, A. A., and Wysocki, C. J. (2005). Preference for human body odors is influenced by gender and sexual orientation. *Psychol. Sci.* **16,** 694–701.
Mateo, J. M., and Johnston, R. E. (2000). Kin recognition and the 'armpit effect': Evidence of self-referent phenotype matching. *Proc. R. Soc. Lond. B Biol. Sci.* **267,** 695–700.
Mateo, J. M., and Johnston, R. E. (2003). Kin recognition by self-referent phenotype matching: Weighing the evidence. *Anim. Cogn.* **6,** 73–76.
McAlonan, K., Cavanaugh, J., and Wurtz, R. H. (2008). Guarding the gateway to cortex with attention in visual thalamus. *Nature* **456,** 391–394.
Miltner, W., Matjak, M., Braun, C., Diekmann, H., and Brody, S. (1994). Emotional qualities of odors and their influence on the startle reflex in humans. *Psychophysiology* **31,** 107–110.
Mineka, S., and Ohman, A. (2002). Phobias and preparedness: The selective, automatic, and encapsulated nature of fear. *Biol. Psychiatry* **52,** 927–937.

Morris, J. S., Ohman, A., and Dolan, R. J. (1998). Conscious and unconscious emotional learning in the human amygdala. *Nature* **393,** 467–470.

Morris, J. S., Ohman, A., and Dolan, R. J. (1999). A subcortical pathway to the right amygdala mediating "unseen" fear. *Proc. Natl. Acad. Sci. USA* **96,** 1680–1685.

Mujica-Parodi, L. R., Strey, H. H., Frederick, B., Savoy, R., Cox, D., Botanov, Y., Tolkunov, D., Rubin, D., and Weber, J. (2009). Chemosensory cues to conspecific emotional stress activate amygdala in humans. *PLoS ONE* **4,** e6415.

Ober, C. (1999). Studies of HLA, fertility and mate choice in a human isolate. *Hum. Reprod. Update* **5,** 103–107.

Ober, C., Weitkamp, L. R., Cox, N., Dytch, H., Kostyu, D., and Elias, S. (1997). HLA and mate choice in humans. *Am. J. Hum. Genet.* **61,** 497–504.

Ober, C., Hyslop, T., and Hauck, W. W. (1999). Inbreeding effects on fertility in humans: Evidence for reproductive compensation. *Am. J. Hum. Genet.* **64,** 225–231.

Ohman, A., and Mineka, S. (2001). Fears, phobias, and preparedness: Toward an evolved module of fear and fear learning. *Psychol. Rev.* **108,** 483–522.

Ohman, A., Flykt, A., and Esteves, F. (2001a). Emotion drives attention: Detecting the snake in the grass. *J. Exp. Psychol. Gen.* **130,** 466–478.

Ohman, A., Lundqvist, D., and Esteves, F. (2001b). The face in the crowd revisited: A threat advantage with schematic stimuli. *J. Pers. Soc. Psychol.* **80,** 381–396.

Olofsson, J. K , Ericsson, E., and Nordin, S. (2008). Comparison of chemosensory, auditory and visual event-related potential amplitudes. *Scand. J. Psychol.* **49,** 231–237.

Olsson, S., Barnard, J., and Turri, L. (2006). Olfaction and identification of unrelated individuals: Examination of the mysteries of human odor recognition. *J. Chem. Ecol.* **32,** 1635–1645.

Pause, B. M., and Krauel, K. (2000). Chemosensory event-related potentials (CSERP) as a key to the psychology of odors. *Int. J. Psychophysiol.* **36,** 105–122.

Pause, B. M., Krauel, K., Sojka, B., and Ferstl, R. (1999). Body odor evoked potentials: A new method to study the chemosensory perception of self and non-self in humans. *Genetica* **104,** 285–294.

Pause, B. M., Krauel, K., Schrader, C., Sojka, B., Westphal, E., Muller-Ruchholtz, W., and Ferstl, R. (2006). The human brain is a detector of chemosensorily transmitted HLA-class I-similarity in same- and opposite-sex relations. *Proc. Biol. Sci.* **273,** 471–478.

Penn, D., and Potts, W. (1998a). How do major histocompatibility complex genes influence odor and mating preferences? *Adv. Immunol.* **69,** 411–436.

Penn, D., and Potts, W. K. (1998b). Chemical signals and parasite-mediated sexual selection. *Trends Ecol. Evol.* **13,** 391–396.

Penn, D. J., Damjanovich, K., and Potts, W. K. (2002). MHC heterozygosity confers a selective advantage against multiple-strain infections. *Proc. Natl. Acad. Sci. USA* **99,** 11260–11264.

Plailly, J., Howard, J. D., Gitelman, D. R., and Gottfried, J. A. (2008). Attention to odor modulates thalamocortical connectivity in the human brain. *J. Neurosci.* **28,** 5257–5267.

Platek, S. M. Keenan, J. P., and Mohamed, F. B. (2005). Sex differences in the neural correlates of child facial resemblance: An event-related fMRI study. *Neuroimage* **25,** 1336–1344.

Poellinger, A., Thomas, R., Lio, P., Lee, A., Makris, N., Rosen, B. R., and Kwong, K. K. (2001). Activation and habituation in olfaction–an fMRI study. *Neuroimage* **13,** 547–560.

Porter, R. H. (1998). Olfaction and human kin recognition. *Genetica* **104,** 259–263.

Porter, R. H., and Moore, J. D. (1981). Human kin recognition by olfactory cues. *Physiol. Behav.* **27,** 493–495.

Potts, W. K., and Wakeland, E. K. (1993). Evolution of MHC genetic diversity: A tale of incest, pestilence and sexual preference. *Trends Genet.* **9,** 408–412.

Prehn, A., Ohrt, A., Sojka, B., Ferstl, R., and Pause, B. M. (2006). Chemosensory anxiety signals augment the startle reflex in humans. *Neurosci. Lett.* **394,** 127–130.

Prehn-Kristensen, A., Wiesner, C., Bergmann, T. O., Wolff, S., Jansen, O., Mehdorn, H. M., Ferstl, R., and Pause, B. M. (2009). Induction of empathy by the smell of anxiety. *PLoS ONE* **4,** e5987.

Roberts, S. C., Havlicek, J., Flegr, J., Hruskova, M., Little, A. C., Jones, B. C., Perrett, D. I., and Petrie, M. (2004). Female facial attractiveness increases during the fertile phase of the menstrual cycle. *Proc. Biol. Sci.* **271**(Suppl. 5), S270–S272.

Rolls, E. T., Critchley, H. D., and Treves, A. (1996). Representation of olfactory information in the primate orbitofrontal cortex. *J. Neurophysiol.* **75,** 1982–1996.

Rouquier, S., Blancher, A., and Giorgi, D. (2000). The olfactory receptor gene repertoire in primates and mouse: Evidence for reduction of the functional fraction in primates. *Proc. Natl. Acad. Sci. USA* **97,** 2870–2874.

Royet, J. P., Koenig, O., Gregoire, M. C., Cinotti, L., Lavenne, F., Le Bars, D., Costes, N., Vigouroux, M., Farget, V., Sicard, G., Holley, A., Mauguiere, F., *et al.* (1999). Functional anatomy of perceptual and semantic processing for odors. *J. Cogn. Neurosci.* **11,** 94–109.

Royet, J. P., Hudry, J., Zald, D. H., Godinot, D., Gregoire, M. C., Lavenne, F., Costes, N., and Holley, A. (2001). Functional neuroanatomy of different olfactory judgments. *Neuroimage* **13,** 506–519.

Russell, M. J. (1976). Human olfactory communication. *Nature* **260,** 520–522.

Sandro Carvalho Santos, P., Augusto Schinemann, J., Gabardo, J., and da Graca Bicalho, M. (2005). New evidence that the MHC influences odor perception in humans: A study with 58 Southern Brazilian students. *Horm. Behav.* **47,** 384–388.

Sato, K. (1977). The physiology, pharmacology, and biochemistry of the eccrine sweat gland. *Rev. Physiol. Biochem. Pharmacol.* **79,** 51–131.

Schaal, B., and Porter, R. H. (1991). "Microsmatic humans" revisited: The generation and perception of chemical signals. *In* "Advances in the Study of Behavior," (P. J. Slater, J. S. Rosenblatt, C. Beer, and M. Milinski, Eds.), Vol. 20, pp. 135–199. Academic Press, Sand Diego.

Schupp, H. T., Ohman, A., Junghofer, M., Weike, A. I., Stockburger, J., and Hamm, A. O. (2004). The facilitated processing of threatening faces: An ERP analysis. *Emotion* **4,** 189–200.

Tooby, J., and Cosmides, L. (1990). The past explains the present—Emotional adaptations and the structure of ancestral environments. *Ethol. Sociobiol.* **11,** 375–424.

Vyas, A., Kim, S. K., Giacomini, N., Boothroyd, J. C., and Sapolsky, R. M. (2007). Behavioral changes induced by toxoplasma infection of rodents are highly specific to aversion of cat odors. *Proc. Natl. Acad. Sci. USA* **104,** 6442–6447.

Wallace, P. (1977). Individual discrimination of humans by odor. *Physiol. Behav.* **19,** 577–579.

Wedekind, C., and Furi, S. (1997). Body odour preferences in men and women: Do they aim for specific MHC combinations or simply heterozygosity? *Proc. R. Soc. Lond. B Biol. Sci.* **264,** 1471–1479.

Wedekind, C., Seebeck, T., Bettens, F., and Paepke, A. J. (1995). MHC-dependent mate preferences in humans. *Proc. R. Soc. Lond. B Biol. Sci.* **260,** 245–249.

Weisfeld, G. E., Czilli, T., Phillips, K. A., Gall, J. A., and Lichtman, C. M. (2003). Possible olfaction-based mechanisms in human kin recognition and inbreeding avoidance. *J. Exp. Child Psychol.* **85,** 279–295.

Weitkamp, L. R., and Ober, C. (1999). Ancestral and recombinant 16-locus HLA haplotypes in the Hutterites. *Immunogenetics* **49,** 491–497.

Wetter, S., Polich, J., and Murphy, C. (2004). Olfactory, auditory, and visual ERPs from single trials: No evidence for habituation. *Int. J. Psychophysiol.* **54,** 263–272.

Whalen, P. J., Rauch, S. L., Etcoff, N. L., McInerney, S. C., Lee, M. B., and Jenike, M. A. (1998). Masked presentations of emotional facial expressions modulate amygdala activity without explicit knowledge. *J. Neurosci.* **18,** 411–418.

Wilson, D. A. (2000). Odor specificity of habituation in the rat anterior piriform cortex. *J. Neurophysiol.* **83,** 139–145.

Wysocki, C. J., and Preti, G. (2000). Human body odors and their perception. *Jpn. J. Taste Smell* **7,** 19–42.

Yamasaki, H., LaBar, K. S., and McCarthy, G. (2002). Dissociable prefrontal brain systems for attention and emotion. *Proc. Natl. Acad. Sci. USA* **99,** 11447–11451.

Yamazaki, K., Beauchamp, G. K., Bard, J., Boyse, E. A., and Thomas, L. (1993). Chemosensory identity and immune function in mice. *In* "Genetics of perception and communications," (C. J. Wysocki and M. R. Kare, Eds.), Vol. 3, pp. 211–225. Dekker, New York.

Yamazaki, K., Beauchamp, G. K., Curran, M., Bard, J., and Boyse, E. A. (2000). Parent-progeny recognition as a function of MHC odortype identity. *Proc. Natl. Acad. Sci. USA* **97,** 10500–10502.

Young, J. M., Friedman, C., Williams, E. M., Ross, J. A., Tonnes-Priddy, L., and Trask, B. J. (2002). Different evolutionary processes shaped the mouse and human olfactory receptor gene families. *Hum. Mol. Genet.* **11,** 535–546.

Zatorre, R. J., Jones-Gotman, M., Evans, A. C., and Meyer, E. (1992). Functional localization and lateralization of human olfactory cortex. *Nature* **360,** 339–340.

Zatorre, R. J., Jones-Gotman, M., and Rouby, C. (2000). Neural mechanisms involved in odor pleasantness and intensity judgments. *NeuroReport* **11,** 2711–2716.

Zhou, W., and Chen, D. (2008). Encoding human sexual chemosensory cues in the orbitofrontal and fusiform cortices. *J. Neurosci.* **28,** 14416–14421.

Zhou, W., and Chen, D. (2009). Fear-related chemosignals modulate recognition of fear in ambiguous facial expressions. *Psychol. Sci.* **20,** 177–183.

CHAPTER TWO

Female Perception of Male Body Odor

Mark J. T. Sergeant

Contents

Abstract

Olfaction is one of the most crucial forms of communication among nonhuman animals. Historically, olfaction has been perceived as being of limited importance for humans, but recent research has documented that not only do humans have sensitive olfactory abilities, but also odors have the potential to influence our physiology and behavior. This chapter reviews research on olfactory communication among humans, focusing on the effects of male bodily odors on female physiology and behavior. The process of body odor production and the detection of olfactory signals are reviewed, focusing on potential sex differences in these abilities. The effects of male body odors on female physiological and behavioral effects of body odors are considered. Finally, with specific regard to female mate choice, evidence regarding the influence of the major histocompatibility complex and fluctuating asymmetry on male olfactory cues is reviewed.

Division of Psychology, Nottingham Trent University, Nottingham, United Kingdom

Vitamins and Hormones, Volume 83
ISSN 0083-6729, DOI: 10.1016/S0083-6729(10)83002-X

I. Olfaction in Humans

A. The importance of olfactory communication

Olfaction is one of the most crucial forms of communication among nonhuman animals. Existing metabolites such as urine, feces, or sweat can be co-opted for transmitting odors, making olfactory signals energetically efficient to produce. Olfactory signals also have the greatest potential range of any method of animal communication and can be transmitted effectively in total darkness and around obstacles (Műller-Schwarze, 1999; Wyatt, 2003). Unlike visual and auditory signals, odors also remain active in the environment for extended periods, providing the opportunity to lay remote signals (e.g., such as those involved in marking territorial boundaries). However, a disadvantage of olfactory signals is their low emission rate, compared to most auditory or visual signals, meaning that rapid changes in physiological state or psychological motivations cannot be directly communicated (Köster, 2002).

Given the importance of olfaction among nonhuman animals, there has recently been considerable speculation on how odors influence human behavior. However, due to the small volume of the human main olfactory bulb, compared to other species, humans were long considered to be *microsmatic*, in which condition olfactory abilities are limited and have minimal impact on social behavior (Stephan *et al.*, 1970). Indeed recent research suggests that among humans between 55% and 65% of olfactory receptor (OR) genes have become nonfunctional during polygenetic development (Gilad *et al.*, 2003). Gilad *et al.* (2004) have suggested that the loss of OR genes in humans is specifically linked to the development of full trichromatic vision; as humans become more reliant on visual stimuli to perceive the environment, the pressure to retain olfactory abilities diminishes.

Within the last few decades, however, human microsmaty has been fundamentally reconsidered. Both the relative size of olfactory structures in the brain and the number of functional OR genes have been recognized as poor predictors of olfactory ability (Laska *et al.*, 2005). Although it is true that humans have lost a considerable number of OR genes, they still possess the ability to discriminate in excess of 10,000 different odorants (Doty, 2001). Gilad *et al.* (2003) are also keen to illustrate that a number of OR-encoding genes have been conserved in humans and other primates, suggesting that they are "OR genes that are essential to all primates and therefore are under selective pressure to remain intact in humans as well" (pp. 3326). Finally, while the volume of the human olfactory bulb is small compared to the rest of the brain, it is also densely connected to many neural regions (Keverne, 1983). Thus, while human olfactory abilities have undoubtedly been reduced during phylogenetic development, their advanced cognitive abilities mean that the olfactory abilities that have been retained may be used more effectively.

B. Body odor production in humans

There are several areas of the human body capable of producing odors that may act as semiochemicals (i.e., a chemical that transmits a specific signal which has the potential to influence physiology and behavior in a recipient; Law and Regnier, 1971). The specific odors produced from each site are dependent upon interactions between skin gland secretions and the number and type of cutaneous microflora present (Wysocki and Preti, 2000). Moist areas of the body, particularly the anogenital region, axillary (underarm) region, feet, and mouth, support the greatest concentrations of microflora and consequently produce the most noticeable forms of human odor (Wysocki and Preti, 2000). In total, humans possess around three million sweat glands on their bodies, which are capable of producing up to 12 l of fluid a day (Millington and Wilkinson, 1983). The three main forms of sweat gland involved in exocrine function are the eccrine, sebaceous, and apocrine (Labows *et al.*, 1982).

Eccrine glands are the dominant type of human skin gland, being distributed over the entire surface of the skin (Szabo, 1963). They primarily serve a thermoregulatory function, delivering aqueous eccrine sweat to the skin for evaporative cooling (Sato *et al.*, 1995). Although the number and distribution of eccrine glands is similar for both sexes, (Szabo, 1963), males are universally reported to produce more eccrine gland sweat than females (Kawahata, 1960; McChance and Puhorit, 1969).

Sebaceous glands are distributed primarily on the upper body and produce a thick oily secretion called sebum, which is primarily formed from cholesterol and cholesterol esters, long-chain fatty acids, squalene, and triglycerides (Agache and Blanc, 1982). Although sebum itself is largely odorless, it does provide some moisture and materials important for the growth and metabolic regulation of cutaneous microflora (Montagna and Parakkal, 1974).

Apocrine glands are the most important type of secretary gland for the production of possible human semiochemicals. They are located primarily in the anogenital and axillary regions and around the areolae. The glands secrete a viscous, oily fluid containing large amounts of cholesterol, proteins, C19-steroid sulfates, and trace levels of C19-volatile steroids (Gower *et al.*, 1994; Spielman *et al.*, 1995). Apocrine gland secretions alter in response to mental and emotional stimulation, reacting, for example, to fear, anger, and sexual arousal (Hurley and Shelley, 1960). Several studies have shown that these changes in affective state can not only be detected by other individuals, but also influence their cognition (Chen and Haviland-Jones, 2000; Chen *et al.*, 2006; Pause *et al.*, 2004).

Both apocrine and sebaceous glands develop fully at puberty and are part of the secondary sexual characteristics of males and females (Hays, 2003). There are significant differences between the sexes in apocrine gland distribution, with females displaying more glands in all anatomical regions studied (Craigmyle, 1984; Homma, 1926). With specific regard to the axillary region (discussed below), females are reported to have a 75% higher number of glands (Brody, 1975), though males are reported to have noticeably larger apocrine glands (Doty *et al.*, 1978; Hurley and Shelley, 1960) which are more active in secretion (Shehadeh and Klingman, 1963; Shelley *et al.*, 1953). While fresh apocrine gland secretions are odorless (Shehadeh and Klingman, 1963), incubation with microflora results in the production of odiferous substances (Austin and Ellis, 2003; Zeng *et al.*, 1992).

The most important anatomical region for the production of human body odor is the axillae (underarms). The presence of apocrine, eccrine, sebaceous, and apoeccrine glands, together with a high density of cutaneous microflora, results in this region being a unique source of human odor labeled the axillary scent organ (Stoddart, 1990; Wysocki and Preti, 2004). The microflora in this region is composed largely of coryneform and coccal bacteria (such as diphtheroids and micrococci, respectively) (Leyden *et al.*, 1981). The axillary microflora of males tends to be dominated by coryneform bacteria, while females tend to have a dominance of micrococci bacteria (Jackman and Noble, 1983). Given cross-cultural findings that male body odor is perceived as more odorous, and more unpleasant, than female body odor (see below), it is significant that dominance by coryneform bacteria is associated with more intense and pungent odor, while dominance by micrococci bacteria is associated with weaker and more acidic body odor (Labows *et al.*, 1982; Rennie *et al.*, 1991).

C. Axillary secretions

Previous analyses of axillary secretions have tended to focus on the presence of certain volatile androgen-derived steroids such as androstenol (5α-androst-16-en-3βol), androstenone (5α-androst-16-en-3-one), and adrostadienone (androsta-4, 16-dien-3-one), which are considered to provide a musky or urinous odor (Gower and Ruparelia, 1993). Androstadienone may be a precursor for the other more odorous 16-androstene steroids (such as androstenone and androstenol), which are created through the actions of axillary microflora (Gower and Ruparelia, 1993). Levels of the 16-androstene steroids are up to 50 times higher in males compared to those in females (Gower and Ruparelia, 1993).

Recent studies, however, have focused on the presence of C_6–C_{11} acids in axillary secretions, of which 3-methyl-2-hexonic acid 3M2H is by far the most abundant (Zeng *et al.*, 1991). 3M2H is present at far higher concentrations than the 16-androstene steroids, and is believed to provide the characteristic odor of axillary sweat (Zeng *et al.*, 1996). Proportionally higher concentrations of (E)-3M2H are expressed in the axillary secretions of males (Zeng *et al.*, 1996). Other odorous substances identified in human axillary secretions include 3-methyl-3-hydroxylhaxenoic acid (HMHA) (Natsch *et al.*, 2003) and 3-methyl-3-sulfanylhexan-1-ol (Troccaz *et al.*, 2004). Possible sex differences in the relative concentration of these compounds have yet to be investigated.

II. Sex Differences in Sensitivity to Body Odor

A. Olfactory sensitivity

Olfactory sensitivity is assessed by examining an individual's olfactory detection thresholds; the lowest concentration of an odorant that is perceivable to the sense of smell. In addition, specific anosmia rates (i.e., the percentage of people unable to smell a specific odorant despite having an otherwise good sense of smell; Amoore, 1977) provide information on sensitivity to a specific compound. Given that body odor is composed of numerous separate compounds, it is necessary to examine olfactory thresholds and ancsmia rates for each separate component of body odor. It should also be noted that many recently discovered constituents such as HMHA and 3-methyl-3-sulfanylhexan-1-ol have yet to be fully investigated, the extant literature only documenting sensitivities to E-3M2H and various 16-androstene steroids.

With regard to E-3M2H, there appears to be no consistent sex differences for specific anosmia rates and olfactory detection thresholds (Baydar *et al.*, 1992; Wysocki, *et al.*, 1993). However, there do appear to be considerable sex differences in both olfactory detection thresholds and specific anosmia rates for 16-androtene steroids. Females have lower olfactory thresholds for both androstadienone (Koelega and Köster, 1974; Lundström *et al.*, 2003) and androstenol (Kloek, 1961). Similarly, specific anosmia rates are higher among males for both androstadienone (Hummel *et al.*, 2005; Lundström *et al.*, 2003) and androstenol (Koelega and Köster, 1974).

In the largest olfactory study ever undertaken, involving an international sample of 1.5 million participants, Wysocki and Gilbert (1989) report that females were significantly more sensitive to androstenone than males, this finding being replicated in all cultures studied (Barber, 1997). Anosmia rates for androstenone have also been extensively investigated and are reported as being considerably higher among males compared to females (Bremner *et al.*, 2003; though see Amoore, 1977).

Given that males secrete proportionately higher levels of the compounds causing body odor, it is intriguing that females possess greater olfactory sensitivity to some of these, noticeably the 16-androstene steroids. Such a pattern of findings could be interpreted as an efficient system for males transmitting semiochemicals that females are specifically sensitive to. However, among humans there is anecdotal evidence that females are in fact more sensitive to *all* odors, rather than possessing a specific sensitivity to potential semiochemicals. The extant literature on this topic, however, is mixed. There are no significant sex differences in olfactory sensitivity to a range of odorants such as n-butanol (a solvent base to perfumes; Koelega, 1970) and pyridine (spoiled-milk odor; Dorries *et al.*, 1989), while other findings suggest that females have lower olfactory detection thresholds for pyridine (a fish like odor) and m-xylene (a sweet smelling odor; Koelega, 1994). It therefore appears that while females are more sensitive to specific odorants, they do not appear to be universally more sensitive to odorants (Brand and Millot, 2001).

B. Female perceptions of male body odor

Rather than focusing on a particular axillary secretion, some studies have examined female reactions to samples of actual human body odor. The majority of these studies have collected samples of body odor, using either a T-shirt or absorbent pads placed in the axillae. A variety of methodological controls are placed on the dietary, hygiene, and sexual behavior of the odor donor in an attempt to minimize the impact of environmental odors. Similar controls are placed on the individuals rating the samples of body odor. Such studies offer an advantage over compound-specific studies (i.e., using synthetically derived compounds for olfactory testing) as they provide a more natural, and arguably more ecologically valid, insight into reactions to human body odor. However, a difficulty with this form of research is that there is no agreed optimum method for collecting odor samples, and many studies fail to use adequate methodological controls.

A number of studies, however, have specifically aimed to examine sex differences in the perceptions of human body odors. In a study by Schleidt *et al.* (1981) body odor samples were both collected from and assessed by a sample of 48 Germans, 50 Italians, and 44 Japanese individuals (total sample size of 142). Exactly half of the sample was composed of females, and the majority of subjects were pairs of males and females in romantic relationships. All of the subjects, both male and female, rated the body odor of males as being less pleasant than that from females. This finding confirms earlier reports of female's body odor being found more pleasant by Hold and Schleidt (1977) and Schleidt (1980).

One of the most comprehensive studies of body odor perceptions to date was undertaken by Chen and Haviland-Jones (1999). Samples of body odor were collected using strict methodological controls from 30 donors reflecting six distinct age and sex groups. Each group was composed of five individuals, and the six groups were *little girls* (aged around 5), *little boys* (aged around 6), *college-age females* (aged around 20), *college-age males* (aged around 23), *older females* (aged around 71) and *older males* (aged around 73). The samples of body odor from these individuals were then rated by 154 males and 154 females (aged around 19). The odor of college-age males was rated as the most unpleasant, intense, and masculine, closely followed by older females. The odor from both groups of children was rated as the most pleasant, least intense, and least masculine. The samples from college-age females and older males were rated in the middle. The ratings given to both groups of children are understandable, as both the sebaceous glands and apocrine glands, which produce many of the substances that characterize human body odor, do not begin to function until after puberty. This results in a weaker odor among children. Similarly, the ratings given to samples from college-age males and females are consistent with the studies outlined above. Chen and Haviland-Jones (1999) suggest that the somewhat unexpected ratings given to the odors of older males and females could be due to changes in the typical sexually dimorphic ratio of estrogen to testosterone that results from old age in Western populations (Hyde, 2005). In other words, the relative increase in estrogens among older males could have given them a more stereotypically female odor, while the relative increase in testosterone among older females could have given them a more stereotypically male odor.

C. Determining sex from body odor

Given the evident differences between the body odor of males and females, a number of researchers have investigated whether humans can accurately discern the sex of an individual based purely on their odor. The findings from these studies have been somewhat mixed. Russell (1976) collected a single sample of male and female body odor via a T-shirt that had been worn for a 24-h period. Twenty-nine subjects (both males and females) were given the task of correctly differentiating between the male and female body sample. Twenty-two subjects (75.8% of the sample) were able to complete this somewhat simplistic task. A more complex study performed by Hold and Schleidt (1977) involved collecting a series of body odor samples from males and females and then presenting subjects with a total of 10 odors to choose from. Based on this methodology, a total of 16 out of 50 subjects (32% of a sample that was again comprised of both males and females) could reliably discern the sex of an odor donor.

In the Schleidt *et al.* (1981) study mentioned above, females from each of the three international samples were significantly more accurate at the task of identifying an odor donor's sex than males, though precise details of their superiority were not given. However, Schleidt *et al.* (1981) noted that both males and females based their responses on the strength of the odor they were rating, with those possessing stronger odors stereotypically rated as males. This is consistent with earlier research by Doty *et al.* (1978) and, intriguingly, when the data from Russell (1976) and Hold and Schleidt (1977) are reexamined, it appears that the sex ascribed to an odor donor was primarily based on the muskiness of an odor. McBurney *et al.* (1977) noted that stronger smelling body odor was more likely to be perceived by both sexes as masculine, with a range of socially undesirable traits (unintelligent and unsophisticated) and socially desirable but masculine traits (being strong and physically active) ascribed to its donor. This strongly suggests that subjects in the aforementioned study employ a stereotypical method to assess odors: those seen as stronger, and potentially more malodorous, are seen as being from males, while those that are weaker, and potentially more pleasant, are seen as being from females.

III. The Physiological and Behavioral Impact of Male Odor on Females

A. Androstenol and androstenone

Research investigating the physiological and behavioral effects of male odor on females has followed one of two approaches. The first is to collect samples of actual body odor and to examine its impact. The second approach involves examining how individuals react to synthetic copies of the compounds present in body odor, most noticeably the 16-androstene steroids androstenol, androstenone, and androstadienone.

Cowley *et al.* (1977) asked 183 male and female participants to wear surgical masks infused with androstenol while evaluating members of the opposite sex. Female, but not male, participants exposed to androstenol provided more positive evaluations of males. Kirk-Smith *et al.* (1978) found that wearing an androstenol infused mask increased the attractiveness ratings given to a series of female photographs by 12 male and 12 female participants. Finally, Cowley and Brooksbank (1991) report that exposure to androstenol influences human social interactions in nonlaboratory settings. 38 male and 38 female participants were given a necklace containing androstenol to wear overnight, allowing the substance to diffuse into the environment, and then kept a record of their social interactions the following day. Female, but again not male, participants reported significantly more social interactions with males, with Cowley and Brooksbank (1991) concluding that the androstenol made the females relaxed and open to social interactions.

With regard to androstenone, there is some evidence that this substance works to attract females in an environmental setting, but only when used at high concentrations. Kirk-Smith and Booth (1980) sprayed varying concentrations of androstenone on chairs in a dentist's waiting room, and observed the pattern of chair choices made by males and females entering the room over the course of several days. A noticeable proportion of females selected chairs that had been treated by very high concentrations of androstenone, while males avoided sitting in the treated chairs.

While the above findings suggest that androstenol and androstenone can potentially enhance female perceptions of males, the findings in this area are contradictory. Using similar methods to Cowley and Brooksbank (1991), Black and Biron (1982) found that exposure to androstenol had no impact on how females evaluated males or the length and intensity of social interactions. Similarly Benton and Wastell (1986) found that androstenol had no effect on females' sexual arousal or responses to erotic prose. The findings for androstenone are equally inconsistent, with some authors reporting that this compound had no effect on females' evaluation of males (Filsinger *et al.*, 1990; McCullough *et al.*, 1981), while others reported that it negatively influenced females' selfperceptions and evaluation of males (Filsinger *et al.*, 1985; Maiworm and Langthaler, 1992). Preti *et al.* (1997) suggest that many of these inconsistent findings may be due to the methodologies employed by researchers, particularly the small number of participants employed and the variable concentrations of 16-androstene steroids used (i.e., some studies used samples at naturally occurring levels while others used samples 1000 times more concentrated).

One phenomenon that has been consistently reported, based on research with strict methodological controls and employing relatively large samples, is that female perceptions of androstenone vary across the menstrual cycle. Hummel *et al.* (1991) report that 35 female participants perceived androstenone negatively during menstruation, with perceptions becoming less negative around ovulation. This change was not observed for other odors (nicotine and phenylethylalcohol) tested in parallel and was not associated with changes in olfactory sensitivity. Grammer (1993) subsequently confirmed this finding using a sample of 289 females; androstenone was again perceived as significantly more positive when the female participants were ovulating. Interestingly, this effect was not observed for females currently taking hormonal contraceptives. This suggests that although female perceptions of androstenone are generally negative, they become less so proximal to ovulation. Both Hummel *et al.* (1991) and Grammer (1993) speculate that as males secrete higher levels of androstenone than females, which provides them with more malodorous body odor, females may be less perturbed by this malodor around ovulation. This may therefore be a mechanism to increase contact between males and females at the optimum moment for conception, aiding the process of human reproduction.

Thorne *et al.* (2003) examined the influence of actual body odor on intersexual contact. Thirty-two females (half using hormonal contraceptives) rated both male vignette characters and faces following exposure to samples of body odor collected from four males. It was found that females rated the male faces and some elements of the male vignette characters, mostly associated with attractiveness, as more positive following exposure to the body odor samples.

B. Androstadienone

A number of recent studies have examined the neuropsychological and behavioral reactions to androstadienone. Savic *et al.* (2001) documented that androstadienone activates the preoptic and ventromedial nucleus of the hypothalamus in females. In a PET study of 10 females exposed to androstadienone, Jacob *et al.* (2001) documented changes in glucose metabolism in several neural regions. Some of these areas are involved in emotional processing and recognition (noticeably the prefrontal cortex and amygdala) and it was suggested that androstadienone could mediate interpersonal interactions. Similar reactions to androstadienone were reported in another PET study of five females by Gulyás *et al.* (2004).

The influence of androstadienone and oestratraenol (an estrogen resembling compound) on individual mood state has also been investigated. Jacob and McClintock (2000) documented that both androstadienone and oestratraenol were found to both maintain a positive mood and prevent a rise in negative mood in females. The opposite effects were observed for males, with both substances increasing negative mood. These findings are in contrast to the sexually dimorphic neurophysiological reactions to these substances reported by Savic *et al.* (2001).

A similar study by Grosser *et al.* (2000) on 40 females was largely consistent with the findings of Jacob and McClintock (2000). Grosser *et al.* (2000) report that exposure resulted in a reduction of nervousness, tension, and other negative emotions and an increase in parasympathetic-like effects (a decrease in respiratory and cardiac frequency and increased body temperature) indicative of a relaxed physiological state. Further research by Jacob *et al.* (2002) examined the comparative effects of androstenol, androstadienone, and a musk deer pheromone muscone (3-methyl-cyclopentadecanone) in a sample of 18 males and 19 females. The effects of androstadienone administered via passive inhalation were unique, preventing both a drop in positive mood and an increase in negative mood. However, in contrast to the earlier research of Jacob and McClintock (2000), the modulating effects of these substances were apparent for both males and females.

A comprehensive review by Bensafi *et al.* (2003) examined both physiological reactions and changes in mood in response to androstadienone and oestratraenol in 12 males and 12 females. No significant effects on mood or sexual arousal were recorded during or following administration of the compounds for either males or females. Androstadienone did, however, produce sexually dimorphic effects in physiological arousal, increasing it in females and, to some degree, decreasing it in males. The most significant changes were in skin conductance, heart rate, and thoratic respiration, which suggested an increase in sympathetic-like effects among females and parasympathetic-like effects in males. Oestratraenol produced no significant reactions in either sex.

Although the above studies seem to indicate that androstadienone and oestratraenol can influence both mood and physiological arousal, the precise pattern of these effects is unclear. Bensafi *et al.* (2004) suggest that some inconsistencies may be due to methodological differences between the above studies such as the relative concentrations of androstadienone employed (i.e., androstadienone may produce dose-dependent effects). To investigate this suggestion, 30 males and 30 females were exposed to both high and low concentrations of androstadienone (50 mg and 2 mg, respectively, diluted in 30 ml of mineral oil) and a control odor (30 ml of mineral oil). Following exposure to high concentrations of androstadienone, positive mood was increased and negative mood was decreased in females, skin conductance increased in females (indicative of sympathetic-like effects) and skin temperature increased in males (indicative of parasympathetic-like effects). No significant effects were documented in response to either low concentrations of androstadienone or the control odor.

Studies of the specific behavioral effects of androstadienone are currently limited. Lundström and Olsson (2005) documented that while nondetectable amounts of androstadienone did modulate psychophysiological arousal and mood in females, in a consistent manner to that described above, it did not change evaluations of male facial attractiveness. Saxton *et al.* (2008) found that female participants gave higher ratings of male attractiveness in a speed-dating context after exposure to androstadienone. However, the effects of this substance were inconsistent across the three studies conducted by Saxton *et al.* (2008).

C. The effects of odor on sexual behavior

Although intriguing, the above studies did not investigate the influence of odors on actual sexual behavior. In one of the few studies of this area, Cutler *et al.* (1998) reported that when a sample of males wore an unidentified blend of chemicals derived from male axillary secretions (commercially marketed as the "pheromone" Athena 10X), they experienced significantly increased sexual interactions with females compared to a control sample of males wearing a placebo substance. Two studies employing a similar methodology and synthesized axillary chemicals also demonstrated increased contact with the opposite sex among premenopausal females (McCoy and Pitino, 2002) and postmenopausal females (Rako and Friebely, 2004).

Although these studies seem to provide strong evidence that axillary secretions can influence actual sexual behavior, they have each received intense criticism (Hays, 2003; Wysocki and Preti, 1998). In none of the above studies was the physical attractiveness or levels of sexual motivations of the experimental and control samples assessed. It is not known whether the increased sexual behavior in the "pheromone" groups was simply due to them containing more attractive or sexually motivated individuals rather than the substances they were wearing. There were also large differences between the samples in terms of their current relationship status, and no attempts were made to statistically control for this. It is quite possible that those subjects in a committed long-term relationship may have had a greater opportunity to interact with members of the opposite sex. Similarly no information was recorded on the subject's ability to interact with the opposite sex in social situations due to geographical location, family commitments, employment, religious conviction, or similar factors.

IV. The Effects of Odor on Mate Choice

A. The major histocompatibility complex

The major histocompatibility complex (MHC) is a group of genes involved in the immunological recognition of self (i.e., the cells of an organism) and nonself (i.e., exogenous cells belonging to invading organisms, usually indicative of infectious diseases) in animal species (Penn and Potts, 1999). Yamazaki *et al.* (1976) first demonstrated that not only do mice signal their MHC characteristics through body odor, but this information can also be used to identify individuals. Similar findings have now been reported for a number of other nonhuman species (). As MHC characteristics are heritable, they provide some indication of genetic similarity (relatedness) to other individuals (Penn and Potts, 1998). Such information helps not only to avoid inbreeding but also, through MHC-dissociative mating, to increase offspring immunocompetence; the offspring of two MHC-dissimilar parents will possess a more varied immune system, providing improved defenses against a wider variety of illnesses (Penn and Potts, 1999).

Human MHC characteristics are correctly referred to as human leukocyte antigen (HLA) characteristics, and are the most polymorphic loci in the human genome (Penn, 2002). The degree of HLA-dissimilarity between a two pair-bonded individuals can have a significant impact on their reproductive success. Couples with a high degree of HLA similarity are less likely to conceive children and more prone to spontaneous abortions (Ober *et al.*, 1998), and have a lower success rate for attempted IVF conceptions (Ho *et al.*, 1994).

Humans express information on their HLA characteristics through body odors, possibly due to individual variation in cutaneous microflora or skin gland secretion (Penn and Potts, 1998). Wedekind *et al.* (1995) first demonstrated that humans are able to discriminate another individual's HLA characteristics through body odor. A total of 49 female participants were presented with body odor samples collected from 44 males of varying HLA-dissimilarity. Odor from males with a greater degree of HLA-dissimilarity received higher hedonic ratings than odors from HLA-similar males. The use of oral contraceptives by females reversed these preferences, so that odors from HLA similar males received higher ratings. Wedekind *et al.* (1995) suggested that this type of contraceptive altered females' hormonal state to mimic pregnancy, under which conditions females may prefer to be around HLA-similar individuals who are reminiscent of kin.

Following the initial study of Wedekind *et al.* (1995), a number of other researchers have documented preferences for the body odor of HLA-dissimilar individuals among populations from Europe (Wedekind and Füri, 1997), North America (Jacob *et al.*, 2002; Thornhill *et al.*, 2002), and South America (Santos *et al.*, 2005). All of these studies documented a preference by female participants for the odors of HLA dissimilar males, with the exception of two studies. Thornhill *et al.* (2002) only documented a general preference among females for HLA heterozygosity in males, whereas Roberts *et al.* (2008) found that preferences were dependent upon a female's relationship status; single women demonstrated a preference for HLA similar males, whereas females in a relationship demonstrated a preference for dissimilar males. Roberts *et al.* (2008) interpreted this finding as indicating that females may use HLA characteristics expressed in odors to seek out dissimilar males for extra-pair copulations, maximizing fitness in any subsequent offspring.

While the above findings demonstrate that humans have the ability to discern HLA characteristics in others, they do not provide direct evidence that HLA-similarity affects mate choice. However, such a possibility can be addressed by examining the degree of HLA-similarity among existing pair-bonded couples. Ihara *et al.* (2000) found no clear evidence that the degree of HLA-dissimilarity between 300 Japanese couples differed from chance. Similarly, Hedrick and Black (1997) examined HLA similarity among 194 couples drawn from 11 South Amerindian tribes. The degree of HLA-dissimilarity between the pair-bonded couples was again not significantly different from chance, suggesting that HLA compatibility was not a significant factor during mate choice. However, Hedrick and Black (1997) did not account for the practice of socially enforced cross-cousin marriages common among some of the tribes studied (Murdock, 1957). Given the heritable nature of HLA characteristics, such marriages to closely related kin would significantly reduce the degree of HLA-dissimilarity among the pair-bonded couples. Research by Ober *et al.* (1997) examined the HLA similarity of 411 American Hutterite couples. The findings demonstrated that couples within the population were less likely to share HLA groupings than chance would predict, suggesting that HLA-dissimilarity did influence mate choice.

B. Fluctuating asymmetry

The deviations an individual shows from perfect bilateral symmetry are referred to as fluctuating asymmetry (FA) (Kowner, 2001). The greater the deviation from perfect symmetry (high FA), the more the individual has been negatively affected by environmental and genetic stresses during ontogeny, such as those caused by inbreeding or deleterious mutations. Therefore, the more symmetrical an individual is (lower FA), the better they have been able to resist these stresses, indicating more effective immune system function (Møller and Swaddle, 1997; Polak, 2003). Symmetry also has a substantial impact on male mating success, with more symmetrical males rated as more facially attractive (Gangestad *et al.*, 1994) and having more sexual partners (Gangestad and Simpson, 2000).

This female preference for more symmetrical males also extends to preferences for body odor. Gangestad and Thornhill (1998) asked 29 female participants to rate samples of body odor collected from 41 male participants with varying degrees of asymmetry. Female participants in the most fertile phase of their menstrual cycle (the proliferative phase) gave higher hedonic ratings to body odor collected from more symmetrical males. During other phases of the menstrual cycle, female participants showed no preferences for male odor based on symmetry. These findings for the variation in female preferences for the odor of symmetrical males have since been confirmed by three additional studies (Rikowski and Grammer, 1999; Thornhill and Gangestad, 1999; Thornhill *et al.*, 2002). Each of these studies also investigated whether males showed any preference for the body odor of symmetrical females. None of the studies documented this. The mechanism by which these differences in FA are expressed in body odor is unclear, though Gangestad and Thornhill (1998) suggest that it may work through altering the concentrations of axillary secretions or cutaneous microflora.

Gangestad and Thornhill (1998) suggest that this preference for symmetrical males around ovulation may reflect an innate desire by females to mate with a male who has "good genes." What this means in practice is that females have more desire for males who would provide strong genetic benefits for any children the female would have; low FA signals a strong functional immune system, which would benefit offspring by making them more resistant to perturbations during ontogeny. Such an explanation would also address why this female olfactory preference emerged around ovulation, as this is the period with the greatest conception risk for females.

V. Conclusions

There are clear sex differences in both the production and perception of body odors. Regarding axillary odors, there are sex differences in the number and type of apocrine gland, type of axillary microflora, and in the secretion levels of 16-androstene steroids. In each instance, the sex differences are such that males will produce more odorous secretions. Given these findings, it is not surprising that male body odor is cross-culturally rated as more intense, and unpleasant, than female odor. Regarding odor perception, there are no consistent sex differences in sensitivity to many body odor constituents, such as 3M2H. With regard to 16-androstene steroids, however, females demonstrate both lower detection thresholds for these substances and show lower anosmia rates than males.

Initial studies suggest that when females were exposed to certain body odor constituents, such as androstenone and androstenol, their perceptions of males became more positive. This in turn appeared to alter both the nature and length of females' social interactions with males. Given the higher levels of these substances in male axillary secretions, it is possible that male body odor could therefore serve as a means to attract females. However, the initial studies of these substances suffered from numerous methodological problems and were contradicted by numerous negative findings. One exception to this seems to be that female hedonic perceptions of androstenone varied across the menstrual cycle, peaking around ovulation, which may serve to increase contact between males and females at the optimum moment for conception. Research examining reactions to androstadienone suggests this substance also effects human behavior, is processed in a sexually dimorphic manner and impacts both mood and physiological function. The precise effects of this substance have yet to be documented however, due to methodological inconsistencies between studies.

Humans possess the ability to express immune system function (HLA characteristics) through body odor, with females able to discriminate HLA-dissimilarity in males. Preferences for HLA-dissimilar males appear to influence mate choice. Symmetry (FA) is also expressed through body odor, with females demonstrating a preference for the odor of more symmetrical males in the proliferative phase of their menstrual cycles. These findings represent some of the strongest evidence to date that humans produce and receive semiochemicals.

REFERENCES

Agache, P., and Blanc, D. (1982). Current status in sebum knowledge. *Int. J. Dermatol.* **21,** 304–315.

Amoore, J. E. (1977). Specific anosmias to 5-alpha-16-en-3-one and omega-pentadecalactone: The ruinous and musky primary odors. *Chem. Senses Flavour* **2,** 401–425.

Austin, C., and Ellis, J. (2003). Microbial pathways leading to steroidal malodour in the axillae. *J. Steroid Biochem. Mol. Biol.* **87,** 105–110.

Barber, C. E. (1997). Olfactory acuity as a function of age and gender: A comparison of African and American samples. *Int. J. Aging Hum. Dev.* **44,** 317–334.

Baydar, A. E., Petrzilka, M., and Schott, M. P. (1992). Perception of characteristic axillary odors. *Perfum. Flavor.* **17,** 2–9.

Bensafi, M., Brown, W., Tsutsui, T., Mainland, J., Johnson, B., Bremner, E., Young, N., Mauss, I., Ray, B., Gross, J., Richards, J., Stappen, I., *et al.* (2003). Sex-steroid derived compounds induce sex-specific effects on autonomic nervous system function in humans. *Behav. Neurosci.* **117,** 1125–1134.

Bensafi, M., Tsutsui, T., Levenson, R. W., and Sobel, N. (2004). Sniffing a human sex-steroid derived compound affects mood and autonomic arousal in a dose-dependent manner. *Psychoneuroendocrinology* **29,** 1290–1299.

Benton, D., and Wastell, V. (1986). Effects of androstenol on human sexual arousal. *Biol. Psychol.* **22,** 141–147.

Black, S., and Biron, C. (1982). Androstenol as a human pheromone: No effect on perceived physical attractiveness. *Behav. Neural Biol.* **34,** 326–330.

Brand, G., and Millot, J. L. (2001). Sex differences in human olfaction: Beyond evidence and enigma. *Q. J. Exp. Psychol.* **54B,** 259–270.

Bremner, E. A., Mainland, J. D., Khan, R. M., and Sobel, N. (2003). The prevalence of androstenone anosmia. *Chem. Senses* **28,** 423–432.

Brody, B. (1975). The sexual significance of the axillae. *Psychiatry* **38,** 278–289.

Chen, D., and Haviland-Jones, J. (1999). Rapid mood change and human odour. *Physiol. Behav.* **68,** 241–250.

Chen, D., and Haviland-Jones, J. (2000). Human olfactory communication of emotion. *Percept. Mot. Skills* **91,** 771–781.

Chen, D., Katdare, A., and Lucas, N. (2006). Chemosignals of fear enhance cognitive performance in humans. *Chem. Senses* **31,** 415–423.

Cowley, J. J., and Brooksbank, B. W. L. (1991). Human exposure to putative pheromones and changes in aspects of social behaviour. *J. Steroid Biochem. Mol. Biol.* **39,** 647–659.

Cowley, J. J., Johnson, A. L., and Brooksbank, B. W. L. (1977). The effect of two odorous compounds on performance in an assessment-of-people test. *Psychoneuroendocrinology* **2,** 159–172.

Craigmyle, M. B. L. (1984). The Apocrine Glands and the Breast. Wiley, New York.

Cutler, W. B., Friedman, E., and McCoy, N. L. (1998). Pheromonal influences on sociosexual behaviour in men. *Arch. Sex. Behav.* **27,** 1–13.

Dorries, K. M., Schmidt, H. J., Beauchamp, G. K., and Wysocki, C. J. (1989). Changes in sensitivity to the odor of androstenone during adolescence. *Dev. Psychobiol.* **22,** 423–435.

Doty, R. L. (2001). Olfaction. *Annu. Rev. Psychol.* **52,** 423–452.

Doty, R. L., Orndorff, M. M., Leyden, J., and Kligman, A. (1978). Communication of gender from human axillary odors: Relationship to perceived intensity and pleasantness. *Horm. Behav.* **16,** 13–22.

Filsinger, E. E., Braun, J. J., and Monte, W. C. (1985). An examination of the effects of putative pheromones on human judgements. *Ethol. Sociobiol.* **6,** 227–236.

Filsinger, E. E., Braun, J. J., and Monte, W. C. (1990). Sex differences in response to the odor of alpha androstenone. *Percept. Mot. Skills* **70,** 216–218.

Gangestad, S. W., and Simpson, J. A. (2000). The evolution of human mating: The role of trade-offs and strategic pluralism. *Behav. Brain Sci.* **23,** 573–644.
Gangestad, S. W., and Thornhill, R. (1998). Menstrual cycle variation in women's preference for the scent of symmetrical men. *Proc. R. Soc. London, Ser. B* **265,** 927–933.
Gangestad, S. W., Thornhill, R., and Yeo, R. A. (1994). Facial attractiveness, developmental stability and fluctuating asymmetry. *Ethol. Sociobiol.* **15,** 73–85.
Gilad, Y., Man, O., Paabo, S., and Lancet, D. (2003). Human specific loss of olfactory receptor genes. *Proc. Natl. Acad. Sci. USA* **100,** 3324–3327.
Gilad, Y., Wiebe, V., Przeworski, M., Lancet, D., and Paabo, S. (2004). Loss of olfactory receptor genes coincides with the acquisition of full trichromatic vision in primates. *Public Libr. Sci.: Biol.* **2,** 120–125.
Gower, D. B. and Ruparelia, B. A. (1993). Olfaction in humans with special reference to odorous 16-androstenes: Their occurrence, perception and possible social, psychological, and sexual impact. *J. Endocrinol.* **137,** 167–187.
Gower, D. B., Holland, K. T., Mallet, A. I., Rennie, P. J., and Watkins, W. J. (1994). Comparison of 16-androstene steroid concentrations in sterile apocrine sweat and axillary secretions: Interconversions of 16-androstenes by the axillary microflora – A mechanism for axillary odour production in man? *J. Steroid Biochem. Mol. Biol.* **48,** 409–418.
Grammer, K. (1993). 5-alpha-anrost -16en-3-on: A male pheromone? A brief report. *Ethol. Sociobiol.* **14,** 201–208.
Grosser, B. I., Monti-Bloch, L., Jennings-White, C., and Berliner, D. L. (2000). Behavioural and elctrophysiological effects of androstadienone, a human pheromone. *Psychoneuroendocrinology* **25,** 289–299.
Gulyás, B., Keri, S., O'Sullivan, B. T., Decety, J., and Roland, P. E. (2004). The putative pheromone androstadienone activates cortical fields in the human brain related to social cognition. *Neurochem. Int.* **44,** 595–600.
Hays, W. S. T. (2003). Human pheromones: Have they been demonstrated? *Behav. Ecol. Sociobiol.* **54,** 89–97.
Hedrick, P. W., and Black, F. L. (1997). HLA and mate selection: No evidence in South Amerindians. *Am. J. Hum. Genet.* **61,** 505–511.
Ho, H. N., Yang, Y. S., Hsieh, R. P., Lin, H. R., Chen, S. U., Chen, H. F., Huang, S. C., Lee, T. Y., and Gill, T. J. 3rd. (1994). Sharing of human leukocyte antigens in couples with unexplained infertility affects the success of in vitro fertilization and tubal embryo transfer. *Am. J. Obstet. Gynecol.* **170,** 63–71.
Hold, B., and Schleidt, M. (1977). The importance of human odor in non-verbal communication. *Z. Tierpsychol.* **43,** 225–238.
Homma, H. (1926). On apocrine sweat glands in white and Negro men and women. *Bull. Johns Hopkins Hosp.* **38,** 365–371.
Hummel, T., Gollisch, R., Wildt, G., and Kobal, G. (1991). Changes in olfactory perception during the menstrual cycle. *Experientia* **47,** 712–715.
Hummel, T., Krone, F., Lundström, J. N., and Bartsch, O. (2005). Androstadienone thresholds in adolescents. *Horm. Behav.* **47,** 306–310.
Hurley, H. J. Jr., and Shelley, W. B. (1960). The Human Apocrone Sweat Gland in Health and Disease. Thomas, Springfield, IL.
Hyde, J. S. (Ed.) (2005). Biological Substrates of Human Sexuality. American Psychological Association, London.
Ihara, Y., Aoki, K., Tokunga, K., Takahashi, K., and Juji, T. (2000). HLA and human mate choice: Tests on Japanese couples. *Anthropol. Sci.* **108,** 199–214.
Jackman, P. J. H., and Noble, W. C. (1983). Normal axillary skin microflora in various populations. *Clin. Exp. Dermatol.* **8,** 259–268.
Jacob, S., and McClintock, M. K. (2000). Psychological state and mood effects of steroidal chemosignals in women and men. *Horm. Behav.* **37,** 57–78.

Jacob, S., Kinnunen, L. H., Metz, J., Cooper, M., and McClintock, M. K. (2001). Sustained human chemosignal unconsciously alters brain function. *NeuroReport* **12,** 2391–2394.

Jacob, S., Garcia, S., Hayreh, D., and McClintock, M. K. (2002). Psychological effects of musky compounds: Comparison of androstadienone with androstenol and muscone. *Horm. Behav.* **42,** 274–283.

Kawahata, A. (1960). Sex differences in sweating. *In* "Essential Problems in Climatic Physiology," (E. H. Oga, K. Ogata, and S. Itoh, Eds.), pp. 169–184. Nakado Publishing, Kyoto.

Keverne, E. B. (1983). Chemical communication in primate reproduction. *In* "Pheromones and Reproduction in Mammals," (J. G. Vandenburgh, Ed.), pp. 79–92. New York, Academic Press.

Kirk-Smith, M., and Booth, D. A. (1980). Effects of androstenone on choice of location in others' presence. *In* "Olfaction and Tastes VII," (H. van der Starre, Ed.), pp. 397–400. IRL Press, London.

Kirk-Smith, M. D., Booth, D. A., Carroll, D., and Davies, P. (1978). Human social attitudes affected by androstenol. *Res. Commun. Psychol. Psychiatry Behav.* **3,** 379–384.

Kloek, J. (1961). The smell of some steroid sex hormones and their metabolites: Reflections and experiments concerning the significance of smell for the mutual relations of the sexes. *Psychiatry, Neurol., Neurochem.* **64,** 309–344.

Koelega, H. S. (1970). Extraversion, sexual arousal and olfactory sensitivity. *Acta Psychol.* **34,** 51–56.

Koelega, H. S. (1994). Sex differences in olfactory sensitivity and the problem of the generality of smell acuity. *Percept. Mot. Skills* **78,** 203–213.

Koelega, H. S., and Köster, E. P. (1974). Some experiments on sex differences in odor perception. *Ann. NY Acad. Sci.* **236,** 234–246.

Köster, E. P. (2002). The specific characteristics of the sense of smell. *In* "Olfaction, Taste and Cognition," (C. Rouby, B. Schaal, D. Dubois, R. Gervais, and A. Holley, Eds.), pp. 27–43. Cambridge University Press, Cambridge.

Kowner, R. (2001). Psychological perspective on human developmental stability and fluctuating asymmetry: Sources, applications, and implications. *Br. J. Psychol.* **92,** 447–469.

Labows, J. N., McGinley, K., and Klingman, A. (1982). Perspectives on axillary odor. *J. Soc. Cosmet. Chem.* **34,** 193–202.

Laska, M., Genzel, D., and Wiser, A. (2005). The number of functional olfactory receptor genes and the relative size of olfactory brain structures are poor predictors of olfactory discrimination performance with enantiomers. *Chem. Senses* **30,** 171–175.

Law, R. H., and Regnier, F. E. (1971). Pheromones. *Annu. Rev. Biochem.* **40,** 533–548.

Leyden, J. J., McGinley, K. J., Hoelzle, E., Labows, J. N., and Klingman, A. M. (1981). The microbiology of the human axillae and its relationship to axillary odor. *J. Invest. Dermatol.* **77,** 413–416.

Lundström, J. N., and Olsson, M. J. (2005). Subthreshold amounts of social odorant affect mood but not behavior, in heterosexual women when tested by a male, but not a female, experimenter. *Biol. Psychol.* **70,** 197–204.

Lundström, J. N., Hummel, T., and Olsson, M. J. (2003). Individual differences in sensitivity to the odor of 4, 16-androstadien-3-one. *Chem. Senses* **28,** 643–650.

Maiworm, R. M., and Langthaler, W. U. (1992). Influence of androstenol and androsterone on the evaluation of men of varying attractiveness levels. *In* "Chemical Signals in Vertebrates VI," (R. L. Doty and D. Muller-Schwarze, Eds.), pp. 575–579. Plenum, New York.

McBurney, D. H., Levine, J. M., and Cavanaugh, P. H. (1977). Psychophysical and social ratings of human body odour. *Pers. Soc. Psychol. Bull.* **3,** 135–138.

McChance, R. A., and Puhorit, G. (1969). Ethnic differences in the response of the sweat glands to pilocarpine. *Nature* **221,** 378–379.

McCoy, N. L., and Pitino, L. (2002). Pheromonal influences on sociosexual behaviour in young women. *Physiol. Behav.* **75,** 367–375.

McCullough, P. A., Owen, J. W., and Pollack, E. I. (1981). Does androstenol affect emotion? *Ethol. Sociobiol.* **2,** 85–88.

Millington, P. E., and Wilkinson, R. (1983). Skin. Cambridge University Press, Cambridge.

Møller, A. P., and Swaddle, J. P. (1997). Asymmetry, Developmental Stability and Evolution. Oxford University Press, Oxford.

Montagna, W., and Parakkal, P. (1974). The Structure and Function of Skin. Academic Press, New York.

Müller-Schwarze, D. (1999). Signal specialization and evolution in mammals. *In* "Advances in Chemical Signals in Vertebrates," (R. E. Johnston, Ed.), pp. 1–14. Kluwer Academic/Plenum Publishers, New York.

Murdock, G. P. (1957). World ethnographic sample. *Am. Anthropol* **59,** 664–687.

Natsch, A., Gfeller, H., Gygax, P., Schmid, J., and Acuna, G. (2003). A specific bacterial aminoacylase cleaves odorant precursors secreted in the human axilla. *J. Biol. Chem.* **278,** 5718–5727.

Ober, C., Weitkamp, L. R., Cox, N., Dytch, H., Kostyu, D., and Elias, S. (1997). HLA and mate choice in humans. *Am. J. Hum. Genet.* **61,** 497–504.

Ober, C., Hyslop, T., Elias, S., Weitkamp, L. R., and Hauck, W. W. (1998). HLA matching and fetal loss: Results of a 10-year prospective study. *Hum. Reprod.* **13,** 33–38.

Pause, B. M., Ohrt, A., Prehn, A., and Ferstl, R. (2004). Positive emotional priming of facial perception in females is diminished by chemosensory anxiety signals. *Chem. Senses* **29,** 797–805.

Penn, D. J. (2002). The scent of genetic compatability: Sexual selection and the major histocompatability complex. *Ethology* **108,** 1–21.

Penn, D. J., and Potts, W. K. (1998). MHC-disassortative mating preferences reversed by cross-fostering. *Proc. R. Soc. London, Ser. B* **265,** 1299–1306.

Penn, D. J., and Potts, W. K. (1999). The evolution of mating preferences and major histocompatability complex genes. *Am. Nat.* **153,** 145–164.

Polak, M. (2003). Developmental Instability: Causes and Consequences. Oxford University Press, Oxford.

Preti, G., Spielman, A. I., and Wysocki, C. J. (1997). Vomeronasal organ and human chemical communication. *In* "Encyclopedia of Human Biology," (R. Dulbecco, Ed.), 2nd edn., Vol. 8, pp. 769–783. Academic Press, New York.

Rako, S., and Friebely, J. (2004). Pheromonal influences on sociosexual behaviour in postmenopausal women. *J. Sex Res.* **41,** 372–380.

Rennie, P. J., Gower, D. G., and Holland, K. T. (1991). In-vitro and in-vivo studies of human axillary odour and cutaneous microflora. *Br. J. Dermatol.* **124,** 596–602.

Rikowski, A., and Grammer, K. (1999). Human body odour, symmetry and attractiveness. *Proc. R. Soc. London, Ser. B* **266,** 869–874.

Roberts, S. C., Gosling, L. M., Carter, V., and Petrie, M. (2008). MHC-correlated odour preferences in humans and the use of oral contraceptives. *Proc. R. Soc. London, Ser. B* **275,** 2715–2722.

Russell, M. J. (1976). Human olfactory communication. *Nature* **260,** 520–522.

Santos, P. S., Schinemann, J. A., Gabardo, J., and Bicalho, M. G. (2005). New evidence that the MHC influences odor perception in humans: A study with 58 Southern Brazilian students. *Horm. Behav.* **47,** 384–388.

Sato, K., Kane, N., Soos, G., and Sato, F. (1995). The eccrine sweat gland: Basic science and disorder of eccrine sweating. *In* "Progress in Dermatology," (A. N. Moshell, Ed.), Vol. 29, pp. 1–11. Dermatology Foundation, Evanston, IL.

Savic, I., Berglund, H., Gulyas, B., and Roland, P. (2001). Smelling of odourous sex hormone-like compounds causes sex-differentiated hypothalamic activation in humans. *Neuron* **31,** 661–668.

Saxton, T. K., Lyndon, A., Little, A. C., and Roberts, S. C. (2008). Evidence that androstadienone, a putative human chemosignal, modulates women's attributions of men's attractiveness. *Horm. Behav.* **54,** 597–601.

Schleidt, M. (1980). Personal odor and nonverbal communication. *Ethol. Sociobiol.* **1,** 225–231.

Schleidt, M., Neumann, P., and Morishita, H. (1981). A cross-cultural study on the attitude towards personal odours. *J. Chem. Ecol.* **7,** 19–31.

Shehadeh, N., and Klingman, A. (1963). The bacteria responsible for axillary odor. *J. Invest. Dermatol.* **41,** 3–10.

Shelley, W. B., Hurley, H. J., and Nichols, A. C. (1953). Axillary odour: Experimental study of the role of bacteria, apocrine sweat, and deodorants. *Arch. Dermatol. Syphiol.* **68,** 430–446.

Spielman, A. I., Zeng, X.-N., Leyden, J. J., and Preti, G. (1995). Proteinaceous precursors of human axillary odor: Isolation of two novel odor binding proteins. *Experientia* **51,** 40–47.

Stephan, H., Bauchot, R., and Andy, O. J. (1970). Data on size of the brain and of various body parts in insectivores and primates. *In* Schaal, B. and Porter, R. H. (1991). Microsmatic humans revisited: The generation and perception of chemical signals. *Adv. Study Behav.*, 20, 135–199.

Stoddart, D. M. (1990). The Scented Ape: The Biology and Culture of Human Odour. Cambridge University Press, Cambridge.

Szabo, G. (1963). The number of eccrine sweat glands in human skin. *In* "Advances in the Biology of Skin," (W. Montagna, R. A. Ellis, and A. F. Silver's, Eds.), pp. 3–10. Pergamon, Oxford.

Thorne, F., Neave, N., Scholey, A., Moss, M., and Fink, B. (2003). Effects of putative male pheromones on female ratings of male attractiveness: Influence of oral contraceptives and the menstrual cycle. *Neuroendocrinol. Lett.* **23,** 291–297.

Thornhill, R., and Gangestad, S. W. (1999). The scent of symmetry: A human sex pheromone that signals fitness. *Evol. Hum. Behav.* **20,** 175–201.

Thornhill, R., Gangestad, S. W., Miller, R., Scheyd, G., McCollough, J. K., and Franklin, M. (2002). Major histocompatability complex genes, symmetry and body scent attractiveness in men and women. *Behav. Ecol.* **14,** 668–678.

Troccaz, M., Starkenmann, C., Niclass, Y., van de Waal, M., and Clark, A. J. (2004). 3- Methyl-3-sulfanyhexan-1-ol as a major descriptor for the human axillae sweat odour profile. *Chem. Biodivers.* **1,** 1022–1035.

Wedekind, C., and Füri, S. (1997). Body odour preferences in men and women: Do they aim for specific MHC combinations or simply heterozygosity? *Proc. R. Soc. London, Ser. B* **264,** 1471–1479.

Wedekind, C., Seebeck, T., Bettens, F., and Paepke, A. (1995). MHC dependent mate preferences in humans. *Proc. R. Soc. London, Ser. B* **260,** 245–249.

Wyatt, T. D. (2003). Pheromones and Animal Behavior: Communication by Smell and Taste. Cambridge University Press, Cambridge.

Wysocki, C. J., and Gilbert, A. N. (1989). National geographic smell survey: Effects of age are heterogeneous. *Ann. NY Acad. Sci.* **561,** 12–28.

Wysocki, C. J., and Preti, G. (1998). Pheromonal influences. *Arch. Sex. Behav.* **27,** 627–629.

Wysocki, C. J., and Preti, G. (2000). Human body odors and their perception. *Jpn. J. Smell Taste* **7,** 19–42.

Wysocki, C. J., and Preti, G. (2004). Facts, fallacies, fears, and frustrations with human pheromones. *Anat. Rec. A* **281,** 1201–1211.

Wysocki, C. J., Zeng, X.-N., and Preti, G. (1993). Specific anosmia and olfactory sensitivity to 3-mthyl-2-hexonic acid: A major component of human axillary odor. *Chem. Senses* **18,** 652–653.
Yamazaki, K., Boyse, E. A., Mike, V., Thaler, H. T., Mathieson, B. J., Abbott, J., Boyse, J., Zayas, Z. A., and Thomas, L. (1976). Control of mating preferences in mice by genes in the major histocompatability complex. *J. Exp. Med.* **144,** 1324–1335.
Zeng, X.-N., Leyden, J. J., Lawley, H. J., Sawano, K., Nohara, I., and Preti, G. (1991). Analysis of characteristic odors from human male axillae. *J. Chem. Ecol.* **17,** 1469–1492.
Zeng, X.-N., Leyden, J. J., Brand, J. G., Spielman, A. I., McGinley, K., and Preti, G. (1992). An investigation of human apocrine gland secretion for axillary odor precursors. *J. Chem. Ecol.* **18,** 1039–1055.
Zeng, X.-N., Leyden, J. J., Spielman, A. I., and Preti, G. (1996). Analysis of characteristic human female odors: Qualitative comparisons to males. *J. Chem. Ecol.* **22,** 237–257.

CHAPTER THREE

Current Issues in the Study of Androstenes in Human Chemosignaling

Jan Havlicek,* Alice K. Murray,[†] Tamsin K. Saxton,[‡] *and* S. Craig Roberts[†]

Contents

* Department of Anthropology, Faculty of Humanities, Charles University, Prague, Czech Republic
[†] School of Biological Sciences, University of Liverpool, Liverpool, UK
[‡] Philosophy, Psychology and Language Sciences, University of Edinburgh, Edinburgh, UK

Vitamins and Hormones, Volume 83
ISSN 0083-6729, DOI: 10.1016/S0083-6729(10)83003-1

Abstract

We review research on the 16-androstenes and their special claim, born originally of the finding that androstenes function as boar pheromones, to be human chemosignals. Microbial fauna in human axillae act upon the 16-androstenes to produce odorous volatiles. Both individual variation and sex differences in perception of these odors suggest that they may play a role in mediating social behavior, and there is now much evidence that they modulate changes in interpersonal perception, and individual mood, behavior, and physiology. Many of these changes are sensitive to the context in which the compounds are experienced. However, many key outstanding questions remain. These include identification of the key active compounds, better quantification of naturally occurring concentrations and understanding how experimentally administered concentrations elicit realistic effects, and elucidation of individual differences (e.g., sex differences) in production rates. Until such issues are addressed, the question of whether the androstenes play a special role in human interactions will remain unresolved.

I. Introduction

The cologne of a potential suitor, the smell of freshly baked bread pumped temptingly into a supermarket: the world is full of odors that are designed to alter our mood, perception, and behavior. Odors have tremendous effects on us, and influence us in unexpected ways. For instance, unsurprisingly, people automatically adjust the spread of their fingers to match the size of an object that they reach out to grasp. Yet present someone with a strawberry (a small item) while exposing them to the odor of an orange (a larger item), and people's grasp widens subtly yet perceptibly—and vice versa (Castiello *et al.*, 2006). These cross-modal modulations are not restricted to motor responses: for example, odors perceived as pleasant influence visual ratings of attractiveness (Demattè *et al.*, 2007), while sweet odors influence ratings of different tastes (Stevenson *et al.*, 1999). Yet when it comes to the question of whether odorous chemicals that are of human origin can systematically influence other humans, the answers tend to be more confused.

Human axillary odor derives in part from a range of compounds known as androstenes. Following early findings that some androstenes constitute pheromones produced in boar saliva, giving rise to classic stereotyped behavior in the form of lordosis (Signoret and du Mesnil du Buisson, 1961), research has attempted to establish whether androstenes affect human behavior in similar ways. Yet the question of whether there is any sense in speaking of human pheromones remains open. Some of those who consider the existence of human pheromones to be an unresolved question do so on the basis of what they see as a shortage of empirical data (e.g., Hays, 2003). The concern of others may be less to do with the specific findings (or lack of them) and more an objection based on definitional semantics, based on a preference to reserve the term "pheromone" for traditional releaser or primer effects (review in Saxton and Havlicek, 2010). Others (e.g., Doty, 2010) refute the suggestion that mammals have pheromones at all, preferring to think of them simply as social chemosignals. In this light, social odors influence behavior in the way that a peacock's train or a human smile might do in the visual domain.

Whether or not they turn out to be pheromones (if these exist in mammals), research continues into the influence of androstenes on human physiology and behavior. Studies have focussed on the production of androstenes in the axillae, the biochemistry and microbiology that influence the origins of human body odor, and the impact of sex differences and puberty on these mechanisms. Others have investigated individual differences in perception, including effects of the menstrual cycle, differences in odor threshold levels, and the effects of sensitization. Finally, some researchers have directed their efforts at understanding whether androstenes impact on human mood, physiology, perception, and behavior. Here we synthesize these different approaches, commenting on problematic areas such as the use of variable methodologies to elucidate relevant effects in humans. We suggest that the lack of a consistent pattern of results may arise through a lack of ecologically valid approaches and an insufficient theoretical framework. We conclude by offering suggestions which may direct future research in this complex and challenging field.

II. Biochemistry of Androstenes

A. Production

The main 16-androstenes occurring in humans are 5α-androst-16-en-3-one (5α-androstenone), 5α-androst-16-en-3α-ol (5α-androstenol), and 4,16-androstadien-3-one (androstadienone). Their metabolism has been extensively studied in pigs, in which they are produced in the Leydig cells in the testes from the precursor pregnenolone (Brooks and Pearson, 1986). In humans, it is thought that these compounds are produced in the adrenal glands and the ovary (Smals and Weusten, 1991) and that their metabolism follows a common steroidogenic pathway (Dufort *et al.*, 2001); however, their detailed metabolism is far from understood. Androstenol has been detected in human urine (Brooksbank and Haslewood, 1961); androstenone (Claus and Alsing, 1976) and androstadienone (Brooksbank *et al.*, 1972) occur in plasma and saliva (Bird and Gower, 1983).

The 16-androstenes are also found in the axillary region, a major source of human body odor (although they represent only a small proportion of the compounds found here (James *et al.*, 2004) and some have argued they contribute relatively little to the character of armpit odor (Natsch *et al.*,

2006)). The axillae are abundant in eccrine and apocrine skin glands. The main function of the eccrine glands, which produce chlorine and magnesium ions and water, is thermoregulation. In contrast, apocrine glands produce a range of chemicals including fatty acids, cholesterol, and 16-androstene steroids. Analysis of fresh apocrine secretion induced by adrenaline injection found that it contained dehydroepiandrosterone, androsterone, and cholesterol (Labows *et al.*, 1979). Other studies detected androstadienone and 5α-androstenone, but no 3α-androstenol (Gower *et al.*, 1994).

Differences in androstene production, for example those associated with age and sex, are important for understanding their potential function. Although information is sparse, levels of 5α-androstenone are on average higher in adult men compared to women (Bird and Gower, 1983), and excretion of androstenol in the urine of prepubertal individuals is negligible compared to postpuberty (Cleveland and Savard, 1964). These findings are indicative of a sexually dimorphic pattern of expression which becomes evident around puberty, a pattern that is characteristic of a trait that is subject to sexual selection (e.g., see Andersson 1986).

B. The role of the skin microflora

Androstenes and other compounds constitute a substrate for axillary bacteria which produce odorous volatiles (Leyden *et al.*, 1981; Savelev *et al.*, 2008). This is evidenced by experimental treatment with a bactericidal agent (Povidone-iodine) leading to a significant decrease in 5α-androst-16-en-one (Bird and Gower, 1982). Similarly, other agents (e.g., Farnesol Plus) which inhibit growth of coryneforms result in a decrease in armpit odor intensity (Haustein *et al.*, 1993).

The axillary microflora consist primarily of *Micrococcus*, *Staphylococcus*, *Propionibacteria*, *Corynebacteria*, and eukaryotic *Malasezia* (Leyden *et al.*, 1981; Rennie *et al.*, 1991; Taylor *et al.*, 2003; Wilson, 2005). The *Corynebacteria* appear to be primarily responsible for the intensity of axillary odor (Rennie *et al.*, 1991), and this is supported by *in vitro* studies showing that coryneform bacteria are of special significance in 16-androstene metabolism (Leyden *et al.*, 1981; Rennie *et al.*, 1991), although only a small subset of coryneforms are able to metabolize these steroids (Austin and Ellis, 2003; Decreau *et al.*, 2003). Early *in vitro* studies using both pure and mixed cultures of coryneforms showed that they are able to metabolize testosterone into various breakdown products including dihydrotestosterone and 17-androstenes; however, 16-androstenes were not detected (Nixon *et al.*, 1984, 1986a,b, 1987). Some *Micrococcus luteus* strains, but not *Staphylococcus* or *Propionibacterium*, were also found to metabolize testosterone (Rennie *et al.*, 1989b). Detailed examination of biochemical pathways shows that coryneforms can transform only precursors containing a C16 double bond (Austin and Ellis, 2003). These molecules include androstadienol and androstadienone, which are

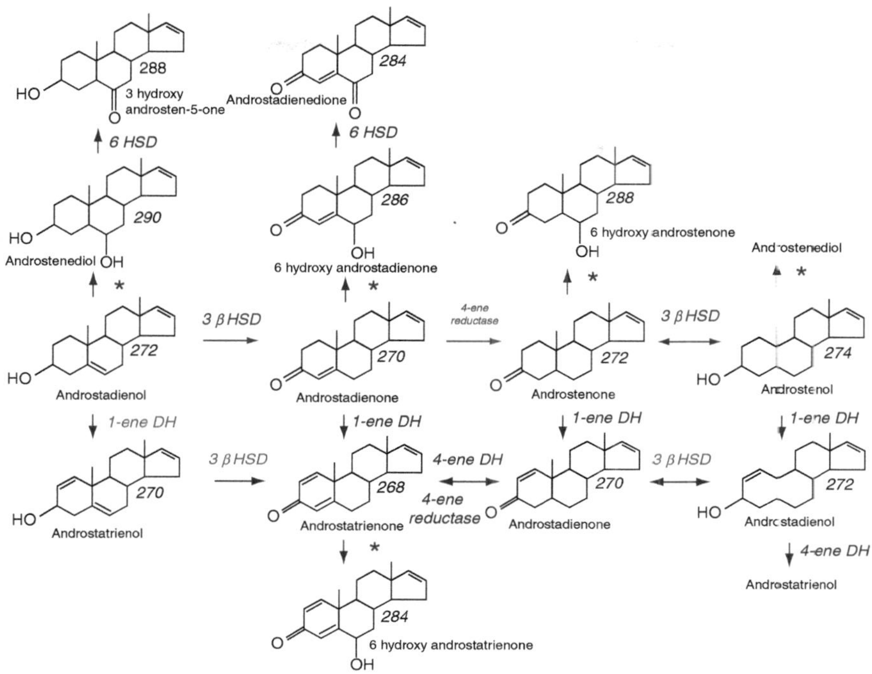

Figure 3.1 Biotransformation of 16-androstenes by corynebacteria (A) axillary isolates. It is important to note that the extent of biotransformation of 16-androstene steroids is likely to be more complex than that presented in this figure, as both α- and β-forms of hydroxylated steroids are probably generated. Key: HSD, hyroxysteroid dehydrogenase; DH, dehydrogenase. *Denotes biotransformations that may involve a number of enzymes (e.g., hydroxylase or dehydroxylase and hydratase activities). Reprinted from *J. Steroid Biochem. Mol. Biol.* 87, Austin and Ellis Microbial pathways leading to steroidal malodour in the axilla. 105-110. (2003) with permission from Elsevier.

subsequently transformed into several different androstenes including 5α-androstenone and 3α-androstenol (Fig. 3.1). There is further evidence for reversible transformations between 5α-androstenone and 3α-androstenol, between 3α-androstenol and androstadienol, and between 5α-androstenone and androstadienone (Rennie *et al.*, 1989a). Another study using androsta-5,16-dien 3β-ol, androsta-4,16-dien 3β-ol, and androsta-5,16-dien 3β-one as substrates for coryneforms found a main reaction at C-3 oxidation which resulted in odorous androsta-4,16-dien-3-one (Decreau *et al.*, 2003).

C. Quantitative assessments of androstene production

Quantitative estimates of axillary extracts find high interindividual variability. Using gas chromatography–mass spectrometry (GC–MS), Nixon *et al.* (1988) found the following concentrations in male axillary hair extracts (in pmol/total axillary hair weight/24 h): androstenone 0–433, androstadienone 0–4103, androstadienol 0–728, 3α-androstenol 0–1752, and 3β-androstenol 0–416. Comparison between the sexes indicates higher levels of androstenone in men (range 5.2–1019 pmol/24 h) than in women (range 1.2–16.6 pmol/24 h, with one outlier of 551 pmol/24 h) (Gower *et al.*, 1985). In another study, male samples contained higher concentrations of dehydroepiandrosterone sulfate, but not androstenol (Preti *et al.*, 1987). Concentrations of androstenol showed cyclic patterns, with a peak in the midfollicular phase of the menstrual cycle in women, and some seasonal fluctuations in men (Preti *et al.*, 1987).

III. Psychophysical Research Using Androstenes

A. Prevalence of specific anosmia

Specific anosmia (Amoore, 1967) is a condition in which an individual with normal olfactory sensitivity is incapable of perceiving a particular odor. A classic example, and thus an extensively studied case, is that of androstenone anosmia. Estimates of prevalence range from 7.6% in females and 44.3% in males (Griffiths and Patterson, 1970), to 46% (Amoore *et al.*, 1977) or 50% (Beets and Theimer, 1970) in all subjects (see Table 3.1 for a more comprehensive overview of anosmia studies). Rates of androstenol anosmia may reach 90% in females and 45% in males (Gower *et al.*, 1985). However, it has been claimed that the interpretation of the term "anosmia," in conjunction with the screening methods employed, may have led to overestimation of rates of nondetection (Bremner *et al.*, 2003). Even after identifying putative nondetectors using standard methods, forced-choice tests showed that these individuals could identify androstenone at rates above chance, despite low confidence in their decision. In light of this, Bremner *et al.* revised downward the rate of androstenone anosmia in a healthy adult population to 1.8–6.0%, considerably lower than previous estimates.

Similar findings have arisen in relation to levels of 16-androstene anosmia. In a study focussing on the laboratory-synthesized compound 5-α-androst-16-an-3-one (androstanone), it was found that previously labeled anosmics were able to detect androstanone under experimental conditions (Van Toller *et al.*, 1983). The authors likened this to the results of a previous study (Schiffman, 1979) in which subjects were hypnotically induced into a state where they could perceive previously undetectable odors, attributing the newfound detection to a form of altered perceptual state. Anosmic subjects from the same study were found to correctly identify androstanone in a secondary detection task in which they were presented with androstanone and told when to expect it. Here they recognized the odor from the

Table 3.1 Reported androstenone nondetection rates

Study	Method/criterion for nondetection	Concentration	*N*[a]	Nondetection rate[a] (%)
Beets and Theimer (1970)	One trial; subjective assessment	Unknown (diluted in alcohol)	F (35), M (65)	11
Griffiths and Patterson (1970)	One trial; subjective assessment of smelling strip	Unknown (800 ng residual evaporated from ether as dilutant)	F (145), M (165)	F (7.6), M (44.3)
Amoore *et al.* (1977)	2/5AFC[b] threshold; lowest conc. with both correct	2.9 ppb solution (water)	764	47
Dorries *et al.* (1989)	Two AFC runoff series; <5 consecutive correct	1.0×10^{-1} (highest conc.); in mineral oil	Not specified	F (24), M (40)
Gilbert and Wysocki (1987) and Wysocki *et al.* (1991)	Scratch and sniff strip; subjective assessment	Not specified	26, 200	F (24), M (33)
Pause *et al.* (1999)	2 AFC staircase; <7 reversals	1.25 mg/ml of 1,2-propanediol (highest); 0.04 μg/ml (lowest)	F (132)	F (10.6)
Stevens and O'Connell (1995)	2/5 runoff series, threshold test; <2 consecutive correct trials	5.4 mM binary dilution series, 12 steps	40	75
Sirota *et al.* (1999)	3AFC runoff series; <4 consecutive correct trials	1.25 mg/ml binary dilution series (mineral oil); 10 steps	M (20)	M (25)
Morofushi *et al.* (2000)	One/two runoff series, threshold test; <4 consecutive correct trials	5 μM to 5 mM in 1.5 ml mineral oil; 10 steps	F (63)	F (22)
Filsinger *et al.* (1984)	Passive exposure; subjective assessment of impregnated paper	1 mg crystal residue evaporated from 1% solution in 100% ethanol	F (102), M (98)	F (9), M (13)

(continued)

Table 3.1 *(continued)*

Study	Method/criterion for nondetection	Concentration	N[a]	Nondetection rate[a] (%)
Bremner *et al.* (2003)	3AFC screening followed by yes/no forced-choice detection	5 mg crystal androstenone; 30 ml of 7.34×10^{-3} M androstenone in light mineral oil	M (33), F (22)	3AFC: 16.3 (no sex differences) FC: 1.8–6.0
Baydar *et al.* (1993)	3AFC staircase, <3 consecutive correct trials	19.36 ppb androstanone diluted with humidified air stream	F (41), M (38)	F (15.8), M (26.8)
Boyle *et al.* (2006) (Expt 1)	3 AFC	Air bubbled through 4 ppm androstenone in propylene glycol, diluted to 80% v/v androstenone	13	0
Knaapila *et al.* (2008)	Scratch-and-sniff: rate from "no odor" (presumed anosmic) to "extremely strong odor"	0.1% solution in diethyl phthalate	917 (twins; 137 without co-twin)	F (17.6), M (21.9)
Kline *et al.* (2007)	2AFC; anosmia defined as ≤50% accuracy	500 ppm (volume/mass)	F (34), M (34)	F (26.5), M (17.6)
Lübke *et al.* (2009)	2AFC single staircase	Highest concentration: 1.25 mg/ml in 1,2-propanediol	M (27)	M (25.9)
Wang *et al.* (2004)	Three-repetition, 2AFC staircase	3.67 mM (0.1% w/v) in silicone oil	58	15.5
Pierce *et al.* (2004)	Rate odor on 1–9 intensity scale (1 = presumed anosmic)	3.67 mM (1×10^{-1}% wt/vol; 1 g/L) androstenone in light mineral oil	F (136), M (122)	F (14.7), M (28.7)

Table on page 45 reprinted with permission from Oxford University Press and taken from Bremner *et al.* (2003). The prevalence of androstenone anosmia. *Chem.Senses* **28,** 423-432 and updated on this page to include further studies.

[a] F denotes female participants, M denotes males, otherwise sex was not specified.

[b] AFC = Alternative forced-choice.

first trial, claiming that they did not respond to the odor initially because they could not give the odor a verbal label. The same subjects exhibited a skin conductance response when exposed to androstanone, despite not consciously detecting its odor (Van Toller *et al.*, 1983).

Worldwide variation in the ability to detect androstenone is apparent (Gilbert and Wysocki, 1987), yet explanations for this have only recently been considered. Boyle *et al.* (2006) attributed this variation to trigeminal interference. The trigeminal system detects chemical irritants in the environment; in doing so, it seems to inhibit olfactory processing of odors (Cain and Murphy, 1980). Most odorants have a trigeminal component (Doty *et al.*, 1978) which is usually concentration-dependent (Cometto-Muniz *et al.*, 1998; Hummel *et al.*, 1992). Accordingly, anosmia variation could be due to trigeminal sensation, which in turn will be dependent upon the concentrations and methodologies of researchers. Indeed, Boyle *et al.* (2006) reported an inverse correlation between androstenone olfactory thresholds and trigeminal sensitivity. Incorporation of trigeminal data might therefore be advantageous in understanding this area of study.

In summary, the number of people who are truly anosmic to androstenone seems to be reliant on many factors. For future studies to control for anosmia occurrence, it seems necessary to establish a standardized method by which it can be reported. Pause *et al.* (1999) showed that altering the conservativeness of methodology resulted in anosmia estimates ranging between 10% and 37%.

B. Thresholds

Olfactory thresholds are usually measured using a geometric concentration scale, consisting of binary dilution steps (see Keller and Vosshall, 2004 for an overview). Early work investigated the idea that sensitivity to androstenone was inherited (Pollack *et al.*, 1982), possibly as a dominant Mendelian trait (Smith, 1974). More recently, twin studies indicate significant heritability (Gross-Isseroff *et al.*, 1992; Knaapila *et al.*, 2008; Wysocki and Beauchamp, 1984) and genetic variation in the odorant receptor OR7D4 has been found to influence both androstenone valence and sensitivity (Keller *et al.*, 2007). However, threshold differences also occur between individuals, between sexes, across the menstrual cycle, and through puberty.

Lundström *et al.* (2003b) identified a bimodal distribution in sensitivity to androstadienone, with a small group of highly sensitive "supersmellers," but their androstadienone threshold did not correlate with those for phenyl ethyl alcohol (PEA, a rose odor), suggesting that androstadienone sensitivity may be different from general olfactory acuity. A similar pattern of bimodal sensitivity can also be found for androstenone (Amoore, 1991). However, Jacob *et al.* (2006) reported not a bimodal, but a multimodal threshold distribution of androstadienone, arguing that thresholds to related axillary steroids are likely to be dependent upon individual variation in exposure history, thereby implying that thresholds are plastic and environmentally influenced, at least to some extent (also see "Sensitization"). This could potentially explain the finding that homosexual men have lower thresholds to androstenone than heterosexual men (Lubke *et al.*, 2009).

Lundström *et al.* (2003b) also reported a tendency for women to have lower thresholds for androstadienone than men, confirming previous observations (Koelega and Koster, 1974). However, there appears to be no sex difference in thresholds to androstenone (Gower *et al.*, 1985).

With regard to the menstrual cycle, Lundström *et al.* (2006) reported that women's sensitivity to androstadienone was higher in the fertile phase than in the luteal phase. They suggested that this was linked to the potential functional role of androstadienone in mate choice (Jacob and McClintock, 2000; Lundström *et al.*, 2003a,b; Savic *et al.*, 2001; Saxton *et al.*, 2008a), and this was also evidenced by the lack of a comparable change in responses to the odor of PEA.

Savic *et al.* (2001) reported a sexually dimorphic effect whereby women, but not men, exhibited anterior hypothalamic activation following exposure to androstadienone (androstenol has similar effects: Savic and Berglund, 2010). Since the anterior hypothalamus plays a significant role during puberty (causing the release of gonadotropins from the pituitary gland), it might be expected that androstadienone thresholds would also change during puberty. Consistent with this prediction, a relatively high proportion of very young children may be able to detect androstenone (Schmidt and Beauchamp, 1988), suggesting a decrease in sensitivity between early childhood and adulthood. Furthermore, a peripubertal decrease in androstenone sensitivity has been reported in men but not in women (Dorries *et al.*, 1989), possibly due to the sexual dimorphism in production discussed above. A similar trend occurs for androstadienone thresholds (Hummel *et al.*, 2005). Furthermore, Chopra *et al.* (2008) reported the same effect not only for androstadienone, but also for 2-methyl, 3-mercapto-butanol (2M3M; a malodorous component of human sweat), using both chemosensory event-related potentials (CSERPs) and psychophysically measured thresholds. The results of the CSERPs were consistent with psychophysical findings, whereby increases in latencies in male pubescents highlighted their higher thresholds to androstadienone.

C. Sensitization

Sensitization is the process of becoming more sensitive to a stimulus. Repeated exposure to an odor normally leads to adaptation and decreased sensitivity; but unusually, the reverse seems to occur for androstenone and androstadienone, a characteristic that contributes to their unique properties. Wysocki *et al.* (1989) noticed that heightened sensitivity could be induced in some individuals by repetitive exposure. They reported that the ability to smell androstenone was induced in 10 of 20 initially insensitive subjects after they had been systematically exposed to androstenone (for 3 min, 3 times a day, for 6 weeks). Their explanation likened the olfactory system to an immune system response, with clonal expression of olfactory receptors occurring by a yet unknown mechanism. Subsequent studies have suggested that other sites mediate these changes, including the olfactory epithelium (Wang *et al.*, 2004; Yee and Wysocki, 2001) and central components of the olfactory system (Mainland *et al.*, 2002).

Similarly, Jacob *et al.* (2006) reported a reduction in thresholds for androstadienone, in both men and women, of more than 4 orders of magnitude (from 3.5×10^{-3} M to 0.3×10^{-6} M) after repetitive exposure (following the same exposure schedule as Wysocki *et al.*, but for 2 weeks only). Using this same methodology, with the addition of CSERP and olfactory-evoked potential (OEP) readings, Boulkroune *et al.* (2007) shed light on gender dimorphisms during this sensitization process. Although they found a decrease in detection thresholds for androstadienone similar to those found by Jacob *et al.*, changes in the later components of the evoked potentials were specific to women and apparently linked to cognitive and perceptual functioning, indicative of a female-specific "learning" component in androstadienone perception. Again, these results are consistent with androstenes bearing characteristics fitting of sexually selected chemosignals.

D. Hedonic perception

A range of studies have investigated how the hedonic perception of androstene compounds differs across time and between individuals. Verbal labels range from being reminiscent of "strong urine" (Ohloff *et al.*, 1983) to "musky" (Jacob *et al.*, 2002) and "unpleasant" (Lundström *et al.*, 2003b), and compounds vary in intensity: androstadienone has been described as a "low-odor androstene" in comparison with androstenone (Pause, 2004). While investigating the effects of repetitive exposure to androstadienone, Jacob *et al.* (2006) reported an additional change in perceived odor quality with increased sensitivity, a result confirmed by Boulkroune *et al.* (2007). Low-sensitivity subjects initially rated androstadienone with a wide range of negative and positive descriptors. Following exposure-induced sensitization, negative adjectives such as "putrid," "vegetable," and "woody" came to predominate. This process was explained in terms of two putative odor channels, one responding to broadly pleasant odors and the other to putrid odors (Jacob *et al.*, 2006), via low- and high-affinity receptors, respectively (Polak, 1973; Stevens and O'Connell, 1995). Thus, exposure to androstadienone in sensitized individuals might activate the high-affinity receptors responsive to putrid odors while the low-affinity receptors remain inactive.

Most studies of hedonics have focussed on changes in odor perception across the menstrual cycle. Hummel *et al.* (1991) investigated the hedonic estimates of several odorants, including androstenone. Only with regard to androstenone did trend analysis reveal a significant change across cycle phase, with more pleasant perceptions at midcycle. Similarly, Grammer (1993) reported that, while females rated androstenone as unattractive, their response became less negative around ovulation.

IV. Psychological Effects

A. Changes in interpersonal perception

A summary of studies describing effects of androstenes on perception, mood, and behavior is provided in Table 3.2. In an early experiment, Cowley *et al.* (1977) asked participants to wear surgical masks impregnated with androstenol, volatile fatty acids, or a control (nontreated) mask. Participants then assessed suitability of three job applicants of each sex who were pictured in photographs accompanied by verbal descriptions. Women exposed to androstenol rated applicants more positively than those wearing masks impregnated with fatty acids; men exposed to androstenol rated applicants more negatively than the control group. A similar technique (i.e., impregnated masks and rating of images) was also used by Kirk-Smith *et al.* (1978), this time with participants rating photographs of people, animals, and buildings. Androstenol exposure caused both women and men to judge female images as more attractive (images of both sexes were also rated as emotionally warmer), but there was no effect on ratings of images depicting animals or buildings (although they found the opposite in a follow-up study: Kirk-Smith and Booth, 1990). More recently, the impregnated mask technique was used to explore the effect of androstenol in a marketing context (Ebster and Kirk-Smith, 2005). Raters judged three magazines regarded by an independent panel as masculine, neutral, and feminine in terms of their philosophy, target audience, and purchasing intention. When exposed to androstenol, men but not women increased their ratings of the masculinity and positivity of the "masculine" journal. Together, these results imply a degree of context specificity, discussed further below.

The impregnated mask technique has been criticized because it exposes experimental participants to far higher androstene concentrations than those found in axillary odor. To avoid this, Black and Biron (1982) aimed to use a more natural setting. In their design, men and women watched a 15-min slide-show, together with a confederate of the opposite sex who had applied androstenol, exaltolide (a synthetic musk), or a nonsmelling substance. Participants afterward judged the confederate's attractiveness. There was no significant effect of androstenol or exaltolide. However, as noted by Filsinger *et al.* (1985), there was a statistical tendency ($p = 0.07$) for confederates to be rated as less attractive by those in the androstenol condition.

Table 3.2 A summary of key studies investigating effects of androstenone, androstenol, and androstadienone on perception, mood, and behavior

Study	Compound[a]	Conc./ Quantity	Target sex[b] (*N*)	Mask[c]	Exposure method	Measure	Main effect[b]
Perception							
Cowley *et al.* (1977)	AL	1 mg/1 ml	F, M (183)	×	Surgical mask	Perception of others	F attributed more positive traits to others, M attributed more negative traits to others.
Kirk-Smith *et al.* (1978)	AL	0.3 mg	F (12), M (12)	×	Surgical mask	Perception of others	F rated more attractive by both sexes.
Black and Biron (1982)	AL	1% in 95% ethanol	F (39), M (39)	×	Confederate's odor	Attractiveness perception	None
Filsinger *et al.* (1984)	AN	1 mg	F (102), M (98)	×	Envelopes	Self and other perception	M rated M more passive. F rated themselves as less sexy
Filsinger *et al.* (1985)	AL, AN	1 mg, 1 mg	F (132), M (122)	×	Envelopes	Self and other perception	AL: M rated M more attractive. AN: F rated M and F less attractive
Kirk-Smith and Booth (1990)	AN	0.25 mg	F (8), M (8)	×	Surgical mask	Perception of others	Rated others as less sexy
Ebster and Kirk-Smith (2005)	AL	1 mg/ml	F (60), M (60)	×	Surgical masks	Product evaluation	M rated men's magazines more masculine and had more positive buying intentions
Saxton *et al.* (2008a)	AND	250 μM	F (22,19,12)	✓	Upper lip	Attractiveness perception	F rated M more attractive
Hummer and McClintock (2009)	AND	250 μM	F (30), M (20)	✓	Upper lip	Perception of emotion	Raters more engaged to emotionally significant stimuli

(continued)

Table 3.2 *(continued)*

Study	Compound[a]	Conc./ Quantity	Target sex[b] (*N*)	Mask[c]	Exposure method	Measure	Main effect[b]
Mood							
Cowley *et al.* (1980)	AL	1 mg/1 ml	F (153)	×	Surgical masks	Mood during the menstrual cycle	Increased irritability during menses
McCollough *et al.* (1981)	AL	2 second spray of Boar Mate	F (161), M (59)	×	Surgical masks	Emotional responsiveness	No effect
Benton (1982)	AL	150 μg	F (18)	×	Upper lip	Mood during the menstrual cycle	F more submissive during middle of menstrual cycle
Jacob and McClintock (2000); Expt 1	AND	250 μM	F (10), M (10)	×	Upper lip	Mood and alertness	Increased positive mood state in F
Jacob and McClintock (2000); Expt 2	AND	250 μM	F (31)	✓	Upper lip	Mood and alertness	Prevention of mood deterioration. Modulatory effect
Jacob *et al.* (2001a)	AND	250 μM	F (44), M (21)	✓	Upper lip	Skin temp, skin conductance, and mood	M increase in positive mood with a F experimenter
Jacob *et al.* (2002)	AND, AL	250 μM	F (18), M (19)	✓	Smelling swab/ upper lip	Mood	Reduced negative mood and increased positive mood
Lundström *et al.* (2003a)	AND	250 μM	F (38,40)	✓	Upper lip	Mood and concentration	Increased feelings of focus

Bensafi *et al.* (2003)	AND	50 mg	F (12), M (12)	×	Jars	Mood	No effect on mood
Bensafi *et al.* (2004a)	AND	50 mg	F (36), M (36)	×	jars	Mood, memory and autonomic function	Maintained positive mood and decreased memory of events in F
Bensafi *et al.* (2004b)	AND	6250 μM, 250 μM	F (30), M (30)	×	Jars	Mood and autonomic function	High concentration increased positive mood and decreased negative mood in F only
Lundström and Olsson (2005)	AND	250 μM	F (37)	✓	Upper lip	Mood and arousal	Increase in psychophysical arousal and mood when experimenter was M
Villemure and Bushnell (2007)	AND	250 μM	F (48)	×	Jars	Pain thresholds and mood	Increased positive mood in F in the absence of pain
Wyart *et al.* (2007)	AND	30 mg	F (21)	×	Jars	Cortisol levels, mood, and physiological arousal	Maintained positive mood and increased sexual arousal
Behavior							
Kirk-Smith and Booth (1980)	AN	3.2 μg, 16 μg, 32 μg	540	×	Sprayed chairs	Preference of seats	F preferred to sit on 3.2 μg or 32 μg sprayed seats. M avoided 32 μg sprayed seats
Gustavson *et al.* (1987)	AL	2.5 mg	480	×	Sprayed Perspex	Choice of toilet cubicle	M avoided sprayed stalls, F had no preference
Cowley and Brooksbank (1991)	AL	1 mg	F (38), M (38)	×	Impregnated necklace	Opposite sex exchanges	F reported more exchanges with males

[a] Compound abbreviations: AN refers to androstenone, AND to androstadienone; AL to androstenol.
[b] Target sex refers to the individuals exposed to the compound (F = female, M = male).
[c] Masking odor: used/not used (in all cases where used, masking odor was eugenol/clove oil).

It is not known whether the short duration of exposure to the compound, and length of time between exposure and rating, could have minimized a possibly transient effect.

Another method for testing the psychological effects of the androstenes was introduced by Filsinger *et al.* (1984, 1985). A male photograph, impregnated with different compounds, was rated by participants on several personality and appearance scales. In their first study, they compared androstenone with three controls: no odor, a negative odor (scatol, a fecal odor), and a positive odor (methyl anthranilate, a fruit odor). This procedure aimed to control for effects based on a possible hedonic quality of androstenone. Men judged the man in the photograph as more passive if they were exposed to androstenone compared with the positive odor; there was no difference in women's ratings. However, women in the androstenone condition rated themselves as less sexy than controls. A follow-up study compared effects of androstenone, androstenol, and exaltolide (Filsinger *et al.*, 1985). Here, photos of both sexes were rated. Men judged male images less positively if exposed to androstenone compared with androstenol and exaltolide. They also rated images of men treated with androstenol as sexier than those assessing unscented photos. Men exposed to all the three compounds rated themselves less sexy than the men in the no-odor condition. Women exposed to androstenone and androstenol, compared with the no-odor condition, rated men as more weak and less sexy; and women in the androstenone condition rated women's photos as less sexy. No effect on self-perception was detected.

Most recently, Hummer and McClintock (2009) tested whether the effects of androstadienone on attention and perception are restricted to social and emotional contexts. They found that inhalation of androstadienone caused men and women to react faster to affective facial expressions but not to neutral faces or nonsocial stimuli (shapes). Similarly, in Stroop tests, androstadienone affected attention to both positive and negative emotional words, but not attention to neutral stimuli.

All of these studies took place under laboratory conditions. To discover whether androstenes might have effects in more naturalistic settings, Saxton *et al.* (2008a) carried out three speed-dating experiments (speed-dating involves a series of time-limited interactions as a means to meet potential partners). In two out of three experiments, women exposed to androstadienone masked in clove oil (to avoid possible detection of androstadienone) rated the men they interacted with as more attractive than did women exposed to clove oil alone (all women met the same men).

B. Changes in mood

As described in the introduction, odors are powerful modulators of affective states, so it is not surprising that researchers have explored the effects of androstenes on mood (see Table 3.2). In an early study, Cowley *et al.*,

(1980) used masks impregnated with androstenol to test changes in mood across the menstrual cycle. Women exposed to androstenol (as compared to no-odor or naphthalene conditions) reported higher levels of irritability and depression during their menstrual bleeding. A similar study found that androstenone elicited higher ratings of alertness and excitability compared to a nonodor control (Kirk-Smith and Booth, 1990). Benton (1982), in contrast, applied androstenol or a control compound every morning to the woman's filtrum, finding that androstenol-exposure induced higher submissiveness self-ratings at midcycle. In a similar vein, Jacob and McClintock (2000) daubed participants' necks and filtrums with androstadienone, estratetraenol, or a control (propylene glycol, in which the steroids were dissolved). Estratetraenol is a steroid substance detected in pregnant women (Thysen *et al.*, 1968), with several physiological effects (Monti-Bloch and Grosser, 1991). At intervals of 6 min, 2 h, 4 h, and 9 h postapplication, participants completed questionnaires on their emotional state. After 6 min, androstadienone and estratetraenol were associated with increased positive mood in women, and decreased mood in men. Androstadienone-exposed women scored higher on some subscales (i.e., "Stimulant," "High") even after 2 h, and experienced lower postexperiment decrease in positive mood.

Another paper compared the effects of androstadienone, androstenol, and muscone (a synthetic steroid) (Jacob *et al.*, 2002), which share similar chemical structure and perceptual qualities. Compounds were first inhaled passively, then applied to the participant's filtrum 25 min later. Androstadienone again prevented a decrease in positive mood (factor "Elation-vigor") compared to both androstenol and muscone, and also prevented an increase in negative mood compared to muscone.

Changes in women's mood due to androstadienone were subsequently confirmed in two experiments by another research group (Lundström *et al.*, 2003a). Here, women reported feeling more focussed following application of androstadienone in eugenol (a synthetic clove odor); results were identical when those women who reliably discriminated androstadienone were excluded. Similarly, Villemure and Bushnell (2007) reported mood changes and increased tolerance of pain following androstadienone exposure (in women but not men).

Other studies suggest that the mood effects of androstadienone could be modulated by various contexts. McCollough *et al.* (1981) induced mood by asking participants to read a passage of erotic fiction, but found no differences in ratings of 11 emotional scales between those exposed (via masks) to androstenol, rose, or a no-odor control. Subsequently, Bensafi *et al.* (2004a) induced emotional reactions by presenting excerpts from happy, sad, arousing, and neutral movies. Exposure to androstadienone while watching a sad movie was associated with positive mood in women and sad mood in men. Androstadienone and estratetraenol were linked with increased arousal in both sexes while watching an erotic movie, but there was no change when participants viewed neutral and funny movies, consistent with previous studies of mood effects in neutral contexts (Bensafi *et al.*, 2003; Hummer and McClintock, 2009).

Finally, another study of emotional contexts found that androstadienone increased positive mood and sexual arousal in women (Wyart *et al.*, 2007). A further development arose when Jacob *et al.* (2001a) noted that mood changes depend on the administrator's sex: women's positive mood in the presence of androstadienone increased in the presence of a male but not a female administrator (see also Lundström and Olsson, 2005).

As some critiques have acknowledged (e.g., Black and Biron, 1982), the key variable in these studies appears to be the concentration of the compound under investigation. The only study on this issue has showed that a high concentration of androstadienone (625 μM) increased positive and decreased "high arousal negative mood" in women in contrast to men, whereas no mood effect at a low concentration (250 μM) was observed (Bensafi *et al.*, 2004b).

C. Behavioral effects

Evidence about context-dependent effects of androstenes on mood change and perception is certainly important, but leaves open the question of whether these effects translate into behavioral changes. To answer this, we should examine evidence on behavioral effects, and in particular those investigated in naturalistic settings. In the first study of this kind, researchers impregnated seats in a dentist's waiting room with androstenone (Kirk-Smith and Booth, 1980). Female patients approached the treated seats, while male patients avoided them. In a second elegant study, researchers impregnated doors of student restroom stalls with ethanol, androstenol, or androsterone (a compound that smells similar to androstenol, but is not a constituent of human body odor), and monitored men's and women's usage (Gustavson *et al.*, 1987). Men but not women avoided cubicles impregnated with androstenol, but not the two controls.

A third group of researchers used a "necklace technique" to test the effect of androstenol and copulines in natural settings (Cowley and Brooksbank, 1991). Participants wore a plastic tube with open ends that had been impregnated with the target substance (0.25 ml chloroform with 1 mg/ml androstenol) as a necklace from the afternoon until the next morning, when they were asked to record details of all their morning social interactions, including sex of their interlocutor, length and depth of the conversation, and details of who initiated the interaction. Women who wore androstenol reported more interactions with men but not with other women, and longer and deeper conversations.

D. Effects on physiology

The research group led by Luis Monti-Bloch in the late 1980s focussed on the question of human vomeronasal organ (VNO) function. One of the substances they used in their experiments was androstadienone. Its application directly into the VNO led to neural activity (measured by an electrovomeronasogram) in men but not in women, whereas application to the main olfactory mucosa did not reveal any such activity (Monti-Bloch and Grosser, 1991; for a detailed overview of key physiclogical studies, see Table 3.3). Another study of women by the same team found electrovomeronasal activity immediately after the application of the substance, together with an increase in skin conductance, decrease in respiration rate and pulse 35 min after the application, and a decrease in negative mood (Grosser *et al.*, 2000). Other studies, reviewed below, did not set out to differentiate whether androstadienone was perceived by the main olfactory organ or the VNO.

Several of the studies reviewed above also assessed physiological changes, and most revealed sex-specific changes. For instance, Jacob *et al.* (2001a) found an increase in skin conductance in women (but not men) following exposure to androstadienone, and that women's skin temperature decreased while it increased in men. These effects were particularly evident in women when the experimenter was male; there was no effect of the experimenter's gender on male participants.

Sex-specific changes were also observed in a study by Bensafi *et al.* (2003), who constructed an overall physiological index to measure arousal. Androstadienone increased arousal in women and decreased it in men. This was mainly due to changes in skin conductance, pulse, and respiration. A follow-up study by the same team, to test the effect of context (Bensafi *et al.*, 2004a), found increases in skin temperature, and a decrease in respiration rates in men but not women, following exposure to androstadienone in the context of an erotic video. In other contexts (induced by viewing a neutral, happy, or sad movie), androstadienone did not induce physiological changes. A second study (Bensafi *et al.*, 2004b) reported that only a high dose (625 μM) and not a low dose (250 μM) of androstadienone was associated with affective and physiological changes. Finally, Wyart *et al.* (2007) suggest that androstadienone raises levels of cortisol in women (men were not tested). The authors also replicated findings of the effects of androstadienone on composite measures of physiological arousal.

E. Brain imaging

If androstenes work as human chemosignals, they should give rise to specific brain responses. This issue has been explored by several brain imaging studies (see Table 3.3). Smelling androstadienone in clove oil activates the right

Table 3.3 A summary of the key studies investigating the effects of androstadienone and androstenone on human physiology and brain function

Study	Compound[a]	Conc.	Target sex[b] (*N*)	Mask[c]	Exposure method	Measure	Main effect[b]
Electrophysiology							
Van Toller *et al.* (1983)	AN	0.6 mg, 6 mg, and 10 mg	M (11) F (16)	×	Smelling strip	Skin conductance	Increased skin conductance in reported anosmics
Grosser *et al.* (2000)	AND	100 pg	F (40)	×	VNO	Tension and autonomic function	Reduction in nervousness, tension, and other negative feelings. Altered autonomic function
Jacob *et al.* (2001a)	AND	250 μM	F (44), M (21)	✓	Upper lip	Skin temperature and skin conductance	Skin temp increases in M and lowered in F Increased skin conductance in both
Bensafi *et al.* (2003)	AND	50 mg	F (12), M (12)	×	Jars	Physiological state	Increased physiological arousal in F but not M
Wyart *et al.* (2007)	AND	30 mg	F (21)	×	Jars	Cortisol levels, mood and physiological arousal.	Increased cortisol levels in saliva and physiological arousal
Brain imaging							
Jacob *et al.* (2001b)	AND	250 μM	F (10)	×	Passive inhalation	FDG—PET scan	Activated the right prefrontal cortex, amygdala, and hypothalamus in F
Savic *et al.* (2001)	AND	200 mg	F (12), M (12)	×	Passive inhalation	PET	Activated anterior-ventral hypothalamus in F

Gulyas *et al.* (2004)	AND	5% solution	F (5)	×	Jars	PET	Activated orbitofrontal cortex, inferior prefrontal cortex and fusiform gyrus
Savic *et al.* (2005)	AND	200 mg	F (12), M (24)	×	Bottles	PET	Activated areas associated with sexual behavior in homosexual M and heterosexual F
Berglund *et al.* (2006)	AND	200 mg	F (24), M (12)	×	Bottles	PET	Lesbian F processed AND more similarly to heterosexual M than heterosexual F.

[a] Compound abbreviations: AN refers to androstenone; AND to androstadienone.
[b] Target sex refers to the individuals exposed to the compound (F = female, M = male).
[c] Masking odor: used/not used (in all cases where used, masking odor was clove oil).

prefrontal cortex, amygdala, and hypothalamus in women (Jacob *et al.*, 2001b). Specific comparisons of the sexes have revealed sex-specific activations: androstadienone (200 mg in crystalline form) activated the anterior-ventral hypothalamus in women, while estratetraenol activated the same brain area in men (Savic *et al.*, 2001). These areas are sexually dimorphic and are presumably involved in sexual behavior, including sexual orientation. A subsequent study showed that homosexual men exhibited activation patterns similar to heterosexual women (Savic *et al.*, 2005). Moreover, heterosexual (but not homosexual) women showed an activation of the hypothalamus after inhalation of androstadienone (Berglund *et al.*, 2006). Interestingly, both compounds activate areas known to be involved in processing odor perception (e.g., amygdala, piriform, orbitofrontal, and insular cortex).

Gulyas *et al.* (2004) compared brain activations in four odor conditions: androstadienone (5% solution in dipropylene glycol), pleasant (gamma-methyl-ionon), unpleasant (methyl-thio-butanoate), and a control (dipropylene glycol). Androstadienone showed activation in the orbitofrontal cortex, inferior prefrontal cortex, and fusiform gyrus, compared to the control, and activation in the inferior prefrontal cortex and superior temporal cortex compared to the pleasant and unpleasant odors. The superior temporal cortex area is known to be involved in face recognition and in mental states connected with social interactions. The inferior prefrontal cortex is activated in social cognitive and emotional processes. Thus, these activational patterns emphasize the potential role of androstenes in social interactions.

V. Discussion

The literature we have reviewed leads us to several overarching questions that we believe remain largely unanswered, but which necessitate satisfactory answers before we can even approach a full understanding of the role of androstenes in human social interactions.

A. What compound(s) are responsible for social function?

Most of the research to date has investigated effects of androstenone, androstenol, or androstadienone. While there is plenty of mixed evidence and conflicting results from these studies, the fact that the majority of studies find some form of effect, and most that investigate a specific effect find somewhat complementary findings, suggests that there is reasonable evidence that androstenes do influence physiology, psychology, and behavior to some degree. However, given that very few studies have compared the effects of two or more of these compounds within the same study, and because most studies use widely varying methodologies, it remains a very difficult task to form a coherent picture.

The selection of the compound of interest (from the three previously mentioned) for different experiments appears, at least to us, somewhat arbitrary. We perceive there to have been a gradual shift in focus of interest from androstenone and androstenol in earlier work to androstadienone more recently. The earlier work was inspired by findings in pigs that androstenone functioned as a releaser pheromone in sexual activity. However, the reason for the shift from androstenone to androstadienone is unclear. In our view, the choice of compound appears to be more akin to the vagaries of fashion than a logical and rational process of falsification. We should hasten to admit that we have not been immune to this ourselves (e.g., in the selection of androstadienone for our speed-dating study Saxton *et al.*, 2008a). However, what is clearly needed in future work is a concerted effort to actively compare the effects of the three compounds within the same experiments. This will enable us to determine the extent to which reported effects are compound-specific or compound-general. This is a question that is critical to the discussion of possible pheromonal effects, since any definition of a pheromone (strict or not) will require us to determine the compound responsible.

What if it emerges that such studies demonstrate that androstene compounds exert comparable effects? Would this mean that they are all pheromones, or none? The answer to this question may depend critically on a greater understanding of the biochemical metabolic pathways involved in the formation of each compound, and in the compound-specific contributions to the chemosignal (discussed below). That is, which of the compounds are actually perceived and contribute to appropriate responses by the signal receivers, and which are simply either precursors or byproducts of the active compound(s)?

We also need to be aware of the possibility that the true functional signal carried in axillary odor may be a mixture of compounds, rather than a single one acting in isolation. At least in vertebrates, almost all chemical signals are composed of compound mixtures, with the precise communicative message being determined by precise ratios of a subsample of key compounds. For example, colony-specific signatures of ants are formed by ratios of different cuticular hydrocarbons (Guerrieri *et al.*, 2009). Similarly in mice, individual variation in urinary odor associated with genes in the major histocompatibility complex, which influences MHC-disassortative mate choice independently of other cues (Roberts and Gosling, 2003), is coded by characteristic ratios of volatile carboxylic acids (Singer *et al.*, 1997). In this light, it is possible that each of the three compounds, at given ratios, contributes to an overall signal. It is also possible that other, yet unknown, compounds are involved. If either of these possibilities turns out to be true, we will have barely begun to understand how the androstenes influence behavior. Also, each of the compounds may have a slightly different effect; for instance, it was reported recently that distinct cuticular hydrocarbons affect species and sex recognition and sex attractiveness in fruit flies (Billeter *et al.*, 2009).

B. What is the relevant concentration to enable social function?

A glance at Tables 3.2 and 3.3 shows the diversity of concentrations which have been used to assess effects of androstenes. To some extent, these are due to the differing intensities of the three most commonly studied compounds—androstadienone is the least intense and thus researchers have tended to use this at a comparably higher concentration than in the case of the other two. Further variation across studies using any given compound is largely due to individual preferences of different researchers, and subsequent studies often tend to copy the chosen concentration. An example is the choice of a concentration of 250 μM, at which Jacob and McClintock (2000) tested the effects of androstadienone and estratetraenol on mood. No justification was given for the use of this concentration, which is far higher than any measured concentration (see section on Quantitative Assessment), but this has since been used by a substantial number of studies (Tables 3.2 and 3.3).

Does the use of substantially higher compound concentrations in experiments invalidate the results? This approach was criticized almost three decades ago by Black and Biron (1982). However, the use of higher concentrations might not alter the nature or direction of an effect, though this awaits testing—indeed, studies that have compared effects at different concentrations within the same study are fewer than those that have compared the effects of different compounds in the same study. Results of a study by Bensafi *et al.* (2004b) support the notion that concentration matters. It will certainly be interesting to see results of studies that test supranormal and substantially reduced concentrations. However, what seems indisputable is that a higher concentration must enhance the likelihood of signal detection, and thus the likelihood of any response. In this regard, it will be interesting to discover what the typical concentrations of relevant compounds are in the headspace surrounding the axillae—the medium in which any natural chemoreception will take place. To date, quantitative measures of concentrations stem from measurements on axillary skin or hair, or from artificially elicited apocrine secretion. At best, this markedly overestimates the concentrations at which potential functionally relevant detection takes place.

Furthermore, supranormal concentrations are likely to introduce potentially anomalous results if they elicit responses in individuals who would not detect or react to more ecologically valid concentrations. As we have outlined, substantial variation in detection thresholds and rates of anosmia are hallmarks of androstene psychophysical research. Detection thresholds vary not just between individuals, but also at different times (e.g., across the menstrual cycle) and depending on the degree of prior exposure. The latter may be relevant, for example, when comparing women who experience male axillary odor on a regular basis, such as via the odor of their male partners, with those who do not (e.g., those without current partners). Indeed, recent studies investigating women's perception of male odors find that partnered women perceive odors in different ways compared with currently single women, whether the effect is concerned with the relationship between odor pleasantness and either male dominance (Havlicek *et al.*, 2005) or MHC-similarity (Roberts *et al.*, 2008).

To fully understand responses to androstenes, we need to take into account these kinds of effects, whether it is by collecting relevant background information (e.g., relationship status) and/or by undertaking some form of psychophysical screening before behavioral/psychological measurement. One example of the benefits of such an approach is the study by Morofushi *et al.* (2000), which found that individual women with higher sensitivity to androstenol were more likely to exhibit synchronization in their menstrual cycles, compared to those who were less sensitive. Without this information, the possible implication of androstenol in cycle synchronization would have been missed.

C. Is individual variation in production, detection, and sensitivity to behavioral change consistent with a signaling function?

As we have described, there is huge diversity in the kinds of effects that have been attributed to the androstenes, and in the consistency of findings within specific experimental paradigms. However, some themes have emerged that bear upon the question that underpins most of the research, namely whether androstenes carry communicative significance. Two of the most important appear to be that there are sex differences in both production and response to androstene compounds, and that the context in which testing occurs is critical to obtaining apparent responses.

Whether or not androstenes are produced at different levels in men and women is clearly a question of fundamental importance. A sex difference would allow us to infer which sex is the signaler, and it appears that this is males, as might be expected from the starting point of the field (and of this chapter): the boar pheromone. Very few studies have produced quantitative estimates of androstene expression in individuals, but the existing evidence (albeit based on a very small sample) suggests that levels are higher in men than women (Gower *et al.*, 1985). This, coupled with the finding that androstene production becomes upregulated around puberty (Cleveland and Savard, 1964), indicates that the signal is likely to be involved in sexual selection. However, what it does not conclusively help us with is the identity of the signal receiver. The nature of chemical communication, in contrast with most visual and acoustic signals, means that this is usually open to question, since the same signal may be used by conspecifics of both sexes in different contexts (see e.g., Gosling and Roberts, 2001).

It is possible, for example, that androstenes are produced by males as part of an intrasexual signaling system linked to competition over access to resources or mates. In light of links between mammalian scent-marking and dominance (Gosling and Roberts, 2001), this explanation resonates particularly well with findings that androstene exposure leads to physiological arousal (Jacob *et al.*, 2001a; but see Bensafi *et al.*, 2003), higher masculinity ratings of male magazines (Ebster and Kirk-Smith, 2005), and avoidance by men but not women of impregnated restroom stalls (Gustavson *et al.*, 1987). However, it seems that females also respond to androstene exposure in a manner consistent with the notion that androstene expression is an intersexual signal. Women exposed to androstenes rate males more positively than controls (androstadienone: Saxton et al., 2008a; but see opposite effect of androstenone: Filsinger et al., 1985), experience more exchanges with men (Cowley and Brooksbank, 1991), and experience heightened physiological arousal (Bensafi *et al.*, 2003). Furthermore, brain imaging studies suggest that smelling androstadienone affects brain activity according to sexual orientation (Savic *et al.*, 2005). Teasing apart the differential responses and sensitivity to androstenes is of utmost importance in understanding their communicative function, and more work is needed to attain a clearer picture of which sex is the principal receiver (although it is possible that a signal selected for communication with one sex might have been co-opted, during evolutionary history, as a signal to the other).

Sensitivity to context is one way to address this, and it is becoming clear that the context in which experiments take place has a large bearing on the nature of the result. Ecological validity in the study of androstenes has been discussed in Saxton *et al.* (2008a,b). Two examples will suffice here. First, in two experiments, Jacob *et al.* (2001a) and Lundström and Olsson (2005) showed that exposure to androstadienone influenced women's mood, but only in a subsample of female participants who were tested by a male experimenter; those tested by a female experimenter experienced no alteration in mood. This again suggests that androstenes function as a signal to women. Second, in contrast with previous experiments in the laboratory that found no effect on women's attributions of male attractiveness (e.g., Black and Biron, 1982), or even reduced them (Filsinger *et al.*, 1985), when these effects were tested in a face-to-face scenario (a speed-dating context), attributions increased as predicted (Saxton *et al.*, 2008a).

If androstenes are produced by men, perhaps mainly to signal to women, what is the information that is being signaled? It is conceivable that androstenes are simply sex-markers, indicating that the signaler is male. However, it seems likely that, in common with other sexually selected signals, the message is more subtle and complex than this, signaling individual variation in male quality and thus suitability as a mate and father. Studies of female perceptions of male axillary odors show that women who express a relatively high preference for androstadienone also have relatively high preferences for masculine male faces; this suggests cross-modal concordance in preference strength for masculine traits (Cornwell *et al.*, 2005). Furthermore, axillary odor pleasantness correlates with psychometric dominance in men (Havlicek *et al.*, 2005) and physical indicators of attractiveness in other sensory modalities (e.g., Rikowski and Grammer, 1999), results that link odor quality with other physical traits that indicate putative male quality. Although the chemical basis for the latter studies is unknown, it seems reasonable in light of Cornwell *et al.*'s results that androstenes could be at least partly responsible for mediating these important behavioral effects. Finally in this regard, differential sensitivity (Lundström *et al.*, 2006) and higher hedonic ratings (Grammer, 1993; Hummel *et al.*, 1991) to androstenes at midcycle, when conception is most likely, also point to an evolutionary adaptation to optimal discrimination of good-quality mates, who would be predicted to have characteristic androstene profiles.

D. To what extent are androstenes special?

What we have discussed thus far assumes that the three androstenes that have been most studied (or others, or a mixture composed of these) are responsible for a set of physiological and/or psychological responses, and that these responses are specific and unique to these compounds. This seems a reasonable conclusion, though it is by no means certain.

One way that this conclusion can be made more plausible is the use of odor controls in experimental designs. It is possible that some of the effects we have reviewed are at least partly due to nonspecific sensory stimulation inherent in the presentation of the androstene odors. Perhaps this is most likely in the measurement of physiological responses such as arousal, but in principle it applies equally to any outcome variable. To circumvent this flaw in design, a number of studies have included odor controls where the control is a nonandrostene. Several studies (e.g., Saxton *et al.*, 2008a) have used clove oil; in this approach, the clove odor is presented together with the androstene, and without it (Saxton *et al.* additionally used a water control). Although this has the additional advantage of acting as a masking odor to prevent experimental participants from detecting the androstene, it means that the androstene is presented within an odor mixture, and in a way that is in no way ecologically valid. Another alternative is to include another condition altogether, ideally another nonandrostene odor that occurs naturally within axillary odor (to enhance ecological validity) or is perceptually similar. For example, Jacob *et al.* (2002) used muscone, a synthetic musky odor, finding that androstadienone, but not muscone (or androstenol), was responsible for maintaining positive mood. Such examples of odor specificity support the idea that androstenes have specific effects and that it is thus a reasonable exercise to focus on these particular compounds, which after all represent only a small proportion of the cocktail of compounds present in axillary odor.

Another way to investigate the specificity of androstene effects could be to use a comparative approach; in other words, to examine the extent to which responses to androstenes are conserved across closely related species (e.g., nonhuman primates), relative to other odor compounds. Laska *et al.* (2005) measured thresholds for androstenone and androstenol in spider monkeys, squirrel monkeys, and pig-tailed macaques. They found that androstenone thresholds are similar to those of humans, yet androstenol thresholds are considerably higher. Although there are no details of sexual dimorphisms in thresholds, nor a comparison involving other, nonandrostene compounds, this kind of research is an appropriate start to what we think could potentially be a fruitful approach.

E. Conclusions

We have outlined a considerable body of research that collectively describes a set of compounds, expressed in natural axillary odor at higher levels in males, which have specific physiological and behavioral effects in other individuals, particularly in females. Put like this, androstenes sound very much like pheromones, according to almost any definition. Despite this, we remain cautious about this conclusion and prefer to use the term chemosignal (or even semiochemical). Reasons for this caution include the facts that it remains unclear which compound or mixture of compounds is responsible for the most potent effects, that we think it far from conclusively demonstrated that any one of these compounds is responsible for the effects as opposed to a generic androstene or odor effect (although there is some limited support for this notion), and that effects remain to be shown at ecologically appropriate concentrations (which are as yet unknown). At another level, we wish to distance ourselves from what we see as the naive search for a human sex pheromone that encapsulates much of the media's coverage of the research described here, and that perhaps represents the motivation of some researchers. The simplistic view of such pheromones, in which involuntary, stereotypical responses are triggered by the faintest whiff of a compound, arises from an uncritical extrapolation from the kind of pheromonal response observed in insects. In contrast to this, our primary concern is that an ecologically appropriate framework, informed by evolutionary approaches where appropriate, should be used to explore and elucidate the action of this group of compounds. Although a good start has been made, we think that this work has some way yet to go.

ACKNOWLEDGMENTS

J. H. was supported by GACR P407/10/1303 grant and Czech Ministry of Education grant 0021620843 at the time of preparing the manuscript. A. K. M. was supported by the BBSRC.

REFERENCES

Amoore, J. E. (1967). Specific anosmia—A clue to the olfactory code. *Nature* **214,** 1095–1098.

Amoore, J. E. (1991). Specific anosmias. *In* "Smell and Taste in Health and Disease," (T. V. Getchell, R. L. Doty, L. M. Bartonshuk, and J. B. Snow, Eds.), pp. 655–664. Raven Press, New York.

Amoore, J. E., Pelosi, P., and Forrester, L. J. (1977). Specific anosmias to 5-alpha-androst-16-en-3-one and omega-pentadecalactone: The urinous and musky primary odors. *Chem. Senses Flavor* **2,** 401–425.

Andersson, M. (1986). Sexual selection. Princeton University Press, Princeton, New Jersey.

Austin, C., and Ellis, J. (2003). Microbial pathways leading to steroidal malodour in the axilla. *J. Steroid Biochem. Mol. Biol.* **87,** 105–110.

Baydar, A., Petrzilka, M., and Schott, M.-P. (1993). Olfactory thresholds for androstenone and Galaxolide: sensitivity, insensitivity and specific anosmia. *Chem. Senses* **18,** 661–668.

Beets, M. G. J., and Theimer, E. T. (1970). Odour similarity between structurally unrelated odorants. *In* "Taste and Smell in Vertebrates," (G. E. W. Wolstenholme and J. Knight, Eds.), pp. 313–323. Churchill, London.

Bensafi, M., Brown, W. M., Tsutsui, T., Mainland, J. D., Johnson, B. N., Bremner, E. A., Young, N., Mauss, I., Ray, B., Gross, J., Richards, J., Stapper, I., *et al.* (2003). Sex-steroid derived compounds induce sex-specific effects on autonomic nervous system function in humans. *Behav. Neurosci.* **117,** 1125–1134.

Bensafi, M., Brown, W. M., Khan, R., Levenson, B., and Sobel, N. (2004a). Sniffing human sex-steroid derived compounds modulates mood, memory and autonomic nervous system function in specific behavioral contexts. *Behav. Brain Res* **152,** 11–22.

Bensafi, M., Tsutsui, T., Khan, R., Levenson, R. W., and Sobel, N. (2004b). Sniffing a human sex-steroid derived compound affects mood and autonomic arousal in a dose-dependent manner. *Psychoneuroendocrinology* **29,** 1290–1299.

Benton, D. (1982). The influence of androstenol-a putatuve human pheromone-on mood throughout the menstrual cycle. *Biol. Psychol.* **15,** 249–256.

Berglund, H., Lindstrom, P., and Savic, I. (2006). Brain response to putative pheromones in lesbian women. *Proc. Natl. Acad. Sci. USA* **103,** 8269–8274.

Billeter, J.-C., Atallah, J., Krupp, J. J., Millar, J. G., and Levine, J. D. (2009). Specialized cells tag sexual and species identity in *Drosophila melanogaster*. *Nature* **461,** 987–989.

Bird, S., and Gower, D. B. (1982). Axillary 5-alpha-androst-16-en-3-one, cholesterol and squalene in men; preliminary evidence for 5-alpha-androst-16-en-3-one being a product of bacterial action. *J. Steroid Biochem. Mol. Biol.* **17,** 517–522.

Bird, S., and Gower, D. B. (1983). Estimation of the odorous steroid, 5-alpha-androst-16-en-3-one, in human saliva. *Experientia* **39,** 790–791.

Black, S. L., and Biron, C. (1982). Androstenol as a human pheromone: No effect on perceived physical attractiveness. *Behav. Neural Biol.* **34,** 326–330.

Boulkroune, N., Wang, L. W., March, A., Walker, N., and Jacob, T. J. C. (2007). Repetitive olfactory exposure to the biologically significant steroid androstadienone causes a hedonic shift and gender dimorphic changes in olfactory-evoked potentials. *Neuropsychopharmacology* **32,** 1822–1829.

Boyle, J. A., Lundström, J. N., Knecht, M., Jones-Gotman, M., Schaal, B., and Hummel, T. (2006). On the trigeminal percept of androstenone and its implications on the rate of specific anosmia. *J. Neurobiol.* **66,** 1501–1510.

Bremner, E. A., Mainland, J. D., Khan, R. M., and Sobel, N. (2003). The prevalence of androstenone anosmia. *Chem. Senses* **28,** 423–432.

Brooks, R. I., and Pearson, A. M. (1986). Steroid hormone pathways in the pig, with special emphasis on boar odor—A review. *J. Anim. Sci.* **62,** 632–645.

Brooksbank, B. L., and Haslewood, G. A. D. (1961). Estimation of androst-16-en-3alpha-ol in human urine. Partial synthesis of androstenol and of its beta-glucosiduronic acid. *Biochem. J.* **80,** 488–496.

Brooksbank, B. W. L., Wilson, D. A. A., and MacSweeney, D. A. (1972). Fate of androsta-4, 16-dien-3-one and the origin of 3α-androst-16-ene in man. *J. Endocrinol.* **52,** 239–251.

Cain, W. S., and Murphy, C. L. (1980). Interaction between chemo-receptive modalities of odor and irritation. *Nature* **284,** 255–257.

Castiello, U., Zucco, G. M., Parma, V., Ansuini, C., and Tirindelli, R. (2006). Cross-modal interactions between olfaction and vision when grasping. *Chem. Senses* **31,** 665–671.

Chopra, A., Baur, A., and Hummel, T. (2008). Thresholds and chemosensory event-related potentials to malodors before, during, and after puberty: Differences related to sex and age. *Neuroimage* **40,** 1257–1263.

Claus, R., and Alsing, W. (1976). Occurrence of 5-alpha-androst-16en-3-one, a boar pheromone, in man and its relationship to testosterone. *J. Endocrinol.* **68,** 483–484.

Cleveland, W. W., and Savard, K. (1964). Studies of excretion of androst-16-en-3alpha-ol. *J. Clin. Endocrinol. Metabol.* **24,** 983.

Cometto-Muniz, J. E., Cain, W. S., and Abraham, M. H. (1998). Nasal pungency and odor of homologous aldehydes and carboxylic acids. *Exp. Brain Res.* **118,** 180–188.

Cornwell, R. E., Boothroyd, L., Burt, D. M., Feinberg, D. R., Jones, B. C., Little, A. C., Pitman, R., Whiten, S., and Perrett, D. I. (2005). Concordant preferences for opposite-sex signals? Human pheromones and facial characteristics. *Proc. Roy. Soc. Lond. B* **271,** 635–640.

Cowley, J. J., and Brooksbank, B. W. (1991). Human exposure to putative pheromones and changes in aspects of social behaviour. *J. Steroid Biochem. Mol. Biol.* **39,** 647–659.

Cowley, J. J., Johnson, A. L., and Brooksbank, B. W. (1977). The effect of two odorous compounds on performance in an assessment-of-people test. *Psychoneuroendocrinology* **2,** 159–172.

Cowley, J. J., Harwey, F., Johnston, A. T., and Brooksbank, B. W. L. (1980). Irritability and depression during menstrual cycle-possible role for an exogenous pheromone? *Irish J. Psychol.* **3,** 143–156.

Decreau, R. A., Marson, C. M., Smith, K. E., and Behan, J. M. (2003). Production of malodorous steroids from androsta-5, 16-dienes and androsta-4, 16-dienes by Corynebacteria and other human axillary bacteria. *J. Steroid Biochem. Mol. Biol.* **87,** 327–336.

Demattè, M. L., Österbauer, R., and Spence, C. (2007). Olfactory cues modulate facial attractiveness. *Chem. Senses* **32,** 603–610.

Dorries, K. M., Schmidt, H. J., Beauchamp, G. K., and Wysocki, C. J. (1989). Changes in sensitivity to the odor of androstenone during adolescence. *Dev. Psychobiol.* **22,** 423–435.

Doty, R. L. (2010). The great pheromone myth. John Hopkins University Press, Baltimore, Maryland.

Doty, R. L., Brugger, W. E., Jurs, P. C., Orndorff, M. A., Snyder, P. J., and Lowry, L. D. (1978). Intranasal trigeminal stimulation from odorous volatiles: Psychometric responses from anosmic and normal humans. *Physiol. Behav.* **20,** 175–185.

Dufort, I., Soucy, P., Lacoste, L., and Luu-The, V. (2001). Comparative biosynthetic pathway of androstenol and androgens. *J. Steroid Biochem. Mol. Biol.* **77,** 223–227.

Ebster, C., and Kirk-Smith, M. (2005). The effect of the human pheromone androstenol on product evaluation. *Psychol. Market.* **22,** 739–749.

Filsinger, E. E., Braun, J. J., Monte, W. C., and Linder, D. E. (1984). Human (*Homo sapiens*) responses to the pig (*Sus scrofa*) sex pheromone 5 alpha-androst-16-en-3-one. *J. Comp. Psychol.* **98,** 219–222.

Filsinger, E. E., Braun, J. J., and Monte, W. C. (1985). An examination of the effects of putative pheromones on human judgments. *Ethol. Sociobiol.* **6,** 227–236.

Gilbert, A. N., and Wysocki, C. J. (1987). The results of the National Geographic Smell Survey. *National Geographic* **172,** 514–525.

Gosling, L. M., and Roberts, S. C. (2001). Scent-marking by male mammals: Cheat proof signals to competitors and mates. *Adv. Stud. Behav.* **30,** 169–217.

Gower, D. B., Bird, S., Sharma, P., and House, F. R. (1985). Axillary 5 alpha-androst-16-en-3-one in men and women: Relationships with olfactory acuity to odorous 16-androstenes. *Experientia* **41,** 1134–1136.

Gower, D. B., Holland, K. T., Mallet, A. I., Rennie, P. J., and Watkins, W. J. (1994). Comparison of 16-androstene steroid concentrations in sterile apocrine sweat and axillary secretions: Interconversions of 16-androstenes by the axillary microflora—A mechanism for axillary odor production in man? *J. Steroid Biochem. Mol. Biol.* **48,** 409–418.

Grammer, K. (1993). 5-Alpha-androst-16en-3-alpha-on—A male pheromone? A brief report. *Ethol. Sociobiol.* **14,** 201–207.

Griffiths, N. M., and Patterson, R. L. (1970). Human olfactory responses to 5-alpha-androst-16-en-3-one- -principal component of boar taint. *J. Sci. Food Agric.* **21,** 4–6.

Gross-Isseroff, R., Ophir, D., Bartana, A., Voet, H., and Lancet, D. (1992). Evidence for genetic determination in human twins of olfactory thresholds for a standard odorant. *Neurosci. Lett.* **114,** 115–118.

Grosser, B. I., Monti-Bloch, L., Jennings-White, C., and Berliner, D. L. (2000). Behavioral and electrophysiological effects of androstadienone, a human pheromone. *Psychoneuroendocrinology* **25,** 289–299.

Guerrieri, F. J., Nehring, V. J., Jørgensen, C. G., Nielsen, J., Galizia, C. G., and d'Ettorre, P. (2009). Ants recognise foes and not friends. *Proc. Roy. Soc. Lond. B* **276,** 2461–2468.

Gulyas, B., Keri, S., O'Sullivan, B. T., Decety, J., and Roland, P. E. (2004). The putative pheromone androstadienone activates cortical fields in the human brain related to social cognition. *Neurochem. Int.* **44,** 595–600.

Gustavson, A. R., Dawson, M. E., and Bonett, D. G. (1987). Androstenol, a putative human pheromone, affects human (*Homo sapiens*) male choice performance. *J. Comp. Psychol.* **101,** 210–212.

Haustein, U. F., Herrmann, J., Hoppe, U., and Engel, W. (1993). Growth inhibition of coryneform bacteria by a mixture of three natural products—Farnesol, glyceryl, monolaurate and phenoxyethenol: HGQ. *J. Soc. Cosmet. Chem.* **44,** 211–220.

Havlicek, J., Roberts, S. C., and Flegr, J. (2005). Women's preference for dominant male odour: Effects of menstrual cycle and relationship status. *Biol. Letts* **1,** 256–259.

Hays, W. S. T. (2003). Human pheromones: Have they been demonstrated? *Behav. Ecol. Sociobiol.* **54,** 89–97.

Hummel, T., Gollisch, R., Wildt, G., and Kobal, G. (1991). Changes in olfactory perception during the menstrual cycle. *Experientia* **47,** 712–715.

Hummel, T. Livermore, A., Hummel, C., and Kobal, G. (1992). Chemosensory event-related potentials in man: Relation to olfactory and painful sensations elicited by nicotine. *Electroenceph. Clin. Neurophysiol.* **84,** 192–195.

Hummel, T., Krone, F., Lundström, J. N., and Bartsch, O. (2005). Androstadienone odor thresholds in adolescents. *Horm. Behav.* **47,** 306–310.

Hummer, T. A., and McClintock, M. K. (2009). Putative human pheromone androstadienone attunes the mind specifically to emotional information. *Horm. Behav.* **55,** 548–559.

Jacob, S., and McClintock, M. K. (2000). Psychological state and mood effects of steroidal chemosignals in women and men. *Horm. Behav.* **37,** 57–78.

Jacob, S., Hayreh, D. J. S., and McClintock, M. K. (2001a). Context-dependent effects of steroid chemosignals on human physiology and mood. *Physiol. Behav.* **74,** 15–27.

Jacob, S., Kinnunen, L. H., Metz, J., Cooper, M., and McClintock, M. K. (2001b). Sustained human chemosignal unconsciously alters brain function. *Chem. Senses* **12,** 2391–2392.

Jacob, S., Garcia, S., Hayreh, D., and McClintock, M. K. (2002). Psychological effects of musky compounds: Comparison of androstadienone with androstenol and muscone. *Horm. Behav.* **42,** 274–283.

Jacob, T. J. C., Wang, L. W., Jaffer, S., and McPhee, S. (2006). Changes in the odor quality of androstadienone during exposure-induced sensitization. *Chem. Senses* **31,** 3–8.

James, A. G., Casey, J., Hyliands, D., and Mycock, G. (2004). Fatty acid metabolism by cutaneous bacteria and its role in axillary malodour. *World J. Microbiol. Biotechnol.* **20,** 787–793.
Keller, A., and Vosshall, L. B. (2004). Human olfactory psychophysics. *Curr. Biol.* **14,** R875–R878.
Keller, A., Zhuang, H. Y., Chi, Q. Y., Vosshall, L. B., and Matsunami, H. (2007). Genetic variation in a human odorant receptor alters odour perception. *Nature* **449,** 468–472.
Kirk-Smith, M. D., and Booth, D. A. (1980). Effect of androstenone on choice of location in others' presence. *Olfaction Taste* **7,** 1–3.
Kirk-Smith, M. D., and Booth, D. A. (1990). The effect of five odorants on mood and assessment of other people. *In* "Chemical Signals in Vertebrates," (D. W. MacDonald, D. Müller-Schwarze, and S. E. Natynczuk, Eds.), pp. 48–54. Oxford University Press, Oxford.
Kirk-Smith, M. D., Booth, D. A., Carroll, D., and Davies, P. (1978). Human social attitudes affected by androstenol. *Res. Commun. Psychol., Psychiatry Behav.* **3,** 379–384.
Kline, J. P., Schwartz, G. E., and Dikman, Z. V. (2007). Interpersonal defensiveness and diminished perceptual acuity for the odor of a putative pheromone: Androstenone. *Biol. Psychol.* **74,** 405–413.
Knaapila, A., Tuorila, H., Silventoinen, K., Wright, M. J., Kyvik, K. O., Cherkas, L. F., Keskitalo, K., Hansen, J., Martin, N. G., Spector, T. D., Kaprio, J., and Perola, M. (2008). Genetic and environmental contributions to perceived intensity and pleasantness of androstenone odor: An international twin study. *Chemosens. Percept.* **1,** 34–42.
Koelega, H. S., and Koster, E. P. (1974). Some experiments on sex differences in odor perception. *Ann. NY Acad. Sci.* **237,** 234–246.
Labows, J. N., Preti, G., Hoelzle, E., Leyden, J., and Kligman, A. (1979). Steroid analysis of human apocrine secretion. *Steroids* **34,** 249–258.
Laska, M., Wieser, A., and Salazar, L. T. H. (2005). Olfactory responsiveness to two odorous steroids in three species of nonhuman primates. *Chem. Senses* **30,** 505–511.
Leyden, J. J., McGinley, K. J., Holzle, E., Labows, J. N., and Kligman, A. M. (1981). The microbiology of the human axilla and its relationship to axillary odor. *J. Invest. Dermatol.* **77,** 413–416.
Lubke, K., Schablitzky, S., and Pause, B. M. (2009). Male sexual orientation affects sensitivity to androstenone. *Chemosens. Percept.* **2,** 154–160.
Lundström, J. N., and Olsson, M. J. (2005). Subthreshold amounts of social odorant affect mood, but not behavior, in heterosexual women when tested by a male, but not a female, experimenter. *Biol. Psychol.* **70,** 197–204.
Lundström, J. N., Goncalves, M., Esteves, F., and Olsson, M. J. (2003a). Psychological effects of subthreshold exposure to the putative human pheromone 4, 16-androstadien-3-one. *Horm. Behav.* **44,** 395–401.
Lundström, J. N., Hummel, T., and Olsson, M. J. (2003b). Individual differences in sensitivity to the odor of 4, 16-androstadien-3-one. *Chem. Senses* **28,** 643–650.
Lundström, J. N., McClintock, M. K., and Olsson, M. J. (2006). Effects of reproductive state on olfactory sensitivity suggest odor specificity. *Biol. Psychol.* **71,** 244–247.
Mainland, J. D., Bremner, E. A., Young, N., Johnson, B. N., Khan, R. M., Bensafi, M., and Sobel, N. (2002). Olfactory plasticity: One nostril knows what the other learns. *Nature* **419,** 802.
McCollough, P. A., Owen, J. W., and Pollak, E. I. (1981). Does androstenol affect emotion? *Ethol. Sociobiol.* **2,** 85–88.
Monti-Bloch, L., and Grosser, B. I. (1991). Effect of putative pheromones on the electrical activity of the human vomeronasal organ and olfactory epithelium. *J. Steroid Biochem. Mol. Biol.* **39,** 573–582.

Morofushi, M., Shinohara, K., Funabashi, T., and Kimura, F. (2000). Positive relationship between menstrual synchrony and ability to smell 5 alpha-androst-16-en-3 alpha-ol. *Chem. Senses* **25,** 407–411.

Natsch, A., Derrer, S., Flachsmann, F., and Schmid, J. (2006). A broad diversity of volatile carboxylic acids, released by a bacterial aminoacylase from axilla secretions, as candidate molecules for the determination of human-body odor type. *Chem. Biodivers.* **3,** 1–20.

Nixon, A., Mallet, A. I., Jackman, P. J. H., and Gower, D. B. (1984). Production of 5-alpha-dihydrotestosterone and 5-beta-dihydrotestosterone by isolated human axillary bacteria. *FEMS Microbiol. Lett.* **25,** 153–157.

Nixon, A., Jackman, P. J. H., Mallet, A. I., and Gower, D. B. (1986a). Metabolism of testosterone by mixed human axillary bacteria. *Biochem. Soc. Trans.* **14,** 773.

Nixon, A., Mallet, A. I., Jackman, P. J., and Gower, D. B. (1986b). Testosterone metabolism by isolated human axillary *Corynebacterium* spp.: A gas-chromatographic mass–spectrometric study. *J. Steroid Biochem.* **24,** 887–892.

Nixon, A., Jackman, P. J. H., Mallet, A. I., and Gower, D. B. (1987). Testosterone metabolism by pure and mixed cultures of human corynebacteria. *FEMS Microbiol. Lett.* **41,** 53–58.

Nixon, A., Mallet, A. I., and Gower, D. B. (1988). Simultaneous quantification of five odorous steroids (16-androstenes) in the axillary hair of men. *J. Steroid Biochem. Mol. Biol.* **29,** 505–510.

Ohloff, G., Maurer, B., Winter, B., and Giersch, W. (1983). Structural and configurational dependence of the sensory process in steroids. *Helv. Chim. Acta* **66,** 192–217.

Pause, B. M. (2004). Are androgen steroids acting as pheromones in humans? *Physiol. Behav.* **83,** 21–29.

Pause, B. M., Rogalski, K. P., Sojka, B., and Ferstl, R. (1999). Sensitivity to androstenone in female subjects is associated with an altered brain response to male body odor. 24th Conference of the German Society of Psychophysiology and its Applications Lubeck, Germany, pp. 129–137.

Pierce, J. D., Cohen, A. B., and Ulrich, P. M. (2004). Responsivity to two odorants, androstenone and amyl acetate, and the affective impact of odors on interpersonal relationships. *J. Comp. Psychol.* **118,** 14–19.

Polak, E. H. (1973). Multiple profile-multiple receptor site model for vertebrate olfaction. *J. Theor. Biol.* **40,** 469–484.

Pollack, M. S., Wysocki, C. J., Beauchamp, G. K., Braun, D., Callaway, C., and Dupont, B. (1982). Absence of HLA association or linkage for variations in sensitivity to the odor of androstenone. *Immunogenetics* **15,** 579–589.

Preti, G., Cutler, W. B., Christensen, C. M., Lawley, H., Huggins, G. R., and Garcia, C.-R. (1987). Human axillary extracts: Analysis of compounds from samples which influence menstrual timing. *J. Chem. Ecol.* **13,** 717–731.

Rennie, P. J., Holland, K. T., Mallet, A. I., Watkins, W. J., and Gower, D. B. (1989a). Interconversion of androst-16-ene steroids by human axillary aerobic coryneform bacteria. *Biochem. Soc. Trans.* **17,** 1027–1028.

Rennie, P. J., Holland, K. T., Mallet, A. I., Watkins, W. J., and Gower, D. B. (1989b). Testosterone metabolism by human axillary bacteria. *Biochem. Soc. Trans.* **17,** 1017–1018.

Rennie, P. J., Gower, D. B., and Holland, K. T. (1991). In-vitro and in-vivo studies of human axillary odour and the cutaneous microflora. *Brit. J. Dermatol.* **124,** 596–602.

Rikowski, A., and Grammer, K. (1999). Human body odour, symmetry and attractiveness. *Proc. Roy. Soc. Lond. B* **266,** 869–874.

Roberts, S. C., and Gosling, L. M. (2003). Genetic similarity and quality interact in mate choice decisions by female mice. *Nat. Genet.* **35,** 103–106.

Roberts, S. C., Gosling, L. M., Carter, V., and Petrie, M. (2008). MHC-correlated odour preferences in humans and the use of oral contraceptives. *Proc. Roy. Soc. Lond. B* **275,** 2715–2722.

Savelev, S. U., Antony-Babu, S., Roberts, S. C., Wang, H., Clare, A. S., Gosling, L. M., Petrie, M., Goodfellow, M., O'Donnell, A. G., and Ward, A. C. (2008). Individual variation in 3-methylbutanal: A putative link between HLA and skin microflora. *J. Chem. Ecol.* **34,** 1253–1257.
Savic, I., and Berglund, H. (2010). Androstenol—A steroid derived odor activates the hypothalamus in women. *PLoS One* **5,** e8651.
Savic, I., Berglund, H., Gulyas, B., and Roland, P. (2001). Smelling of odorous sex hormone-like compounds causes sex-differentiated hypothalamic activations in humans. *Neuron* **31,** 661–668.
Savic, I., Berglund, H., and Lindstrom, P. (2005). Brain response to putative pheromones in homosexual men. *Proc. Natl. Acad. Sci. USA* **102,** 7356–7361.
Saxton, T. K., and Havlicek, J. (2010). A brief introduction to "human pheromones". *In* "Pheromones: Theories, Types and Uses," (I. M. Gregory, Ed.). Nova Science Publishers, New York.
Saxton, T. K., Lyndon, A., Little, A. C., and Roberts, S. C. (2008a). Evidence that androstadienone, a putative human chemosignal, modulates women's attributions of men's attractiveness. *Horm. Behav.* **54,** 597–601.
Saxton, T. K., Little, A. C., and Roberts, S. C. (2008b). Ecological validity in the study of human pheromones. *In* "Chemical Signals in Vertebrates XI," (J. L. Hurst, R. J. Beynon, S. C. Roberts, and T. D. Wyatt, Eds.), pp. 111–120. Springer, New York.
Schiffman, S. S. (1979). Preference: A multidimensional concept. *In* "Preference Behaviour and Chemoreception," (J. H. A. Kröeze, Ed.), pp. 63–81. Information Retrieval Ltd., London.
Schmidt, H. J., and Beauchamp, G. K. (1988). Adult-like odor preferences and aversions in 3-year-old children. *Child Dev.* **59,** 1136–1143.
Signoret, J. P., and du Mesnil du Buisson, F. (1961). Étude du comportement de la truie en oestrus. Proceedings of the 4th International Congress on Animal Reproduction 2, pp. 171–175.
Singer, A. G., Beauchamp, G. K., and Yamazaki, K. (1997). Volatile signals of the major histocompatibility complex in male mouse urine. *Proc. Natl. Acad. Sci. USA* **94,** 2210–2214.
Sirota, P., Davidson, B., Mosheva, T., Benhatov, R., Zohar, J., and Gross-Isserroff, R. (1999). Increased olfactory sensitivity in first episode psychosis and the effect of neuroleptic treatment on olfactory sensitivity in schizophrenia. *Psychiatr. Res.* **86,** 143–153.
Smals, A. G., and Weusten, J. J. (1991). 16-Ene-steroids in the human testis. *J. Steroid Biochem. Mol. Biol.* **40,** 587–592.
Smith, C. (1974). Concordance in twins: Methods and interpretation. *Am. J. Hum. Genet.* **26,** 454–466.
Stevens, D. A., and O'Connell, R. J. (1995). Enhanced sensitivity to androstenone following regular exposure to pemenone. *Chem. Senses* **20,** 413–419.
Stevenson, R. J., Prescott, J., and Boakes, R. A. (1999). Confusing tastes and smells: How odours can influence the perception of sweet and sour tastes. *Chem. Senses* **24,** 627–635.
Taylor, D., Daulby, A., Grimshaw, S., James, G., Mercer, J., and Vaziri, S. (2003). Characterisation of the microflora of the human axilla. *Int. J. Cosmet. Sci.* **25,** 137–145.
Thysen, B., Elliott, W. H., and Katzman, P. A. (1968). Identification of estra-1, 3, 5 (10), 16-tetraen-3-ol (estratetraenol) from the urine of pregnant women. *Steroids* **11,** 73–87.
Van Toller, C., Kirk-Smith, M., Wood, N., Lombard, J., and Dodd, G. H. (1983). Skin conductance and subjective assessments associated with the odor of 5-alpha-androstan-3-one. *Biol. Psychol.* **16,** 85–107.
Villemure, C., and Bushnell, M. C. (2007). The effects of the steroid androstadienone and pleasant odorants on the mood and pain perception of men and women. *Eur. J. Pain* **11,** 181–191.
Wang, L. W., Chen, L. X., and Jacob, T. (2004). Evidence for peripheral plasticity in human odour response. *J. Physiol.* **554,** 236–244.
Wilson, M. (2005). Microbial Inhabitants of Humans. Cambridge University Press, Cambridge.

Wyart, C., Webster, W. W., Chen, J. H., Wilson, S. R., McClary, A., Khan, R. M., and Sobel, N. (2007). Smelling a single component of male sweat alters levels of cortisol in women. *J. Neurosci.* **27,** 1261–1265.
Wysocki, C. J., and Beauchamp, G. K. (1984). Ability to smell androstenone is genetically-determined. *Proc. Natl. Acad. Sci. USA* **81,** 4899–4902.
Wysocki, C. J., Dorries, K. M., and Beauchamp, G. K. (1989). Ability to perceive androstenone can be acquired by ostensibly anosmic people. *Proc. Natl. Acad. Sci. USA* **86,** 7976–7978.
Wysocki, C. J., Pierce, J. D., and Gilbert, A. N. (1991). Geographic, cross-cultural, and individual variation in human olfaction. *In* "Smell and Taste in Health and Disease," (T. V. Getchell, R. L. Doty, L. M. Bartoshuk, and J. B. Snow, Eds.), pp. 287–314. Raven Press, New York.
Yee, K. K., and Wysocki, C. J. (2001). Odorant exposure increases olfactory sensitivity: Olfactory epithelium is implicated. *Physiol. Behav.* **72,** 705–711.

CHAPTER FOUR

Mammary Odor Cues and Pheromones: Mammalian Infant-Directed Communication about Maternal State, Mammae, and Milk

Benoist Schaal

Contents

Abstract

Neonatal mammals are exposed to an outstandingly powerful selective pressure at birth, and any mean to alleviate their localization effort and accelerate acceptance to orally grasp a nipple and ingest milk should have had advantageous consequences over evolutionary time. Thus, it is essential for females to display a biological interface structure that is sensorily conspicuous and executively easy for their newborns. Females' strategy to increase the

Research Group on Developmental Ethology and Cognitive Psychology, Center for Taste and Smell Science, CNRS, Dijon, France

Vitamins and Hormones, Volume 83
ISSN 0083-6729, DOI: 10.1016/S0083-6729(10)83004-3

conspicuousness of nipples could only exploit the newborns' most advanced and conserved sensory systems, touch and olfaction, and selection has accordingly shaped tactilely and olfactorily conspicuous mammary structures. This evolutionary modification has worked either by affecting structural features of mammaries or indirectly by affecting maternal behavioral propensities to create olfactory traces on them. These predictions are considered here in mammalian cases that have received empirical attention among marsupials, rodents, lagomorphs, ungulates, carnivores, and primates. It appears that broadcasting chemical cues and/or signals from the mammae is a pan-mammalian reproductive strategy to pilot neonatal arousal, motivation and attraction to the mother, provide assistance in localizing and orally grasping the mammae, and boost up learning. But the ways by which these chemical cues are produced and assembled on the mammae are both diverse between species and complex within species, offering an outstanding opportunity for comparative analyses in chemical communication.

I. Introduction: Sensory Guidance to the Milk Resource for Inexperienced, Fragile Newborns

After having taken its primal breaths, the first challenge of any newborn mammal is to reach the source of milk as promptly as possible. The speediness of this first suckling is vital as it conditions mother-to-newborn transmission not only of hydration, nutriments, calories but also of passive immunization, safe bacterial colonization, growth factors, peptides active on several behaviorally important functions (e.g., pain relief, memory, sleep induction), and last but not least, sensory information. This latter informative aspect about the nurturing context, the mother, mammary cues, and milk is often overlooked, although it unavoidably impinges on the developing organism in its current and future competence.

Since antiquity scholars have attempted to question the processes underlying this first response of newborn mammals toward their mother and milk. The earliest empirical record about neonatal attraction to milk is probably Galen's (130–200). Exposing a goat kid to wine, oil, honey, milk, and various cereals and fruits, he noted that "... it snuffled at each vessel ..., and after having sniffed them all, absorbed the milk," to conclude "that animals' natures do not need to be taught" (Daremberg, 1856). Darwin (1872) also acknowledged that "There is no greater difficulty in understanding how young mammals have instinctively learned to suck the breast ..." Weaving evolutionary and developmental issues into this oxymoron-*instinctively learned*, Darwin recognized that lactation and sucking imply a conundrum of morphological, physiological, cognitive, and behavioral arrangements in both sides of the mammalian mother–young relationship.

These arrangements extend from gland structure and position to all steps of performance from the female's lactational synthetic processes and nursing acceptance to the neonate's sucking competence and absorptive abilities. Selective pressure operates thus on both partners in the dyad, leading to optimization of milk production and provision in females and milk access and exploitation by neonates.

Young mammals are exposed to an outstandingly powerful selective pressure at the occasion of two early developmental bottlenecks, birth and weaning, periods that concentrate physiological, cognitive, behavioral, and social challenges to their viability. Therefore, any means that could alleviate neonatal localization effort and accelerate the acceptance to orally grasp a nipple should have had advantageous consequences over evolutionary time. Here, the emphasis will be on the birth transition. In face of "predictable" threats to neonatal viability and evolved properties of milk to counteract them, it is essential for females to display an interface structure that is sensorily conspicuous and executively easy for their newborns. Nipples or teats, the milk outlet structures of the maternal body which infants have to obligatorily contact for survival, may thus be expected to be the locus of evolutionary sculpting for sensory advertisement.

The organization of the mother–infant relationship is extremely diverse among mammals, ultimately determined by ecological constraints, evolved reproductive strategies, social structure of mother–infant exchanges (exclusivity, quality, and duration of interactions), level of neonatal autonomy, and pace of development during and beyond the lactation period (Clutton-Brock, 1991). However, diversity can always be reduced to shared mechanisms: first, in terms of the sensory resource that is mobilized in mediating mother–neonate exchanges and second, in terms of the generality of maternal effects, viz. the transmission of information about the environment that females create around their offspring during fetal and postnatal development. Here, we describe one strategy by which mammalian females have shaped the sensory ecology of their progeny and fine-tuned their neural, cognitive, and behavioral development.

II. Evolution and General Functions of Mammary Odor Cues

Several hypotheses have been proposed to represent the macroevolutionary advent of lactation in mammals, emphasizing various sources of selective pressures supposed to have enforced the mother–infant bond. In their scenario to the evolution of lactation in tetrapods (cf. Long, 1969; Oftedal, 2002), Darwin (1872) and others after him (Bresslau, 1907; Gregory, 1910) have proposed that offspring *nutrition* and *hydration* were the *primum movens* toward the advent of lactation in endothermic therapsid reptiles. Accordingly, protolactation was believed to have emerged by the way of augmented exocrine secretions from ventral skin glands that co-occurred with the elaboration of highly vascularized abdominal incubation structures; passively absorbed through the egg shell or actively ingested by neonates, these secretions may have had a survival advantage, driving progressive specialization of the production apparel (hypertrophied mammae, orally graspable nipples/teats) and of the secretion (colostrum, milk) in females, and of intake competence (sucking behavior, digestive processes, learning) in the offspring (Oftedal, 2002). Blackburn *et al.* (1989) ameliorated this scenario in adding the *protective function* afforded by lacteal secretions under the selective pressure of microbial predation on both offspring and females. Finally, Graves and Duvall (1983), and before them Gregory (1910), proposed that secretions originating from the mammary field may have carried sensory properties bearing specialized *communicative function*. This latter function was expressed in terms of offspring → mother attraction and facilitation to locate mammary areas, hence providing litter cohesion, physical protection, and optimized milk intake.

In the sequential ordering of the evolutionary appearance of these nonexclusive functions, it does not seem unreasonable to speculate that the communicative function of protolacteal secretions, because it warrants infant → mother contact, has either antedated protective and nutritive-hydrational functions, at least in viviparous species, or it has emerged as a result of coevolving neonatal learning abilities. From empirical evidence in extant mammals (see below), both unconditional and conditional ways to acquire the communicative value of mammary odor do function in newborns. But all sources of mammary messages may not have evolved under the same functional demand. While some of them may be seen as bearing an exclusive communicative function (e.g., the inguinal glands of several ungulates), others may be secondary to local requirements for the preservation of nipple functionality against the heavy stress that offspring wield on it. For example, the evolutionary specialization of suckable mammary appendages has co-opted exocrine structures which secretions: (i) protect the skin and ductal entries from bacterial invasion, (ii) favor the creation of the airtight seal indispensable to the extractive efficacy of suction, and (iii) relieve friction effects due to sucking neonates. Such local exocrine specializations in typical nipple structures were best described to date in lagomorph and primate females (Schaal *et al.*, 2008b, 2009; see below).

Once dependence on milk was evolutionarily engaged in the reproduction of radiating mammals, the critical nature of immediately postnatal intake of colostrum certainly become the strongest selective pressure that drove mammalian females to evolve nipples/teats that were easily locatable and orally graspable by inexperienced newborns. In that process, the females' strategy to increase the conspicuousness of nipples could only exploit the newborns' most advanced sensory systems. Although the whole range of sensory systems could theoretically be exploited to support the female → young transfer of milk, the most basic, and hence most conserved, ways could only rely on somesthesis and chemoreception. Some species give birth to neonates which sensorium is limited to these modalities (e.g., sightless newborns in monotremes, marsupials, altricial rodents, or carnivores), while other species bear newborns which behavior is controlled by all the senses, including hearing and vision (such as ungulates or some precocial rodents that are sensorily and physiologically/motorically precocial, or primates that are sensorily precocial, but motorically altricial). Thus, touch and olfaction appear to be *the* sensory channels that are most universally "exploitable" by females to shape infant-directed information sources about maternal and lactational state, about the location of the source of milk, and about milk itself.

Accordingly, one may predict that evolutionary pressure on mammalian females has worked in the direction of shaping tactilely[1] and olfactorily conspicuous mammary structures. This evolutionary modification may have worked either directly by affecting structural features of mammaries or indirectly by affecting maternal behavioral propensities to create olfactory traces on mammary structures. Selective pressure may also be expected to have oriented chemical communication pertaining to milk transfer toward specialized signals, using processes based on redundancy, noticeability, repertoire size, and alerting potency of odorants (Müller-Schwarze, 1999). Here, we will consider these predictions in mammalian cases that have received more or less in-depth empirical attention regarding the involvement of odor cues and pheromones in the regulation of the nursing/sucking relationship.

III. What Is in a Scent? Informational Intricacy in Mammary Odor

Mammary glands are specialized tubuloalveolar structures that have evolved to synthesize colostrum and milk. Depending on species, they are distributed on the pectoral-ventral-inguinal regions of the females' body, generally as bilateral pairs of glands, ranging in number from 2 (e.g., primates) up to 22 or more (in certain insectivores; Raynaud, 1969). They are morphologically diverse, ranging from nippleless ventral spots in monotremes (Cowie, 1984), whereof milk is excreted from separate gland tubes associated with hair, to structures of flat (rat, mice) or more or less prominent or pendulous appearance in marsupial and eutherian mammals. These more elaborate mammary structures are equipped each with an

[1] The behavioral impact of tactile, textural, and thermal cues will be kept out of the present discussion.

outlet, the *papilla mammae*, or nipple or teat,[2] where the galactophores converge in one or several apical ostia (see Raynaud, 1969). In this chapter, emphasis will be given to the chemoperceptual properties that mammary areas broadcast to newborns.

Beyond their tactile and textural properties, mammary structures of mammals aggregate a variety of intricate sources of potentially odorous substrates. These exocrine sources originate from mammary structures and extramammary processes. Mammary sources are mainly represented by the colostrum and milk, which carry intrinsic odor qualities that depend on maternal factors (e.g., lactational stage, dietary and aerial ecology, stress, physical activity). Other mammary substrates are secreted or excreted by glands distributed on, and adjacent to, the skin of the mammary structure or of the nipple/teat itself. The whole range of elementary skin glands is indeed represented in the areola–nipple region, including eccrine, apocrine, and sebaceous glands. In some species, the mammary area is additionally endowed with sophisticated glandular specializations, working either in close functional link with lactation (e.g., human Montgomery's glands, MG) or seemingly throughout reproductive life (e.g., ovine inguinal glands).

The substrates secreted or excreted locally onto the nipple–areolar skin can be mingled with substrates brought here from extramammary sources. The nature of these exogenous substrates is variable according to species. In some rodents and carnivores, parturient females actively lick their abdomen and nipple-lines, potentially spreading there a mix of urogenital and amniotic fluids, blood, saliva, and all kinds of secretions from oral or facial glands. Later on, females nursing altricial neonates alternate licking them and their own ventral fur, possibly mixing infant-specific substrates (e.g., urine, feces, glandular secretions from anal or urogenital sources) with her own substrates (saliva). Reciprocally, newly born mammals first stain the maternal nipple–areolar region with a mix of amniotic fluid and saliva, and thereafter with mixed saliva and milk coagulate, and possibly other substrates originating from the facial area (e.g., secretions of lachrymal, nasal, facial, or ear glands; remnants of dietary compounds).

To further expand this chemosensory scramble, all these mammary and extramammary substrates may be handled by surface processes, such as the catabolic action of salivary enzymes or of the local microflora. Finally, local thermal conditions may differentiate emitted odor compounds as a function

[2] The English terminology regarding the mammary milk outlet can vary in different traditions. While common language dictionaries do equate the use of "nipple" and "teat" (e.g., Oxford Concise Dictionary; Webster Dictionary), usage tends to reserve the term "nipple" for humans and "teat" for other mammals. However, anatomists differentiate "nipples" as skin appendages at the tip of which *primary* milk ducts exit directly, and "teats" as structures on which a *secondary* canal opens, formed as a sinus or an enlarged cistern into which primary milk ducts converge (Long, 1969). In general nipples are smaller structures (as in rats, mice, cats, dogs, or primates), while teats have greater dimensions (as in ewes and cows). The milk outlets of marsupials are also named "teat" rather than "nipple" (M. A. Renfree, personal communication). Here, we will generally follow the anatomical tradition.

of their vapor pressure. In that line, it may be noted that mammary structures are generally situated in highly vascularized regions bearing higher surface temperature. Considering the intricacy of these multiple sources of biological substrates and local ecological conditions (heat, humidity, epidermal texture, pilosity, commensal microflora), the mammary-based chemistry that females present to their offspring is expected to be commensurably complex.

This complexity of mammary stimuli can be split first along physical and chemical criteria, such as volatility, polarity, solubility, functional moieties, stability, and multicomponentiality. For example, volatile and involatile fractions of mammary secretions lead to either detection from a distance or to the need of direct contact for perception to occur. Involatile proteins, lipids, or hydrocarbon may in this way act as carriers or precursors of volatile ligands. The involatile fraction in a secretion/excretion has indeed the potential to protract the emission duration of associated volatile compounds. Such intrinsic or extrinsic differences in volatility may be linked to contrastive sensory impact, such as ephemeral alarm-like effects depending on high volatility/high diffusibility compounds, while longer lasting attractant effects rely on heavier, often more polar compounds (Alberts, 1992; Müller-Schwarze, 1999, 2006). But, involatile compounds are also increasingly recognized to work as chemosignals, bringing even more complexity to the field of chemical communication. For example, in mice, main urinary proteins (MUPs) encode individual identity (Hurst *et al.*, 2001).

A second big divide in the complexity of the mammary odor mixture is between individual-specific and species-specific compounds. Whereas some odor compounds may reflect idiosyncratic traits of the female (e.g., her atmospheric environment, diet, level of stress, physiological state, health and parasite load, lactational age) or of the young (diet, physiological state, sex, age), others may carry higher level categories of meanings (e.g., species/genus; kin, group, or population identity). Depending on the type of behavioral test used to assess responses, a neonate's ability to extract individual or supraindividual meanings can be evidenced from a same substrate. For example, rabbit or human newborns reveal that conspecific milk can transmit odor cues bearing differentiable meanings related either to the individual mother or to any lactating female of the species (Coureaud *et al.*, 2002; Schaal, 2005). In the same way, lambs are strongly reactive to inguinal gland secretions, but much more when they come from their mother (Vince and Ward, 1984).

A third divide in the complexity of social odors in general, and in mammary odors in particular, pertains to the notions of cue versus signal. This distinction has been repeatedly proposed (e.g., Dusenberry, 1992; Hauser, 1996; Maynard-Smith and Harper, 2003) to separate informative elements—*cues*—considered to incidentally derive from normal life sustenance processes in the emitter, from informative elements—*signals*—which "alter the behavior of other organisms, which evolved because of that effect, and which are effective because the receiver's response has also evolved" (Maynard-Smith and Harper, 2003: 3). While cues may be lastingly "on," signals can be switched "on–off" according to emitter's behavior or condition (Hauser, 1996). Mammary odor cues would include informative compounds derived from maternal physiology (hormonal state, stress) or metabolism (diet, wastes) without additional cost involved to produce them, whereas mammary odor signals would designate informative compounds that exploit specific response biases in the receiver and evolved for a specific signaling function. This would imply that, in the context of complex mammary odor mixtures, rare signals will unavoidably be embedded in a system of abundant cues. Thus, undoing odor signals from the affluence of confounded odor cues are expectedly a difficult achievement. Once chemically identified, odor stimuli may be classified as pheromones if they satisfy a set of necessary criteria. A first definition of the concept (Karlson and Lüscher, 1959), based on empirical evidence from insects, was minimalist in terms of such criteria in including "substances, which are secreted outside by an individual and received by a second individual of the same species, in which they release a specific reaction, for example, a definite behavioral or developmental process." Accordingly, any chemosensory factor exchanged between conspecifics could be argued to act as a pheromone. To avoid a latent confusion about the nature of the cues involved as well as about the nature of elicited responses in mammals, Beauchamp *et al.* (1976) have proposed a set of criteria in an attempts to resize the concept of pheromone so that it better matches the cognitive complexity underlying mammalian behavior (see also Doty, 2003; Johnston, 2000). These criteria imply that: (1) the candidate compound(s) is (are) chemically "simple," in the sense that the active fraction is composed of one molecular compound or a very small set of chemicals in a given ratio; (2) the candidate compound(s) release(s) unambiguous responses in a receiver which are morphologically invariant in a same context, and obvious in terms of adaptive function; (3) these responses are elicited in a selective way, thus should be tested against reference compounds; (4) the species specificity of these responses should be established; and (5) finally, the coupling between the candidate signal and the response should minimally or not at all depend on previous exposure and learning. Thus, in principle, the concept of pheromone would imply that early neonatal responsiveness to the candidate compounds cannot be ascribed to prenatal induction by direct exposure, to facilitated learning during the natal process, or to rapid learning immediately after birth. Accordingly, to keep its meaningfulness to the concept of pheromone, a candidate secretion, excretion, or any mixture of odor factors bearing repeatable behavioral and/or physiological effects on newborns (e.g., the excretion of a gland, abdominal skin secretions, milk, saliva) should not be baptized "pheromone." If they verify some of the above criteria without going into chemical identification, such mixtures could be considered "candidate secretions for pheromonal mediation" (Doty, 2003). The term pheromone should be set aside to designate *clearly identified* chemical compounds that have undergone systematic screening of the above operational criteria. This is the rule that we will adopt in the following presentation of mammary semiochemistry.

The chemosensory complexity of mammary-based odors has been mostly investigated in milk, the mammary substrate that appears most practical to comply with classical chemoanalytic techniques. Milk is however physically, chemically, and biochemically multifaceted, and the fraction(s) responsible for its chemosensory activity are extremely tricky to characterize. A first step in reducing this huge complexity of milk has been to limit the analysis to compounds collectable in its headspace. But even then the profile of volatiles from milk remains exquisitely complex, leading to gas chromatographic (GC) tracings ranging from more than 150 peaks (e.g., in ovine milk: Moio *et al.*, 1996; in rabbit milk: Schaal *et al.*, 2003) to 20–40 peaks (in human milk, e.g., Büttner, 2007; Shimoda *et al.*, 2000). In addition, to such volatile compounds, numerous nonvolatile compounds may be chemosensorily active by themselves or act as carriers of volatile compounds (e.g., Beynon *et al.*, 2008; Murakami *et al.*, 1998). To disentangle the behavioral activity of these potential cues and signals in milk is a complicated enterprise, and it has so far been successfully carried out in only few mammalian species.

IV. Pan-Mammalian Distribution of Mammary Odor Cues and Signals

In this section, we will attempt to synthesize observations and experimental facts on mammary odor cues and signals in different mammalian orders. From the outset, it appears that the coverage of the topic is surprisingly scarce, and hence very heterogeneous across taxa. While some orders were left out for reasons of rarity, accessibility, or practicality, others could be studied more extensively because they comprised species that were kept in captivity or domesticated.

The contribution of olfaction to the success of mammalian neonates' quest for the mammae and milk will be assessed in different taxa in applying the following set of criteria: (1) The evidence for use of nasal chemoreception in the orientation toward the mother, specifically toward her mammary area; whenever possible, this will include a succinct anatomical view on the development of nasal chemosensory structures, observations on nasal investigation and suckling, and the impact on them of impairing olfaction through anosmization or through alteration of odor emission. (2) The evidence for scent structures situated on or around the mammary areas, or for significant olfactory indices produced endogenously (in lacteal secretions) or exogenously (by local spreading of extramammary substrates); the extractability of corresponding odor cues from the mammary area for separate experimental restitution to neonates will be considered here. (3) The evidence for neonatal learning of mammary-related odor cues to specify the mechanisms that explain the olfactory control over nipple-search and sucking, and to understand whether a given secretion or odorant may have gained its reinforcing value through prior prenatal or postnatal experience, thus in principle excluding it from being categorized as a pheromone. (4) Finally, the evidence for pheromones, in the form of well-identified compounds embedded among mammary odor cues; pheromones will be considered here as signals distinct from ordinary, learned odor cues in following the operational criteria outlined in the previous section.

A. Marsupials

Relatively little investigation has been devoted to the sensory regulation of the early steps of mother–young relationship in marsupials (e.g., Renfree *et al.*, 1989; Russell, 1982). The sensory control of the newborn's unassisted move from the urogenital orifice to the marsupium, which depends on the type of maternal behavior (Russell, 1982), has not been well studied until recently. The first stage of the climb into the pouch is in response to negative geotropism (Cannon *et al.*, 1976; Lyne *et al.*, 1959), responding to signals that are probably sensed by the otoliths in the semicircular canals (Hughes and Hall, 1984). However, the second stage appears to be driven by chemosensory cues when the pouch young changes direction to enter down into the pouch and attach to one of the available teats.

1. Odor-mediation of mammary localization and of sucking

Early studies suggested that olfactory structures are well developed in newborn *Didelphis* (Langworty, 1928) and *Dasyurus* (Hill and Hill, 1955), whereas more recently the olfactory tract beyond the olfactory bulbs was described as being too immature on the day of birth to sustain behavioral guidance (Ashwell *et al.*, 2008; Chuah *et al.*, 1997; but see Lin *et al.*, 1988). In contrast, it is now established that the main and accessory olfactory systems are developed well enough to support the processing of chemostimuli (in the tammar wallaby; Schneider *et al.*, 2008, 2009). Nevertheless the ultimate check of chemosensory functionality lays in the behavioral outcome following odor stimulation. The first direct evidence shows indeed that newborn tammar wallabies, when simultaneously exposed on a tanned fur to a cotton swab carrying a saline wash of the maternal pouch and a control saline swab, are significantly attracted up toward the former (Schneider *et al.*, 2009); in addition, when contacting the maternal pouch stimulus, such newborns alter the pattern and direction of their actions, either digging into the fur or changing from upward to downward direction of movements, both being suggested to ease their entry into the pouch (Schneider *et al.*, 2009). After finding the pouch entrance in 1–3 min, neonatal macropodid marsupials need an additional 2–5 min to attach to a teat (Renfree *et al.*, 1989). Thus, despite their extreme altricial stage of development, marsupial newborns are exceptionally skilled at speedily finding a teat.

2. Mammary odor sources

Macropodidae are endowed with highly active sebaceous and apocrine glands in the abdominal, pouch, and perimammary regions (Raynaud, 1969). Mykytowycz and Nay (1964: 215) suggest their secretion "may aid the embryo in its movement from the cloaca to the teat after birth." This was also suggested for other species (e.g., *Petaurus breviceps*; Schulze-Westrum, 1965). Glands within the pouch skin produce a brown waxy substance that is removed through the preparturient females' avid self-licking (Renfree *et al.*, 1989). It is a sign of imminent parturition that females self-lick their urogenital orifice: in the tammar wallaby, females direct then 50% of their licking activity to that orifice, while 40% is targeted to the region between it and the pouch (Renfree *et al.*, 1989). This licking may be involved in wetting the fur, in laying down a scent-trail, or in arousing the pouch young, as it was observed that the mother licked "over and ahead of the young in four out of six closely observed 'climbs'" (Renfree *et al.*, 1989: 330). The potential importance of this maternal salivary deposit is suggested in experiments where females were anesthetized during parturition, this treatment leading to more protracted times for newborns to reach the pouch (Renfree *et al.*, 1989; Sharman and Calaby, 1964). It is expectable that macropodid females spread such salivary cues through active licking in the space between the urogenital opening and the teats inside the pouch. As much licking goes on around the urogenital orifice, compounds emitted there (e.g., fetal fluids, blood, secretions/excretions from the urogenital tract) might be mixed with saliva. Thus, in real-life conditions, it cannot be ruled out that maternal licking, and related salivary cues, may be responsible for the attraction of newborn tammar wallabies to the maternal pouch (Schneider *et al.*, 2009). Her licking upward from the urogenital area may create a gradient of urogenital/amniotic odors directed toward the pouch–lacteal area, and conversely her licking downward from the pouch may create a gradient of pouch–lacteal odors toward the urogenital area, both gradients resulting in a progressive transition in odor cues from familiar odors carried in fetal fluids to presumably less familiar odors carried in the pouch–teat region.

The teats themselves may contribute to chemosensory guidance cues to the young within the pouch. In macropodids, the tip of the teats is endowed with a "bud" or "bulbous swelling" developing on 1 or 2 days before parturition (Renfree *et al.*, 1989; Sharman and Calaby, 1964). It is not excluded that attractive cues may be released from this "bud," but so far no histological evidence is noted at this level (e.g., Garcia and Gonçalves, 1984). However, colostrum may be expressed 2 days before birth (Schneider *et al.*, 2009) providing potential odor cues that are ready-to-work for the neonate. Finally, the pouch young attaches to one teat for the next weeks of development in the pouch, lips becoming sealed over days 3–4 around the teat which enlarges in the oral cavity and affixes the young (e.g., Hartman, 1952). If removed after the establishment of this lip–teat seal, pouch young do not easily reattach to a teat, although displacement experiments during the very first days shows reattachment ability. For example, 1-day-old newborns of red kangaroos removed from the first selected teat reattach to another teat in the same pouch (Merchant and Sharman, 1966). However, cross-fostering to females from different species appears to result in losses or nonoptimal growth, suggesting some degree of species-specificity in unidentified sensory, morphological, or physiological factors at the teat or pouch levels (Merchant and Sharman, 1966; but the foster species and the age when such experiments are done are decisive, cf. Trott *et al.*, 2003; Menzies *et al.*, 2007).

3. Evidence for learning of mammary-related odor cues

Although marsupials represent very appealing mammalian models to analyze manifestations of odor learning at "embryonic" stages of development, this line of research has not yet been pursued.

4. Evidence for pheromones

In the same line, in some of the species studied so far for their well-developed main and accessory olfactory systems (e.g., the tammar wallaby; Schneider *et al.*, 2009), systematic research for unconditional signals might prove productive.

B. Rodents

The bulk of rodent studies on the topic have been conducted in the laboratory rat, mouse, and gerbil. Investigations conducted on these models, although not fully conclusive as yet, were seminal in stimulating research on the sensory mechanisms going on around milk acquisition in other mammalian neonates.

1. Odor-mediation of mammary localization and of sucking

Anatomical and neurophysiological evidence indicates relative immaturity of the main olfactory system, but more advanced accessory olfactory system at birth in the rat (e.g., Teicher *et al.*, 1984). Nevertheless profuse evidence for highly competent odor-guided behavior is available in newborn rats and mice (see reviews in Alberts, 1976, 1981; Blass, 1990; Blass and Teicher, 1980;

Rosenblatt, 1983). Newborn rat pups generally prefer the odor emitted by any lactating females over similar odor from virgin females, indicating that lactation correlates with the release of attractive cues (Galef and Muskus, 1979). Rat pups express indeed searching and oral grasping of a nipple when put in contact with the abdomen of an anesthetized lactating rat (Hofer *et al.*, 1976; Teicher and Blass, 1977). Further, they attach faster to unfamiliar females that are matched in postpartum age with their own dam than to such females of different lactational age, suggesting the operation of some time-specific olfactory or tactile features of the nipples (Holloway *et al.*, 1978).

The seminal role of olfaction in neonatal rats' or mice's nipple-finding and grasping is attested through its abolishment by bulbar lesion (Kovach and Kling, 1967; McClelland and Cowley, 1982; Singh and Tobach, 1975; Teicher *et al.*, 1978), by $ZnSO_4$ peripheral denervation (Hofer *et al.*, 1976), or by genetic disruption inducing early dysfunction in olfactory transduction (e.g., Wong *et al.*, 2000). Further, washing the abdomen of a lactating rat results in a drastic reduction of nipple seizing performance in rat pups (aged 9 and 14 days, Hofer *et al.*, 1976; or 2–28 days, Teicher and Blass, 1976; cf. Small,1899, for early evidence). Thus, a substance emitted from the abdominal skin of lactating rats appears to govern the pups' localizatory and oral seizing performance. Similar results in just-born mice indicate that the olfactory effect of nipples is maximal when pups are deposited with their nose over them, and decreases with increasing distance from them (Hongo *et al.*, 2000). Hence, it may appear that a detectable mammary odor factor is more concentrated on and immediately (up to 2 mm) around nipples. When the nipples of lactating mice are washed (with water), this gradual pattern of pup response is eliminated (Hongo *et al.*, 2000).

2. Mammary odor sources

As mentioned above, an active odor factor is emitted on the ventral skin of lactating dams that attracts rat or mouse pups and elicits orientation and mouthing. In mice, this substrate appears most active at short range, suggesting low volatility (Hongo *et al.*, 2000). The exact source of these substrates is not well understood, but it is acknowledged that nipples are important (but see Singh and Hofer, 1978). When rat nipples were washed using organic solvents, the resulting solution vacuum distillated, and the distillate then applied on a nipple rendered inactive by prior washing, pups resumed oral grasping of it (Teicher and Blass, 1976, 1977). The histological sources of potentially active odor factors on the nipple remain unclear. Rat and mouse nipples are endowed with apical sebaceous glands opening into the ductal ostia (Toyoshima *et al.*, 1998a,b), these glands reaching maximal size from the end of gestation and during lactation. It may be noted also that the surface texture of the nipple changes drastically during lactation (Toyoshima *et al.*, 1998a), offering a network of wrinkles that favor the sequestration of mammary and nonmammary substrates, and that shelter local microflora. In the gerbil (*Meriones unguiculatus*), females bear a ventral gland of sebaceous nature the size of which peaks during lactation (Wallace *et al.*, 1973). The secretion of this ventral gland is attractive to male or female adult gerbils, regardless of their exposure to it during development (Blum *et al.*, 1975), but its behavioral impact in nursing is not known.

Milk is another expectable candidate to mediate the release of odorant factors on nipples. Current data *seem* to disconfirm this contention, however. When rat milk was applied on prewashed, inactive nipples, normal nipple attachment response could not be restored in 8- to 9-day-old pups (Singh and Hofer, 1978); it may not be excluded that by that age, rat pups are less responsive to conspecific milk cues or that composition changes in milk (e.g., Luckey *et al.*, 1954) or in pup saliva may have occurred. Alternately, it cannot be excluded that the odor factor in rat milk, if any, rapidly evanesces after milking and the related behavioral activity may have gone before testing (see below the ephemeral impact of the mammary pheromone (MP) in rabbit milk).[3] However, when female rats which nipples were rendered inactive through prewashing received an injection of oxytocin the nipple grasping performance of pups was reinstated (Singh and Hofer, 1978), indicating that an active odor factor might be externalized abdominally under endocrine control. This same effect was replicated when oxytocin was administered to rats whose nipples were ligated (Singh and Hofer, 1978), suggesting that milk as well as nipples themselves were not the unique sources of compounds eliciting grasping in rat pups. Thus, the *current* evidence suggests that milk appears not to bear the strongest effect in releasing oral grasping of nipples in rat newborns. A renewed research effort is clearly needed here. Ongoing investigations in our own group indicate indeed that neonatal mice are well responsive to the odor of fresh mouse milk (Al Ain *et al.*, 2010).

Based on the observation that rat females self-lick during gestation, parturition, and lactation (Roth and Rosenblatt, 1966), it was hypothesized that a mix of saliva and amniotic fluid could be spread ventrally, specifically on the nipple-lines. Positive reactions toward birth fluids were indeed noted in rat and mouse newborns (Hepper, 1987; Kodama, 1990, 2002; Kodama and Smotherman, 1997). The impact of birth fluids was empirically assessed in the context of nursing (Teicher and Blass, 1977): if nipples made inactive

[3] It may be noted that numerous research on rat pup responsiveness to milk odor has paradoxically used cow's milk or cow's milk-based formulas rather than conspecific milk (e.g., Ackerman and Shindledecker, 1978; Cheslock et al., 2000; Johanson and Hall, 1979; Johanson et al., 1984; Koffman et al, 1998; Petrov et al., 1997; Robinson and Smotherman, 1994; Smotherman and Robinson, 1994; Smotherman et al., 1997; Terry and Johanson, 1987). Although olfactory differences of both types of milks are acknowledged, they are considered to present "enough similarities in their composition to be perceived as being similar by pups" (Terry and Johanson, 1987: 328). Beyond practical considerations, the choice of cow's milk-base cream ("half and half") may be justified as a model stimulus for developmental analyses of nutritional regulations or of reward systems. The response pattern of newborn rats to the sensory properties of this heterospecific stimulus may, however, not be generalizable to rat milk.

by prior washing were thereafter painted with amniotic fluid, oral seizing performance recovered at subnormal levels; in the same way, applying saliva of a parturient or lactating dam reinstated pups' nipple grasping (Teicher and Blass, 1977) or elicited arousal and attraction (Sullivan *et al.*, 1986; see also Block *et al.*, 1981, for gerbils). In the normal course of events, newly born rat pups certainly also deposit amniotic fluid blended with saliva during their searching motions over their mother's abdominal fur. Pup saliva alone, as well as pup salivary gland extract, was indeed also efficient in restoring attachment to nipples that were prewashed (Pedersen and Blass, 1981). Finally, when rodent females groom, they spread a range of secretions from their oral–facial area (e.g., Harderian glands) over their face, paws, and ventral fur (Thiessen *et al.*, 1976). They lick then their pups' anogenital area, consuming their urine (Friedman and Bruno, 1976), and lick next their own ventrum, leaving there pup secretions/excretions, originating in urine, or in anal or preputial glands. Thus, in these species, a medley of anogenital glandular or urinary volatile and involatile compounds (e.g., lipocalins, such as MUPs) could be deposited on the nipple-lines (although pure urine from lactating dams appeared only weakly effective; Teicher and Blass, 1976, 1977). It is interesting to note that such involatile proteins are releasable in mammary, parotid, sublingual, submaxillary, and lachrymal glands (Shahan *et al.*, 1987), which secretions are all potentially involved in mother–pup relationships; they could indeed carry or constitute cues that are common to milk, saliva, or other facial or nasal sources.

Thus, at least in the rat, the *current evidence* suggests that the biological substrates that direct mammary localization and that drive nipple grasping might originate from extramammary rather than from mammary sources, through the conveyance of females and newborns themselves. However, much more in-depth research is needed here, especially pertaining to the olfactory activity of conspecific colostrum/milk for neonates.

3. Learning of mammary-related odor cues

Neonatal rodents are adept odor learners and have accordingly been the focus of abundant work unraveling underlying neural and cognitive processes (e.g., Leon, 1992; Moriceau and Sullivan, 2004; Wilson and Sullivan, 1994). Findings on rodent odor learning in the context of the interactions with the dam and exposure to nipples and milk can be summarized as follows (for reviews, cf. Alberts, 1981; Alberts and Gubernick, 1984; Brake *et al.*, 1986; Rosenblatt, 1983): (1) Rat and mice pups acquire experimental odorants painted on the female's abdominal/mammary area, which leads to reasonably infer that they might learn natural odor cues in much the same way. (2) Odor learning is functional from birth onward (e.g., Miller and Spear, 2008, 2010), and it becomes more efficient with age, as a function of maturation and experience; thus, nipple grasping, already well functional right at birth, becomes more attuned during the first hours or days due to the rapid establishment of sensory incentives and to neuromotor training (Armstrong *et al.*, 2006; Bouslama *et al.*, 2005; Dollinger *et al.*, 1978; Rosenblatt, 1983). (3) Neonatal olfactory abilities are already largely molded by prenatal induction, in terms of both sensitivity and preferences (Molina *et al.*, 1995; Schaal and Orgeur, 1992; Smotherman and Robinson, 1987; Youngentob *et al.*, 2007), and this fetal sensory preparation goes in parallel with a relative continuity of chemosensory cues before and after birth (Pedersen and Blass, 1982; Schaal, 2005; Schaal and Orgeur, 1992); specifically, in the case of the rat, the amniotic odor is made directly disponible onto the nipple-lines by maternal self-licking activity (Teicher and Blass, 1977), and milk accumulates odor cues derived from the gestating female's general metabolism and diet (Capretta and Rawls, 1974; Galef and Henderson, 1972; Galef and Sherry, 1973). (4) Multiple, redundant reinforcing agents are at work to potentiate the rapid learning of odor cues in neonates; maternal and infant behavior afford numerous reinforcers such as mere general contact or targeted stimulation (anogenital licking), warmth, the exercise of sucking, postingestive (taste of milk) and postabsorptive (gastric filling, satiety) factors which separately favor the learning of any associated odor cue, their concurrent action being even more efficient (Brake *et al.*, 1986); milk itself through its flavor supports the establishment of learned odor associations (e.g., Brake, 1981). (5) Finally, some compounds in biological secretions may potentiate the learning of co-occurring odor cues: for example, presenting simultaneously an aversive orange scent with the odor of maternal saliva reverses the value of the orange odor into attraction in rat pups (Sullivan *et al.*, 1986); thus odor–odor interactions involving saliva or other behaviorally active compounds emitted from, or conveyed to, the nipples (e.g., colostrum/milk or amniotic fluid; cf. Arias and Chotro, 2007) might rapidly alter the meaning of circumstantially associated odor cues in neonatal rodents. It is clear from the above points in this paragraph that the fast and highly efficient odor learning of fetal and neonatal rodents will make it very difficult to characterize predisposed odor signals, especially pheromones which, by the operational definition adopted here, imply no or minimal experiential induction.

4. Evidence for pheromones

Do newborn rodents respond to odor stimuli from mammary secretions before direct exposure to them? So far this issue does not seem to have been directly addressed using conspecific stimuli (e.g., see Cheslock *et al.*, 2000, using cow's milk). However, extramammary sources, viz. pup saliva, pup salivary gland extract, and nipple wash extract, appear to be reliable elicitors of newborn rat nipple grasping; accordingly these excretions were subjected to GC–MS, with the aim to pinpoint dimethyl disulfide (DMDS), a compound that was *a priori* targeted as a potentially active compound based on evidence from other species (female attractant in male hamster; Singer *et al.*, 1976). Synthetic DMDS (concentration not indicated) was indeed shown to be effective in eliciting nipple grasping in 3- to 5-day-old pups; however, its releasing potency was low (about 50%) relative to that of olfactorily intact nipples (Pedersen and Blass, 1981). Thus, DMDS may be only partially responsible for the release of normal nipple grasping activity in rat pups, and unknown compounds from the natural mixture coating nipples may carry additional impact. It may be noted that in these studies rat pups were aged 3–5 days, implying that the activity of DMDS may derive from extensive exposure during nursing prior to testing. Nevertheless, DMDS appears special because it has the power to elicit responsiveness already in the fetus where it has the effect to reduce responsiveness to aversive perioral stimulation. This effect is mediated by opioidergic brain processes that suggest unconditional reward properties of DMDS from the fetal period onward (Smotherman and Robinson, 1992). Although data are not shown (Blass, 1990), DMDS is reported not to be detected in amniotic fluid, leading to the logical conclusion that its behavioral salience might not depend on prenatal exposure. Thus, until DMDS is further assessed for responsiveness in newly born pups, it may tentatively be considered as a signal from pup saliva that facilitates nipple attachment. To be categorized as a pheromone, its species-specificity remains to be established and its action would need further testing for unspecific arousal effects against reference compounds. Other sulfur-containing volatiles identified in adult rat breath may bear precocious activity, among which are carbon disulfide and carbonyl sulfide. The former was shown to work as an attractant in subadult rats and mice (Bean *et al.*, 1989; Galef *et al.*, 1988), but these compounds have not yet been assayed with neonates and nurslings in these species.

Finally, it is not to be excluded that a lactating rat dams' avid licking of pups' anogenital area and consumption of their urine (Gubernick and Alberts, 1983) may result in the spreading on/around nipples of traces of urinary and urinary tract glandular compounds of semiochemical interest. This mammary distribution of "foreign" substrates may concern, for example, (i) dodecyl propionate, a compound emitted in neonatal rats' preputial secretions and that releases females' licking behavior (Brouette-Lahlou *et al.*, 1991a,b); (ii) MUPs that themselves bear behavioral activity in adult mice; and/or (iii) active MUP-bound ligands known to carry pheromonal effects in young mice (Jemiolo *et al.*, 1987, 1989); in that line, 2-hexanone, 2-heptanone, 4-heptanone, previously shown to promote puberty onset (Jemiolo *et al.*, 1987, 1989), could already affect the responsiveness or physiological state of neonatal or preweaning pups (e.g., Drickamer, 1988). To our knowledge, this has not been tested so far. At last, in the Mongolian gerbil, the sebum obtained from the ventral gland was shown to be attractive for adults, and therein phenylacetic acid was suspected to carry this effect (Thiessen *et al.*, 1974); again, neonatal responsiveness to the entire secretion and to the purported pheromone waits testing. Taken together, extant literature does not clearly establish that rodent females emit from their mammary structures *infant*-directed pheromones that might release immediate responses in offspring or prime their physiological development.

C. Lagomorphs

In that mammalian order, the most complete understanding of odor-based neonatal behavior stems from studies in the European rabbit (*Oryctolagus cuniculus*). Data on odor-guided neonatal behavior from other logomorph taxa (hares, pikas) do apparently lack.

1. Odor-mediation of mammary localization and of sucking

The female rabbit visits her nest once a day to nurse for only 3–5 min (Zarrow *et al.*, 1965), her arrival triggering an intense rush of the litter under her. They display then a typical pattern of probing and searching that generally ends in orally grasping a nipple (Hudson and Distel, 1983; Schley, 1976). This successful nipple grasp, habitually achieved in less than 15 s, is mediated by perioral somesthesis and olfaction (vision and audition being nonfunctional during week 1). When nasal chemoreception is suppressed by bulbectomy or peripheral $ZnSO_4$ anosmization, pups' ability to locate nipples is lost (Schley, 1977, 1979). Further, when altering the source of active cues in a lactating rabbit by washing her abdominal fur, pups are delayed in finding nipples (Müller, 1978). Finally, covering nipples with an airtight film disrupts typical searching behavior, but at various rates depending on the degree and location of the obstruction created on the nipple (Coureaud *et al.*, 2001; Hudson and Distel, 1983).

2. Mammary odor sources

Female rabbits, particularly when lactating, are potent to release searching and oral grasping in pups exposed to their ventral fur (Coureaud and Schaal, 2000; Hudson and Distel, 1984, 1990; Schley, 1976). The same result is reached when exposing pups to excised nipples from lactating versus nonlactating females (Moncomble *et al.*, 2005). Thus, a major source of behaviorally active compounds on rabbit females' belly appear to be the nipples themselves. Currently, little is known on the histological origin of the odor cues, and several odor emission mechanisms may be considered (Moncomble *et al.*, 2005). First, increased keratinization on the nipple epidermis in lactating females supports higher release of lipids derived from epidermal apoptosis. Second, well-developed sebaceous glands are located at the lower part of the nipple, excreting sebum that may be involved in some intrinsic signaling function or acting by its ability to sequester odor-active milk compounds. By washing these surface cues away on excised nipples, pup grasping responses are reduced or abolished. Third, it cannot be excluded that nipple attraction to rabbit pups depends on milk volatiles invisibly oozing from the nipple. Fresh rabbit milk is indeed a powerful releaser of pups' searching–grasping response (Coureaud *et al.*, 2002; Keil *et al.*, 1990; Müller, 1978; Schaal *et al.*, 2003). The behavioral activity of rabbit milk fades, however, within 30 min after collection and resting at ambient temperature (Keil *et al.*, 1990). But, interestingly, in the same conditions the odor of excised nipples from lactating rabbits does not fade away (Moncomble, 2006), suggesting that surface compounds either bear intrinsic behavioral activity or do preserve the activity of some trace remnants of milk or of pup saliva left on the nipple surface.

The compounds that render rabbit milk behaviorally active to neonate pups appear to originate either from environmental sources (viz. diet) transferred into milk or from *de novo* secretion processes in the mammary tract. Both sources of behavioral activity are not exclusive. The intramammary source of active compounds is attested by an experiment that compared the activity of milk samples collected either from the alveolae, from the duct below the nipple, or right after ejection (Moncomble *et al.*, 2005). Only ejected milk was behaviorally efficient, designating the terminal part of the milk ducts as the possible source of active compound(s). Histological analyses reveal indeed that nipple milk ducts of lactating rabbits form an enlarged, extremely tortuous sinus lined with a secretory epithelium (Moncomble, 2006). This convoluted structure suggests an exchange surface optimizing the release of ductal secretions into flowing milk. Alternatively, some involatile or bound substances carried in milk might be oxidized when contacting air, instantaneously releasing volatile compounds.

3. Learning of mammary-related odor cues

Rabbit pups are remarkably fast in learning odors associated with suckling. A series of studies looked for the sensory cues and the reinforcing processes that could come to control searching and oral seizing of nipples by pups. For example, Ivanistkii (1962) described the precocious learning of artificial odorants (e.g., cologne, camphor) painted on the mother's ventral fur. By representing these same odorants outside the nursing context on the experimenter's own hand, he showed that from the first day after birth rabbit pups can learn in only one session a nonspecific odorant associated with searching–sucking activity. Ivanitskii also showed a developmental change in the sucking-induced associative odor learning, which was easiest to establish on days 1–10. These data were further refined by Hudson and her collaborators (Allingham *et al.*, 1999; Hudson, 1985; Kindermann *et al.*, 1994) who established that nursing-induced learning was selective, relatively stable, restricted to a limited period (first 5 days after birth), and dependent on the exertion of sucking (Hudson *et al.*, 2002). Thus, any arbitrary odor cue present on the nipple surface can become meaningful within a single suckling episode. Furthermore, rabbit neonates are born with extensive odor experience gained *in utero* (Bilko *et al.*, 1994; Hudson *et al.*, 1999) and show ability to use such fetal information as directional cues

(Coureaud *et al.*, 2002). Thus, as highlighted above in rodents, prenatal and neonatal olfactory acquisitions may hamper the characterization of potential predisposed, viz. experience-independent, odor signaling processes.

4. Evidence for pheromones

Rabbit pups efficiently locate and grasp a nipple when deposited on the abdomen of any lactating doe. The same response is elicited by milk obtained from any female (Coureaud and Schaal, 2000; Keil *et al.*, 1990). This behavioral activity was present in the milk effluvium, directing analyses toward the volatile fraction of milk. Using a combination of GC–MS and olfactometry, the analysis of the headspace of fresh rabbit milk resulted in the identification of a compound, 2-methyl-but-2-enal (2MB2), accounting for the behavioral effect of whole milk (Schaal *et al.*, 2003). This compound being as efficient as fresh rabbit milk to elicit searching–grasping motions, it was considered a candidate for pheromonal mediation. To assess whether this compound could effectively be classified as a pheromone, it was submitted to systematic tests verifying the five criteria specified in Section III.

Regarding criterion 1, 2MB2 is the chemically "simplest" possible stimulus (viz., monomolecular); its activity is extraordinarily strong in eliciting searching–grasping actions, but it cannot be excluded that additional, not yet identified, compounds from milk could act in the same direction. As to criterion 2, the macroscopic structure of pup responses is not differentiable between pure 2MB2 and entire milk, indicating that a single key-compound from milk can mimic the response elicited by milk itself. Further, 2MB2 is highly efficient to trigger the typical searching–grasping responses regardless of the mode of presentation (at least during the first 10 days after birth). The selective activity of the compound (criterion 3) was ascertained first by comparing pup responsiveness to 40 odorants that are present or not in rabbit milk: these reference odorants being ineffective at any concentration (Coureaud *et al.*, 2003), the behavioral activity of 2MB2 appears to be selective and devoid of nonspecific arousal effects. Further, the activity of 2MB2 was limited within a range of concentrations extending over 5 log units (10^{-9}–10^{-5} g/ml; Coureaud *et al.*, 2004), giving leeway for intensitive fluctuations of the signal. The species-level generality of the releasing potency of 2MB2 (criterion 4) was positively established through its independence from maternal diet and genetic background (Coureaud *et al.*, 2008; Schaal *et al.*, 2003), and its complete inactivity in newborn rats, mice, cats, and even closely related brown hares (*Lepus europaeus*; Schaal *et al.*, 2003). Finally, pup responsiveness to 2MB2 appeared to develop independently from previous exposure to it (criterion 5). To acquire its behavioral efficacy, 2MB2 does indeed not require contingent labor-related arousal, suckling, ingestion of milk, or contact with the mother: pups taken away from the mother immediately after birth displayed maximal response to it at the very first presentation. Furthermore, 2MB2 being efficient in fetuses delivered 1–2 days before term, and chemical analyses having failed to detect it in amniotic fluid and blood plasma from lactating females, its behavioral activity does not appear to derive from prenatal experience (Schaal *et al.*, 2003). Accordingly, current data indicate that the 2MB2 requires neither prenatal nor postnatal exposure to become functionally specified. These results allowed qualifying 2MB2 from rabbit milk as a pheromone, in the sense of the operational redefinition of the concept by Beauchamp *et al.* (1976) and Johnston (2000). As 2MB2 appears to be produced somewhere in the mammary tract, presumably in the final portion of the nipple to be emitted in milk, it was named "mammary pheromone."

In addition to the fulfillment of a set of physical, chemical, or biological criteria, any candidate pheromone should further be demonstrated to be involved in mutually beneficial functions. The involvement of the MP in the reciprocity of the rabbit doe and her litter is straightforward at the general level: (i) on the offspring side, it elicits immediate arousal of the litter and recruitment of directional behavior when the female enters the nest, favoring searching/grasping of a nipple and ingesting milk; (ii) on the females' side, the MP may be a signal that boosts tactile stimulations from pups known to trigger and sustain lactational physiology. So far, data indicate that those individual pups that do not react to the MP on postnatal day 1 have lower survival chances during the following 4 weeks (Coureaud *et al.*, 2007), suggesting that the initial responsiveness to it is linked with long-term viability. Another point of functional interest is the restricted period of effectiveness of the MP that closely matches the period when pups need to contact nipples, viz. between birth and weaning (Coureaud *et al.*, 2008). Finally, the MP triggers automatic responses that ensure that pups are ready to search/grasp a nipple at any time during the first few postnatal days; MP-induced oral grasping is then compulsory at each presentation, and it is only subsequently (after day 5)that it comes to be increasingly controlled by circadian or postingestive factors (Montigny *et al.*, 2006).

D. Ungulates

Among ungulates, the process of locating the mammary gland is generally considered to be a matter of learning by trial and error (e.g., Lent, 1974; Wood-Gush *et al.*, 1986). But, although diversely according to species, olfaction appears to be involved in the localization of the mammae. Behavioral observations and experiments were essentially conducted in the domestic representatives of the *Suidae* (*Sus scrofa*) and *Bovinae* (*Ovis aries*). Newborns in these families are precocial, generally following the female immediately after delivery (lamb) or after a period of nesting (piglet). Neonatal behavior in these species is thus mainly under visual and auditory control. Nevertheless, interactions at close range, especially those involved in the initial localization of the mammary area and establishment of social recognition, appear to be coregulated by nasal chemoreception (Gonzalez-Mariscal and Poindron, 2002; Poindron *et al.*, 1993).

1. Odor-mediation of mammary localization and sucking

The main activity of newly born piglets is nosing over the mother's body, favoring concurrent somesthetic and chemosensory inputs. They react to the odor of the sow's ventrum in general, and after several suckling episodes appear guided toward teats previously used by littermates (Jeppesen, 1982a; Morrow-Tesch and McGlone, 1990b). Flushing an anesthetic into the nose of newly born piglets strongly impairs their ability to locate a teat and to begin sucking, attesting for the involvement of nasal chemoreception (Morrow-Tesch and McGlone, 1990a; Tanaka *et al.*, 1998). Also washing the sow's ventrum with organic solvents considerably increased the just-born piglets' latency to orally grasp a teat and to suck (Morrow-Tesch and McGlone, 1990b). Within the first postnatal hours (McBride, 1963), and more consistently over the first week (Hemworth *et al.*, 1976), piglets develop preferential relationships with one or several specific teats, leading to a given "teat-order"; this ordering could be experimentally mimicked using a surrogate sow made of a row of artificial teats (Jeppesen, 1982a). As the odor surrounding the teats was suggested to be one important factor in the establishment of this teat-order (McBride, 1963), this was tested using the surrogate sow which allowed to deodorize or invert teat positions. This experiment ascertained the impact of odors in individual teat preference of piglets: although nursling pigs may use thermal, tactile, auditory, and visual cues from the sow, as well as such cues from littermates, in the control of real sucking performance, the surrogate sow experiment indicates that they may deposit an individually distinctive odor mark on one or several teats (Jeppesen, 1982b).

Regarding lambs, they stand on their feet within an hour after birth, begin searching for the udder in moving around the ewe, with eventual sucking success. Before effective teat location, lambs nuzzle, lick and bunt actively under the ewe's flanks (Vince, 1993), so that differential tactile and odor qualities are sampled and mammary-related odor cues can be encoded. Although somesthesis and vision appear decisive in achieving sucking within 60 min of testing, lambs momentarily deprived of olfactory abilities through a nasal spray of anesthetic take significantly more time to suck (Vince *et al.*, 1987). Thus, despite the blatant dominance of visual/auditory cues in orientation to, and recognition of, the mother, olfactory cues are of importance for initial mammary localization activities in pig and sheep newborns. This impact might be more or less short-lived, however, depending on the species. Lambs, for example, very sharply decrease their responsiveness to mammary-related odors once they have experienced the first suckling cycles (Vince and Ward, 1994).

2. Mammary odor sources

In the domestic pig, washing the sow's abdomen with organic solvents hinders the piglets' teat localization performance, an indication of altered mammary odor cues. The source and nature of these cues have been insufficiently scrutinized so far. In one study (Morrow-Tesch and McGlone, 1990b), piglets exposed in paired-choice tests to either mammary substrates (viz., colostrum, milk, teat washings) and maternal feces, invariably display preference for fecal odors; as a sow's teats are often tainted with fecal matters, this odor predominates in the nursing environment and may rapidly gain salience as an associative cue. In this fecal odor background, piglets anoint teats with their own odor mark conveyed by unknown biological substrates (amniotic fluid? saliva?) that can contribute to create olfactorily individualized nipples.

In other ungulate families (e.g., *Caprinae, Antilopinae, Cephalophinae*), clearly circumscribed scent glands are located in the immediate vicinity of the udder (Schaffer, 1940; Schwalbe, 1898). These inguinal glands were best described in *Ovis* (Malkmus, 1888; Masselin, 1930; Schaffer, 1940). They are bilaterally located as pockets at the external base of the udder, and secrete an intensely smelling (to humans) wax that tends to spread downward to the teats. Newborn lambs are exceedingly reactive to the odor of this inguinal wax. When exposed to it, they show strong arousal responses in terms of positive directional head movements and of accelerated heart and respiration rates (Vince and Ward, 1984). The odor of inguinal wax elicits stronger responses than the odors of wool or milk, but it appeared to be differentiated in individual terms: maternal wax was more reactogenic than the wax of an unfamiliar ewe (Vince and Billing, 1986).

Although current analyses remain limited, newborn ungulates react distinctively to conspecific milk odor (and flavor). Newly born lambs exhibit a general reaction to ovine milk odor, in terms of attraction to a cloth impregnated with ovine milk as compared to a scentless, humid cloth (Schaal and Orgeur, unpublished data). Ovine milk (Moio *et al.*, 1993, 1996) and colostrum (Rietdorf, 2002) carry indeed a wealth of volatile ethyl esters, aldehydes, and ketones, which derive from intrinsic mammary processes, as well as from metabolites derived from the lactating ewe's diet (Desage *et al.*, 1996; Viallon *et al.*, 2000). Lambs react selectively to dietary odorants transferred into ovine milk (Schaal *et al.*, 1994). Further, evidence from ovine fetuses (last week of gestation) suggests that milks from different lactational stages are chemosensorily differentiable; their orofacial responses to oral infusions are contrasted for: (1) ovine colostrum versus ovine milk and (2) ovine milk versus bovine milk (Robinson *et al.*, 1995), indicating subtle abilities to differentiate conspecific milks differing in age-appropriateness to the tested animal or milks from different species. There is also evidence that *Bos taurus* calves are highly activated (nonnutritive sucking) after the ingestion of small amounts of bovine milk or bovine milk-based replacers (de Passillé *et al.*, 1997; Rushen and de Passillé, 1995). The precise sensory base of such postingestive effects of bovine milk to calves is not understood so far, although there is an indication that the lactose content is a key (de Passillé and Rushen, 2006). These studies raise the potential importance of oral chemoreception in the processing of milk properties by newborns. Finally, the response of piglets to conspecific milk remains ambiguous (Morrow-Tesch and McGlone, 1990b) and has not been adequately investigated so far. When simultaneously exposed in a three-choice testing arena to milk and amniotic fluid (both from mother) and water, piglets orient nearly equally to either biological stimulus (Parfet and Gonyou, 1991). In lambs, selective responsiveness to own amniotic fluid (as opposed to the same fluid from another lamb; Schaal *et al.*, 1995a) and undifferentiated attraction to amniotic fluid odor paired with colostrum odor indicate that prenatal effects could be involved in the reactogenic value of colostrum (Schaal, 2005).

3. Learning of mammary-related odor cues

Learning of odors associated with the mother has been largely shown in neonatal ungulates. For example, a newborn black-tailed deer artificially fed with a surrogate scented with ischiadic gland secretion of male *Antilocapra* for 15 days showed a preference for (1) a dummy carrying *Antilocapra* scent (compared to a dummy scented with black-tailed or mule deer odors) at 2 and 4 weeks; (2) an *Antilocapra* female rather than a conspecific female at 2, 5 months of age, indicating selective treatment and long-term memorization of an odor associated with nursing in this species (Müller-Schwarze and Müller-Schwarze, 1971). Neonatal ungulates are also sensitive to odor exposure through milk, which volatile profile reflects the aromatic profile of the lactating female's diet (Desage *et al.*, 1996; Moio *et al.*, 1996). Milk-related learning was first shown in lambs aged 2–3 days given 50 days a replacer flavored with either garlic or onion; such early exposure influenced intake preference for a nonmilk food that was congruently flavored (Nolte and Provenza, 1992). Similar results were obtained in lambs and in piglets for flavors naturally transferred into milk from the maternal diet (Campbell, 1976; Schaal *et al.*, 1994). Finally, as dietary flavors accumulate in the fetal environment (Nolte *et al.*, 1992; Schaal *et al.*, 1995c), ungulate newborns are exposed in advance to odor cues to be reencountered in colostrum/milk as well as presumably in skin secretions or gland excretions. Such a prenatal influence has been scrutinized in lambs (Schaal *et al.*, 1995a; Simitzis *et al.*, 2008) and in piglets (Langendijk *et al.*, 2007; Oostindjier *et al.*, 2009; Tien and Preston, 2008). Finally, even in the absence of experimental adulteration of the perinatal odor environment, positive responsiveness to prenatal odor substrates was noted in lambs and piglets, namely toward amniotic fluid or the placenta (Grubb, 1974; Parfet and Gonyou, 1991; Schaal *et al.*, 1995a;

Vince, 1992). In addition, when exposed to amniotic fluid and colostrum/milk in a paired-choice test, lambs and piglets display equivalent orientation responses (Parfet and Gonyou, 1991; Schaal, 2005). Thus, amniotic and mammary substrates may carry common sensory or motivational properties, and fetal ungulates may in this way create an anticipatory template for mammary or milk odor cues (Schaal, 2005). Such perinatal overlap in chemical constituents could be mediated by more or less volatile compounds (Rietdorf, 2002) as well as by involatile compounds (e.g., olfactory-binding proteins; Guiraudie-Capraz *et al.*, 2005).

4. Evidence for pheromones

To the best of our knowledge, no evidence for any mammary-related pheromone is available in any ungulate. One candidate substrate worthy of empirical attention for its potential to embed a pheromonal candidate(s) is the inguinal wax of the domestic sheep. However, before further studies are undertaken, the behavioral evidence for unconditional and species-specific responsiveness of lambs to inguinal wax odor should be ascertained. Inguinal wax samples from tested lambs' own mother do not indeed elicit the same investigatory impact than samples taken from unrelated ewes (Vince and Billing, 1986), indicating the lambs' ability to detect in it individual-specific as well as species-specific cues. It may be noted that a mixture of inguinal wax, infraorbital secretion, and wool from rams have the same potency than the entire ram to stimulate the onset of estrus in anoestrus ewes (Knight and Lynch, 1980). Thus, behaviorally active compounds in inguinal wax may be investigated for their releasing effect, as well as for potential priming effects. A first chemical study of postparturient ovine inguinal wax indicates a very complex mixture of volatile and nonvolatile compounds, among which at least 155 could be identified (Rietdorf, 2002). Qualitative and quantitative variations in these compounds from inguinal gland secretion are presumably underlying its individual discriminability by lambs (Vince and Billing, 1986). The other biological substrate worthy of detailed chemoethological enquiry in ungulates is colostrum/milk. It is noteworthy that such fluids are already strongly and discriminatively reactogenic in near-term ovine fetuses (Robinson *et al.*, 1995), indicating that they are rewarding before any opportunity for direct exposure. The chemical and chemosensory bases of such inborn responsiveness awaits investigation.

E. Carnivores

Among carnivores, *Felidae* and *Canidae* were most studied regarding offspring reliance on mother- and mammary-related odor cues. Limited behavioral observations on pup–mother odor exchanges around mammaries were also made in pinnipeds (e.g., *Otariidae*: Marlow, 1975).

1. Odor-mediation of mammary localization and sucking

Newborn kittens trace nipples in nuzzling over the fur until they reach the mammary area; search-like motions allow then fitting lips to a nipple to engage sucking (Rosenblatt, 1971). The whole sequence is controlled by tactile, olfactory, and taste processes (Blass *et al.*, 1988). According to Ewer (1959), kittens solicit nipples unevenly, posterior nipples being more often sucked than anterior ones potentially due to differential milk productivity or attractive odor cues emitted or deposited there. However, more recent evidence indicates no differential nipple quality (Hudson *et al.*, 2009). In 1 or 2 days, newborn *Felidae* tend to show a relative nipple constancy (for one or two adjacent nipples), which stability decreases after the first month (domestic cats: Ewer, 1959; Hudson *et al.*, 2009; Schaal *et al.*, 2007; snow leopard: McVittie, 1978; mountain lion: Pfeiffer, 1980; for further discussion, cf. Mermet *et al.*, 2007; Schneirla *et al.*, 1963).

Sensory explanations for such preferential nipple choice remain uncertain in cats (as opposed to piglets), although it is suggested to be based on distinct nipple odor or on multimodal cues supporting recognition of maternal body shape or of neighboring siblings (Ewer, 1959, 1961; Hudson *et al.*, 2009; Rosenblatt, 1983). The role played by olfaction in the cat–kitten relationship and in the selection of preferred nipples was first examined by impeding it. Thus, kittens' nipple search behavior was hindered by obstructing nostrils, and reinstated after freeing them (Larsson and Stein, 1984); further, before vision/hearing become functional, damage to the olfactory bulbs or olfactory mucosae clearly alters nipple localization performance (Kovach and Kling, 1967; Shuleikina-Turpaeva, 1986). Second, washing the mammary areas with organic solvents affects kittens' nipple searching/grasping behavior (Blass *et al.*, 1988): after washing the queen's mammary area, kittens become restless, but return to calm state when put on an unwashed abdominal area on the same female. Rosenblatt (1972) also reports that washing the mammary areas does not break off the kittens' sucking proneness, but that it does disrupt preference for a particular nipple. However, after washing, kittens progressively resume their selective choice of nipples, suggesting that an individualized odor signal emitted or conveyed on/around the nipple is rapidly restored. A final way to tell apart the impact of olfactory cues and tactile/thermal/visual cues related to maternal morphology or sibling identity in nipple selection is to displace individual kittens from their biological mother to an unfamiliar female (Ewer, 1961; Raihani *et al.*, 2009). In such tests, kittens do not grasp unfamiliar nipples corresponding to the position of those they preferentially sucked on their own mother, indicating clear disturbance. When returned to their mother, they reattached to their particular nipple(s) within a minute (Ewer, 1961). Thus, kittens' selective nipple grasping/sucking can only be based on nipple-specific chemosensory cues. Comparable detailed information regarding the involvement of mammary odor cues in suckling does not seem to be available in *Canidae* or any other carnivore (cf. below).

2. Mammary odor sources

To date, mammary odor *sources* in carnivores have received scant attention and no recent analyses dedicated to mammary and nipple morphology/histology could be found (for early studies, cf. Gisler, 1922; Kaeppeli, 1918). Sometimes contradictory hypotheses have been advanced, essentially centered on kitten attraction to a preferred nipple. Ewer (1959, 1961) suggested that grasping of a nipple during the very first nursing appears hardly triggered by an odor cue, as pups are seen moving across teats several times without change in response; accordingly, nipple odor was speculated to gain meaning when it is engaged in incentive value through association with milk reward (Rosenblatt, 1983). Others report that newborn kittens express active searching over a lactating cat's abdominal fur, but not over the belly of a female rabbit or dog (Prechtl, 1952); similarly, newborn puppies express avoidance of the odor of a cat belly, whereas they are attracted to the ventral odor of an unfamiliar lactating bitch, and even more to that of their own mother (Kassil and Gulina, 1986). As this differentiation is evident before any milk intake in cat and dog newborns (Kassil and Gulina, 1986; Raihani *et al.*, 2009), one may hypothesize the operation of a species-specific system of behaviorally active odor cues emanating from the ventral/mammary region. Thus, any lactating cat/dog emits an attractive odor profile that carries both species- and individually differentiable fractions. It is interesting to note that the ventral odor of the bitch, collected daily between prepartum day 5 and postpartum day 1, becomes more attractive to puppies on days 2 and 1 prepartum and on day 1 postpartum (Kassil and Gulina, 1986), suggesting the emission of increasingly attractive compounds from the very end of gestation and incepting lactation.

Odor cues supporting nipple searching–grasping behavior in kittens or puppies might be produced locally, through abdominal or nipple skin gland secretions, or through colostrum/milk. So far, these mammary substrates do not seem to have been subjected to systematic assays in newborns. Cat and dog females actively self-lick, and lick their offspring, namely to consume their urine and feces for several weeks postpartum (Rheingold, 1963; Rosenblatt *et al.*, 1963). By such self-licking, females' may abdominally distribute traces of extramammary substrates (e.g., amniotic fluid, urine, secretions from facial glands, remnants of offspring urine or feces, secretions from supracaudal glands, etc.). Compounds in these extramammary substrates, that have strong chemosensory impact (in cats, proteins bearing a characteristic catty odor are excreted in urine, such as felinine or cauxin; Hendriks *et al.*, 1995; Miyazaki *et al.*, 2008), could be spread abdominally. The behavioral impact of such well-characterized proteins has not been assayed on newborn cats. Further, neonatal cats and dog may smear maternal abdominal fur and nipples with their own fluids (e.g., amniotic fluid, saliva, milk coagulate, urine). Both maternal and infantile odor substrates may mingle by concurrent mother/offspring actions, and spread over the nipple epidermis as well as entrapped in surrounding hair (e.g., Blass *et al.*, 1988, in kittens; Kassil and Gulina, 1986, in puppies). A sequence of odor cues could therefore take place in space and time, beginning with amniotic substrates mixed with infantile saliva, followed with colostrum, and then milk coagulate mixed with infantile saliva. These contributions may be further mixed with secretions from offspring plantar glands (of eccrine and or sebaceous nature; Schaffer, 1940) deposited while they express bilateral treading movements with forefeet. Thus, a continuous updating of mother-general and offspring-individual odor mosaic might take place around the mammaries in carnivores. These different, potentially time-ordered, sources of odor cues remain speculative and offer a rich area for future behavioral and chemical analyses.

3. Learning of mammary-related odor cues

Carnivore newborns, at least those of the few species studied so far, readily learn to associate odor stimuli to various reinforcers (Rosenblatt, 1983; Stanley *et al.*, 1970). But neonatal learning has been little addressed in the nursing context, with a notable exception that highlights the cognitive sophistication of kitten. To understand the source of effects in the nursing kitten, Rosenblatt (1971, 1972, 1983) designed a surrogate consisting in a pair of latex nipples embedded in artificial fur, each nipple being cued by distinct scents (cologne, wintergreen) and differentially rewarded (nonspecific milk formula vs. nothing). Before nipple choice tests, kittens were trained from birth to suck in presence of one of the odorants. After the end of conditioning (i.e., days 2–6), daily searching duration on either nipple was recorded. From day 3, nuzzling time was longer on the milk-delivering nipple than on the dry nipple, indicating nipple selection based on its individual odor. The hypothesis of a kitten-made odor trail to the nipple was addressed by washing different areas of the surrogate's fur around the nipples and/or the nipples themselves: kittens not only learned the odor contingent with the reinforcing nipple, but they could encode the mammary odor mosaic. When one element of this olfactory mosaic was missing, kittens could rely on the remaining cues to perform the entire searching–grasping sequence to the target nipple; but disturbance of all odor cues compromised nipple attachment. Transposed in the context of natural nursing, these findings with the surrogate would suggest that kittens' nipple grasping is guided by sequential odor cues either in the mother's abdominal fur or on/around nipples (Rosenblatt, 1983). Finally, the fact that several artificial odorants can induce selective behaviors underscores sophisticated odor processing abilities in cat newborns. Converging results on odor learning in the context of nursing are available in newborn puppies that are easily "imprinted" to an artificial odor painted on nipples (e.g., Fox and Himwich, 1965; Kassil and Gulina, 1986), suggesting similar learning abilities of natural mammary odorants. Finally, the direction of postnatal odor reactivity of neonatal cats/dogs toward conspecific mammary substrates may be influenced by fetal odor experience resulting from maternal odor transfer (Becques *et al.*, 2010; Hepper and Wells, 2006; Wells and Hepper, 2006); similar odor-active compounds derived from the mother's diet may pass into the amniotic and mammary compartments, and facilitate offspring acceptance of congruently flavored colostrum.

4. Evidence for pheromones

Although mammary-related odor cues trigger arousal and afford guidance to carnivore neonates, so far no strong evidence for mammary-related pheromones is available. Some claims have been made about the characterization of behaviorally active odor compounds, in the form of a mixture of fatty acids from the abdomen of lactating cats and dogs (Pageat and Gaultier, 2003). However, precise qualitative and quantitative chemical data about these compounds in felids and canids remain to be disclosed in *ad hoc* peer-reviewed journals, and their pheromonal properties (species generality, species specificity, unconditioned responsiveness) need to be substantiated in repeatable conditions.

F. Primates

The nursing relationship has been little studied in nonhuman primates from the perspective of the sensory processes which control it. Current data essentially stem from human studies.

1. Odor-mediation of mammary localization and sucking

Darwin's (1877) first intuition that human infants might use, among other cues, mammary odor to orient their head toward the mother's breast was confirmed a century later by a series of experiments that assessed neonatal responses to odors emitted from the breasts of lactating women. It came out that whole-breast odor collected on a cotton pad reduces arousal in active newborns (Nishitani *et al.*, 2009; Schaal, 1986; Schaal *et al.*, 1980; Sullivan and Toubas, 1998) and increases it in somnolent ones (Russell, 1976; Soussignan *et al.*, 1997; Sullivan and Toubas, 1998). Breast odor also elicits positive head turning (Macfarlane, 1975; Makin and Porter, 1989; Schaal *et al.*, 1980) and stimulates oral activity (Russell, 1976; Soussignan *et al.*, 1997) and breathing pattern (Doucet *et al.*, 2009). It may further stimulate neonatal directional crawling (Varendi and Porter, 2001). When the lactating breast is olfactorily altered by intrusive washing (with water and detergent) or by more gentle disruption through masking, human neonates show clear alterations in their behavior. They appear to take more time, with less success, in reaching the washed breast than the olfactorily intact breast (Varendi *et al.*, 1994). When the breast is merely covered with an airtight plastic film, newborns display less attraction and mouthing responses, less visual attention, and more rapid onset of crying (Doucet *et al.*, 2007). Finally, early observations showed that painting alien, intense odorants on the nipple released aversion and crying in infants (Kroner, 1882; Preyer, 1885). Thus, *Homo* newborns are clearly affected by odor cues emitted from their mother's breasts.

2. Mammary odor sources

The human nipple/areolar region is supplied with all known types of skin gland. The nipple abounds in apocrine and sebaceous glands with ducts opening on its tip and giving off secretions during lactation (Montagna and MacPherson, 1974; Perkins and Miller, 1926). Eccrine sweat glands and large sebaceous glands can also be found on the areolae (Montagna and MacPherson, 1974), the surface of which is additionally dotted with small prominences (Morgagni's corpuscles) that host underlying MG (Montgomery, 1837), composed of sebaceous glands coalesced with miniature mammary acini (Montagna and Yun, 1972; Smith *et al.*, 1982; Vorherr, 1974). A quantitative assessment of MG prevalence, distribution, and patent activity in 121 postparturient women engaging breastfeeding (Doucet *et al.*, 2010b; Schaal *et al.*, 2006) indicated that 97% of (Caucasian) women bore more than 1 MG per areola, and 83%, from 1 to 20 units per areola. These MG can give off a latescent fluid that is visible in about 1 out of 5 women. This polymorphism in MG number/activity may be balanced in part by their nonrandom distribution on the areolae: secretory MG appear indeed most localized over the upper and lateral areolar quadrants, the zones toward which infants' nose are typically directed during nursing (Doucet *et al.*, 2010b; Schaal *et al.*, 2006).

Colostrum and milk released from main lactiferous ducts add their intrinsic olfactory qualities to the areolae. The quality/intensity of lacteal secretions are in part influenced by odorous compounds transferred from maternal diet. Empirical evidence that food aromas or experimental odorants easily pass into milk has been obtained by regularly sampling milk after mothers ingested them (Hausner *et al.*, 2008; Mennella and Beauchamp, 1991a,b, 1996; Schaal, 2005); subsequent odor changes of milk are detectable to infants who modify their sucking pattern and consumption accordingly. In the same way, maternally inhaled odorants (e.g., combusting tobacco) can also be transferred into milk (Mennella and Beauchamp, 1998). Other potential contributions to the mammary area are imported from extramammary sources, conveyed by the newborn and the mother. Regarding the newborn's contribution, such extraneous sources labeling the areolae may be vaginal secretions and blood, amniotic fluid and vernix caseosa covering the skin of the newly born infant; tears, mucus, saliva, and saliva–milk coagulate spread at first sucking episodes. Finally, mothers may add some artificial scent as they often smear their areolae with locally prescribed emollient creams (e.g., Delaunay-El Allam *et al.*, 2006, 2010).

Taken together, these varied sources of mammary substrates create a multifaceted and dynamic areolar odor blend. The lipid fraction from keratinizing epidermis, sebum originating from free sebaceous glands and from MG, as well as fatty acids from milk, may act as odor fixatives that improve the chemical and temporal stability of the olfactory complex formed on the areolae. The intricate arrangement of sebaceous and lacteal sources within the MG may favor the mingling of sebum and areolar milk secretion during sucking episodes. In addition, local biochemical and thermal processes may act on the selective release of given compounds or categories of compounds from the mixture. Namely, salivary enzymes deposited by the suckling infant may speed up the release of odor-active compounds (Büttner, 2002), or areolar skin temperature fluctuations may differentiate volatiles having contrasted vapor pressures.

The complexity of the human areolar–nipple area in terms of multiplicity/intricacy of sources of biological substrates renders the isolation of active odor cues/signals uneasy. A recent study (Doucet *et al.*, 2007) attempted to evaluate whether morphologically differentiable areas of the breast could be related to distinct behavioral effects in newborns. These areas were "fractionated" in applying an odor-free plastic film directly onto the breast, various openings in it allowing to subtract the areolar odor contribution from the whole-breast odor and to separate the areolar odor from that of the nipple or of oozing colostrum/milk. The behavioral impact of the isolated areola was tested in positioning waking newborns next to such a selectively masked breast in an unconstrained nursing posture before a feed. Natural odor cues from the lactating breast modulated arousal states and promoted appetitive oral activity in 3 day olds in terms of mouth opening, tongue protrusion, rooting (see also Koepke and Bigelow, 1997, for similar results in a similar situation). The infants responded similarly to whole breast versus areola versus nipple versus milk odors, suggesting equivalent attractive potencies, all equaling that of human milk. Such behavioral uniformity of breast stimuli may be caused either by overlapping compounds due to shared exocrine sources or cross-contamination, or by perceptually distinct compounds having acquired similar attractiveness due to similar conditions of reward (Delaunay-El Allam *et al.*, 2006). In a finer grained study (Doucet *et al.*, 2009), 3-day-old newborns were directly exposed to native MG secretion and to its components, milk and sebum (from forehead; both stimuli not from their own mother). Neonatal reactivity to these areolar odor cues was also tested against several control stimuli (e.g., solvent, vanilla, fresh cow's milk, cow's milk-based formula). It came out that pure MG secretion equaled fresh human milk in reactogenic potency regarding the respiratory variable, but it had higher activity than human milk, sebum, and all other reference stimuli, in the elicitation of oral–facial responses.

Mainstream lacteal secretions, colostrum and transitional milk, were also tested separately as sources of active odor cues for infants ranging in age from minutes to weeks after birth. The odors of colostrum (from postpartum days 1–2) and milk (from postpartum days 3–4) were shown to elicit reliable positive head-turning responses (Marlier and Schaal, 2005; Marlier *et al.*, 1998). They were also reported to be strong activators of facial and oral responses (mouthing, protruding tongue, rooting) indicative of their attractive value to infants born at gestational term (Russell, 1976; Soussignan *et al.*, 1997) or preterm (Bingham *et al.*, 2003a, 2007). The sucking pattern of infants aged 10–14 days, fed formula since birth, was quantified while being exposed to the odors of their mother's fresh milk, their familiar formula, and a neutral control (water) during a regular formula feed. It resulted that, during the first minute of exposure, the infants exposed to their mother's milk odor evinced higher sucking frequency and positive pressure, leading to a higher sucking efficiency index (i.e., milliliters milk transferred per minute; Mizuno and Ueda, 2004). Further, preliminary data indicate that the odor of colostrum or milk elicits cortical activation, but its specificity remains to be established in comparison to reference odorants (as assessed by EEG or near-infrared spectroscopy; Bartocci *et al.*, 2000; Yasumatsu *et al.*, 1994). Finally, the odor of human milk has been shown in some studies to dampen pain responses more than control stimuli (water or formula; although sucrose appears more efficient; e.g., Mellier *et al.*, 1997; Nishitani *et al.*, 2009; Örs *et al.*, 1999; Rattaz *et al.*, 2005; Upadhyay *et al.*, 2004). The gist of the above results is that odors from human lacteal secretions are clearly detectable to infants aged from about 2 months before term to more than 1 month postbirth, and that they have a particular behavioral effects in terms of arousal, general attraction, appetitive actions, and self-regulatory responses.

Nevertheless, available studies are heterogeneous in many ways (infant age, sampling-conservation methods, design and reliability of testing). For example, it may be noted that, as in the case of rabbit milk described above, the time elapsing between milk sampling and odor testing has a clear influence on the attractive potency of milk odor to newborns: while milk odor remains attractive after standing 30 min at ambient temperature, its attractiveness is significantly reduced after 3 h of ambient storage (Couegnas, 2003). Thus, future efforts toward behavioral assaying and chemoanalysis of lacteal odors will have to take care of the conditions of milk sampling, conditioning, and conservation (cf. Spitzer and Büttner, 2009). So far, only a handful of attempts have been run to chemically characterize the volatile compounds of human milk (Bingham *et al.*, 2003b; Büttner, 2007; Pellizari *et al.*, 1982; Shimoda *et al.*, 2000; Stafford *et al.*, 1976), colostrum, or areolar secretion of MG (Schaal *et al.*, 2008b). Although these analyses found a variety of common odorous compounds ($n = 109$: Shimoda *et al.*, 2000; $n = 5$: Bingham *et al.*, 2003b; $n = 28$:

Büttner, 2007), underlying methods are so diverse (pooled vs. individual milk samples; fresh vs. frozen; solvent extracted vs. headspace sampled with stir bar sorptive extraction; compared to formula milk or UHT treated cow's milk) that no clear view can be drawn. More standardized studies are thus needed to built a representation of the volatile compounds (and their precursors) of milks from diverse ethnic-cultural backgrounds, of their chemical overlap, and of their specificity regarding the milk of other selected mammals. Such a comparative approach should also investigate compounds of lacteal secretions that might overlap (or not) with extra-mammary substrates of semiochemical interest in the nursing situation (such as amniotic fluid and infant saliva).

3. Learning of mammary-related odor cues

As in the other species described above, human newborns exhibit prompt learning of artificial odorants associated with the breast (Delaunay-El Allam *et al.*, 2006, 2010; Schleidt and Genzel, 1990), suggesting that the natural odor of the lactating breast might be acquired in the same way. But merely exposing newborns to an odorant without planned reward or delivering them an odor in association with touch-induced arousal suffices to familiarize them to previously irrelevant stimuli (Balogh and Porter, 1986; Sullivan *et al.*, 1991). Such odor encoding in human infants may be exceedingly rapid after birth (i.e., within the first 30 min; Romantshik *et al.*, 2007), and may last over a year (Delaunay-El Allam *et al.*, 2010). Thus, in natural nursing conditions, the odors of the breast, of milk or of areolar secretion may acquire their meaning through associative learning (e.g., Mizuno *et al.*, 2004). Additional odor sources that the infant might detect while nursing could also be acquired in this way, as for example, the mother's salivary or breath odors, or the scent of her neck or axillae (cf. Cernoch and Porter, 1985; Schaal *et al.*, 1980).

However, newborn infants who were never exposed to their mother's breast or to human milk (viz. bottle-fed) exhibit clear attraction and appetence for their odor (Makin and Porter, 1989; Marlier and Schaal, 2005). Similarly, the odor of MG secretion is reactogenic to neonates that were bottle-fed since birth, indicating that their behavioral activity does not depend on postnatal exposure. Based on the current evidence, it cannot be ruled out that the odors of these mammary secretions/excretions are acquired indirectly during fetal life. First, the amniotic and mammary compartments both constitute metabolic dead-ends, gathering numerous, potentially odorous, compounds from the maternal diet or aerial ecology, and leading to relative transnatal olfactory continuity (Schaal, 2005). The acquisition of such dietary aromas has repeatedly been shown in the human fetus, inducing preferential memories that can be evidenced days to months after birth (Faas *et al.*, 2000; Hepper, 1995; Mennella *et al.*, 2001; Schaal *et al.*, 1998, 2000). The same mechanism of transnatal continuity is at work for hormones and their odorous metabolites (e.g., androstenone) which are transferred into the amniotic fluid (e.g., Hartmann *et al.*, 2010) and found as well in human milk (Büttner, 2007), and to which neonates are strongly responsive (Doucet *et al.*, 2010a). Second, newborns maintain for at least several days their reactivity to stimuli they were exposed to before delivery: they react to the odor of amniotic fluid (Schaal *et al.*, 1995b; Varendi *et al.*, 1996), and even more to the odor of their own amniotic fluid (Schaal *et al.*, 1998). When amniotic fluid was experimentally painted on the breast, as expectedly occurs when the freshly born infant first faces it, it is preferred to a breast without amniotic staining (Varendi *et al.*, 1997). In sum, human infants are able to early engage odors into learned repertoires of salient sensory cues related to the mother and breast, and this operates even before birth.

4. Evidence for pheromones

So far no evidence for a compound that would qualify as a pheromone is at hand in primate, viz. human, mother → infant communication. However, in humans, two mammary-related substrates, colostrum/milk and the secretion from the areolar MG, are valuable candidates for systematic analyses: they elicit reliable behavioral and psychophysiological responses that appear general (i.e., elicited by secretions from unfamiliar, unrelated females), species-specific (i.e., differentiable from heterospecific secretions), and dissociable from nonspecific arousal effects caused by any odorant. In addition, their behavioral activity does not derive from postnatal experience to breast-related stimuli, although the role of prenatal induction cannot be excluded so far. Clearly, further investigation is needed to confirm these first results, and to substantiate whether mainstream milk and MG secretions convey redundant or distinct odor information to infants. These mammary secretions may now be subjected to chemical analyses to pin down compounds that can be brought to systematic behavioral assaying with human newborns.

V. Regulation of Mammary Odor Cues and Pheromones

A. Emission in females

The emission rate or activity of mammary chemical signals fluctuates intraindividually along lactation and at each nursing episode. For example, the mixture of abdominal odor cues of lactating rabbits or cats is more efficient to release pup searching in early rather than late lactation (Coureaud *et al.*, 2001; Hudson and Distel, 1984; Raihani *et al.*, 2009). Little is known about the endocrine control of such abdominal odor cues, and whether it operates in anticipation of the engagement of nursing behavior or only in response to the sensory awareness of offspring. In rabbit females, sucking-related tactile stimulation of the nipples triggers prolactin and oxytocin release that controls milk production and ejection (Summerlee *et al.*, 1986), and affects the tonic release of sebum (Wales and Ebling, 1971). In rats, an injection of oxytocin reinstates the attractivity of lactating females' abdomen after experimental disruption by washing (Singh and Hofer, 1978). The endocrine effects of sucking-related somesthesis increase up to 15–20 days postpartum, and then progressively drop with approaching weaning (Summerlee *et al.*, 1986), providing a basis for long-term variation in mammary-related chemoemission. In the rabbit, the pup reactivity to the complex odor of milk and to the pure MP follows fluctuations comparable to those noted with whole abdominal odor cues: when 2-day-old pups are exposed to the odor of fresh rabbit milk from either postpartum day 2 or 23 (weaning: day 30), the behavioral activity of milk declines between both sampling times, and MP concentration in the milk effluvium drops accordingly (Coureaud *et al.*, 2006). Thus, the MP in milk or related compounds in abdominal cues may be involved in the postnatal course of young → female interactions. In women, lactation-related variations in the olfactory attractiveness of the breast for infants remain poorly understood. Increased sebaceous productivity of areolar MG may be effective in late pregnancy and early lactation (Burton *et al.*, 1973), leading to presumable variations in the amount/composition of areolar secretions. If MG support any sort of communicative function, one may expect an enhanced secretory output right after delivery and then before ensuing nursing bouts. More women tend indeed to show more secretory MG on postpartum days 1–3 than on days 15 or 30 (Schaal *et al.*, 2006), but more conclusive data are needed here.

Mammary odor cues also appear to vary qualitatively and/or quantitatively in the shorter term of the nursing cycle. Abdominal odor cues of lactating rabbits are more efficient to release pup searching in prenursing rather than postnursing conditions (Coureaud *et al.*, 2001). Nursing-related variations in lactogenic hormones may indeed favor milk emission at the nipple (and in humans at the lactiferous component of MG) and stimulate the secretory activity of skin glands. Infant attraction to the mammae may also be influenced by thermal changes due to local metabolic activity or to specialized responses. For example, in humans the areolar dermis is underlain with a vascular complex, Haller's vascular plexus (Mitz and Lalardie, 1977). An acute vasodilatation of this structure may confer a higher temperature to the areolar surface as compared to adjacent skin, hence, maximizing evaporation of odorants oozing from the MG, and optimizing odor release in synchrony with the demanding infant (Vuorenkoski *et al.*, 1969).

To sum up, the best studied case of the rabbit highlights that the production and/or emission of mammary odor cues are under the tonic control of gonadal steroids and lactogenic hormones. This leads to the externalization of odor cues at the very end of gestation and around birth, when pups' reactivity to it is at its zenith. Then, the attractant potency of the mammary odor mixture appears to drop, and the release of the well-characterized MP is abolished near weaning. Thus, when weaning begins, rabbit females may control pup motivation to suckle in reducing MP emission. Within the peaking period of lactation, the timely control of mammary chemosignalization is presumably modulated by rhythmic processes (e.g., Montigny *et al.*, 2006) and by infant-related distal and proximal stimuli.

B. Reception by newborns

With advancing lactation and changing needs of offspring the decrease in the female's emission of mammary odor signals may be echoed in changes of neonatal reactivity to them. This is presently best documented in rabbit pups for the MP. The MP potency to release neonatal responses decreases progressively over the preweaning period, indicating the intervention of unknown endogenous and exogenous regulatory factors. The rate of response of domestic pups to the MP goes indeed through several stages, beginning with a first drop (from above 90% to ~80% respondents) around postnatal days 8–11 that coincides with eye opening (~day 10–11) and corresponds to the reorganization of the pups' perceptual balance (Montigny, 2008). A second drop in responsiveness (from ~80% to ~40%) occurs between days 11 and 21, when pups become increasingly mobile, localize the female visually, initiate suckling, and progressively begin to ingest solid food. Finally, a major drop is seen after the third week, when the typical searching–seizing response to the MP vanishes completely (Coureaud *et al.*, 2008; Montigny, 2008).

The rabbit pup response to mammary/milk signals is also developmentally regulated by circadian and metabolic processes. Pup reactivity to the MP round the clock changes as a function of milk intake. On day 2, they react automatically at any time to the MP, without influences from prior milk intake or other emerging circadian factors (Montigny *et al.*, 2006). But by day 5, and more so by day 10, this reliable response to the MP becomes restricted to prenursing hours. These data make clear that, with changing metabolic needs and incoming visual information, sucking behavior progressively escapes control by the MP. This shift from automatic to prandially controlled response to the MP is of particular significance in the context of the rare milk-resource access evolved by *Oryctolagus* females. Such response variations over time to the MP may warrant that rabbit offspring are first tethered to the mammae, and then progressively disinvest them as nonmilk foods can be orally and digestively processed. This progressive phenomenon of shifting control from chemosensory to other senses awaits investigations in other mammalian newborns.

VI. Conclusions and Prospects

This chapter suggests that, at least in the representative species of extant mammalian groups surveyed above, aspects of maternal morphology, physiology, and behavior were evolutionarily selected to render the mammary areas conspicuous for newborns. This apparently universal strategy of mammalian females to advertise mammaries relies on informative means that match the earliest developing perceptual and behavioral abilities of newborn organisms, their common sensory denominator being somesthesis and chemoreception. Accordingly, broadcasting some sort of chemical cues and/or signals from the mammae is a suitable pan-mammalian reproductive strategy to pilot neonatal arousal, motivation, and attraction to the mother; to provide assistance in localizing and orally seizing the mammae; and to boost up well-timed learning. However, the ways by which these chemical cues are produced and assembled on the mammary area appear in the same time diverse between species and complex within species.

The interspecies diversity in mammary chemical signalization to newborns, based on the few species scrutinized to date, can be reduced to a common system composed of (1) a female subsystem of semiochemicals emitted in, on, or around the mammae, from nonspecialized skin glands, from specialized scent glands, and/or from the mammary gland itself through lacteal secretions; (2) a neonatal subsystem of semiochemicals resulting from the unavoidable contact-related deposit of extramammary substrates, generally from oral–facial sources (mainly saliva, or other oral/perioral cues); (3) finally, an additional female subsystem of extramammary semiochemicals results from the propensities to leave oral–facial substrates (salivary cues) as a consequence of self- and/or offspring-centered care (licking). The actuality of these different subsystems of cues and signals depends on species-specific patterns of nursing behavior and neonate position in the altricial–precocial continuum. While semiochemical subsystems 1 and 2 are basic to the normal performance of milk transfer in any mammalian mother–infant unit, subsystem 3 is restricted to those species whose females self-lick during pregnancy-lactation.

Within a same species, the mammary semiochemical system appears complex in terms of distinct, co-occurring sources of odorous substrates and in terms of the dynamic interplay of the semiochemical subsystems during the nursing cycle and along the unfolding female–young relation until weaning. The cues created by subsystems 1 and 2 are temporally ordered in the early development of the mother–young unit. Subsystem 1 logically works in advance of the initial suckling episode, from the end of pregnancy under endocrine control, preparing the mammary papilla for the nursing-naïve newborn. In species having adopted subsystem 3, females are also often involved in applying extramammary cues on the nipples in advance of the very first nursing. In the days/weeks following the initiation of nursing, the relative saliency of these different semiochemical subsystems depends on the species considered: in some species, newborns rely exclusively on maternal cues (subsystem 1), while in others their overmark maternal cues (due to the operation of subsystems 1 and 3) in bringing their own semiochemicals to the situation (subsystem 2). This latter case is best illustrated in cat and pig newborns.

As mentioned previously, the mammalian females' strategy to olfactorily advertise their mammaries is obviously conditional upon coevolved neonatal means to sense these cues and signals, and to aptly react to them. The most conserved, and hence universally exploitable, sensory abilities are perioral–oral somesthesis and chemosensation, but later developing systems (audition, vision) are rapidly involved in perception in species bearing sensorily precocial newborns or when they become functional in altricial newborns (Gottlieb, 1971). The mammary semiochemical system capitalizes on the full range of neonatal anticipatory and concurrent means of chemosensory processing by at least three mechanisms (Schaal *et al* ., 2009): (1) exploiting the transnatal continuity in chemosensory cues (using odorous metabolites transferred *in utero* as cues in colostrum/milk; using amniotic cues by directly spreading them over the mammae), (2) affording predisposed stimuli which unconditionally affect neonatal arousal and responsiveness, and (3) presenting a range of unanticipated, circumstantial odorants that are rapidly turned into meaningful cues by the multiple, redundant rewards beget by the nursing situation.

While cognitive mechanisms 1 and 3 are common to all mammalian mother–newborn units studied so far, mechanism 2 has been evidenced so far in only one species (i.e., the MP of the rabbit). In addition, these different mechanisms work interactively over the first postnatal days; various stimuli present on the mammaries can indeed bootstrap the immediate learning of novel stimuli in neonates by way of their primary (rabbit MP; Coureaud *et al.*, 2006) or secondary reinforcing properties (rat amniotic fluid or saliva; Arias and Chotro, 2007; Sullivan *et al.*, 1986), leading potentially to the rapid amplification of a novel, locally valid repertoire of meaningful cues toward the mammae and the maternal organism (e.g., Coureaud *et al.*, 2009; Patris *et al.*, 2008). But, in addition to such odor–odor potentiated learning, nursing-related odors should be considered in a wider, multimodal context, as they may also potentiate the acquisition of nonolfactory stimuli. For example, in human newborns the breast odor elicits longer durations of eye-opening (Doucet *et al.*, 2007), making the brain disponible to maternal visual cues. Another example is that of highly visual newborn ungulates (sheep) that are also powerfully aroused by mammary odor cues (Vince and Billing, 1986); once the mammary position is found, probably aided by these odor cues, and rewarded by sucking, lambs may encode it spatially and completely shift from olfactory to visual control. This intermodal potentiation may operate in few sucking episode, as the lambs' response to these odors cues drops sharply after the first suckling episodes (Vince and Billing, 1984). Clearly, over evolutionary time, mammalian females can only have exploited, and hence selected, these multiple cognitive mechanisms in their neonates to optimize viability and adaptive responsiveness in progeny (Alberts, 1987; Schaal, 2005; Schaal *et al.*, 2009).

The above review brings convincing evidence that neonatal mammals can develop a repertoire of learned odor *cues* derived from intra- and extramammary sources, but it indicates only rare cases of evolved odor *signals*, viz. pheromones, that control nursing. The best documented case so far for such a mammary-based pheromone is the European rabbit, *Oryctolagus* (Schaal *et al.*, 2008a). This imbalance certainly is a result of absence of evidence, rather than evidence of absence, and pleas for more intensive research in an area that bears great potential to advance our knowledge on mammalian communication, chemoreception, and especially pheromones. It is a vital imperative for mammalian neonates to detect sensory cues from mother, mammae, and milk, and it is accordingly expectable that neonates are evolutionarily designed to do it right at birth. Thus, testing neonatal animals with odor stimuli they may be canalized to detect may be a productive way to identify new pheromones, as well as to uncover strategies of females to produce odor messages and to facilitate their sensing by neonates. In fact, newborn mammals may allow the strongest corroboration of the concept of pheromone in its renewed formulation by Beauchamp *et al.* (1976) and more recently by others (e.g., Doty, 2003; Johnston, 2000). Newborns (especially those of the altricial type) are generally restricted in sensory abilities, specialized in responsiveness, limited in their repertoire of odor memories, and they are highly motivated to approach the attachment figure or salient sensory traits "disembodied" from her. Finally, in many species, newborns are easy to handle (although it is not always the case of maternal females). In fact, probably the most complete demonstration to date of a mammalian pheromone, according to the operational criteria of Beauchamp *et al.*, has advantageously made use of the newborn of a readily available species.

Empirical emphasis on newborns may also help to assess the validity of categorizing stimuli into evolved *signals* and ontogenetically acquired *cues* (cf. Section II). Both kinds of stimuli are often considered as functionally equivalent, bringing arguments to some authors who propose to clear any distinction between pheromonal signals and circumstantially learned odor cues. However, under adequate experimental circumstances, there is evidence that this is not the case. When mixtures containing species-specific stimuli and mixtures containing individual-specific stimuli are presented concurrently, neonates do not treat them as equivalent. For example, human infants deprived from birth of direct exposure to mother's breast/milk exhibit a clear preference for human milk odor over the odor of their formula milk that yet brought them recurrently to satiation (Marlier and Schaal, 2005). In the same line, when paired with human milk odor, a camomile odor associated with nursing from birth does not surpass milk in attractiveness for human newborns (Delaunay-El Allam *et al.*, 2006), indicating that the most dominant or the most recent smell is not obligatorily the most attractive in a relative preference test. Thus, mammalian female–neonate units may be particularly suited models to uncover whether, when, why, and how the chemoreceptive system establishes the relative salience of social odor stimuli.

The scarcity of our knowledge on the chemosensory regulation of nursing behavior in mammalian species is amazing when one considers its vital importance in neonatal survival and initial social development. Renewed interest in that topic, after the considerable work of developmental psychobiologists in the years 1970–1980 (e.g., Alberts, 1981, 1987; Blass and Teicher, 1980; Rosenblatt, 1983), would certainly be rewarding to further understand the proximate mechanisms and development of chemoemission and chemoreception in readily accessible mammalian species (laboratory rodents, domestic ungulates and carnivores, humans). This should boost interest in more "exotic" species for which we have positive indications of neonatal odor-guided behavior in the nursing context (e.g., marsupials, insectivores, pinniped carnivores, nonhuman primates) or for which such indications seem lacking (e.g., monotremes, proboscidians, cetaceans). This would be of the uppermost interest for comparative and phylogenetic analyses of a communicative convergence that is seminal in the evolutionary success of the mammalian radiations. Between species, differences in mammary signalization and in neonatal reception/integration of such signals are now worthy of consideration in the light of corresponding life history variables.

ACKNOWLEDGMENTS

I gratefully thank Ingrid Jakob and Marilyn Renfree for offering their time and energy to comment on the chapter; Ben Pitcher and Isabelle Charrier for providing useful references; Wittko Francke, Andrea Büttner, Dominique Langlois, Matthias Rietdorf, and Gunnar Weibchen for their work relative to the chemical bases of mammary signals; and my colleagues and students in Dijon and abroad, Syrina Al-Ain, Gérard Coureaud, Sébastien Doucet, Karine Durand, Claire Fenech, Ingrid Jakob, Elisabeth Hertling, André Holley, Anne-Sophie Moncomble, Delphine Montigny, Pierre Orgeur, Bruno Patris, Heiko Rödel, and Robert Soussignan, for their past and continued collaboration in unraveling the behavior of mammalian neonates.

REFERENCES

Ackerman, S. H., and Shindledecker, R. (1978). A method for artificial feeding of motherless 2-week-old rat pups. *Dev. Psychobiol.* **11,** 385–391.

Al Ain, S., Chraiti, A., Patris, B., and Schaal, B. (2010). An exploration of mammary odour cues in newborn mice. Annual Meeting of the European Chemoreception Research Organisation (Avignon, France).

Alberts, J. R. (1976). Olfactory contributions to behavioral development in rodents. *In* "Mammalian Olfaction: Reproductive Processes and Behavior," (R. L. Doty, Ed.). Academic Press, New York.

Alberts, J. R. (1981). Ontogeny of olfaction: Reciprocal roles of sensation and behavior in the development of perception. *In* "Development of Perception: Psychological perspectives," (R. N. Aslin, J. R. Albert, and M. R. Petersen, Eds.). Vol. 1. Academic Press, New York.

Alberts, J. R. (1987). Early learning and ontogenetic adaptation. *In* "Perinatal development: A psychobiological perspective," (N. A. Krasnegor, E. M. Blass, M. A. Hofer, and W. P. Smotherman, Eds.), pp. 11–37. Academic Press, Orlando, FA.

Alberts, A. C. (1992). Constraints on the design of chemical communication systems in terrestrial vertebrates. *Am. Nat.* **139,** 562–589.

Alberts, J. R., and Gubernick, D. G. (1984). Early learning as ontogenetic adaptation for ingestion by rats. *Learn. Motiv.* **15,** 334–359.

Allingham, K., Brennan, P. A., Distel, H., and Hudson, R. (1999). Expression of c-Fos in the main olfactory bulb of neonatal rabbits in response to garlic as a novel and conditioned odour. *Behav. Brain Res.* **104,** 157–167.

Arias, C., and Chotro, M. G. (2007). Amniotic fluid can act as an appetitive unconditioned stimulus in preweanling rats. *Dev. Psychobiol.* **49,** 139–149.

Armstrong, C. M., DeVito, L. M., and Cleland, T. A. (2006). One-trial associative odor learning in neonatal mice. *Chem. Senses* **31,** 343–349.

Ashwell, K. W., Marotte, L. R., and Cheng, G. (2008). Development of the olfactory system in a wallaby (*Macropus eugenii*). *Brain Behav. Evol.* **71,** 216–230.

Balogh, R. D., and Porter, R. H. (1986). Olfactory preferences resulting from mere exposure in human neonates. *Infant Behav. Dev.* **9,** 395–401.

Bartocci, M., Winberg, J., Ruggierro, C., Bergqvist, L. L., Serr, G., and Lagercrantz, H. (2000). Activation of olfactory cortex in newborn infants after odor stimulation: A functional near-infrared spectroscopy study. *Pediatr. Res.* **48,** 18–23.

Bean, N. J., Galef, B. G., and Mason, R. J. (1989). At biologically significant concentrations, carbon disulfide both attracts mice and increases their consumption of bait. *J. Wildlife Manag.* **52,** 502–507.

Beauchamp, G. K., Doty, R. L., Moulton, D. G., and Mugford, R. A. (1976). The pheromone concept in mammals: A critique. *In* "Mammalian Olfaction, Reproductive Processes, and Behavior," (R. L. Doty, Ed.), pp. 143–160. Academic Press, New York.

Becques, A., Larose, C., Gouat, P., and Serra, J. (2010). Effects of pre- and postnatal olfactogustatory experience on early preferences at birth and dietary selection at weaning in kittens. *Chem. Senses* **35,** 41–45.

Beynon, R. J., Hurst, J. L., Turton, M. J., Robertson, D. H. L., Armstrong, S. D., Cheetham, S. A., Simpson, D., MacNicoll, A., and Humphries, R. E. (2008). Urinary lipocalins in Rodenta: Is there a generic model. *In* "Chemical signals in Vertebrates," (J. L. Hurst, R. J. Beynon, S. C. Roberts, and T. D. Wyatt, Eds.), Vol. 11, pp. 37–49. Springer Science, New York.

Bilko, A., Altbäcker, V., and Hudson, R. (1994). Transmission of food preference in the rabbit: The means of information transfer. *Physiol. Behav.* **56,** 907–912.

Bingham, P. M., Abassi, S., and Sivieri, E. (2003a). A pilot study of milk odor effect on nutritive sucking by premature infants. *Arch. Pediatr. Adolesc. Med.* **157,** 72–75.

Bingham, P. M., Sreven-Tuttle, D., Lavin, E., and Acree, T. (2003b). Odorants in breast milk. *Arch. Pediatr. Adolesc. Med.* **157,** 1031.

Bingham, P., Churchill, D., and Ashikaga, T. (2007). Breast milk odor via olfactometer for tube-fed, premature infants. *Behav. Res. Meth.* **39,** 630–634.

Blackburn, D. G., Hayssen, V., and Murphy, C. J. (1989). The origins of lactation and the evolution of milk: A review with new hypotheses. *Mammal. Rev.* **19,** 1–26.

Blass, E. M. (1990). Suckling: Determinants, changes, mechanisms, and lasting impressions. *Dev. Psychol.* **26,** 520–533.

Blass, E. M., and Teicher, M. H. (1980). Suckling. *Science* **210,** 15–22.

Blass, E. M., Shuleikina-Turpaeva, K., and Luschekin, V. (1988). Sensory determinants of nipple-attachment behavior in 2–4-day-old kittens. *Dev. Psychobiol.* **21,** 365–370.

Block, M. L., Volpe, L. C., and Hayes, M. J. (1981). Saliva as a chemical cue in the development of social behavior. *Science* **211,** 1062–1064.

Blum, S. L., Balsiger, D., Ricci, J. S., and Spiegel, D. K. (1975). Effects of early exposure to ventral gland odor on physical and behavioral development and adult social behavior in Mongolian gerbils. *J. Comp. Physiol. Psychol.* **81,** 1210–1219.

Bouslama, M., Durand, E., Chauvière, L., ven den Bergh, O., and Gallego, J. (2005). Olfactory classical conditioning in newborn mice. *Behav. Brain Res.* **86,** 19–27.

Brake, S. C. (1981). Suckling infant rats learn a preference for a novel olfactory stimulus paired with milk delivery. *Science* **211,** 506–508.

Brake, S. C., Shair, H., and Hofer, M. A. (1986). Exploiting the nursing niche: The infant's sucking and feeding in the context of the mother–infant interaction. *In* "Handbook of Behavioral Neurobiology," (E. M. Blass, Ed.), Vol. 9, pp. 347–388. Plenum Press, New York.

Bresslau, E. (1907). Die Entwicklung des Mammarapparates der Monotremen, Marsupialier, und einiger Placentalier. Ein Beitrag zur Phylogenie der Säugethiere. I. Entwicklung und Ursprung des Mammarapparates von Echidna. *Semon's Zool. Forschungreis.* **4,** 459–518.

Brouette-Lahlou, I., Amouroux, R., Chastrette, F., Cosnier, J., Stoffelsma, J., and Vernet-Maury, E. (1991a). Dodecyl propionate, attractant from rat pup preputial gland: Characterization and identification. *J. Chem. Ecol.* **17,** 1343–1354.

Brouette-Lahlou, I., Vernet-Maury, E., and Chanel, J. (1991b). Is rat-dam licking behavior regulated by pups' preputial gland secretion? *Anim. Learn. Behav.* **19,** 177–184.

Burton, J. L., Shuster, S., Cartlidge, M., Libman, L. J., and Martell, U. (1973). Lactation, sebum excretion and melanocyte-stimulating hormone. *Nature* **243,** 349–350.

Büttner, A. (2002). Influence of human saliva on odorant concentrations. 2. *J. Agric. Food Chem.* **50,** 7105–7110.

Büttner, A. (2007). A selective and sensitive approach to characterize odour-active and volatile constituents in small-scale human milk samples. *Flavour Fragr. J.* **22,** 465–473.

Campbell, R. G. A. (1976). Note on the use of a feed flavour to stimulate the feed intake of weaner pigs. *Anim. Prod.* **23,** 417–419.

Cannon, J. R., Bakker, H. R., Bradshaw, S. D., and McDonald, I. R. (1976). Gravity as the sole navigational aid to the newborn quokka. *Nature* **259,** 42.

Capretta, P. J., and Rawls, L. H. (1974). Establishment of a flavour preference in rats: Importance of nursing and weaning experience. *J. Comp. Physiol. Psychol.* **86,** 670–673.

Cernoch, J. M., and Porter, R. H. (1985). Recognition of maternal axillary odors by infants. *Child Dev.* **56,** 1593–1598.

Cheslock, S. J., Varlinskaya, E. I., Petrov, E. S., and Spear, N. E. (2000). Rapid and robust olfactory conditioning with milk before suckling experience: Promotion of nipple attachment in the newborn rat. *Behav. Neurosci.* **114,** 484–495.

Chuah, M. I., Tennent, R., and Teague, R. (1997). Developmental anatomy of the primary olfactory pathway in the opossum (*Monodelphis domestica*). *Histol. Histopathol.* **12,** 799–806.

Clutton-Brock, T. H. (1991). The Evolution of Parental Care. Princeton University Press, Princeton, NJ.

Couegnas, A. (2003). L'odeur du lait humain: stabilité de son pouvoir attractif chez le nouveau-né. Unpublished MSc Report, University of Burgundy, Dijon.

Coureaud, G., and Schaal, B. (2000). Attraction of newborn rabbits to abdominal odors of adult conspecifics differing in sex and physiological state. *Dev. Psychobiol.* **36,** 271–281.

Coureaud, G., Schaal, B., Langlois, D., and Perrier, G. (2001). Orientation responses of newborn rabbits to odors emitted by lactating females: Relative effectiveness of surface and milk cues. *Anim. Behav.* **61,** 153–162.

Coureaud, G., Schaal, B., Hudson, R., Orgeur, P., and Coudert, P. (2002). Transnatal olfactory continuity in the rabbit: Behavioral evidence and short-term consequence of its disruption. *Dev. Psychobiol.* **40,** 372–390.

Coureaud, G., Langlois, D., Perrier, G., and Schaal, B. (2003). A single key-odorant accounts for the pheromonal effect of rabbit milk: Further test of the mammary pheromone's activity against a wide sample of volatiles from milk. *ChemoEcology* **13,** 187–192.

Coureaud, G., Langlois, D., Sicard, G., and Schaal, B. (2004). Newborn rabbit reactivity to the mammary pheromone: Concentration–response relationship. *Chem. Sens.* **29,** 341–350.

Coureaud, G., Moncomble, A. S., Montigny, D., Dewas, M., Perrier, G., and Schaal, B. (2006). A pheromone that rapidly promotes learning in the newborn. *Curr. Biol.* **16,** 1956–1961.

Coureaud, G., Fortun-Lamothe, L., Langlois, D., and Schaal, B. (2007). The reactivity of neonatal rabbits to the mammary pheromone as a probe for viability. *Animal* **1,** 1026–1032.

Coureaud, G., Rödel, H., Kurz, C. A., and Schaal, B. (2008). Age dependent responsiveness to the mammary pheromone in domestic and wild rabbits. *ChemoEcology* **18,** 52–59.

Coureaud, G., Jouhanneau, M., and Schaal, B. (2009). Impact of pheromone-induced odour learning on the sucking success of rabbit newborns. 31st International Ethological Conference (Rennes, France).

Cowie, A. T. (1984). Lactation. *In* "Reproduction in Mammals," (C. R. Austin and R. V. Short, Eds.), Vol. 3, pp. 195–231. Cambridge University Press, Cambridge, UK.

Daremberg, C. (1856). Œuvres anatomiques, physiologiques et médicales de Galien, Vol. 2, Paris.

Darwin, C. (1872). The Origin of Species by Means of Natural Selection or the Preservation of Favoured Races in the Struggle for Life. 6th edn. New American Library, New York.

Darwin, C. (1877). A biographical sketch of an infant. *Mind* **7,** 285–294.

de Passillé, A. M., and Rushen, J. (2006). What components of milk stimulate sucking in calves? *Appl. Anim. Behav. Sci.* **101,** 243–252.

de Passillé, A. M., Rushen, J., and Janzen, M. (1997). Some aspects of milk that elicit non-nutritive sucking in the calf. *Appl. Anim. Behav. Sci.* **53,** 167–173.

Delaunay-El Allam, M., Marlier, L., and Schaal, B. (2006). Learning at the breast: Preference formation for an artificial scent and its attraction against the odor of maternal milk. *Infant Behav. Dev.* **29,** 308–321.

Delaunay-El Allam, M., Soussignan, R., Patris, B., Marlier, I., and Schaal, B. (2010). Long-lasting memory for an odor acquired at the mother's breast. *Dev. Sci.*

Desage, M., Schaal, B., Orgeur, P., Soubeyran, J., and Brazier, J. L. (1996). Gas chromatographic-mass spectrometric method to characterise the transfer of dietary odorous compounds into plasma and milk. *J. Chromatogr. B* **678,** 205–211.

Dollinger, M. J., Holloway, W. R., and Denenberg, V. H. (1978). Nipple attachment in rats during the first 24 hours of life. *J. Comp. Physiol. Psychol.* **92,** 619–626.

Doty, R. L. (2003). Mammalian pheromones: Fact or fantasy? *In* "Handbook of Olfaction and Gustation," (R. L. Doty, Ed.), 2nd edn., pp. 345–383. Marcel Dekker, New York.

Doucet, S., Soussignan, R., Sagot, P., and Schaal, B. (2007). The smellscape' of mother's breast: Effects of odor masking and selective unmasking on neonatal arousal, oral and visual responses. *Dev. Psychobiol.* **49,** 129–138.

Doucet, S., Soussignan, R., Sagot, P., and Schaal, B. (2009). The secretion of areolar (Montgomery's) glands from lactating women elicits selective, unconditional responses in neonates. *PLoS ONE* **4,** e7579.

Doucet, S., Hartmann, C., Dittrich, R., Soussignan, R., Schaal, B., and Büttner, A. (2010a). Human neonatal responses to androstenone. Annual Meeting of the American Chemosensory Society (St Petersburg, FA).

Doucet, S., Soussignan, R., Sagot, P., Schaal, B. (2010b). The areolar glands in postparturient women and their links with breastfeeding, lactation onset and early infant growth, submitted for publication.

Drickamer, L. C. (1988). Puberty-influencing chemosignals in house mice: Ecological and evolutionary considerations. *In* "Chemical Signals in Vertebrates," (D. Duvall, D. Müller-Schwarze, and R. M. Siverstein, Eds.), Vol. 4, pp. 441–455. Plenum, New York.

Dusenberry, D. B. (1992). Sensory Ecology: How Organisms Acquire and Respond to Information. WH Freeman, New York.

Ewer, R. F. (1959). Suckling behaviour in kittens. *Behaviour* **15,** 146–162.

Ewer, R. F. (1961). Further observations on suckling behaviour in kittens, together with some general considerations of the interrelations of the innate and acquired responses. *Behaviour* **17,** 247–260.

Faas, A. E., Sponton, E. D., Moya, P. R., and Molina, J. C. (2000). Differential responsiveness to alcohol odor in human neonates. Effects of maternal consumption during gestation. *Alcohol* **22,** 7–17.

Fox, M. W., and Himwich, W. A. (1965). Olfactory imprinting: A measure of early learning in the neonate dog. *Proc. Fed. Amer. Soc. Exp. Biol.* **24,** 522.

Friedman, M. I., and Bruno, J. P. (1976). Exchange of water during lactation. *Science* **197,** 409–410.

Galef, B. G., and Henderson, P. W. (1972). Mother's milk: A determinant of the feeding preferences of weaning rat pups. *J. Comp. Physiol. Psychol.* **78,** 213–219.

Galef, B. G., and Muskus, P. A. (1979). Olfactory mediation of mother–young contact in Long-Evans rats. *J. Comp. Physiol. Psychol.* **93,** 708–716.

Galef, B. G., and Sherry, D. F. (1973). Mother's milk: A medium for the transmission of cues reflecting the flavour of mother's diet. *J. Comp. Physiol. Psychol.* **83,** 374–378.

Galef, B. G., Mason, J. R., Pretty, G., and Bean, N. J. (1988). Carbon disulfide: A semiochemical mediating socially-induced diet choice in rats. *Physiol. Behav.* **42,** 119–124.

Garcia, P. J., and Gonçalves, R. P. (1984). Histological and ultrastructural observations of the attachment between the oral cavity of the fetus and the nipple of the mother opossum (*Didelphis azurae*). *Ant. Anz. (Jena)* **157,** 151–157.

Gisler, E. (1922). Die Entwicklung der Milchdrüse bei der Katze. Doctoral dissertation, University of Zürich.

Gonzalez-Mariscal, G., and Poindron, P. (2002). Parental care in mammals: Immediate internal and sensory factors of control. *In* "Hormones, Brain and Behavior," (D. W. Pfaff, A. M. Etgen, S. E. Fahrbach, R. Moss, and R. T. Rubin, Eds.), Vol. 1, pp. 215–298. Elsevier Science, New York.

Gottlieb, G. (1971). Ontogenesis of sensory function in birds and mammals. *In* "The Biopsychology of Development," (E. Tobach, L. R. Aronson, and E. Shaw, Eds.). Academic Press, New York.

Graves, B. M., and Duvall, D. (1983). A role for aggregation pheromons in the evolution of mammal like reptile lactation. *Am. Nat.* **122,** 835–839.

Gregory, W. K. (1910). The orders of mammals. *Bull. Am. Mus. Nat. Hist.* **27,** 1–524.

Grubb, P. (1974). Social organization of Soay sheep and the behaviour of ewes and lambs. *In* "Island Survivors: The Ecology of the Soay Sheep of St Kilda," (P. A. Jewell, C. Milner, and J. M. Boyd, Eds.), pp. 131–159. Athlone Press, London.

Gubernick, D. J., and Alberts, J. R. (1983). Maternal licking of young: Resource exchange and proximate controls. *Physiol. Behav.* **31,** 593–601.

Guiraudie-Capraz, G., Slomianny, M. C., Pageat, P., Malosse, C., Cain, M. H., Orgeur, P., and Nangnan-Le Meillour, P. (2005). Biochemical and chemical supports for a transnatal olfactory continuity through sow maternal fluids. *Chem. Senses* **30,** 241–251.

Hartman, C. G. (1952). Opossums. University of Texas Press, Austin, TX.

Hartmann, C., Doucet, S., Dittrich, R., Schaal, B., and Buettner, A. (2010). Identification of odor active substances in human amniotic fluid. Annual meeting of the American Chemosensory Society (St Petersburg, FA, 25–29 May).

Hauser, M. D. (1996). The Evolution of Communication. MIT Press, Cambridge, M.A.

Hausner, H., Bredie, W., Molgaard, C., Petersen, M. A., and Moller, P. (2008). Differential transfer of dietary flavour compounds into human breast milk. *Physiol. Behav.* **95,** 118–124.

Hemworth, P. H., Winfield, C. G., and Mullaney, P. D. (1976). A study of the development of teat-order in piglets. *Appl. Anim. Ethol.* **2,** 225–233.

Hendriks, W. H., Moughan, P. J., Tarttelin, M. F., and Woolhouse, A. D. (1995). Felinine: A urinary amino acid of Felidae. *Comp. Biochem. Physiol.* **112B,** 581–588.

Hepper, P. G. (1987). The amniotic fluid: An important priming role in kin recognition. *Anim. Behav.* **35,** 1343–1346.

Hepper, P. G. (1995). Human fetal "olfactory" learning. *Int. J. Prenat., Perinat. Psychol. Med.* **7,** 147–151.

Hepper, P. G., and Wells, D. L. (2006). Perinatal olfactory learning in the domestic dog. *Chem. Senses* **31,** 207–212.

Hill, J. P., and Hill, W. C. O. (1955). The growth stages of the native cat (*Dasyurus viverrinus*) together with observations on the anatomy of the newborn young. *Trans. Zool. Soc. London* **135,** 349–452.

Hofer, M. A., Shair, H., and Singh, P. J. (1976). Evidence that maternal ventral skin substance promote suckling in infant rats. *Physiol. Behav.* **17,** 131–136.

Holloway, W. R., Dollinger, M. J., and Denenberg, V. H. (1978). Differential nipple attachment by the neonatal rat. *Behav. Biol.* **24,** 428–441.

Hongo, T., Hakuba, A., Shiota, K., and Naruse, I. (2000). Suckling dysfunction caused by defects in the olfactory system in genetic arhinencephaly mice. *Biol. Neonate* **78,** 293–299.

Hudson, R. (1985). Do newborn rabbits learn the odour stimuli releasing nipple-search behavior? *Dev. Psychobiol.* **18,** 575–585.

Hudson, R., and Distel, H. (1983). Nipple location by newborn rabbits: Evidence for pheromonal guidance. *Behaviour* **82,** 260–275.

Hudson, R., and Distel, H. (1984). Nipple-search pheromone in rabbits: Dependence on season and reproductive state. *J. Comp. Physiol. A* **155,** 13–17.

Hudson, R., and Distel, H. (1990). Sensitivity of female rabbits to changes in photoperiod as measured by pheromone emission. *J. Comp. Physiol. A* **167,** 225–230.

Hudson, R., Schaal, B., and Bilko, A. (1999). Transmission of olfactory information from mother to young in the European rabbit. *In* "Mammalian Social Learning: Comparative and Ecological Perspectives," (H. O. Box and K. R. Gibson, Eds.), pp. 141–157. Cambridge University Press, Cambridge, UK.

Hudson, R., Labra-Cardero, D., and Mendoza-Solovna, A. (2002). Suckling, not milk, is important for the rapid learning of nipple-search odours in newborn rabbits. *Dev. Psychobiol.* **41,** 226–235.

Hudson, R., Raihani, G., Gonzalez, D., Bautista, A., and Distel, H. (2009). Nipple preference and contests in suckling kittens of the domestic cat are unrelated to presumed nipple quality. *Dev. Psychobiol.* **51,** 322–332.

Hughes, R. L., and Hall, L. S. (1984). Embryonic development in the common brushtail possum *Trichosurus vulpecula*. *In* "Possums and Gliders," (A. P. Smith and I. D. Hume, Eds.), pp. 197–212. Australian Mammal Society, Sydney, Australia.

Hurst, J. L., Payne, C. E., Nevison, C. M., Marie, A. D., Humphries, R. E., Robertson, D. H., Cavaggioni, A., and Beynon, R. J. (2001). Individual recognition in mice mediated by major urinary proteins. *Nature* **414,** 631–634.

Ivanistkii, A. M. (1962). The morphophysiological investigation of development of conditioned alimentary reactions in rabbits during ontogenesis. Experimental Studies of Higher Nervous Activity in Man and Animals. Works of the Institute of Higher Nervous Activity, Moscow, Physiological Series. Vol. 4, pp. 126–141. Israel Program for Scientific Translations Ltd, Jerusalem.

Jemiolo, B., Andreolini, F., Wiesler, D., and Novotny, M. (1987). Variations in mouse (*Mus musculus*) urinary volatiles during different periods of pregnancy and lactation. *J. Chem. Ecol.* **13,** 1941–1956.

Jemiolo, B., Andreolini, F., Xie, T. M., Wiesler, D., and Novotny, M. (1989). Puberty-affecting synthetic analogs of urinary chemosignals in the house mouse, *Mus domesticus*. *Physiol. Behav.* **46,** 293–298.

Jeppesen, L. E. (1982). Teat-order in groups of piglets reared on an artificial sow. I. Formation of teat-order and influence of milk yield on teat preference. *Appl. Anim. Ethol.* **8,** 335–345.

Jeppesen, L. E. (1982). Teat-order in groups of piglets reared on an artificial sow. II. Maintenance of teat-order with some evidence for the use of odour cues. *Appl. Anim. Ethol.* **8,** 347–350.

Johanson, I. B., and Hall, W. G. (1979). Appetitive learning in 1-day-old rat pups. *Science* **205,** 419–421.

Johanson, I. B., Polefrone, J. M., and Hall, W. G. (1984). Appetitive conditioning in neonatal rats: Conditioned ingestive responding to stimuli paired with oral infusion of milk. *Dev. Psychobiol.* **17,** 357–381.

Johnston, R. E. (2000). Chemical communication and pheromones: The types of chemical signals and the role of the voméronasal system. *In* "The Neurobiology of Taste and Smell," (T. E. Finger, W. L. Silver, and D. Restrepo, Eds.), pp. 101–127. Wiley, New York.

Kaeppeli, F. (1918). Über Zitzen- und Zisternenverhältnisse de Haussäugetiere. Doctoral dissertation, University of Zürich.

Karlson, P., and Lüscher, M. (1959). "Pheromones": A new term for a class of biologically active substances. *Nature* **183,** 55–56.

Kassil, V. G., and Gulina, L. K. (1986). Role of smell in the food-seeking activity of newborn puppies. *Fisiol. Zh. SSSR Im IM Sechenova* **72,** 437–444.

Keil, W., von Stralendorff, F., and Hudson, R. (1990). A behavioral bioassay for analysis of rabbit nipple-search pheromone. *Physiol. Behav.* **47,** 525–529.

Kindermann, U., Hudson, R., and Distel, H. (1994). Learning of suckling odours by newborn rabbits declines with age and suckling experience. *Dev. Psychobiol.* **2,** 111–122.

Knight, T. W., and Lynch, P. R. (1980). Sources of ram pheromones that stimulate ovulation in the ewe. *Anim. Reprod. Sci.* **13,** 133–136.

Kodama, N. (1990). Preference for amniotic fluid in newborn mice. Annual Meeting of the International Society for Developmental Psychobiology, Cambridge, UK.

Kodama, N. (2002). Effects of odor and taste of amniotic fluid and mother's milk on body movements in newborn mice. *Dev. Psychobiol.* **41,** 310.

Kodama, N., and Smotherman, W. P. (1997). Effects of amniotic fluid on head movement in cesarean delivered rat pups. *Dev. Psychobiol.* **30,** 255.

Koepke, J. E., and Bigelow, A. E. (1997). Observations on newborn suckling behavior. *Infant Behav. Dev.* **20,** 93–98.

Koffman, D. J., Petrov, E. S., Varlinskaia, E. I., and Smotherman, W. P. (1998). Thermal, olfactory, and tactile stimuli increase oral grasping of an artificial nipple by the newborn rat. *Dev. Psychobiol.* **33,** 317–326.

Kovach, J. K., and Kling, A. (1967). Mechanisms of neonate sucking behaviour in the kitten. *Anim. Behav.* **15,** 91–101.
Kroner, T. (1882). Über die Sinnesempfindungen des Neugeborenen. *Bresslauer ärztl. Ztschr.* **4,** 37–58.
Langendijk, P., Bolhuis, J. E., and Laurensen, B. F. A. (2007). Effects of pre- and postnatal exposure to garlic and anisseed flavour on pre- and postweaning feed intake in pigs. *Livest. Prod. Sci.* **108,** 284–287.
Langworty, O. R. (1928). The behavior of pouch young opossums correlated with the myelinization of tracts in the nervous system. *J. Comp. Neurol.* **46,** 201–240.
Larsson, M. A., and Stein, B. E. (1984). The use of tactile and olfactory cues in neonatal orientation and localization of the nipple. *Dev. Psychobiol.* **17,** 423–436.
Lent, P. C. (1974). Mother–infant relationships in Ungulates. *In* "The behavior of ungulates and its relations to management," (V. Geist and F. Walther, Eds.), Vol. 1, pp. 13–55. IUCN, Morges, Switzerland.
Leon, M. (1992). Neuroethology of olfactory preference development. *J. Neurobiol.* **23,** 1557–1573.
Lin, P. J. J., Phelix, C., and Krause, W. J. (1988). An immunohistochemical study of olfactory epithelium in the opossum before and after birth. *Z. Mikrosk.-Anat. Forsch. (Leipzig)* **102,** 272–282.
Long, C. A. (1969). The origin and evolution of mammary glands. *Bioscience* **19,** 519–523.
Luckey, T. D., Mende, T. J., and Pleasants, J. (1954). The physical and chemical characterization of rats' milk. *J. Nutr.* **54,** 345–359.
Lyne, A. G., Pilton, P. E., and Sharman, G. B. (1959). Oestrous cycle, gestation period and parturition in the marsupial *Trichosurus vulpecula. Nature* **183,** 622–623.
Macfarlane, A. J. (1975). Olfaction in the development of social preferences in the human neonate. *Ciba Found. Symp.* **33,** 103–117.
Makin, J. W., and Porter, R. H. (1989). Attractiveness of lactating females' breast odors to neonates. *Child Dev.* **60,** 803–810.
Malkmus, B. (1888). Die rudimentäre Beuteltasche des Schaffe. *Arch. Wiss.-Prakt. Tierhlk.* **14,** 1–24.
Marlier, L., and Schaal, B. (2005). Human newborns prefer human milk: Conspecific milk odor is attractive without postnatal exposure. *Child Dev.* **76,** 155–168.
Marlier, L., Schaal, B., and Soussignan, R. (1998). Bottle-fed neonates prefer an odor experienced in utero to an odor experienced in the feeding context. *Dev. Psychobiol.* **33,** 133–145.
Marlow, B. J. (1975). The comparative behaviour of the Australian sea lions *Neophoca cinerea* and *Phocarctos hookeri* (*Pinnipedia, Otariidae*). *Mammalia* **39,** 159–230.
Masselin, J. N. (1930). Recherche sur la structure et la biologie des glandes odorantes du mouton. *Ann. Anat. Pathol.* **7,** 766–776.
Maynard-Smith, J., and Harper, D. (2003). Animal Signals. Oxford University Press, Oxford, UK.
McBride, G. (1963). The "teat-order" and communication in young pigs. *Anim. Behav.* **11,** 53–56.
McClelland, R. J., and Cowley, J. J. (1982). The effect of lesions of the olfactory bulbs on the growth and behavior of mice. *Physiol. Behav.* **9,** 319–324.
McVittie, R. (1978). Nursing behavior of snow leopard cubs. *Appl. Anim. Ethol.* **4,** 159–168.
Mellier, D., Bezard, S., and Caston, J. (1997). Etudes exploratoires des relations intersensorielles olfaction-douleur. *In* "L'odorat chez l'enfant: perspectives croisées," (B. Schaal, Ed.), pp. 98–111. Presses Universitaires de France (Enfance), Paris.
Mennella, J. A., and Beauchamp, G. K. (1991a). Maternal diet alters the sensory qualities of human milk and the nursling's behavior. *Pediatrics* **88,** 737–744.

Mennella, J. A., and Beauchamp, G. K. (1991b). The transfer of alcohol to human milk: Effects on flavor and the infant's behavior. *New Engl. J. Med.* **325,** 981–985.

Mennella, J. A., and Beauchamp, G. K. (1996). The human infants' responses to vanilla flavors in human milk and formula. *Infant Behav. Dev.* **19,** 13–19.

Mennella, J. A., and Beauchamp, (1998). Smoking and the flavor of milk. *New Engl. J. Med.* **339,** 1559–1560.

Mennella, J. A., Jagnow, C. P., and Beauchamp, G. K. (2001). Prenatal and postnatal flavor learning by human infants. *Pediatrics* **107,** 1–6.

Menzies, B. R., Shaw, A. B. G., Terry, A., Fletcher, A., and Renfree, M. B. (2007). Perturbed growth and development in marsupial young after reciprocal cross-fostering between species. *Reprod. Fertil. Dev.* **19,** 976–983.

Merchant, J. C., and Sharman, G. B. (1966). Observations on the attachment of marsupial pouch young to the teats and of the rearing of pouch young by foster-mothers of the same or different species. *Aust. J. Zool.* **14,** 593–609.

Mermet, N., Coureaud, G., MCGrane, S., and Schaal, B. (2007). Odour-guided social behavior in newborn and young cats. *ChemoEcology* **17,** 187–199.

Miller, S. S., and Spear, N. E. (2008). Olfactory learning in the rat neonate soon after birth. *Dev. Psychobiol.* **50,** 554–565.

Miller, S. S., and Spear, N. E. (2010). Mere odor exposure learning in the rat neonate immediately after birth and 1 day later. *Dev. Psychobiol.* **52,** 343–351.

Mitz, V., and Lalardie, J. P. (1977). A propos de la vascularisation et de l'innervation sensitive du sein. *Senologia* **2,** 33–39.

Miyazaki, M., Yamashita, T., Taira, H., and Suzuki, A. (2008). The biological function of cauxin, a Major Urinary Protein of the domestic cat (*Felis catus*). *In* "Chemical signals in Vertebrates," (J. L. Hurst, R. J. Beynon, S. C. Roberts, and T. D. Wyatt, Eds.), Vol. 11, pp. 51–60. Springer Science, New York.

Mizuno, K., and Ueda, A. (2004). Antenatal olfactory learning influences infant feeding. *Early Hum. Dev.* **76,** 83–90.

Mizuno, K., Mizuno, N., Shinohara, T., and Noda, M. (2004). Mother–infant skin-to-skin contact after delivery results in early recognition of own mother's milk odour. *Acta Paediatr.* **93,** 1640–1645.

Moio, L., Dekimpe, J., Etevent, P., and Addeo, F. (1993). Neutral volatile compounds in the raw milks from different species. *J. Dairy Res.* **60,** 199–213.

Moio, L., Rillo, L., Ledda, A., and Addeo, (1996). Odorous constituents of ovine milk in relationship to diet. *J. Dairy Sci.* **79,** 1322–1331.

Molina, J. C., Chotro, M. G., and Domíngez, H. D. (1995). Fetal alcohol learning resulting from alcohol contamination of the prenatal environment. *In* "Fetal Development. A Psychobiological Perspective," (J. P. Lecanuet, W. P. Fifer, N. E. Krasnegor, and W. P. Smotherman, Eds.). Lawrence Erlbaum, Hillsdale, NJ.

Moncomble, A. S. (2006). De la prise de lait à l'ingestion non lactée chez le lapin: analyses éthologiques, histologiques et chimiques de sources odorantes significatives pour le lapereau nouveau-né. Unpublished doctoral thesis, University of Burgundy, Dijon.

Moncomble, A. S., Coureaud, G., Quennedey, B., Langlois, D., Perrier, G., Brossut, R., and Schaal, B. (2005). The mammary pheromone of the rabbit: Where does it come from? *Anim. Behav.* **69,** 29–38.

Montagna, W., and MacPherson, E. E. (1974). Some neglected aspects of the anatomy of human breasts. *J. Invest. Dermatol.* **63,** 10–16.

Montagna, W., and Yun, J. S. (1972). The glands of Montgomery. *Br. J. Dermatol.* **86,** 126–133.

Montgomery, W. F. (1837). An Exposition of the Signs and Symptoms of Pregnancy, the Period of Human Gestation, and Signs of Delivery. Sherwood, Gilber, and Piper, London.

Montigny, D. (2008). Fonctions adaptatives immédiates et différées de la phéromone mammaire chez le lapereau. Unpublished Doctoral thesis: University of Paris 13, Villetaneuse, France.

Montigny, D., Coureaud, G., and Schaal, B. (2006). Shift from automatism to prandial control in the response of newborn rabbits to the mammary pheromone. *Physiol. Behav.* **89,** 742–749.

Moriceau, S., and Sullivan, R. M. (2004). Unique neural circuitry for neonatal olfactory learning. *J. Neurosci.* **24,** 1182–1189.

Morrow-Tesch, J., and McGlone, J. J. (1990a). Sensory systems and nipple attachment behavior in neonatal piglets. *Physiol. Behav.* **47,** 1–4.

Morrow-Tesch, J., and McGlone, J. J. (1990b). Sources of maternal odors and the development of odor preferences in baby pigs. *J. Anim. Sci.* **68,** 3563–3571.

Müller, K. (1978). Zum Saugverhalten von Kaninchen unter besonderer Berücksichtigung des Geruchsvermögen. Unpublished doctoral dissertation, University of Giessen, Germany.

Müller-Schwarze, D. (1999). Signal specialization and evolution in mammals. *In* "Chemical Signals in Vertebrates," (R. E. Johnston, D. Müller-Schwarze, and P. W. Sorensen, Eds.), pp. 1–14. Klüwer-Plenum, New York.

Müller-Schwarze, D. (2006). Chemical Ecology of Vertebrates. Cambridge University Press, Cambridge, UK.

Müller-Schwarze, D., and Müller-Schwarze, C. (1971). Olfactory imprinting in a precocial mammal. *Nature* **229,** 55–56.

Murakami, K., Lagarde, M., and Yuki, Y. (1998). Identification of minor proteins of human colostrum and mature milk by 2-dimensional electrophoresis. *Electrophoresis* **19,** 2521–2527.

Mykytowycz, R., and Nay, T. (1964). Studies of the cutaneous glands and hair follicles of some species of macropodidae. *CSIRO Wildl. Res.* **9,** 200–217.

Nishitani, S., Miyamura, T., Tagawa, M., Sumi, M., Takase, R., Doi, H., Moriuchi, H., and Shinohara, K. (2009). The calming effect of a maternal breast milk odor on the human newborn infant. *Neurosci. Res.* **63,** 66–71.

Nolte, D. L., and Provenza, F. D. (1992). Food preferences in lambs after exposure to flavours in milk. *Appl. Anim. Behav. Sci.* **32,** 617–620.

Nolte, D. L., Provenza, F. D., Callan, R., and Panter, K. E. (1992). Garlic in the ovine fetal environment. *Physiol. Behav.* **52,** 1091–1093.

Oftedal, O. T. (2002). The mammary gland and its origin during synapsid evolution. *J. Mamm. Gland Biol. Neoplasia* **7,** 225–251.

Oostindjier, M., Bolhuis, J. E., van den Brand, H., and Kemp, B. (2009). Prenatal flavor exposure affects flavor recognition and stress-related behavior of piglets. *Chem. Senses* **34,** 775–787.

Örs, R., Özek, E., Baysoy, G., Cebeci, D., Bilgen, H., Türküner, M., and Basaran, M. (1999). Comparison of sucrose and human milk on pain response in newborns. *Eur. J. Pediatr.* **158,** 63–66.

Pageat, P., and Gaultier, E. (2003). Current research in canine and feline pheromones. *Vet. Clin. Small Anim. Pract.* **33,** 187–211.

Parfet, K. A. R., and Gonyou, H. W. (1991). Attraction of newborn piglets to auditory, visual, olfactory, and tactile stimuli. *J. Anim. Sci.* **69,** 125–133.

Patris, B., Perrier, G., Schaal, B., and Coureaud, G. (2008). Pheromone-induced odour learning in newborn rabbits: Implications for the development of social preferences. *Anim. Behav.* **76,** 305–314.

Pedersen, P. A., and Blass, E. M. (1981). Olfactory control over suckling in albino rats. *In* "Development of perception, Psychobiological perspectives. Audition Somatic Perception and the Chemical Senses," (R. N. Aslin, J. R. Alberts, and M. R. Petersen, Eds.), Vol. 1, pp. 359–381. Academic Press, New-York.

Pedersen, P. A., and Blass, E. M. (1982). Prenatal and postnatal determinants of the 1st suckling episode in albino rats. *Dev. Psychobiol.* **15,** 349–355.

Pellizari, E. D., Hartwell, T. D., Harris, B. S. H. III, Waddell, R. D., Whitaker, D. A., and Erickson, M. D. (1982). Purgeable organic compounds in mother's milk. *Bull. Environ. Contam. Toxicol.* **28,** 322–328.

Perkins, O. M., and Miller, A. M. (1926). Sebaceous glands in the human nipple. *Am. J. Obstet.* **11,** 789–794.

Petrov, E. S., Varlinskaia, E. I., and Smotherman, W. P. (1997). The newborn rat ingests fluids through a surrogate nipple: A new technique for the study of early suckling behavior. *Physiol. Behav.* **112,** 901–906.

Pfeiffer, S. (1980). Role of the nursing order in social development of mountain lion kittens. *Dev. Psychobiol.* **13,** 47–53.

Poindron, P., Nowak, R., Lévy, F., Porter, R. H., and Schaal, B. (1993). Development of exclusive mother–young bonding in sheep and goats. *Oxf. Rev. Reprod. Biol.* **15,** 311–364.

Prechtl, H. F. R. (1952). Angeborene Bewegungsweisen junger Katzen. *Experientia* **8,** 220–221.

Preyer, W. (1885). Die Seele des Kindes. (French translation) Editions Alcan, Paris.

Raihani, G., Gonzalez, D., Arteaga, L., and Hudson, R. (2009). Olfactory guidance of nipple attachment and suckling in kittens of the domestic cat: Inborn and learned responses. *Dev. Psychobiol.* **51,** 662–671.

Rattaz, C., Goubet, N., and Bullinger, A. (2005). The calming effect of a familiar odor on full-term newborns. *Dev. Behav. Pediatr.* **26,** 86–92.

Raynaud, A. (1969). Mamelles. *In* "Traité de Zoologie," (P. P. Grassé, Ed.), Vol. 16 (4), pp. 1–147. Masson, Paris.

Renfree, M. B., Fletcher, T. P., Blanden, D. R., Lewis, P. R., Shaw, G., Gordon, K., Short, R. V., Parer-Cook, E., and Parer, D. (1989). Physiological and behavioural events around the time of birth in macropodid marsupials. *In* "Kangaroos, Wallabies, and Rat-Kangaroos," (G. Grigg, P. Jarman, and I. Hume, Eds.), pp. 324–337. Surrey Beatty and Sons, New South Wales, Australia.

Rheingold, H. (1963). Maternal behavior in the dog. *In* "Maternal Behavior in Mammals," (H. L. Rheingold, Ed.), pp. 169–202. Wiley, New York.

Rietdorf, M. (2002). Identifizierung und Synthese flüchtiger Substanzen aus Säugetieren. University of Hamburg, Germany, Doctoral dissertation.

Robinson, S. R., and Smotherman, W. P. (1994). Behavioral effects of milk in the rat fetus. *Behav. Neurosci.* **108,** 1139–1149.

Robinson, S. R., Wong, C. H., Robertson, S. S., Nathanielsz, P. W., and Smotherman, W. P. (1995). Behavioral responses of the chronically instrumented sheep fetus to chemosensory stimuli presented in utero. *Behav. Neurosci.* **109,** 551–562.

Romantshik, O., Porter, R. H., Tillmann, V., and Varendi, H. (2007). Preliminary evidence of a sensitive period for olfactory learning by human newborns. *Acta Paediatr.* **96,** 372–376.

Rosenblatt, J. S. (1971). Suckling and home orientation in the kitten. A comparative developmental study. *In* "The Biopsychology of Development," (E. Tobach, L. R. Aronson, and E. Shaw, Eds.), pp. 345–410. Academic Press, New York.

Rosenblatt, J. S. (1972). Learning in newborn kittens. *Sci. Am.* **227,** 18–25.

Rosenblatt, J. S. (1983). Olfaction mediates developmental transitions in the altricial newborn of selected species of mammals. *Dev. Psychobiol.* **16,** 347–375.

Rosenblatt, J. S., Tobach, E., and Schneirla, T. C. (1963). Maternal behavior in the cat. *In* "Maternal Behavior in Mammals," (H. L. Rheingold, Ed.), pp. 122–168. Wiley, New York.

Roth, L., and Rosenblatt, J. S. (1966). Changes in self-licking during pregnancy in the rat. *J. Comp. Physiol. Psychol.* **63,** 397–400.

Rushen, J., and de Passillé, A. M. (1995). The motivation of non-nutritive sucking in calves, *Bos Taurus*. *Anim. Behav.* **49,** 1503–1510.
Russell, M. J. (1976). Human olfactory communication. *Nature* **260,** 520–522.
Russell, E. M. (1982). Patterns of parental care and parental investment in marsupials. *Biol. Rev.* **57,** 423–486.
Schaal, B. (1986). Presumed olfactory exchanges between mother and neonate in humans. *In* "Ethology and Psychology," (J. Le Camus and J. Cosnier, Eds.), pp. 101–110. Privat, I.E.C., Toulouse.
Schaal, B. (2005). From amnion to colostrum to milk: Odor bridging in early developmental transitions. *In* "Prenatal Development of Postnatal Functions," (B. Hopkins and S. P. Johnson, Eds.), pp. 51–102. Praeger, London.
Schaal, B., and Orgeur, P. (1992). Olfaction in utero: Can the rodent model be generalized? *Quart. J. Exp. Psychol.* **44B,** 245–278.
Schaal, B., Montagner, H., Hertling, E., Bolzoni, D., Moyse, R., and Quichon, R. (1980). Olfactory stimulations in mother–infant relations. *Reprod. Nutr. Dev.* **20,** 843–858.
Schaal, B., Orgeur, P., and Porter, R. H. (1994). Short-term flavour preference induced by dietary flavours transferred into mother's milk. *Infant Behav. Dev.* **17**(ICIS issue), 927.
Schaal, B., Orgeur, P., and Arnould, C. (1995a). Olfactory preferences in newborn lambs: Possible influence of prenatal experience. *Behaviour* **132,** 351–365.
Schaal, B., Marlier, L., and Soussignan, R. (1995b). Responsiveness to the odor of amniotic fluid in the human neonate. *Biol. Neonate* **67,** 397–406.
Schaal, B., Orgeur, P., Desage, M., and Brazier, J. (1995c). Transfer of the aromas of the pregnant and lactating mother's diet to fetal and neonatal environments in the sheep. *Chem. Senses* **20,** 93–94.
Schaal, B., Marlier, L., and Soussignan, R. (1998). Olfactory function in the human foetus: Evidence from selective neonatal responsiveness to the odor of amniotic fluid. *Behav. Neurosci.* **112,** 1438–1449.
Schaal, B., Marlier, L., and Soussignan, R. (2000). Human foetuses learn odors from their pregnant mother's diet. *Chem. Senses* **25,** 729–737.
Schaal, B., Coureaud, G., Langlois, D., Giniès, C., Sémon, E., and Perrier, G. (2003). Chemical and behavioural characterisation of the rabbit mammary pheromone. *Nature* **424,** 68–72.
Schaal, B., Doucet, S., Sagot, P., Hertling, E., and Soussignan, R. (2006). Human breast areolae as scent organs: Morphological data and possible involvement in maternal-neonatal coadaptation. *Dev. Psychobiol.* **48,** 100–110.
Schaal, B., Coureaud, G., Mermet, N., McGrane, S., and Udé, L. (2007). Impact of maternal odours on the feeding behavior of kittens. Unpublished report. Centre Européen des Sciences du Goût, Dijon.
Schaal, B., Coureaud, G., Moncomble, A. S., Langlois, D., and Perrier, G. (2008a). Many common odour cues and (at least) one pheromone shaping the behaviour of young rabbits. *In* "Lagomorph Biology: Evolution, Ecology and Conservation," (P. C. Alves, N. Ferrand, and K. Hackländer, Eds.), pp. 189–209. Springer Verlag, Berlin.
Schaal, B., Doucet, S., Soussignan, R., Rietdorf, M., Weibchen, G., and Francke, W. (2008b). The human breast as a scent organ: Exocrine structures, secretions, volatile components, and possible functions in breastfeeding interactions. *In* "Chemical Signals in Vertebrates, Vol. 11," (J. L. Hurst, R. J. Beynon, S. C. Roberts, and T. D. Wyatt, Eds.), pp. 325–335. Springer Verlag, Berlin.
Schaal, B., Coureau, G., Doucet, S., Delaunay-El Allam, M., Moncomble, A. S., Montigny, D., Patris, B., and Holley, A. (2009). Olfactory mammary signalisation in females and neonatal odour processing: Ways evolved in rabbit and human. *Behav. Brain Res.* **200,** 346–358.
Schaffer, J. (1940). Die Hautdrüsenorgane des Säugetiere. Urban Schwarzenberg, Berlin.

Schleidt, M., and Genzel, C. (1990). The significance of mothers perfume for infants in the first weeks of life. *Ethol. Sociobiol.* **11,** 145–154.

Schley, P. (1976) Untersuchungen zur künstlichen Aufzucht von Hauskaninchen. Habilitationsschrift, University of Giessen, Germany.

Schley, P. (1977). Die Ausschaltung des Geruchsvermögens und sein Einfluss auf das Saugverhalten von Jungkaninchen. *Berl. Münch. Tierärztl. Wochenschr.* **90,** 382–385.

Schley, P. (1979). Olfaction and suckling behavior in young rabbits. *In* "Proceedings of the 1st World Lagomorph Conference," (K. Myers and C. D. MacInnes, Eds.), pp. 291–294. University of Guelph, Guelph, Canada.

Schneider, N. Y., Fletcher, T. P., Shaw, G., and Renfree, M. B. (2008). The vomeronasal organ of the tammar wallaby. *J. Anat.* **213,** 93–105.

Schneider, N. Y., Fletcher, T. P., Shaw, G., and Renfree, M. B. (2009). The olfactory system of the tammar wallaby is developed at birth and directs the neonate to its mother's pouch odours. *Reproduction* **138,** 849–857.

Schneirla, T. C., Rosenblatt, J. S., and Tobach, E. (1963). Maternal behavior in the cat. *In* "Maternal Behaviour in Mammals," (H. L. Rheingold, Ed.), pp. 122–168. Wiley, New York.

Schulze-Westrum, T. G. (1965). Innerartliche Verständigung durch Düfte beim Gleitbeutler, *Petaurus breviceps* papuanus Thomas (Marsupialia Phalangeridae). *Z. Vergl. Physiol.* **50,** 151–220.

Schwalbe, G. (1898). Über die vermeintlichen offenen Mammartaschen bei Huftieren. *Morphol. Arb.* **8,** 341–364.

Shahan, K., Denaro, M., Gilmartin, M., Shi, Y., and Derman, E. (1987). Expression of 6 mouse major urinary protein genes in the mammary, parotid, sublingual, submaxillary, and lachrymal glands and in the liver. *Mol. Cell. Biol.* **7,** 1947–1954.

Sharman, G. B., and Calaby, J. H. (1964). Reproductive behaviour in the red kangaroo, *Megaleia rufa,* in captivity. *CSIRO Wildl. Res.* **9,** 58–85.

Shimoda, Y. T., Ishikawa, H., Hayakawa, I., and Osajima, Y. (2000). Volatile compounds of human milk. *J. Fac. Agr., Kyushu. Univ.* **45,** 199–206.

Shuleikina-Turpaeva, K. V. (1986). Sensory organization of alimentary behaviour in the kitten. *Adv. Study Behav.* **16,** 1–37.

Simitzis, P. E., Delogeorgis, S. G., Bizelis, J. A., and Fegeros, K. (2008). Feeding preferences in lambs influenced by prenatal flavour exposure. *Physiol. Behav.* **93,** 529–536.

Singer, A. G., Acosta, W. C., O'Connell, R. J., and Thiessen, D. D. (1976). Dimethyl disulfide: An attractant heromone in hamster vaginal secretion. *Science* **191,** 948–950.

Singh, P. J., and Hofer, M. A. (1978). Oxytocin reinstates maternal olfactory cues for nipple orientation and attachment in rat pups. *Physiol. Behav.* **20,** 385–389.

Singh, P. J., and Tobach, E. (1975). Olfactory bulbectomy and nursing behavior in rat pups. *Dev. Psychobiol.* **8,** 151–164.

Small, W. S. (1899). Notes on the psychic development of the young white rat. *Am. J. Psychol.* **11,** 80–100.

Smith, D. M., Peters, T. G., and Donegan, W. L. (1982). Montgomery's areolar tubercle. A light microscopic study. *Arch. Pathol. Lab. Med.* **106,** 60–63.

Smotherman, W. P., and Robinson, S. R. (1987). Psychobiology of fetal experience in the rat. *In* "Perinatal development: A Psychobiological Perspective," (N. A. Krasnegor, E. M. Blass, M. A. Hofer, and W. P. Smotherman, Eds.), pp. 39–60. Academic Press, Orlando, FL.

Smotherman, W. P., and Robinson, S. R. (1992). Dimethyl disulfide mimics the effect of milk on fetal behavior and responsiveness to cutaneous stimuli. *Physiol. Behav.* **52,** 761–765.

Smotherman, W. P., and Robinson, S. R. (1994). Milk as the proximal mechanism for behavioral change in the newborn. *Acta Paediatr. Suppl.* **374,** 64–70.

Smotherman, W. P., Goffman, D., Petrov, E. S., and Varlinskaia, E. I. (1997). Oral grasping of a surrogate nipple by the newborn rat. *Dev. Psychobiol.* **31,** 3–17.

Soussignan, R., Schaal, B., Marlier, L., and Jiang, T. (1997). Facial and autonomic responses to biological and artificial olfactory stimuli in human neonates: Re-examining early hedonic discrimination of odors. *Physiol. Behav.* **62,** 745–758.

Spitzer, J., and Büttner, A. (2009). Characterization of aroma changes in human milk during storage at − 19 °C. *Food Chem.* 10.1016/j.foodchem.2009.10.015.

Stafford, M., Horning, M. G., and Zlatkis, A. (1976). Profiles of volatile metabolites in body fluids. *J. Chromatogr. B* **126,** 495–502.

Stanley, W. C., Bacon, W. E., and Fehr, C. (1970). Discriminated instrumental learning in neonatal dogs. *J. Comp. Physiol. Psychol.* **70,** 335–343.

Sullivan, R. M., and Toubas, P. (1998). Clinical usefulness of maternal odor in newborns: Soothing and feeding preparatory responses. *Biol. Neonate* **74,** 402–408.

Sullivan, R. M., Hofer, M. A., and Brake, S. C. (1986). Olfactory-guided orientation in neonatal rats is enhanced by a conditioned change in behavioral state. *Dev. Psychobiol.* **19,** 615–623.

Sullivan, R. M., Taborsky, S. B., Mendoza, R., Itano, A., Leon, M., Cotman, C. W., *et al.* (1991). Olfactory classical conditioning in neonates. *Pediatrics* **87,** 511–517.

Summerlee, A. J., Paisley, A. C., O'Byrne, K. T., Fairhall, K. M., Robinson, I. C., and Fletcher, J. (1986). Aspects of the neuronal and endocrine components of reflex milk ejection in conscious rabbits. *J. Endocrinol.* **108,** 143–149.

Tanaka, T., Ochiai, N., Tanida, H., and Yoshimoto, T. (1998). The role of visual, auditory, and olfactory stimuli in teat seeking behavior of piglets. *Anim. Sci. Technol. (Jpn.)* **69,** 854–860.

Teicher, M. H., and Blass, E. M. (1976). Suckling in the newborn rat: Eliminated by nipple lavage, reinstated by pup saliva. *Science* **193,** 422–425.

Teicher, M. H., and Blass, E. M. (1977). First suckling response in the newborn albino rat: The roles of olfaction and amniotic fluid. *Science* **198,** 635–636.

Teicher, M. H., Flaum, L. E., Williams, M., Eckert, S. J., and Lumia, A. R. (1978). Survival, growth and suckling behavior of neonatally bulbectomized rats. *Physiol. Behav.* **21,** 553–561.

Teicher, M. H., Shaywitz, B. A., and Lumia, A. R. (1984). Olfactory and vomeronasal system mediation of maternal recognition in the developing rat. *Dev. Brain Res.* **12,** 97–110.

Terry, L. M., and Johanson, I. B. (1987). Olfactory influences on the ingestive behavior of infant rats Dev. *Psychobiology* **20,** 313–332.

Thiessen, D. D., Regnier, F. E., Rice, M., Goodwin, M., Issacks, N., and Lawson, N. (1974). Identification of a ventral scent marking pheromone in the male Mongolian gerbil (*Meriones unguiculatus*). *Science* **184,** 83–84.

Thiessen, D. D., Clancy, A., and Goodwin, M. (1976). Harderian pheromone in the Mongolian gerbil (*Meriones unguiculatus*). *Chem. Ecol.* **2,** 231–238.

Tien, D. V., and Preston, T. R. (2008). Pre- and post-natal exposure to duckweed affects postweaning familiarity and intake in Large White and Mong Cai pigs. Proceedings of the SAREC Workshop, Hue University, Hue City, Vietnam.

Toyoshima, Y., Ohsako, S., Nagano, R., Matsumoto, M., Hidaka, S., and Nishinakagawa, H. (1998a). Histological changes in mouse nipple tissue during the reproductive cycle. *J. Vet. Med. Sci.* **60,** 405–411.

Toyoshima, Y., Ohsako, S., Matsumoto, M., Hidaka, S., and Nishinakagawa, H. (1998b). Histological and morphometrical studies on the rat nipple during the reproductive cycle. *Exp. Anim.* **47,** 29–36.

Trott, J. F., Simpson, K. J., Moyle, R. L. C., Hearn, C. M., Shaw, G., Nicholas, K. R., Marilyn, B., and Renfree, M. B. (2003). Maternal regulation of milk composition, milk production, and pouch young. Development during lactation in the Tammar Wallaby (*Macropus eugenii*). *Biol. Reprod.* **68,** 929–936.

Upadhyay, A., Aggarwal, R., Narayan, S., Joshi, M., Paul, V. K., and Deorari, A. K. (2004). Analgesic effect of expressed breast milk in procedural pain in term neonates: A randomized, placebo-controlled, double-blind trial. *Acta Paediatr.* **93,** 518–522.

Varendi, H., and Porter, R. H. (2001). Breast odour as the only maternal stimulus elicits crawling towards the odour source. *Acta Paediatr.* **90,** 372–375.

Varendi, H., Porter, R. H., and Winberg, J. (1994). Does the newborn baby find the nipple by smell? *Lancet* **344,** 989–990.

Varendi, H., Porter, R. H., and Winberg, J. (1996). Attractiveness of amniotic odor: Evidence for prenatal olfactory learning? *Acta Paediatr.* **85,** 1223–1227.

Varendi, H., Porter, R. H., and Winberg, J. (1997). Natural odour preferences of newborn infants change over time. *Acta Paediatr.* **86,** 985–990.

Viallon, C., Martin, B., Verdier-Metz, I., Pradel, P., Garel, J. P., Coulon, J. B., and Berdagué, J. L. (2000). Transfer of monoterpenes and sesquiterpenes from forage into milk fat. *Lait* **80,** 635–641.

Vince, M. A. (1992). Personal communication (letter of February 11, 1992).

Vince, M. A. (1993). Newborn lambs and their dams: The interaction that leads to sucking. *Adv. Study Behav.* **22,** 239–268.

Vince, M. A., and Billing, A. E. (1986). Infancy in the sheep: The parts played by sensory stimulation in bonding between the ewe and lamb. *In* "Advances in Infancy Research," (L. P. Lipsitt and C. Rovee-Collier, Eds.), Vol. 4, pp. 2–37. Ablex, Norwood, NJ.

Vince, M. A., and Ward, T. M. (1984). The responsiveness of newly born Clunforest lambs to odor sources in the ewe. *Behaviour* **87,** 117–127.

Vince, M. A., Lynch, J. J., Mottershead, B. E., Green, G. C., and Elwin, R. L. (1987). Interaction between normal ewes and newly born lambs deprived of visual, olfactory and tactile sensory information. *Appl. Anim. Behav. Sci.* **19,** 119–136.

Vorherr, H. (1974). The Breast. Morphology, Physiology, and Lactation. Academic Press, New York.

Vuorenkoski, V., Wasz-Hockert, O., Koivisto, E., and Lind, J. (1969). The effect of cry stimulus on the temperature of the lactating breast of primipara. *Experientia* **25,** 1286–1287.

Wales, N. A., and Ebling, F. J. (1971). The control of apocrine glands of the rabbit by steroid hormones. *J. Endocrinol.* **51,** 763–770.

Wallace, P., Owen, K., and Thiessen, D. D. (1973). The control and function of maternal scent marking in the Mongolian gerbil. *Physiol. Behav.* **10,** 463–466.

Wells, D. L., and Hepper, P. G. (2006). Prenatal olfactory learning in the domestic dog. *Anim. Behav.* **72,** 681–686.

Wilson, D. A., and Sullivan, R. M. (1994). Neurobiology of associative learning in the neonate: Early olfactory learning. *Behav. Neural Biol.* **61,** 1–18.

Wong, S. T., Trinh, K., Hacker, B., Chan, G. C., Lowe, G., Gaggar, A., Xia, Z., Gold, G. H., and Storm, D. R. (2000). Disruption of the type III adenyl cyclise gene leads to peripheral and behavioral anosmia in transgenic mice. *Neuron* **27,** 487–497.

Wood-Gush, D. G. M., Carson, K., Lawrence, A. B., and Moser, H. A. (1986). Parental behaviour in ungulates. *In* "Parental Behaviour," (W. Sluckin and M. Herbert, Eds.), pp. 85–115. Blackwell, Oxford, UK.

Yasumatsu, K., Uchida, S., Sugano, H., and Suzuki, T. (1994). The effects of the odour of milk and orange on the spectral power of EEG in infants. *J. Univ. Occup. Environ. Health (Jpn.)* **16,** 71–83.

Youngentob, S. L., Kent, P. F., Sheehe, P. R., Molina, J. C., Spear, N. E., and Youngentod, L. M. (2007). Experience-induced fetal plasticity: The effect of gestational ethanol exposure on the behavioral and neurophysiologic olfactory response to ethanol odor in early postnatal and adult rays. *Behav. Neurosci.* **121,** 1293–1305.

Zarrow, M. X., Denenberg, V. H., and Anderson, C. O. (1965). Rabbit: Frequency of suckling in the pup. *Science* **150,** 1835–1836.

CHAPTER FIVE

Exposure to Female Pheromones During Pregnancy Causes Postpartum Anxiety in Mice

Caroline M. Larsen *and* David R. Grattan

Contents

Abstract

The postpartum period is associated with an increased incidence of pathological anxiety, exerting a substantial burden on both the mother and the baby. We have shown that pharmacological suppression of prolactin in early pregnancy decreases maternal neurogenesis to cause postpartum anxiety. The present data demonstrate that physiological suppression of prolactin secretion through

Centre for Neuroendocrinology and Department of Anatomy and Structural Biology, University of Otago, Dunedin, New Zealand

Vitamins and Hormones, Volume 83
ISSN 0083-6729, DOI: 10.1016/S0083-6729(10)83005-5

exposure to unfamiliar female pheromones throughout pregnancy prevented the normal postpartum attenuation of anxiety in mice, resulting in high anxiety relative to postpartum controls. Female pheromone-exposed mice also showed severely impaired maternal behavior in an anxiogenic situation. Mice exposed to female pheromones had decreased serum prolactin levels in early pregnancy, resulting in an ablation of the normal increase of neurogenesis on day 7 of pregnancy. These data demonstrate that low serum prolactin levels in early pregnancy, whether induced pharmacologically or as a physiological consequence of exposure to unfamiliar female pheromones, result in failure to show the normal adaptive decrease in anxiety after birth. This provides new insight into possible mechanisms that might underlie postpartum anxiety in women.

During the postpartum period, there is an increased incidence of dysfunctional mood disorders (Munk-Olsen *et al.*, 2006; Stowe and Nemeroff, 1995), with pathological anxiety, the most common (Britton, 2005, 2007; Matthey *et al.*, 2003; Wenzel *et al.*, 2003). Postpartum anxiety can severely affect the mother–infant relationship (Manassis *et al.*, 1994), and have long-lasting adverse effects on cognitive, emotional, and other aspects of infant development (Barnett *et al.*, 1991; O'Connor *et al.*, 2002). Postpartum mood disorders are also associated with an increased incidence of child abuse (Fraser *et al.*, 2000), and increased conflict in marital relationships leading to a higher rate of separation and divorce (Boyce and Stubbs, 1994; Lovestone and Kumar, 1993). Attempts to understand the mechanisms underlying postpartum mood disorders have been impeded by the lack of an animal model that induces anxiety or depression postpartum, while retaining the unique hormonal characteristics and social stresses of gestation (NIH, USA, PA-09-174, 2009).

The anterior pituitary hormone prolactin is critically involved in a number of adaptive responses in the maternal brain (Grattan *et al.*, 2008). We have recently shown that pharmacological suppression of prolactin very early in pregnancy in mice decreased adult neurogenesis in the maternal brain during pregnancy and induced anxiety postpartum, potentially providing a novel model of postpartum mood disorders. The aim of this study was to determine whether more subtle physiological changes in prolactin during pregnancy, such as might occur in response to stress or infection (Brunton *et al.*, 2008), might also alter mood and behavior postpartum. Exposure to pheromones alters levels of prolactin and neurogenesis in virgin female mice (Larsen *et al.*, 2008; Mak *et al.*, 2007). Therefore, we hypothesized that exposure to pheromones during pregnancy might similarly influence prolactin secretion during pregnancy, thereby inducing changes in mood postpartum. We exposed pregnant mice to male, female, or no pheromones throughout pregnancy and subsequently assessed anxiety on day 2 postpartum on an elevated plus maze (EPM) and in the light–dark box (LDB), well-characterized models of rodent anxiety. To determine whether pheromone exposure would change essential postpartum behaviors, we also examined maternal behavior, both in the home cage and in a clean novel cage (as an anxiogenic challenge; Larsen and Grattan, 2010). Finally, to identify possible mechanisms of pheromone action, pheromone-induced changes in prolactin secretion and levels of neurogenesis in the subventricular zone (SVZ) were analyzed.

I. Materials and Methods

A. Subjects

Maternally naive virgin or day 1 pregnant C57BL/6J mice (6–9 weeks old) were either housed in 32 × 16 × 18 cm individual cages or in 28 × 54 × 18 cm split cages with another male, or a female, allowing pheromonal, visual, and olfactory contact without permitting physical contact (Larsen *et al.*, 2008; all groups $n = 6$). Some females were paired with males, and were considered day 1 pregnant when mating was confirmed by sperm being present in a vaginal smear, at which time they were transferred into the cages, as above. Pheromones are bound to major urinary proteins, and hence placing urine-soaked bedding in with the female will expose her to pheromones without the confounding effects of a companion. To confirm that effects seen were due to pheromones, additional groups were exposed to urine-soaked sawdust obtained from another mouse for 23 days prior to behavioral testing (Larsen *et al.*, 2008). Virgin female and day 1 pregnant control groups had 0.5 g of clean sawdust placed in the cage daily for 23 days. After initial studies revealed an effect of female pheromones on anxiety and maternal behavior, all subsequent studies were undertaken using only female pheromones (i.e., without the male pheromone group). Mice were housed under a 12-h light–dark cycle, with *ad libitum* access to food and water. The University of Otago Animal Ethics Committee approved all experiments.

B. Anxiety testing

Day 2 postpartum or virgin females were assessed for anxiety on the EPM and the LDB, as previously described (Larsen and Grattan, 2010). All testing was carried out between 9.30 and 10.30 a.m. in the room where the animals were usually housed. To avoid habituation to stress, the animals were not handled prior to the experiment. Elevated plus maze (EPM): To assess anxiety, the mouse was placed on the central platform facing an open arm, and allowed to roam at will for 5 min. All arm entries and exits were recorded. Once a mouse had all 4 paws on an arm of the maze, it was counted as having entered that arm, while placing 2 paws out of an arm was counted as an exit. Light–dark box (LDB): The LDB had an enclosed dark box (18 × 27 × 27 cm; black perspex sides, bottom and top, approx 30 lux) separated by a partition with a hole (6 cm) from a light box (27 × 27 × 27 cm; clear perspex, with a transparent cover with ventilation holes in it; lit 56 cm from above with a 100 W light bulb, approx 753 lux). Mice were placed at the entrance to the dark box and allowed to roam at will for 5 min. All entries and exits to the light or dark box were recorded. Once a mouse had all 4 paws within a box it was counted as having entered that box, while placing 2 paws out of a box was counted as an exit. To further evaluate the role of prolactin in female pheromone-induced anxiety, pheromone-exposed pregnant mice were injected s.c. with prolactin (50 μg of purified ovine prolactin in saline) at 4.30 p.m. from day 1 to day 3 of pregnancy (to mimic the early pregnancy surges in prolactin).

C. Maternal behavior testing

Day 2 postpartum mice had their pups removed from the home cage. Immediately, three foster pups were placed into the cage and maternal behaviors recorded. To assess maternal behavior in an anxiogenic situation, another group of postpartum day 2 females were placed into a clean novel cage into which three foster pups had been placed, and any behavior recorded (as described previously, Larsen and Grattan, 2010). Full maternal behavior was defined as being when the mouse had gathered all three pups to a nest and was crouching over them. Testing was continued for a maximum of 120 min. Testing was performed between 9.30 and 11.30 a.m.

D. Serum prolactin levels in early pregnancy

Pregnant mice, either exposed to no pheromones or female pheromones, were sacrificed for collection of trunk blood every 4 h from 9 a.m. on day 1 of pregnancy to 9 p.m. on day 4 of pregnancy for measurement of prolactin by radioimmunoassay using NIH reagents, as described previously (Larsen *et al.*, 2008). Sensitivity was 2 ng/ml, and all samples were run in a single assay, with an intra-assay % C.V. 2.5%.

E. Neurogenesis

Virgin female mice, or day 7 pregnant mice exposed to female or no pheromones, were injected with bromodeoxyuridine (BrdU), as reported previously (Larsen *et al.*, 2008). Briefly, BrdU (Sigma) was injected every 2 h from 5 a.m. to 3 p.m. (6 injections of 12 mg/100 g of body weight, dissolved in phosphate buffer). Mice were then perfused with 4% paraformaldehyde at 5 p.m. BrdU-labeled cells were detected using immunohistochemistry (mouse monoclonal anti-BrdU, 1:200, Dako, Carpinteria, CA). Dual label immunofluorescence histochemistry was performed to determine whether the BrdU-labeled cells were neurons using doublecortin as a marker (goat antidoublecortin, 1:100, Santa Cruz). For quantification, the SVZ was observed under 20× magnification, and BrdU-immunoreactive cells counted in a systematic manner after a random start, such that all labeled nuclei were counted in 1-in-6 serial sections (120 μm apart) for a total of 14 sections throughout the SVZ (approximately Bregma +1.94–3.9 mm). Data are presented as the total counts collected, and are not corrected for the total number of sections.

F. Statistical analysis

The data are expressed as mean ± SEM. The amount of time on the open arms is expressed as a percentage of total time on the open and closed arms (open time/(open + closed time) × 100). Data were compared by ANOVA and Fishers PLSD, $P < 0.05$ was used as the level of significance.

II. Results

A. Exposure to unfamiliar female pheromones throughout pregnancy increased anxiety in postpartum mice

As has been previously reported (Maestripieri and D'Amato, 1991; Larsen and Grattan, 2010), postpartum females spent significantly more time on the open arms of the EPM than virgin controls (Fig. 5.1A and B, $^{+}P < 0.05$), indicative of reduced anxiety. In contrast, postpartum females exposed to female pheromones for the duration of pregnancy, either by split-cage housing with a virgin female (Fig. 5.1A, $^{\star}P < 0.05$), or by exposure to urine-soaked bedding (Fig. 5.1B, $^{\star}P < 0.05$), were significantly more anxious on the EPM compared to postpartum controls. In contrast, there was no effect of exposure to male pheromones on anxiety on the EPM in postpartum females (Fig. 5.1A and B). Data from the LDB showed a similar increase in postpartum anxiety in the female pheromone-exposed animals. Postpartum mice exposed to female pheromones had a significant increase in the amount of time spent in the dark chamber of the LDB, and a decreased latency to enter the dark chamber of the LDB compared to postpartum controls (Fig. 5.1C, $^{\star}P < 0.05$). The data show that female pheromone exposure for the duration of pregnancy induces postpartum anxiety.

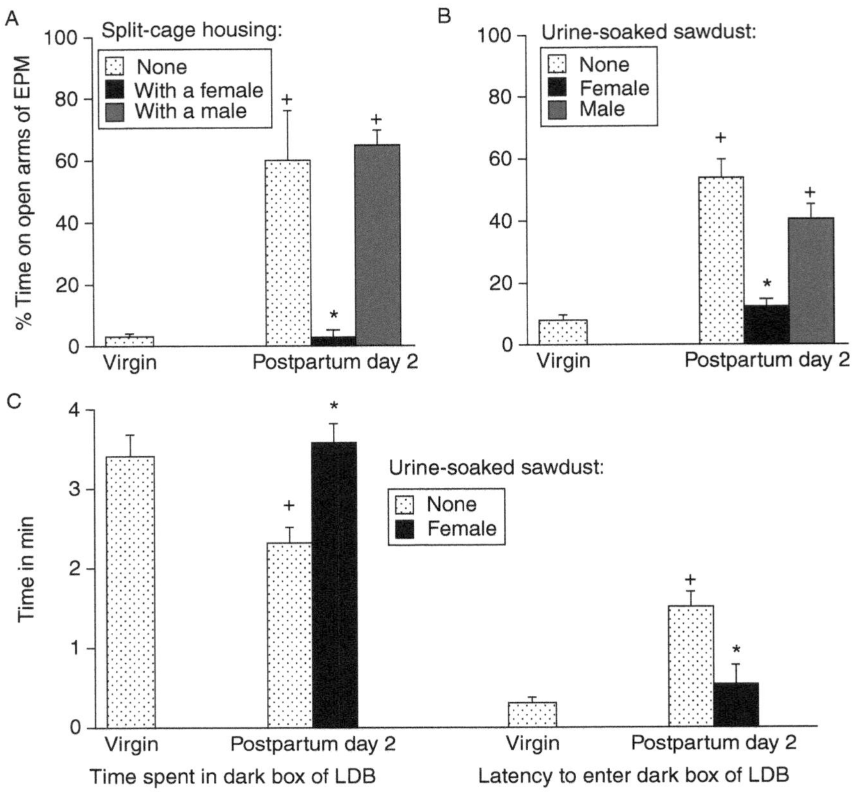

Figure 5.1 Female pheromone exposure throughout pregnancy increases anxiety. Elevated plus maze (EPM). Day 2 postpartum controls spent significantly more time on the open arms of an EPM compared to virgin mice ($^{+}P < 0.05$). Mice exposed to female pheromones for the duration of pregnancy, either by split-cage housing (A), or by exposure to urine-soaked bedding (B), spent significantly less time on the open arms of the EPM compared to day 2 postpartum controls ($^{\star}P < 0.05$), and therefore displayed a significant increase in anxiety. In contrast, exposure to male pheromones throughout pregnancy had no effect. Light–Dark Box (LDB). Postpartum controls had an increased latency to enter the dark chamber of the LDB, and spent significantly less time in the dark chamber of the LDB compared to virgin controls (C, $^{+}P < 0.05$). Mice exposed to female pheromones for the duration of pregnancy had a decreased latency to enter the dark chamber of the LDB, and spent significantly more time in the dark chamber of the LDB, displaying a significant increase in anxiety compared to postpartum controls (C, $^{\star}P < 0.05$).

B. Anxious postpartum females displayed impaired maternal behavior

To determine whether pheromone-induced postpartum anxiety affected maternal behavior, maternal behavior was examined using a pup retrieval paradigm in pheromone-exposed mice. As reported previously, in the

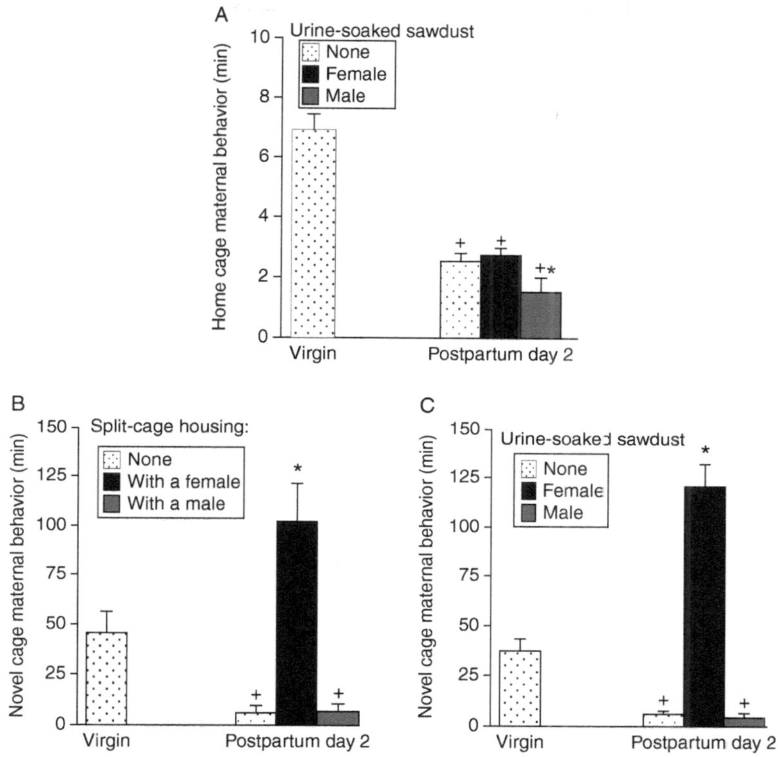

Figure 5.2 Female pheromone exposure throughout pregnancy inhibits postpartum maternal behavior in an anxiogenic situation. Maternal behavior in a home cage. Day 2 postpartum mice were significantly faster to express maternal behavior to foster pups compared to virgin controls (A, $^{+}P < 0.05$). Exposure to female pheromones had no effect, either by split-cage housing (data not shown), or by exposure to urine-soaked bedding (A), while mice exposed to male pheromones for the duration of pregnancy expressed maternal behavior more rapidly to foster pups compared to all other groups (A, $^{\star}P < 0.05$). Maternal behavior in a novel cage. Both day 2 postpartum controls, and male pheromone-exposed females, were significantly faster to express maternal behavior to foster pups than virgin controls (B and C, $^{+}P < 0.05$). Day 2 postpartum mice exposed to female pheromones for the duration of the pregnancy displayed significantly impaired maternal behavior to foster pups in an anxiogenic situation compared to both the male pheromone-exposed mice and the individually housed controls (B and C, $^{\star}P < 0.05$).

home cage, postpartum females were significantly faster to express maternal behavior compared to virgin controls (Fig. 5.2A, $^{+}P < 0.05$), and females exposed to male pheromones throughout pregnancy were significantly faster to express maternal behavior than postpartum controls (Fig. 5.2A, $^{\star}P < 0.05$; Larsen *et al.*, 2008). Maternal behavior in mice exposed to female pheromones was not significantly different compared to postpartum controls when tested in the home cage (Fig. 5.2A). In the anxiogenic situation of a novel cage, all groups tested took significantly longer to express full maternal behavior compared to that in the home cage. Both day 2 postpartum control mice and male pheromone-exposed females remained significantly faster to express full maternal behavior compared to virgin controls, yet, there was now no significant difference between these two groups (Fig. 5.2B and C, $^{+}P < 0.05$). In contrast, however, female pheromone-exposed mice placed in an anxiogenic situation (novel cage) displayed dramatically impaired maternal behavior to foster pups (Fig. 5.2B and C, $^{\star}P < 0.05$). The female pheromone-exposed mice investigated the pups occasionally, but did not gather them to their nest, or sit with the pups. Instead, they made a nest some distance away from the pups and either took significantly longer to express full maternal behavior or, in the majority of animals, did not express full maternal behavior at all within the designated 120-min observation period.

C. Exposure to female pheromones decreased serum prolactin levels in early pregnancy

To test the hypothesis that changes in prolactin secretion during pregnancy might underlie the pheromone-induced alterations in mood postpartum, levels of serum prolactin during early pregnancy were measured by radioimmunoassay. Although the previously described pattern of twice daily prolactin surges in early pregnancy was maintained (Fig. 5.3, $^{+}P < 0.05$; Larsen and Grattan, 2010), serum prolactin levels in pregnant mice exposed to female pheromones were significantly lower than those of controls at many time points on days 1–3 of pregnancy (Fig. 5.3, $^{\star}P < 0.05$; # urine-soaked sawdust added at 9 a.m. daily). From day 5 of pregnancy there were not any significant differences between the two groups.

D. The role of suppressed prolactin in mediating pheromone-induced postpartum anxiety

To test whether the decreased serum prolactin in early pregnancy induced by exposure to female pheromones was specifically responsible for inducing postpartum anxiety, we injected pheromone-exposed mice with prolactin at 5 p.m. daily from day 1 to day 3 of pregnancy. Animals were subsequently tested for anxiety on day 2 postpartum, approximately 3 weeks after hormone treatment. Remarkably, restoring normal prolactin levels in early pregnancy completely prevented the increased anxiety seen in postpartum mice exposed to female pheromones throughout pregnancy (Fig. 5.4). This implies that prolactin in early pregnancy is specifically

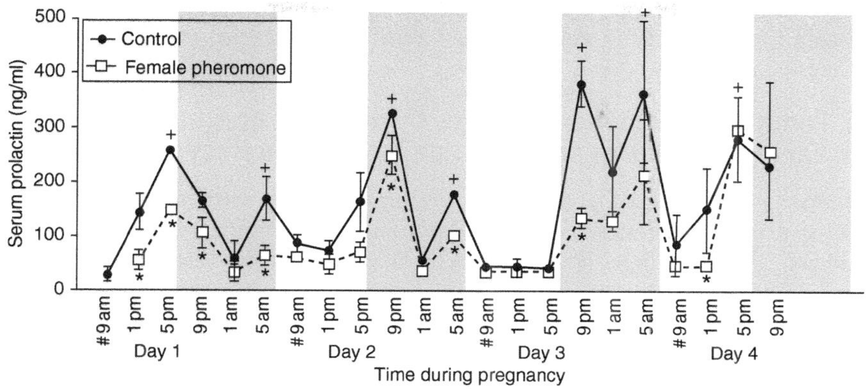

Figure 5.3 Serum prolactin levels from day 1 to day 2 of pregnancy. Pregnant mice had a twice daily surge in serum prolactin levels with an afternoon peak just prior to lights off at 6 p.m. and a smaller nocturnal peak approximately 1 h before lights on ($^+P < 0.05$). Pregnant mice had urine-soaked sawdust placed in the cage at 9 a.m. daily throughout pregnancy ($^\#P < 0.05$). Pregnant mice exposed to female pheromones showed significantly decreased serum prolactin levels at many time points from day 1 to 3 of pregnancy, compared to pregnant controls ($^\star P < 0.05$). From day 5 of pregnancy there were no significant differences between the groups (data not shown).

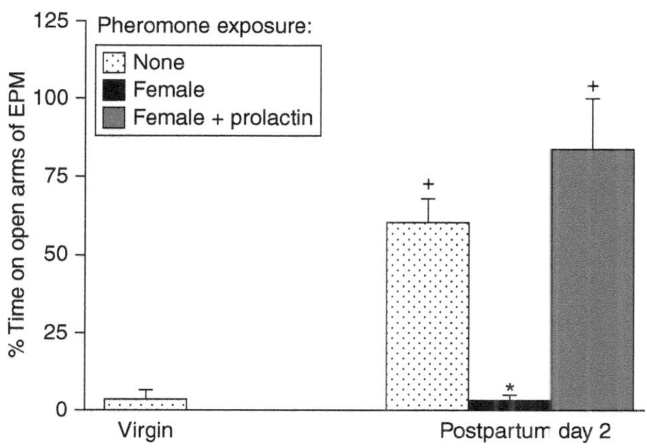

Figure 5.4 Restoration of prolactin prevents the female pheromone-induced increase in anxiety postpartum. Day 2 postpartum controls spent significantly more time on the open arms of an EPM compared to virgin mice ($^+P < 0.05$). Mice exposed to female pheromones for the duration of pregnancy by exposure to urine-soaked bedding spent significantly less time on the open arms of the EPM compared to day 2 postpartum controls ($^\star P < 0.05$), and therefore displayed a significant increase in anxiety. Female pheromone-exposed pregnant mice injected with prolactin from day 1 to day 3 of pregnancy had no significant differences in anxiety compared to postpartum controls.

required for adaptive responses that occur in the maternal brain during pregnancy and become evident as behavioral changes postpartum.

E. Female pheromone exposure throughout pregnancy decreased neurogenesis on day 7 of pregnancy

One known action of prolactin in the brain during early pregnancy is an increase in neurogenesis in the SVZ of the maternal brain (Larsen and Grattan, 2010; Shingo *et al.*, 2003), and we have previously shown that pharmacological suppression of prolactin during early pregnancy led to a decrease in neurogenesis in this region (Larsen and Grattan, 2010). Therefore, we examined whether this was also affected by exposure to female pheromones during pregnancy. Decreased serum prolactin in early pregnancy, induced by exposure to female pheromones, significantly reduced levels of neurogenesis in the SVZ on day 7 of pregnancy compared to postpartum controls, reducing the numbers of BrdU-labeled cells to that of a virgin nonpregnant mouse (Fig. 5.5A, $^{*}P < 0.05$). There were no significant differences in the percentage of BrdU-labeled cells in the SVZ that were double labeled with doublecortin, a neuronal marker, between any of the groups (Fig. 5.5B).

III. Discussion

Day 2 postpartum mice displayed decreased anxiety on the EPM compared to virgin mice, consistent with previous experimental findings (Larsen and Grattan, 2010; Maestripieri and D'Amato, 1991). In contrast, female pheromone exposure throughout pregnancy significantly increased anxiety on day 2 postpartum. In women, postpartum anxiety can impair maternal responsiveness to, and care of the infant (Barnett *et al.*, 1991; Fraser *et al.*, 2000; O'Connor *et al.*, 2002). In a similar manner, mice exposed to female pheromones for the duration of pregnancy also displayed dramatically impaired responsiveness to, and an extreme lack of care for pups when placed in an anxiogenic situation. The combined syndrome of an increase in anxiety together with impairment of maternal behavior suggests that exposing mice to female pheromones throughout pregnancy provides a novel model for studying postpartum mood disorders. Importantly, this approach is completely noninvasive, and retains the unique characteristics of gestation.

We have previously shown that pharmacological suppression of serum prolactin levels, solely in early pregnancy, can initiate increased postpartum anxiety over 2 weeks later (Larsen and Grattan, 2010). The results shown here indicate that postpartum anxiety caused by female pheromone exposure is also induced by low prolactin during early pregnancy. Moreover,

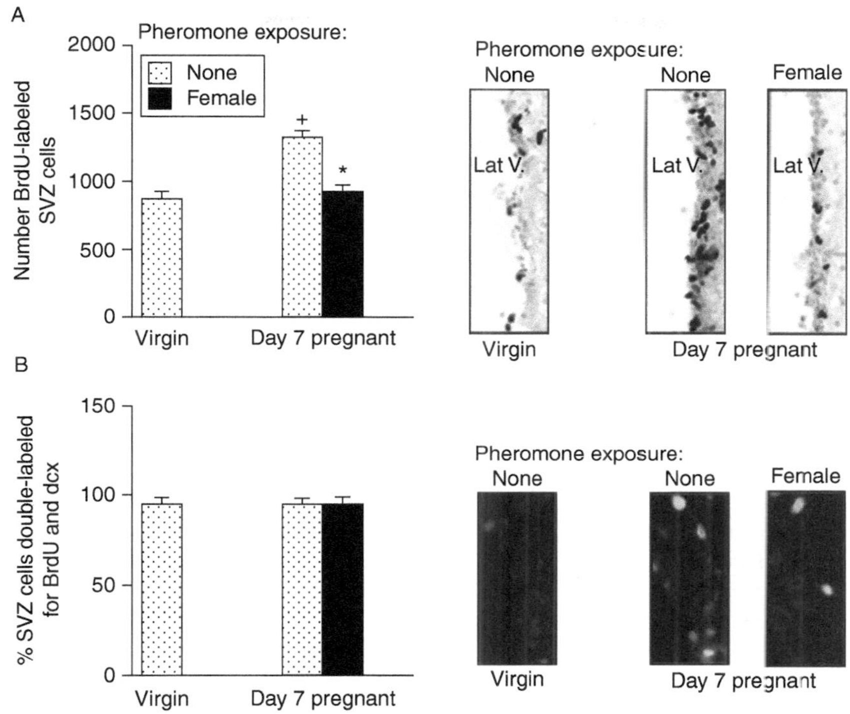

Figure 5.5 Female pheromone exposure throughout pregnancy decrease neurogenesis on day 7 of pregnancy. (A). Day 7 pregnant mice had a significant increase in the number of BrdU-labeled cells in the subventricular zone (SVZ) compared to virgin controls ($^{+}P < 0.05$). Day 7 pregnant females exposed to female pheromones for 7 days showed a significant decrease in BrdU-labeled cells in the SVZ compared to controls ($^{\star}P < 0.05$). Micrographs show representative images from the SVZ, with black staining representing BrdU-labeled cells (Lat. V.: lateral ventricle). (B) There were no significant differences between pheromone-exposed or control mice, in the percentage of BrdU-labeled cells that coexpressed Dcx. Representative merged images immunoreactive for BrdU (green) and Dcx (red) in the lateral ventricle of the SVZ in each group are shown. (For interpretation of the references to color in this figure legend, the reader is referred to the Web version of this chapter.)

reminiscent of the pharmacological suppression of prolactin, injections of prolactin to restore serum prolactin levels in early pregnancy in pheromone-exposed mice completely prevented the pheromone-induced increase in anxiety. This suggests that the pheromone-induced decrease in prolactin in early pregnancy is the mechanism underlying the induction of postpartum anxiety.

In our previous work using pharmacological suppression of prolactin, we identified a potential role for the increase in SVZ neurogenesis on mood postpartum (Larsen and Grattan, 2010). In the present study, serum prolactin levels in mice exposed to female pheromones during pregnancy were significantly lower than in pregnant controls, but they were still higher than basal levels seen in virgin mice, and higher than the levels seen in mice when prolactin was suppressed pharmacologically (Larsen and Grattan, 2010). Nevertheless, the decrease in prolactin induced by female pheromone exposure was sufficient to completely suppress the pregnancy-induced increase in neurogenesis in the SVZ. These data support the hypothesis that increased neurogenesis in the SVZ is important for adaptive changes in mood postpartum. Extensive work has linked impaired neurogenesis in other brain regions to the development of mood disorders (Duman *et al.*, 2001), but how the increase in SVZ neurogenesis during pregnancy moderates mood postpartum remains unclear.

The implication of our data is that any physiological or pathophysiological factor that might influence prolactin levels or neurogenesis during pregnancy could lead to development of mood disorders. Previous studies examining the hormonal regulation of mood during the peripartum period have predominantly focused on acute changes in hormones at that time, and no clear role of hormones in the control of mood has emerged. The present data support the hypothesis that levels of hormones in early pregnancy are crucial for euthymic mood postpartum. Hence, factors influencing hormones early in pregnancy, such as stress, nutrition, or medication, might have an important and previously unsuspected impact on mood in the postpartum period.

REFERENCES

Barnett, B., Schaafsma, M. F., Guzman, A. M., and Parker, G. B. (1991). Maternal anxiety: A 5-year review of an intervention study. *J. Child Psychol. Psychiatry* **32,** 423–438.

Boyce, P. M., and Stubbs, J. M. (1994). The importance of postnatal depression. *Med. J. Aust.* **161,** 471–472.

Britton, J. R. (2005). Pre-discharge anxiety among mothers of well newborns: Prevalence and correlates. *Acta Paediatr.* **94,** 1771–1776.

Britton, J. R. (2007). Maternal anxiety: Course and antecedents during the early postpartum period. *Depress. Anxiety* .

Brunton, P. J., Russell, J. A., and Douglas, A. J. (2008). Adaptive responses of the maternal hypothalamic-pituitary-adrenal axis during pregnancy and lactation. *J. Neuroendocrinol.* **20,** 764–776.

Duman, R. S., Nakagawa, S., and Malberg, J. (2001). Regulation of adult neurogenesis by antidepressant treatment. *Neuropsychopharmacology* **25,** 836–844.

Fraser, J. A., Armstrong, K. L., Morris, J. P., and Dadds, M. R. (2000). Home visiting intervention for vulnerable families with newborns: Follow-up results of a randomized controlled trial. *Child Abuse Negl.* **24,** 1399–1429.

Grattan, D. R., Steyn, F. J., Kokay, I. C., Anderson, G. M., and Bunn, S. J. (2008). Pregnancy-induced adaptation in the neuroendocrine control of prolactin secretion. *J. Neuroendocrinol.* **20,** 497–507.

Larsen, C. M., and Grattan, D. R. (2010). Prolactin-induced mitogenesis in the subventricular zone of the maternal brain during early pregnancy is essential for normal postpartum behavioral responses in the mother. *Endocrinology* **151,** 3805–3814.

Larsen, C. M., Kokay, I. C., and Grattan, D. R. (2008). Male pheromones initiate prolactin-induced neurogenesis and advance maternal behavior in female mice. *Horm. Behav.* **53,** 509–517.

Lovestone, S., and Kumar, R. (1993). Postnatal psychiatric illness: The impact on partners. *Br. J. Psychiatry* **163,** 210–216.

Maestripieri, D., and D'Amato, F. R. (1991). Anxiety and maternal aggression in house mice (*Mus musculus*): A look at interindividual variability. *J. Comp. Psychol.* **105,** 295–301.

Mak, G. K., Enwere, E. K., Gregg, C., Pakarainen, T., Poutanen, M., Huhtaniemi, I., and Weiss, S. (2007). Male pheromone-stimulated neurogenesis in the adult female brain: Possible role in mating behavior. *Nat. Neurosci.* **10,** 1003–1011.

Manassis, K., Bradley, S., Goldberg, S., Hood, J., and Swinson, R. P. (1994). Attachment in mothers with anxiety disorders and their children. *J. Am. Acad. Child Adolesc. Psychiatry* **33,** 1106–1113.

Matthey, S., Barnett, B., Howie, P., and Kavanagh, D. J. (2003). Diagnosing postpartum depression in mothers and fathers: Whatever happened to anxiety? *J. Affect. Disord.* **74,** 139–147.

Munk-Olsen, T., Laursen, T. M., Pedersen, C. B., Mors, O., and Mortensen, P. B. (2006). New parents and mental disorders: A population-based register study. *JAMA* **296,** 2582–2589.

NIH (USA, PA-09-174, 2009). Womens Mental Health in Pregnancy and the Postpartum Period.

O'Connor, T. G., Heron, J., Golding, J., Beveridge, M., and Glover, V. (2002). Maternal antenatal anxiety and children's behavioural/emotional problems at 4 years. Report from the Avon Longitudinal Study of Parents and Children. *Br. J. Psychiatry* **180,** 502–508.

Shingo, T., Gregg, C., Enwere, E., Fujikawa, H., Hassam, R. Geary, C., Cross, J. C., and Weiss, S. (2003). Pregnancy-stimulated neurogenesis in the adult female forebrain mediated by prolactin. *Science* **299,** 117–120.

Stowe, Z. N., and Nemeroff, C. B. (1995). Women at risk for postpartum-onset major depression. *Am. J. Obstet. Gynecol.* **173,** 639–645.

Wenzel, A., Haugen, E. N., Jackson, L. C., and Robinson, K. (2003). Prevalence of generalized anxiety at eight weeks postpartum. *Arch. Womens Ment. Health* **6,** 43–49.

CHAPTER SIX

Major Urinary Protein Regulation of Chemical Communication and Nutrient Metabolism

Yingjiang Zhou *and* Liangyou Rui

Contents

Abstract

The major urinary protein (MUP) family members contain a conserved β-barrel structure with a characteristic central hydrophobic pocket. They are secreted by the liver and excreted into the urine. MUPs bind via their central pockets to volatile pheromones or other lipophilic molecules, and regulate pheromone transportation in the circulation, excretion in the kidney, and release into the air from urine marks. MUPs are highly polymorphic, and the MUP profiles in urine function as individual identity signatures of the owners. The MUP signatures are detected by the main and accessory olfactory systems and trigger adaptive behavioral responses and/or developmental processes. Circulating MUPs serve

Department of Molecular & Integrative Physiology, University of Michigan Medical School, Ann Arbor, Michigan, USA

Vitamins and Hormones, Volume 83

ISSN 0083-6729, DOI: 10.1016/S0083-6729(10)83006-7

as a metabolic signal to regulate glucose and lipid metabolism. Recombinant MUP1 markedly ameliorates hyperglycemia and glucose intolerance in mice with type 2 diabetes. MUP1 suppresses hepatic gluconeogenesis and promotes energy expenditure in skeletal muscle by stimulating mitochondrial biogenesis and function. MUPs are unique members of the lipocalin superfamily that mediate both chemical and metabolic signaling.

I. Introduction

Animals as well as human beings have evolved a variety of communication mechanisms to exchange information. Chemical communication plays a key role in regulating both behavioral and physiological responses in the animal kingdom. Individuals generate scent substances which are excreted into the environment via sweat, urine, and feces. These scent substances serve as chemical signals and are perceived by conspecifics to trigger adaptive behavioral and physiological responses in the receivers (Brennan and Kendrick, 2006; Tirindelli *et al.*, 2009). Most scent substances are unstable, volatile small molecules and bind to their cognate protein carries. These carries not only extend the lifetime but also regulate the release of the scent substances (Hurst, 2009; Tirindelli *et al.*, 2009). The major urinary protein (MUP) family proteins bind to, concentrate, and stabilize many volatile scent substances (e.g., pheromones), thereby controlling both pheromone transportation in circulation and pheromone release into the air from urine scent marks (Brennan and Kendrick, 2006; Hurst, 2009; Tirindelli *et al.*, 2009). Additionally, MUPs themselves may serve as chemical signals to convey their owners' identity information to conspecifics (Chamero *et al.*, 2007). Recent studies reveal that the MUP family members also regulate nutrient metabolism independently of chemical signaling (Hui *et al.*, 2009; Zhou *et al.*, 2009). Nutrient metabolism provides energy supply to power behavioral and physiological activities. Therefore, the MUP family members appear to coordinate behavioral response and energy metabolism by serving as both chemical and metabolic signals.

II. MUP Structure and Polymorphism

MUPs belong to the lipocalin superfamily (Cavaggioni and Mucignat-Caretta, 2000; Finlayson *et al.*, 1965). The lipocalin family members have relatively low similarity in their amino acid sequences; however, their tertiary structures are extremely conserved with a characteristic β-barrel consisting of eight β-strands (Bocskei *et al.*, 1992). Most lipocalin family members bind, via their central hydrophobic pockets formed by these eight

β-strands, to small lipophilic molecules, including fatty acids, steroids, retinol, and pheromones (Schlehuber and Skerra, 2005).

A. MUPs bind to pheromones via their central β-barrel cavities

The MUP family members were initially discovered in urine as a group of small proteins with molecular weights around 18 kD (Finlayson *et al.*, 1965; Lane and Neuhaus, 1972). MUPs are mainly synthesized in the liver and secreted into the bloodstream (Shaw *et al.*, 1983). Due to their small sizes, MUPs are efficiently filtered through the glomeruli and excreted into the urine (Kimura *et al.*, 1991). The isoelectric points of MUPs in urine vary from 4.6 to 5.3 (Bocskei *et al.*, 1992; Clissold and Bishop, 1982). Each individual adult male mouse excretes approximately 8–14 different MUP isoforms in urine (Hurst, 2009).

MUP tertiary structures have been extensively studied by both X-ray crystallography and NMR spectroscopy (Bocskei *et al.*, 1992; Darwish Marie *et al.*, 2001; Lucke *et al.*, 1999; Timm *et al.*, 2001; Zidek *et al.*, 1999). The structures of both endogenous and recombinant MUP1 protein have been characterized (Bocskei *et al.*, 1991; Timm *et al.*, 2001). The MUP family members contain a characteristic eight antiparallel β-strands that are linked by seven loops to form a β-barrel (Bocskei *et al.*, 1992; Darwish Marie *et al.*, 2001; Lucke *et al.*, 1999; Timm *et al.*, 2001; Zidek *et al.*, 1999). The first loop is a large Ω-loop that functions as a dynamic lid of the β-barrel, and the other six are typical short β-hairpin (Timm *et al.*, 2001). The interior of the β-barrel forms a hydrophobic pocket that binds directly to hydrophobic pheromones.

The affinity of different MUP isoforms for pheromones varies. For instance, MUP4 has a 23-fold higher affinity for ($\pm$)-2-sec-butyl-4,5-dihydrothiazole than MUP1 but has a fourfold lower affinity for 6-hydroxy-6-methyl-3-heptanone than MUP1 (Darwish Marie *et al.*, 2001; Sharrow *et al.*, 2002). The affinity for pheromones is determined by the amino acids of the binding pockets (Darwish Marie *et al.*, 2001; Sharrow *et al.*, 2002). A single amino acid substitution in the binding pocket can result in a dramatic change in the affinity of an MUP family member (Darwish Marie *et al.*, 2001). The binding of pheromones to MUPs not only protects against pheromone decomposition in blood and urine but also sustains pheromone action by slowly releasing MUP-bound volatile pheromones into the air from urine marks. Therefore, MUP expression levels control pheromone levels in blood and urine (Sharrow *et al.*, 2002).

B. MUPs are highly polymorphic

MUP expression is sexually dimorphic in rodents, and the levels of MUPs are much higher in males than in females (Geertzen *et al.*, 1973; Lane and Neuhaus, 1972). Androgen potently stimulates MUP expression, resulting in male-dominant expression and excretion of MUPs (Johnson *et al.*, 1995; Kurtz and Feigelson, 1977). MUPs are synthesized mainly in the liver and excreted into the urine (Finlayson *et al.*, 1965; Shaw *et al.*, 1983). MUP synthesis accounts for 3.5–4% of total hepatic protein synthesis in adult male mice (Berger and Szoka, 1981). Urinary MUPs mediate chemical signaling in conspecifics (Tirindelli *et al.*, 2009). The MUP family members are also expressed in the submaxillary, lachrymal, nasal, parotid, mammary glands, and hypothalami; however, the function of extrahepatic MUPs is unknown (Cavaggioni and Mucignat-Caretta, 2000; De Giorgio *et al.*, 2009; Shaw *et al.*, 1983).

The MUP family proteins are encoded by multiple paralogous genes clustered on chromosome 4 in mice and chromosome 5 in rats (Hastie *et al.*, 1979). Rat MUPs are also called α_{2U}-globulins (Lane and Neuhaus, 1972). The amino acid sequences of MUPs are 65% identical between mice and rats (Cavaggioni and Mucignat-Caretta, 2000). The mouse genome contains 21 *MUP* genes and additional 21 *MUP* pseudogenes (Logan *et al.*, 2008). The *MUP* genes and pseudogenes have been independently evolved from a single ancestral gene (Logan *et al.*, 2008). The *MUP* genes contain six coding exons, and the pseudogenes contain premature stop codons due to an insertion or deletion. The *MUP* genes and pseudogenes are classified into two groups. The first group consists of six *MUP* genes (e.g., *MUP1*, *MUP2*, *MUP18*, *MUP24*, *MUP25*, and *MUP26*) and five pseudogenes (Logan *et al.*, 2008). The cDNA sequences of these six *MUP* genes are 82–94% identical. The second group consists of the remaining 15 *MUP* genes and 16 pseudogenes (Logan *et al.*, 2008; Mudge *et al.*, 2008). The cDNA sequences of these 15 *MUP* genes are >97% identical.

The *MUP* genes are extremely polymorphic in wild or outbred mice (Cheetham *et al.*, 2009; Finlayson *et al.*, 1965; Robertson *et al.*, 2007). Each individual adult male mouse normally expresses 8–14 different MUP isoforms; therefore, the number of MUP expression patterns is extremely expanded due to MUP polymorphism (Beynon *et al.*, 2002; Evershed *et al.*, 1993; Hurst, 2009). Polymorphic *MUP* genes serve as a specific genetic marker of individual identity, and the MUP profiles in urine are recognized as an individual identity signature of the owners by conspecific receivers (Cheetham *et al.*, 2007; Hurst *et al.*, 2001; Sherborne *et al.*, 2007).

III. MUP Regulation of Chemical Communication

Pheromones are diverse, biologically active substances that are excreted to the outside by individuals. Pheromones are detected by conspecifics and trigger specific behavioral, physiological, and/or developmental responses in the receivers, including aggression, mating, territory marking, estrous cycles, and pregnancy (Hurst, 2009; Tirindelli *et al.*, 2009).

A. MUPs function as volatile pheromone carriers

Many pheromones are small volatile organic molecules which are unstable in aqueous environments (e.g., blood and urine) (Hurst and Beynon, 2004; Stowers and Marton, 2005). The MUP family members bound via their center hydrophobic cavities to a variety of pheromones (Bocskei *et al.*, 1992; Peele *et al.*, 2003; Sharrow *et al.*, 2002). The MUP-pheromone physical interactions protect against pheromone destruction during both transportation in the bloodstream and excretion into the urine. Additionally, free volatile pheromone molecules are quickly evaporated into the air from scent urine marks. MUPs not only facilitate pheromone transportation as pheromone carries but also prolong pheromone lifetime by slowly releasing their bound pheromones into the air from scent marks (Humphries *et al.*, 1999; Hurst *et al.*, 1998).

B. MUPs act as pheromones to directly regulate behavioral and physiological responses

Interestingly, the MUP1 protein moiety is sufficient to activate sensory neurons in the vomeronasal organ (VNO) and to trigger ovulation (More, 2006). Recombinant MUP1 promotes intermale aggression in the absence of pheromones (Chamero *et al.*, 2007). Moreover, purified MUP1 directly stimulates Gαo-coupled V2R receptors in VNO neuron cultures (Chamero *et al.*, 2007). Therefore, MUPs also act as involatile pheromones in addition to as pheromone carriers.

C. The MUP profiles serve as an individual identity signature

MUPs and their bound pheromones profoundly modulate the behaviors and development of conspecifics. Urine from intact but not castrated males promotes male aggression (Mugford and Nowell, 1970). Males advertise their social status to attract females via urinary pheromones (Bronson and Caroom, 1971; Jemiolo *et al.*, 1991). MUPs accelerate female puberty and promote ovulation (More, 2006; Mucignat-Caretta *et al.*, 1995). The urine scents of unfamiliar males block pregnancy in recently mated females (Bruce, 1959), and MUPs bind to the volatile pheromones involved in pregnancy block (Peele *et al.*, 2003). The polymorphic patterns of MUPs serve as an individual identity signature in urine marks (Hurst and Beynon, 2004; Hurst *et al.*, 2001). Females use the MUP signatures to recognize individual scent owners, preferentially associated with heterozygous males, and avoid inbreeding (Cheetham *et al.*, 2007; Thom *et al.*, 2008).

Pheromones are believed to stimulate sensory neurons in VNO when animals make nasal contact with scent marks (Breer *et al.*, 2006; Halpern and Martinez-Marcos, 2003; Meredith, 1994). Each pheromone activates a specific subset of sensory neurons that convey unique signals to the brain (Dulac and Torello, 2003). VNO neurons project to the accessory olfactory bulb, and the second-order neurons in the accessory olfactory bulb project to amygdala that innervates hypothalamic neurons either directly or indirectly (Tirindelli *et al.*, 2009). In contrast, the airborne volatile odorants are believed to stimulate sensory neurons in the main olfactory epithelium which project to the main olfactory bulb (Tirindelli *et al.*, 2009). The second-order neurons in the main olfactory bulb project to higher centers in the brain, including the piriform cortex and the cortical amygdala (Tirindelli *et al.*, 2009). However, recent studies suggest that both the vomeronasal and the main olfactory systems are involved in pheromone detection (Hurst, 2009).

IV. MUP Regulation of Nutrient Metabolism

Behavioral and developmental responses are powered by energy derived from nutrient metabolism. It is not surprising that many factors simultaneously regulate both behaviors and metabolism. Glucose and fatty acids are the primary fuel substrates to power cellular activity that underlies behavioral and developmental responses. Animals have evolved a sophisticated neuroendocrine system that maintains glucose and lipid homeostasis. For instance, a rise in blood glucose derived from ingested food stimulates pancreatic β-cells to secrete insulin. Insulin in return reduces blood glucose levels by stimulating glucose uptake into skeletal muscle and adipose tissue as well as by suppressing glucose production from the liver (Saltiel and Kahn, 2001). In contrast, a fall in blood glucose during fasting stimulates the secretion of counterregulatory hormones (e.g., glucagon and catecholamines) which increase blood glucose levels by stimulating liver glucose production (Jiang and Zhang, 2003). Therefore, blood glucose homeostasis is maintained mainly by a balance between insulin and counterregulatory hormones. Impaired ability of insulin to decrease blood glucose (insulin resistance) is the primary risk factor for the development of type 2 diabetes. Insulin sensitivity is regulated by multiple humoral factors, including MUP1.

A. MUP1 is involved in nutrient sensing

Recent studies show that the expression and secretion of MUP1 are regulated by nutrient signals. Fasting markedly reduced MUP1 expression in the liver, which is reversed by refeeding (Hui *et al.*, 2009). The liver plays a key role in nutrient sensing and metabolism. In agreement with this observation, caloric restriction also dramatically reduces MUP1 expression in mouse livers (Dhahbi *et al.*, 2004; Miller *et al.*, 2002). The expression of other MUP family members, including MUP4 and MUP5, is also suppressed in calorie-restricted mice (Dhahbi *et al.*, 2004). Interestingly, MUP1 deficiency is associated with obesity and type 2 diabetes. Two groups reported independently that hepatic MUP1 expression and circulating MUP1 levels are markedly reduced in mice with either genetic (leptin receptor-deficient *db/db*) or dietary fat-induced obesity (Hui *et al.*, 2009; Zhou *et al.*, 2009). Interestingly, MUP1 is also expressed in several extrahepatic tissues, and MUP1 expression is similarly reduced in both adipose tissues and the hypothalamus in response to nutrient deprivation (De Giorgio *et al.*, 2009; van Schothorst *et al.*, 2006). Adipocytes and hypothalamic neurons are also key players in nutrient sensing. These observations suggest that MUP1 and/or the other MUP family members are likely involved in the nutrient sensing process, and defects in MUP-mediated nutrient sensing might contribute to the development of metabolic diseases, including type 2 diabetes.

B. MUP1 regulates nutrient metabolism in multiple tissues

There are multiple lines of evidence supporting an important role of MUP1 in glucose metabolism. In mice with either genetic (*db/db*) or dietary-induced type 2 diabetes, liver-specific overexpression of MUP1 markedly reduces hyperglycemia and glucose intolerance (Zhou *et al.*, 2009). Similarly, chronic administration of purified recombinant MUP1 proteins also ameliorates hyperglycemia and improves glucose intolerance in *db/db* mice (Hui *et al.*, 2009). The MUP1 therapy also improves systemic insulin sensitivity in diabetic mice (Hui *et al.*, 2009; Zhou *et al.*, 2009). Interestingly, rosiglitazone (a potent PPARγ agonist) and resveratrol (a natural product abundant in grape skins), two chemically distinct compounds that decrease hyperglycemia and glucose intolerance in diabetic mice, also stimulate MUP1 expression in the liver (Baur *et al.*, 2006; Hui *et al.*, 2009).

MUP1 treatment enhances insulin signaling in the skeletal muscle but not the liver of diabetic mice, suggesting that skeletal muscle is a physiological target of MUP1 (Hui *et al.*, 2009). Moreover, recombinant MUP1 directly suppresses glucose production in primary hepatocyte cultures independently of insulin (Zhou *et al.*, 2009). Additionally, liver-specific overexpression of MUP1 markedly decreases triglyceride levels in the livers of *db/db* mice (Zhou *et al.*, 2009). Therefore, MUP1 may also regulate hepatic glucose and lipid metabolism in an autocrine and/or paracrine fashion. Interestingly, MUP1 expression is also regulated by nutrients in adipose tissue and the hypothalamus, suggesting that MUP1 may regulate the metabolic activity of these two tissues in a similar autocrine and/or paracrine manner (De Giorgio *et al.*, 2009; van Schothorst *et al.*, 2006).

C. MUP1 regulates metabolism by multiple mechanisms

MUP1 reduces blood glucose levels at least in part by suppressing the hepatic gluconeogenic program (Zhou *et al.*, 2009). In both animals and primary hepatocyte cultures, recombinant MUP1 markedly inhibits the expression of phosphoenolpyruvate carboxykinase (PEPCK) and glucose-6-phosphatase (G6Pase), two rate-limiting enzymes for gluconeogenesis (Zhou *et al.*, 2009). Insulin is well known to suppress hepatic gluconeogenesis; however, MUP1 suppresses hepatic glucose production independently of insulin, suggesting that MUP1 regulates the hepatic gluconeogenic program by a novel mechanism (Zhou *et al.*, 2009). Hepatic gluconeogenesis is abnormally elevated in type 2 diabetes, thus significantly contributing to hyperglycemia and glucose intolerance (Ali and Drucker, 2009; Jiang and Zhang, 2003). Type 2 diabetes is associated with a marked reduction in MUP1 expression, suggesting that reduced expression of hepatic MUP1 contributes to abnormally elevated hepatic gluconeogenesis (Hui *et al.*, 2009; Zhou *et al.*, 2009).

Chronic MUP1 treatment also decreases the levels of plasma lipids in *db/db* mice (Hui *et al.*, 2009; Zhou *et al.*, 2009). Moreover, liver-specific overexpression of MUP1 results in a marked reduction in hepatic lipid levels, presumably due to suppression of lipogenic genes in the liver, including the *stearoyl-CoA desaturase-1*, *fatty acid synthase*, *carbohydrate response element binding protein*, and *peroxisome proliferator-activated receptor-γ* (*PPARγ*) genes (Zhou *et al.*, 2009). Chronic administration of purified recombinant MUP1 also decreases lipid levels in the skeletal muscles of *db/db* mice (Hui *et al.*, 2009). Together, these observations suggest that MUP1 regulates both glucose and lipid metabolism in multiple tissues.

MUP1 improves insulin sensitivity in the skeletal muscle at least in part by increasing energy expenditure (Hui *et al.*, 2009). Chronic administration of purified MUP1 proteins increases energy expenditure, body temperature, and ambulatory locomotion in *db/db* mice (Hui *et al.*, 2009). MUP1 increases not only mitochondrial biogenesis but also the capacity of mitochondrial oxidative phosphorylation (Hui *et al.*, 2009). MUP1 promotes mitochondrial biogenesis and function specifically in the skeletal muscle but not other tissues (e.g., adipose tissues and livers) of *db/db* mice (Hui *et al.*, 2009). An increase in mitochondrial content and function is likely to result in an increase in fatty acid β-oxidation and a decrease in lipid levels in skeletal muscles, thereby ameliorating lipotoxicity and insulin resistance in MUP1-treated mice with type 2 diabetes.

Recombinant MUP1 inhibits the hepatic gluconeogenic program directly in primary hepatocyte cultures, suggesting that MUP1 regulates metabolic function in the liver by activating its own cognate receptors (Zhou *et al.*, 2009). Additionally, in animals, circulatory MUP1 binds to, concentrates, and slowly releases various lipophilic molecules (Cavaggioni and Mucignat-Caretta, 2000; Sharrow *et al.*, 2002). These lipophilic molecules may be bioactive and regulate nutrient metabolism; therefore, MUP1 may also regulate metabolism indirectly by controlling the stability, concentrations, and/or activity of these bioactive lipophilic molecules.

V. Conclusions and Future Directions

MUPs belong to the lipocalin superfamily whose tertiary structure contains a conserved β-barrel with a characteristic central hydrophobic pocket. The MUP family members are expressed mainly by the liver and secreted into the bloodstream (Fig. 6.1). Various pheromones and other small lipophilic molecules bind to the central pockets of MUPs and are transported through the circulation. MUPs are excreted into the urine in the kidney, and urinary MUPs prolong pheromone lifetime by slowing the release of MUP-bound pheromones into the air from urine scent marks. MUPs are highly

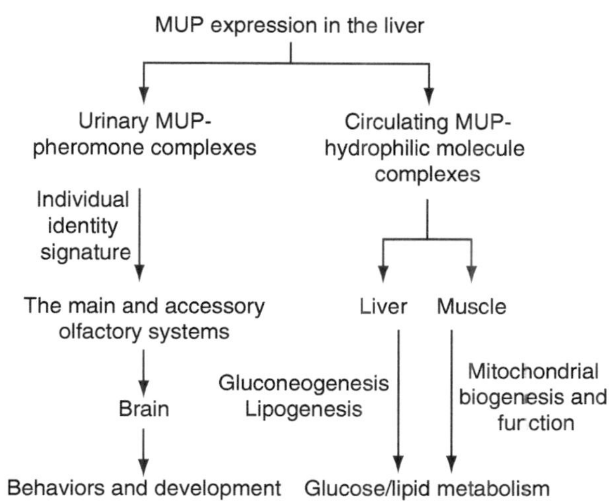

Figure 6.1 A model of MUP action. The MUP family members are expressed mainly by the liver and secreted into the bloodstream. MUPs bind to various volatile pheromones or other lipophilic small molecules and regulate the transportation and bioactivity of these small molecules. MUPs and MUP-bound pheromones are excreted into the urine and detected by the main and accessory olfactory systems of conspecifics. MUPs are highly polymorphic, and the MUP profiles in urine are recognized as an identity signature of the owners by receivers. Additionally, circulating MUPs and MUP-bound bioactive molecules also regulate metabolism by suppressing the hepatic gluconeogenic and/or lipogenic programs as well as by promoting mitochondrial biogenesis and function and insulin sensitivity in skeletal muscles.

polymorphic, and the urinary MUP profiles are recognized as an individual identity signature of the scent owners by conspecifics. MUPs and MUP-bound pheromones are detected by both the main and the accessory olfactory systems. These two systems act coordinately to convey the information about the individual identity of signalers to the brain of conspecific receivers and to trigger behavioral responses and/or developmental processes. However, it remains completely unclear how the MUP detection system and the central nervous system extract the individual identify information encoded in the MUP profiles. Circulating MUPs may play an important role in regulating nutrient metabolism. MUPs, particularly MUP1, suppress the hepatic gluconeogenic and lipogenic programs. MUP1 also promotes mitochondrial biogenesis and oxidative phosphorylation in skeletal muscles, thus increasing energy expenditure and insulin sensitivity. However, it is unclear whether MUP1 regulates metabolism directly through its own cognate receptors or indirectly by controlling the stability, the release, and/or the activity of MUP-bound small molecules. It also remains unclear whether hypothalamic and adipose MUP1, whose expression is regulated by nutrients, regulates metabolism. Additionally, the therapeutic potential of MUP1 in treating type 2 diabetes and metabolic disorders remains to be determined.

ACKNOWLEDGMENTS

This study was supported by RO1 DK 065122 and RO1 DK073601 from NIH.

REFERENCES

Ali, S., and Drucker, D. J. (2009). Benefits and limitations of reducing glucagon action for the treatment of type 2 diabetes. *Am. J. Physiol. Endocrinol. Metab.* **296,** E415–E421.

Baur, J. A., Pearson, K. J., Price, N. L., Jamieson, H. A., Lerin, C., Kalra, A., Prabhu, V. V., Allard, J. S., Lopez-Lluch, G., Lewis, K., Pistell, P. J., Poosala, S., *et al.* (2006). Resveratrol improves health and survival of mice on a high-calorie diet. *Nature* **444,** 337–342.

Berger, F. G., and Szoka, P. (1981). Biosynthesis of the major urinary proteins in mouse liver: A biochemical genetic study. *Biochem. Genet.* **19,** 1261–1273.

Beynon, R. J., Veggerby, C., Payne, C. E., Robertson, D. H., Gaskell, S. J., Humphries, R. E., and Hurst, J. L. (2002). Polymorphism in major urinary proteins: Molecular heterogeneity in a wild mouse population. *J. Chem. Ecol.* **28,** 1429–1446.

Bocskei, Z., Findlay, J. B., North, A. C., Phillips, S. E., Somers, W. S., Wright, C. E., Lionetti, C., Tirindelli, R., and Cavaggioni, A. (1991). Crystallization of and preliminary X-ray data for the mouse major urinary protein and rat alpha-2u globulin. *J. Mol. Biol.* **218,** 699–701.

Bocskei, Z., Groom, C. R., Flower, D. R., Wright, C. E., Phillips, S. E., Cavaggioni, A., Findlay, J. B., and North, A. C. (1992). Pheromone binding to two rodent urinary proteins revealed by X-ray crystallography. *Nature* **360,** 186–188.

Breer, H., Fleischer, J., and Strotmann, J. (2006). The sense of smell: Multiple olfactory subsystems. *Cell. Mol. Life Sci.* **63,** 1465–1475.

Brennan, P. A., and Kendrick, K. M. (2006). Mammalian social odours: Attraction and individual recognition. *Philos. Trans. R. Soc. Lond. B Biol. Sci.* **361,** 2061–2078.
Bronson, F. H., and Caroom, D. (1971). Preputial gland of the male mouse; Attractant function. *J. Reprod. Fertil.* **25,** 279–282.
Bruce, H. M. (1959). An exteroceptive block to pregnancy in the mouse. *Nature* **184,** 105.
Cavaggioni, A., and Mucignat-Caretta, C. (2000). Major urinary proteins, alpha(2U)-globulins and aphrodisin. *Biochim. Biophys. Acta* **1482,** 218–228.
Chamero, P., Marton, T. F., Logan, D. W., Flanagan, K., Cruz, J. R., Saghatelian, A., Cravatt, B. F., and Stowers, L. (2007). Identification of protein pheromones that promote aggressive behaviour. *Nature* **450,** 899–902.
Cheetham, S. A., Thom, M. D., Jury, F., Ollier, W. E., Beynon, R. J., and Hurst, J. L. (2007). The genetic basis of individual-recognition signals in the mouse. *Curr. Biol.* **17,** 1771–1777.
Cheetham, S. A., Smith, A. L., Armstrong, S. D., Beynon, R. J., and Hurst, J. L. (2009). Limited variation in the major urinary proteins of laboratory mice. *Physiol. Behav.* **96,** 253–261.
Clissold, P. M., and Bishop, J. O. (1982). Variation in mouse major urinary protein (MUP) genes and the MUP gene products within and between inbred lines. *Gene* **18,** 211–220.
Darwish Marie, A., Veggerby, C., Robertson, D. H., Gaskell, S. J., Hubbard, S. J., Martinsen, L., Hurst, J. L., and Beynon, R. J. (2001). Effect of polymorphisms on ligand binding by mouse major urinary proteins. *Protein Sci.* **10,** 411–417.
De Giorgio, M. R., Yoshioka, M., and St-Amand, J. (2009). Feeding induced changes in the hypothalamic transcriptome. *Clin. Chim. Acta* **406,** 103–107.
Dhahbi, J. M., Kim, H. J., Mote, P. L., Beaver, R. J., and Spindler, S. R. (2004). Temporal linkage between the phenotypic and genomic responses to caloric restriction. *Proc. Natl. Acad. Sci. USA* **101,** 5524–5529.
Dulac, C., and Torello, A. T. (2003). Molecular detection of pheromone signals in mammals: From genes to behaviour. *Nat. Rev. Neurosci.* **4,** 551–562.
Evershed, R. P., Robertson, D. H., Beynon, R. J., and Green, B. N. (1993). Application of electrospray ionization mass spectrometry with maximum-entropy analysis to allelic 'fingerprinting' of major urinary proteins. *Rapid Commun. Mass Spectrom.* **7,** 882–886.
Finlayson, J. S., Asofsky, R., Potter, M., and Runner, C. C. (1965). Major urinary protein complex of normal mice: Origin. *Science* **149,** 981–982.
Geertzen, H. G., Ouderaa, F. J.v., and Kassenaar, A. A. (1973). Isolation and metabolism of male sex-dependent urinary protein from rats. *Acta Endocrinol. (Copenh)* **72,** 197–208.
Halpern, M., and Martinez-Marcos, A. (2003). Structure and function of the vomeronasal system: An update. *Prog. Neurobiol.* **70,** 245–318.
Hastie, N. D., Held, W. A., and Toole, J. J. (1979). Multiple genes coding for the androgen-regulated major urinary proteins of the mouse. *Cell* **17,** 449–457.
Hui, X., Zhu, W., Wang, Y., Lam, K. S., Zhang, J., Wu, D., Kraegen, E. W., Li, Y., and Xu, A. (2009). Major urinary protein-1 increases energy expenditure and improves glucose intolerance through enhancing mitochondrial function in skeletal muscle of diabetic mice. *J. Biol. Chem.* **284,** 14050–14057.
Humphries, R. E., Robertson, D. H., Beynon, R. J., and Hurst, J. L. (1999). Unravelling the chemical basis of competitive scent marking in house mice. *Anim. Behav.* **58,** 1177–1190.
Hurst, J. L. (2009). Female recognition and assessment of males through scent. *Behav. Brain Res.* **200,** 295–303.
Hurst, J. L., and Beynon, R. J. (2004). Scent wars: The chemobiology of competitive signalling in mice. *Bioessays* **26,** 1288–1298.
Hurst, J. L., Robertson, D. H. L., Tolladay, U., and Beynon, R. J. (1998). Proteins in urine scent marks of male house mice extend the longevity of olfactory signals. *Anim. Behav.* **55,** 1289–1297.

Hurst, J. L., Payne, C. E., Nevison, C. M., Marie, A. D., Humphries, R. E., Robertson, D. H., Cavaggioni, A., and Beynon, R. J. (2001). Individual recognition in mice mediated by major urinary proteins. *Nature* **414,** 631–634.

Jemiolo, B., Xie, T. M., and Novotny, M. (1991). Socio-sexual olfactory preference in female mice: Attractiveness of synthetic chemosignals. *Physiol. Behav.* **50,** 1119–1122.

Jiang, G., and Zhang, B. B. (2003). Glucagon and regulation of glucose metabolism. *Am. J. Physiol. Endocrinol. Metab.* **284,** E671–E678.

Johnson, D., Al-Shawi, R., and Bishop, J. O. (1995). Sexual dimorphism and growth hormone induction of murine pheromone-binding proteins. *J. Mol. Endocrinol.* **14,** 21–34.

Kimura, H., Odani, S., Nishi, S., Sato, H., Arakawa, M., and Ono, T. (1991). Primary structure and cellular distribution of two fatty acid-binding proteins in adult rat kidneys. *J. Biol. Chem.* **266,** 5963–5972.

Kurtz, D. T., and Feigelson, P. (1977). Multihormonal induction of hepatic alpha2u-globulin mRNA as measured by hybridization to complementary DNA. *Proc. Natl. Acad. Sci. USA* **74,** 4791–4795.

Lane, S. E., and Neuhaus, O. W. (1972). Multiple forms of 2 u, a sex-dependent urinary protein of the adult male rat. *Biochim. Biophys. Acta* **263,** 433–440.

Logan, D. W., Marton, T. F., and Stowers, L. (2008). Species specificity in major urinary proteins by parallel evolution. *PLoS ONE* **3,** e3280.

Lucke, C., Franzoni, L., Abbate, F., Lohr, F., Ferrari, E., Sorbi, R. T., Ruterjans, H., and Spisni, A. (1999). Solution structure of a recombinant mouse major urinary protein. *Eur. J. Biochem.* **266,** 1210–1218.

Meredith, M. (1994). Chronic recording of vomeronasal pump activation in awake behaving hamsters. *Physiol. Behav.* **56,** 345–354.

Miller, R. A., Chang, Y., Galecki, A. T., Al-Regaiey, K., Kopchick, J. J., and Bartke, A. (2002). Gene expression patterns in calorically restricted mice: Partial overlap with long-lived mutant mice. *Mol. Endocrinol.* **16,** 2657–2666.

More, L. (2006). Mouse major urinary proteins trigger ovulation via the vomeronasal organ. *Chem. Senses* **31,** 393–401.

Mucignat-Caretta, C., Caretta, A., and Cavaggioni, A. (1995). Acceleration of puberty onset in female mice by male urinary proteins. *J. Physiol.* **486**(Pt 2), 517–522.

Mudge, J. M., Armstrong, S. D., McLaren, K., Beynon, R. J., Hurst, J. L., Nicholson, C., Robertson, D. H., Wilming, L. G., and Harrow, J. L. (2008). Dynamic instability of the major urinary protein gene family revealed by genomic and phenotypic comparisons between C57 and 129 strain mice. *Genome Biol.* **9,** R91.

Mugford, R. A., and Nowell, N. W. (1970). Pheromones and their effect on aggression in mice. *Nature* **226,** 967–968.

Peele, P., Salazar, I., Mimmack, M., Keverne, E. B., and Brennan, P. A. (2003). Low molecular weight constituents of male mouse urine mediate the pregnancy block effect and convey information about the identity of the mating male. *Eur. J. Neurosci.* **18,** 622–628.

Robertson, D. H., Hurst, J. L., Searle, J. B., Gunduz, I., and Beynon, R. J. (2007). Characterization and comparison of major urinary proteins from the house mouse, *Mus musculus* domesticus, and the aboriginal mouse, *Mus macedonicus*. *J. Chem. Ecol.* **33,** 613–630.

Saltiel, A. R., and Kahn, C. R. (2001). Insulin signalling and the regulation of glucose and lipid metabolism. *Nature* **414,** 799–806.

Schlehuber, S., and Skerra, A. (2005). Lipocalins in drug discovery: From natural ligand-binding proteins to "anticalins". *Drug Discov. Today* **10,** 23–33.

Sharrow, S. D., Vaughn, J. L., Zidek, L., Novotny, M. V., and Stone, M. J. (2002). Pheromone binding by polymorphic mouse major urinary proteins. *Protein Sci.* **11,** 2247–2256.

Shaw, P. H., Held, W. A., and Hastie, N. D. (1983). The gene family for major urinary proteins: Expression in several secretory tissues of the mouse. *Cell* **32,** 755–761.

Sherborne, A. L., Thom, M. D., Paterson, S., Jury, F., Ollier, W. E., Stockley, P., Beynon, R. J., and Hurst, J. L. (2007). The genetic basis of inbreeding avoidance in house mice. *Curr. Biol.* **17,** 2061–2066.

Stowers, L., and Marton, T. F. (2005). What is a pheromone? Mammalian pheromones reconsidered. *Neuron* **46,** 699–702.

Thom, M. D., Stockley, P., Jury, F., Ollier, W. E., Beynon, R. J., and Hurst, J. L. (2008). The direct assessment of genetic heterozygosity through scent in the mouse. *Curr. Biol.* **18,** 619–623.

Timm, D. E., Baker, L. J., Mueller, H., Zidek, L., and Novotny, M. V. (2001). Structural basis of pheromone binding to mouse major urinary protein (MUP-I). *Protein Sci.* **10,** 997–1004.

Tirindelli, R., Dibattista, M., Pifferi, S., and Menini, A. (2009). From pheromones to behavior. *Physiol. Rev.* **89,** 921–956.

van Schothorst, E. M., Keijer, J., Pennings, J. L., Opperhuizen, A., van den Brom, C. E., Kohl, T., Franssen-van Hal, N. L., and Hoebee, B. (2006). Adipose gene expression response of lean and obese mice to short-term dietary restriction. *Obesity (Silver Spring).* **14,** 974–979.

Zhou, Y., Jiang, L., and Rui, L. (2009). Identification of MUP1 as a regulator for glucose and lipid metabolism in mice. *J. Biol. Chem.* **284,** 11152–11159.

Zidek, L., Stone, M. J., Lato, S. M., Pagel, M. D., Miao, Z., Ellington, A. D., and Novotny, M. V. (1999). NMR mapping of the recombinant mouse major urinary protein I binding site occupied by the pheromone 2-sec-butyl-4, 5-dihydrothiazole. *Biochemistry* **38,** 9850–9861.

CHAPTER SEVEN

Chemosensory Function of the Amygdala

Nicolás Gutiérrez-Castellanos,* Alino Martínez-Marcos,[†,1] Fernando Martínez-García,[‡] *and* Enrique Lanuza*

Contents

Abstract

The chemosensory amygdala has been traditionally divided into two divisions based on inputs from the main (olfactory amygdala) or accessory (vomeronasal amygdala) olfactory bulbs, supposedly playing different and independent functional roles detecting odors and pheromones, respectively. Recently, there has been increased anatomical evidence of convergence inputs from the main and

* Laboratori de Neurobiologia Funcional i Comparada, Departament de Biologia Cel·lular i Parasitologia, Facultat de Ciències Biològiques, Universitat de València, Dr. Moliner, 50, Burjassot, València, Spain

† Laboratorio de Neuroanatomía Humana, Departamento de Ciencias Médicas, Facultad de Medicina, Centro Regional de Investigaciones Biomédicas, Universidad de Castilla-La Mancha, Albacete, Spain

‡ Laboratori de Neurobiologia Funcional i Comparada, Departament de Biologia Funcional i Antropologia Física, Facultat de Ciències Biològiques, Universitat de València, Dr. Moliner, 50, Burjassot, València, Spain

1 Present address: Fac. Medicina Ciudad Real (UCLM). Avda. MOledores S/N. 13071 Ciudad Real

Vitamins and Hormones, Volume 83
ISSN 0083-6729, DOI: 10.1016/S0083-6729(10)83007-9

accessory bulbs in some areas of the amygdala, and this is correlated with functional evidence of interrelationships between the olfactory and the vomeronasal systems. This has lead to the characterization of a third division of the chemosensory amygdala, the mixed chemosensory amygdala, providing a new perspective of how chemosensory information is processed in the amygdaloid complex, in particular in relation to emotional behaviors. In this chapter, we analyze the anatomical and functional organization of the chemosensory amygdala from this new perspective. Finally, the evolutionary changes of the chemosensory nuclei of the mammalian amygdala are discussed, paying special attention to the case of primates, including humans.

Abbreviations

AAD	anterior amygdaloid area, dorsal
AAV	anterior amygdaloid area, ventral
ac	anterior commissure
acp	posterior limb of the anterior commissure
ACo	anterior cortical nucleus of the amygdala
Acb	nucleus accumbens
AHiA	amygdalo-hippocampal area
AHN	anterior hypothalamic nucleus
AOB	accessory olfactory bulb
APir	amygdalo-piriform transition area
AV	anteroventral thalamic nucleus
BAOT	nucleus of the accessory olfactory tract
BLA	basolateral nucleus of the amygdala, anterior part
BLP	basolateral nucleus of the amygdala, posterior part
BLV	basolateral nucleus of the amygdala, ventral part
BMA	basomedial nucleus of the amygdala, anterior part
BMP	basomedial nucleus of the amygdala, posterior part
BSTIA	bed nucleus of the stria terminalis, intra-amygdaloid part
BSTLP	bed nucleus of the stria terminalis, lateral division, posterior part
BSTMPI	bed nucleus of the stria terminalis, medial division, intermediate part
BSTMPL	bed nucleus of the stria terminalis, medial division, posterolateral part
BSTMPM	bed nucleus of the stria terminalis, medial division, posteromedial part
BSTS	bed nucleus of the stria terminalis, supracapsular part

BST	bed nucleus of the stria terminalis
CA	ammon's horn of the hippocampus
CeA	central amygdala
cp	cerebral peduncle
CPu	caudate putamen
CxA	corticoamygdaloid transition
DEn	dorsal endopiriform nucleus
DG	dentate gyrus
f	fornix
fi	fimbria
I	intercalated nuclei of amygdala
ic	internal capsule
ICj	islands of Calleja
IPAC	interstitial nucleus of the posterior limb of the anterior commissure
LA	lateral nucleus of the amygdala
LEnt	lateral entorhinal cortex
LGP	lateral globus pallidus
LPO	lateral preoptic area
Me	medial amygdala
MeA	anterior medial amygdala (MeAV: ventral; MeAD: dorsal)
MeP	posterior medial amygdala (MePV: ventral; MePD: dorsal)
MPO	medial preoptic area
MxCA	mixed chemosensory amygdala
NLOT	nucleus of the lateral olfactory tract
opt	optic tract
Pir	piriform cortex
PMd	dorsal premammillary nucleus
PMv	ventral premammillary nucleus
PLCo	posterior lateral cortical nucleus of the amygdala
PMCo	posterior medial cortical nucleus of the amygdala
PVA	paraventricular thalamic nucleus, anterior part
S	subiculum
SI	substantia innominata
sm	stria medularis
st	stria terminalis
Tu	olfactory tubercle
VEn	ventral endopiriform nucleus
VMHdm	ventromedial nucleus of the hypothalamus, dorsomedial part

VMHvl	ventromedial nucleus of the hypothalamus, vl: ventrolateral part
VP	ventral pallidum

I. Introduction

The term pheromone (from Greek φέρω phero "to bear" + hormone from Greek όρμή—"impetus") was first described in 1959 by Karlson and Luscher to name chemical substances secreted by some insects for intraspecific communication that were able to induce behavioral or physiological responses in conspecifics (Karlson and Luscher, 1959). Since then, several examples of this kind of substances in different species (including mammals) have been described, where they act as biologically relevant triggers for social and sexual interactions (Wyatt, 2003).

Most mammals possess two chemosensory organs, the olfactory epithelium and the vomeronasal organ. By analyzing the effects of lesions of both systems in hamsters, Powers and Winans (1975) suggested that the vomeronasal system could be fundamental for intersexual communications and mating. It was hypothesized that the vomeronasal system could detect signals with intrinsic biological relevance, specially related to reproduction, and relay this information through the accessory olfactory bulb (AOB) and the amygdala to the hypothalamus (Winans and Scalia, 1970), providing a mechanistic explanation for several phenomena apparently controlled by chemical signals, such as the Bruce's (Bruce and Parrott, 1960), Vandenbergh's (Vandenbergh, 1967), and Whitten's (Whitten, 1956) effects.

Anatomical studies during the early1970s generated the "dual olfactory hypothesis" (Raisman, 1972; Scalia and Winans, 1975; Winans and Scalia, 1970), according to which the olfactory (olfactory epithelium–main olfactory bulb (MOB)–olfactory amygdala) and vomeronasal (vomeronasal organ–AOB–vomeronasal amygdala) systems constituted parallel axis through the forebrain involved in different functions. The main olfactory system would be responsible of long-distance detection of volatile substances, whereas the vomeronasal system would be responsible of short-distance detection of nonvolatile substances (including pheromones) using active pumping mechanisms (Meredith and O'Connell, 1979).

More recent functional and anatomical data modify this view (Baxi *et al.*, 2006; Brennan and Zufall, 2006; Halpern and Martínez-Marcos, 2003; Martínez-García *et al.*, 2009; Restrepo *et al.*, 2004; Zufall and Leinders-Zufall, 2007). A number of reports demonstrate that the olfactory epithelium is able to detect pheromones (Lin *et al.*, 2004), whereas volatile odorants are detected by both olfactory and vomeronasal epithelia (Trinh and Storm, 2004). Consequently, odors and pheromones activate both the main and accessory olfactory bulbs (Xu *et al.*, 2005). Although it is largely accepted that olfactory and vomeronasal pathways run parallel and reach nonoverlapping areas in the amygdala (Shipley *et al.*, 2004), even the earliest reports suggested areas of the amygdala where olfactory and vomeronasal inputs could converge (Scalia and Winans, 1975). This point has been recently reanalyzed (Kang *et al.*, 2009; Martínez-Marcos, 2009; Pro-Sistiaga *et al.*, 2007, 2008) demonstrating the existence of mixed chemosensory–recipient cortical structures within the amygdala.

The chemosensory function of the amygdala, however, has been partially neglected in favor of a role on emotional learning associated to fear (LeDoux, 2000). In fact, it has even been proposed that the amygdala is a heterogeneous structure without anatomical or functional entity, as the chemosensory division of the amygdala would be independent of centers involved in emotional learning (Swanson and Petrovich, 1998). In this chapter, we review the connectivity, neurochemistry, and behavioral data obtained mainly in rodents to propose instead that the chemosensory amygdala processes emotional traits of olfactory and/or vomeronasal stimuli, thus supporting the functional and anatomical unity of the amygdaloid complex. In addition, the data reviewed below open new perspectives to unravel how the amygdaloid complex endows chemosensory inputs with emotional meaning.

II. Compartmentalization of the Chemosensory Amygdala

From a functional point of view, the amygdala can be divided into a chemosensory division (cortical amygdala and medial extended amygdala) that receives direct projections from the main and accessory olfactory bulbs (Martínez-Marcos, 2009), and a multimodal division, deep to the cortical amygdala (Martínez-García *et al.*, 2007), which receives inputs from sensory and associative cortical areas and is composed of the lateral, basolateral, and basomedial nuclei. This scheme is similar to the one that the American neuroanatomist J.B. Johnston proposed more than 85 years ago (Johnston, 1923), which considered a corticomedial division (cortical, medial, and central nuclei) and a basolateral division (basal and lateral nuclei), based on evolutionary and developmental considerations. Current views of the amygdaloid compartmentalization differ from Johnston's in the classification of the central nucleus of the amygdala as part of an additional amygdaloid division, the central extended amygdala, which is related to the basolateral rather than to the corticomedial division (Martínez-García *et al.*, 2008).

In this chapter, we focus on the chemosensory (or corticomedial) division of the amygdala of rodents, including the vomeronasal-recipient division of

Table 7.1 Olfactory, vomeronasal, or mixed chemosensory inputs delineate different subdivisions of the chemosensory amygdala of mammals

Chemosensory amygdaloid subdivision	Amygdaloid nuclei
Olfactory amygdala	Posterolateral cortical nucleus (PLCo)
	Amygdalo-piriform transition area (APir)
Vomeronasal amygdala	Posteromedial cortical nucleus (PMCo)
	Posteromedial bed nucleus of the stria terminalis (BSTMPM)
Mixed chemosensory amygdala	
Olfactory predominance	Anterior cortical nucleus (ACo)
	Corticoamygdaloid transition area (CxA)
	Nucleus of the lateral olfactory tract (NLOT)
Vomeronasal predominance	Medial amygdala (Me)
	Bed nucleus of the accessory olfactory tract (BAOT)
	Anterior amygdaloid area (AA)

bed nucleus of the stria terminalis as part of the medial extended amygdala (Martínez-García *et al.*, 2008; Mohedano-Moriano *et al.*, 2007; Newman, 1999). In the chemosensory amygdala, we distinguish (see Table 7.1) structures receiving projections from the MOB (olfactory amygdala), from the AOB (vomeronasal amygdala), or receiving convergent inputs from both bulbs (mixed chemosensory amygdala, MxCA). As we will see, current data suggest that the amygdalo-hippocampal area (also called posterior nucleus of the amygdala; see Canteras *et al.*, 1992) is strongly related to the vomeronasal amygdala even if it does not receive direct inputs from the AOB (see below).

In this chapter (see Fig. 7.1, Table 7.1), we follow the nomenclature of Paxinos and Franklin (2001) for the mouse amygdala, which somewhat differs from that proposed by other authors in the rat (Pitkanen *et al.*, 1997; Pitkanen, 2000; Swanson, 2004).

A. Olfactory amygdala

1. Posterolateral cortical nucleus

The description of the olfactory input to the posterolateral cortical nucleus of the amygdala was already reported in early works based on the exhaustive dissection of the lateral olfactory tract in rats and rabbits (Allison, 1953; Negus, 1956). Later, using the technique of axonal degeneration after electrolytic lesions (Fink and Heimer, 1967), Scalia and Winans (1975) described the projection from the MOB to this posterior cortical region of the amygdala. The posterolateral cortical nucleus—also named the periamygdaloid cortex (Pitkanen, 2000)—is a pallial derivative probably originated from the embryonic lateral pallium

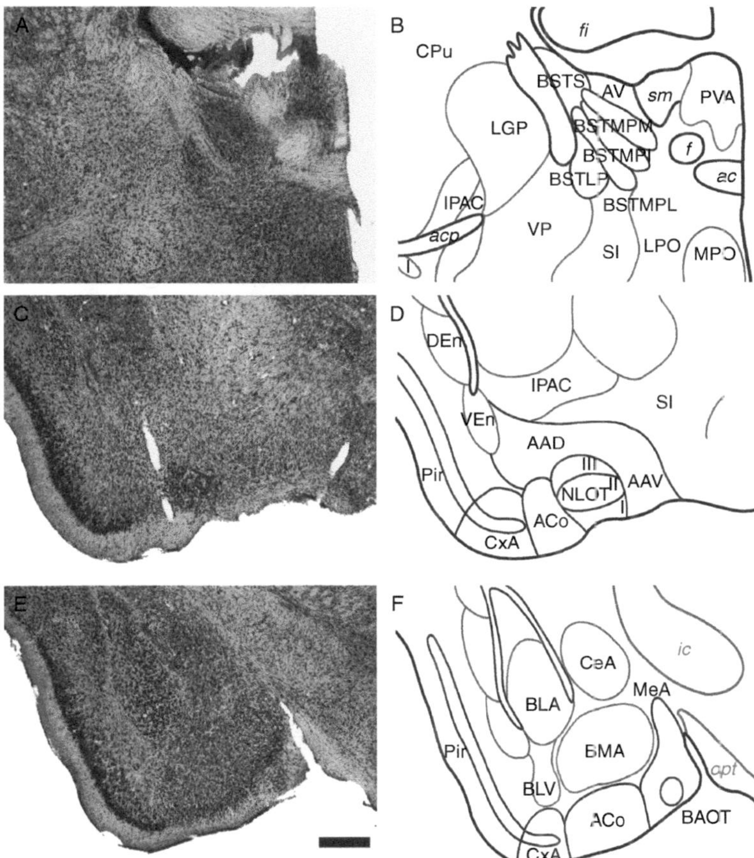

Figure 7.1 Coronal Nissl-stained sections of the mouse extended and anterior amygdala (A, C, and E) and the respective schematic interpretation of the cytoarchitectonical boundaries of the chemosensory nuclei of the amygdala (B, D, and F). For abbreviations, see list. Calibration bar: 500 μm.

(Medina *et al.*, 2004). It is located superficially, next to the caudal piriform cortex (Pir), as part of the posterior cortical amygdala (Fig. 7.2(A)–(D)). It shows a clear layering (Fig. 7.2(A)–(D)), with a molecular layer I in which the axons from the MOB terminate in its superficial half (sublayer Ia). This zone is calretinin-positive (Fig. 7.3(D)–(E)), in agreement with descriptions of calretinin immunoreactivity of mitral cells in the olfactory bulb (Wouterlood and Hrtig, 1995). Layer I also receives inputs from other amygdaloid and extra-amygdaloid inputs, mainly from chemosensory centers (Canteras *et al.*, 1992; Pitkanen, 2000). Deep to layer I, a distinct dense celled layer II can be recognized, where most of the projection cells are located (Ubeda-Bañon *et al.*, 2007). The deepest layer of the

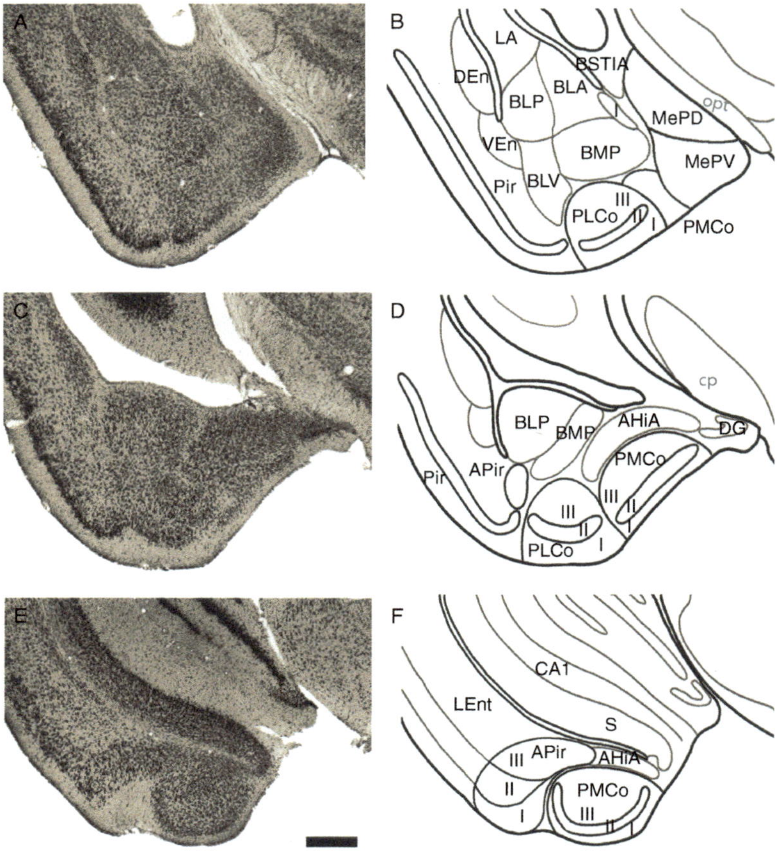

Figure 7.2 Coronal Nissl-stained sections of the mouse posterior amygdala (A, C, and E) and the respective schematic interpretation of the cytoarchitectonical boundaries of the chemosensory nuclei of the amygdala (B, D, and F). For abbreviations, see list. Calibration bar: 500 μm. (See Color Insert.)

nucleus (layer III) contains abundant loosely arranged cell bodies, many of which also belong to projection neurons (Canteras *et al.*, 1992; Ubeda-Bañon *et al.*, 2007). A number of the putative interneurons of layer II and III are immunoreactive for calretinin (Fig. 7.3(D)–(E)), calbindin, or parvalbumin (Kemppainen and Pitkanen, 2000). Only a few interneurons in PLCo, in fact in the cortical amygdala as a whole, have been observed to be positive for somatostatin and NPY (Real *et al.*, 2009).

2. Amygdalo-piriform transition area

The amygdalo-piriform transition area (APir) appears at the level of the posterior amygdala separating it from the caudal edge of the Pir (Fig. 7.2(C) and (D)). Layer II of the APir constitutes an indentation of the olfactory cortex that apparently bridges the cortical amygdala with the posterior

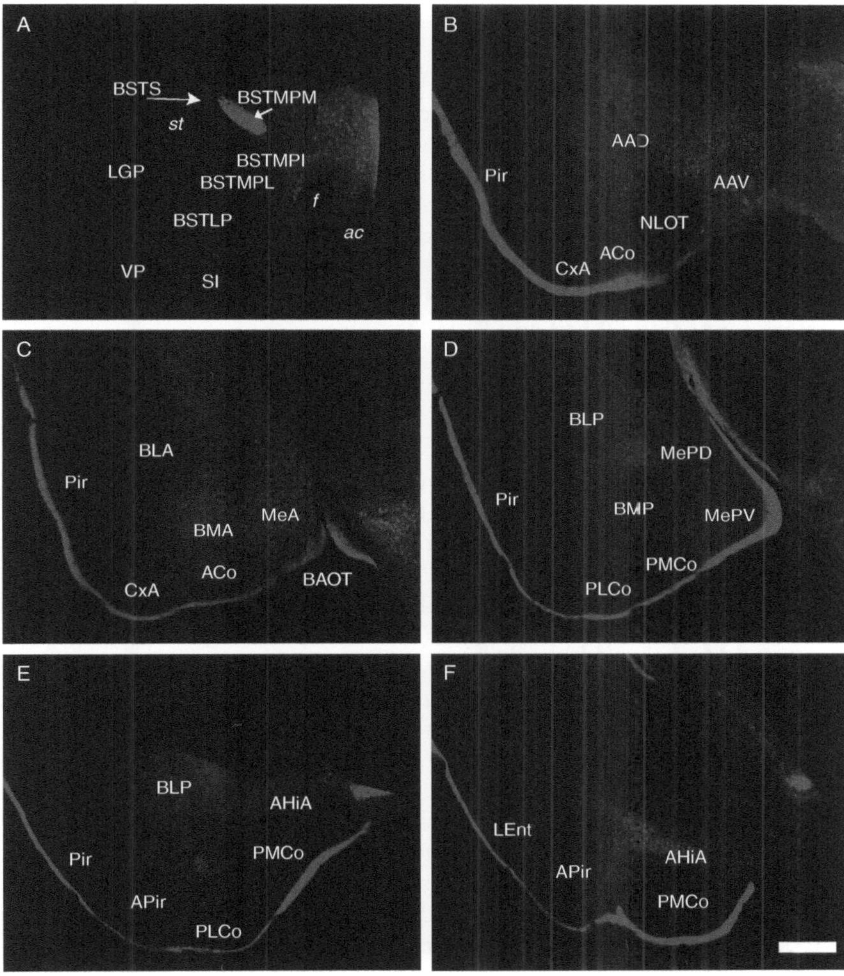

Figure 7.3 Photomicrographs of transverse sections (A, rostral; F, caudal) of a mouse brain showing the immunofluorescence detection of calretinin in the olfactory and vomeronasal projections to the chemosensory amygdala. For abbreviations, see list. Calibration bar: 500 μm. (See Color Insert.)

basolateral amygdala. Caudally, at the levels in which the Pir has disappeared in frontal sections, the APir enlarges considerably and becomes surrounded by the lateral entorhinal cortex (LEnt) (laterally) and the posteromedial amygdalo-hippocampal transition area, with which it shows an apparent continuity (Fig. 7.2(E) and (F)). In the rat, the APir has been divided into medial and lateral divisions, with the medial division being further subdivided into anterior and posterior portions (Jolkkonen *et al.*, 2001; Santiago and Shammah-Lagnado, 2005).

It is controversial whether the APir has a superficial part receiving olfactory input. Some authors consider the APir a deep structure (Paxinos and Franklin, 2001), while others consider that the APir extends up to the pial surface in a region of the caudal amygdala where the molecular layer is specially thick, located between the caudal edge of the Pir and the posteromedial cortical nucleus (PMCo) of the amygdala (Jolkkonen *et al.*, 2001; Santiago and Shammah-Lagnado, 2005). Calretinin immunoreactivity suggests that this thickened molecular layer would indeed receive a direct olfactory input (Fig. 7.3(E) and (F)).

B. Vomeronasal amygdala

1. Posteromedial cortical nucleus

The PMCo of the amygdala was among the first amygdaloid structures reported to receive inputs from the AOB (Winans and Scalia, 1970). It is a pallial structure, possibly derived from the ventral pallium (Martínez-García *et al.*, 2007; Medina *et al.*, 2004). The PMCo displays a special layering with a molecular layer I receiving vomeronasal projections (Fig. 7.5(E) and (F)) that is positive for calretinin (Fig. 7.3(E) and (F)), neuropilin (Fig. 7.4(D)), and acetylcholinesterase (Paxinos and Franklin, 2001). As explained above, calretinin appears to be a marker of chemosensory inputs (Wouterlood and Hrtig, 1995), whereas neuropilin and acetylcholinesterase appear to be specific markers for the vomeronasal pathway (Fig. 7.4(D)). Layer I also receives extra- and intra-amygdaloid projections (Canteras *et al.*, 1992; Kemppainen *et al.*, 2002; our unpublished data in mice). Layer II shows a relatively low cell density, as compared with the adjoining PLCo, and displays small cell bodies. In contrast, layer III neurons show larger cell bodies with polymorphic morphology. The inner limits of layer III are not easy to delineate. Projections from these layers have been reported to the ventral striatum (Ubeda-Bañon *et al.*, 2008). The histochemical detection of vesicular zinc is helpful to trace the boundary between layers II and III (Kemppainen *et al.*, 2002).

2. Posteromedial part of the medial bed nucleus of the stria terminalis

The bed nucleus of the stria teminalis (BST) is a very complex structure, highly compartmentalized, the posterior part of the medial division of which is usually included in the medial extended amygdala. Specifically, the posteromedial part of the medial BST (BSTMPM) receives direct inputs from the AOB (Scalia and Winans, 1975). The BSTMPM is a group of homogenous, densely packed, and darkly stained cells (with acidophilic colorants) (Fig. 7.1(A) and (B)). As in the case of the PMCo, the BSTMPM shows a remarkable immunoreactivity for calretinin (Fig. 7.3(A)) and neuropilin-2 (Fig. 7.4(A)) that apparently coincides with the termination of the afferent from the AOBs (von Campenhausen and Mori, 2000).

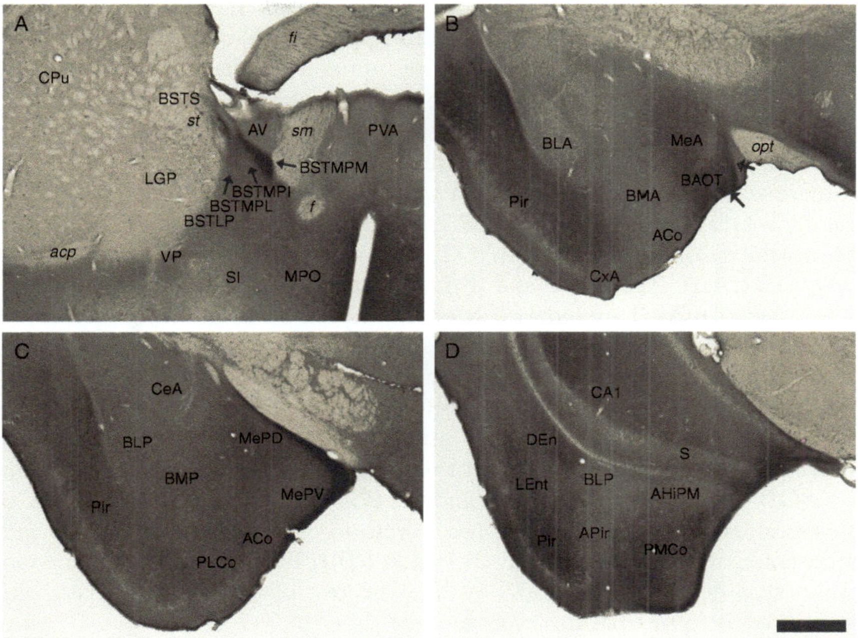

Figure 7.4 Brightfield photomicrographs of transverse sections (A, rostral; D, caudal) of a mouse brain showing the immunohistochemical detection of neuropilin-2 in the chemosensory amygdala, where it specifically labels the projections coming from the AOB. For abbreviations, see list. Calibration bar: 500 μm. (See Color Insert.)

Recent reports indicate that vomeronasal inputs to the BSTMPM arise from the anterior part of the AOB, thus conveying information from neurons of the vomeronasal organ expressing V1R receptors (Mohedano-Moriano *et al.*, 2007). The projections of the BSTMPM to the hypothalamus and other areas have been traced in the rat (Dong and Swanson, 2004). These anatomical data indicate that the regions of the amygdala processing information arising from V1R vomeronasal receptors (BSTMPM) and those receiving mainly V2R inputs show differential projections to the hypothalamus (Mohedano-Moriano *et al.*, 2008).

C. Mixed chemosensory amygdala with olfactory predominance

1. Anterior cortical nucleus

The anterior cortical nucleus (ACo) of the amygdala is the largest structure of the MxCA and shows a clear olfactory predominance (Pro-Sistiaga *et al.*, 2007). At rostral levels of the amygdala, the ACo is located between the other two amygdaloid structures showing mixed chemosensory inputs, namely the corticoamygdaloid transition area (CxA) and the nucleus of the lateral olfactory tract (NLOT). The inputs from the main (major) and accessory (minor) olfactory bulbs show a differential laminar distribution, with olfactory axons terminating superficial to vomeronasal afferents (Fig. 7.5(B) and (C)). This differential lamination of the olfactory and vomeronasal inputs is also found in the CxA and NLOT. More caudally, the ACo enlarges considerably and is situated lateral to the bed nucleus of the accessory olfactory tract (BAOT) and adjacent to the anterior medial amygdala (MeA; Fig. 7.1(E) and (F)). At caudal levels, it is located between the posterior medial amygdala (PMe) and the PLCo (Fig. 7.2(A) and (B)).

The ACo receives its olfactory afferent throughout layer Ia, where it again matches the immunoreactivity for calretinin. The vomeronasal projection (from the AOB) is quantitatively minor and only reaches the most anterior part of nucleus (Pro-Sistiaga *et al.*, 2007) where it terminates in deep layer I (layer Ib). In contrast to other regions receiving inputs from the AOBs (e.g., layer Ia of PMCo and the BSTMPM), this layer of the ACo shows weak immunoreactivity for calretinin (Fig. 7.3(B) and (C)) and appears negative for neuropilin-2 (Fig. 7.4(B)). Deep to layer I, the ACo shows two cell layers (II and III), like the rest of cortical amygdala, but lamination is somewhat more diffuse.

2. Corticoamygdaloid transition area

The CxA is located between the Pir and the ACo (rostrally) (Fig. 7.1(E) and (F)) or the anterior PLCo (caudally). Like other portions of the olfacto-recipient cortex, it shows a quite neat trilayered structure. Layer I receives a superficial (Ia) olfactory input coinciding with the immunoreactivity for calretinin (Fig. 7.3(B) and (C)). Deep to the olfactory innervation, layer Ib receives a minor vomeronasal afferent (Pro-Sistiaga *et al.*, 2007), which seems weakly immunoreactive for neuropilin-2 (Fig. 7.4(B)). The cell layers (II and III) contain projecting neurons. Although the boundary of the CxA with the Pir is not clearly distinguishable in Nissl preparations, the CxA shows a weak acetylcholinesterase reactivity (Paxinos and Franklin, 2001) and a moderately dense dopaminergic innervation (Paxinos *et al.*, 1999) that allow an easy delineation of this structure.

3. Nucleus of the lateral olfactory tract

The NLOT is a superficial nucleus of the amygdala present at rostral levels, supposedly accompanying the fibers of the lateral olfactory tract (thus its name). It is located between the ventral portion of the anterior amygdala and the ACo. In Nissl-stained sections, the NLOT stands out as a portion of the anterior edge of the cortical amygdala with a conspicuous molecular layer I, a thickened layer II showing a nearly circular profile in frontal sections, and a layer III containing loosely organized cells (Fig. 7.1(C) and (D)). The developmental origins of the

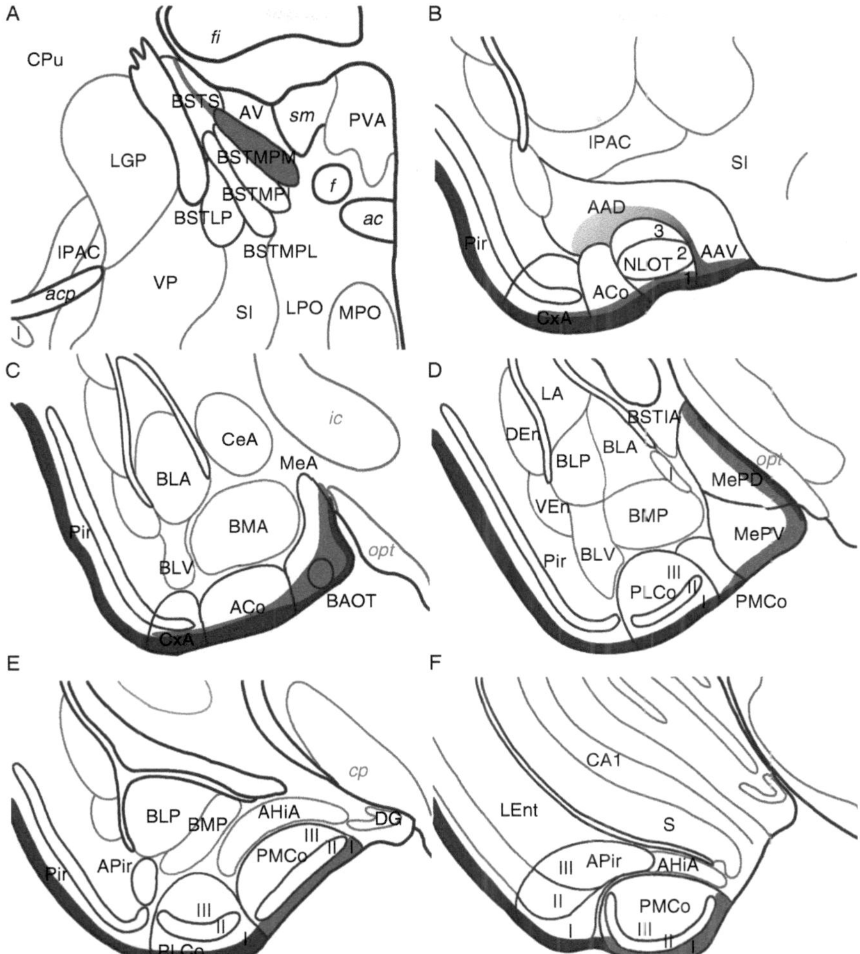

Figure 7.5 Schematic representation of the olfactory (in red) and vomeronasal (in blue) pathways in rodents to the cortical and extended amygdala originated, respectively, by the MOB and AOB. The segregation or integration of both types of information is indicated, delimiting the olfactory, vomeronasal, or mixed chemosensory centers of the amygdala. For abbreviations, see list. (See Color Insert.)

NLOT are heterogeneous. The cells of layer II originate from a region of the neuroepithelium lining the ventral aspect of the caudolateral recess of the lateral ventricle, whose properties recall the embryonic dorsal pallium. From there, layer II NLOT cells migrate rostrally through the caudal amygdaloid stream (Remedios *et al.*, 2007) to become sandwiched between layers I and III that originate from of the rostral pallial neuroepithelium. The NLOT is easily delineated thanks to its high reactivity for the histochemistry of acetyl cholinesterase (Paxinos and Franklin, 2001).

Two sublayers can be distinguished within layer I. Sublayer Ia (superficial) contains the fibers from the MOB, whereas fibers arising in the AOB run through the limit between layers Ia and Ib, where they have been shown to be presynaptic to dendritic elements (Pro-Sistiaga *et al.*, 2007), thus providing a vomeronasal input to a traditional olfactory structure (Fig. 7.5(B)). In contrast to other portions of the olfactory amygdala, layer Ia of the NLOT shows only low-to-moderate immunoreactivity for calretinin (Fig. 7.3(B)). In contrast, like in other regions of the vomeronasal amygdala, the portion of layer I receiving the input from the AOB (sublayer Ib) shows an intense immunoreactivity for neuropilin-2 (not shown).

Neurons of layer II originate the main projections of the NLOT to the olfactory amygdala, as well as a major projection to the olfactory tubercle (Tu) and islands of Calleja (ICj) (Luskin and Price, 1983; Price, 1987) or the dwarf cells of the Tu (Santiago and Shammah-Lagnado, 2004). Remarkably, layer III neurons contribute significantly to the connections of the NLOT (Ottersen, 1980; Santiago and Shammah-Lagnado, 2004).

D. Mixed chemosensory amygdala with vomeronasal predominance

1. Medial amygdala

The medial nucleus of the amygdala was soon recognized as a target of the vomeronasal projections of the AOB (Winans and Scalia, 1970). However, as suggested in early reports in different mammals (Scalia and Winans, 1975) and confirmed recently in rats (Pro-Sistiaga *et al.*, 2007) and mice (Kang *et al.*, 2009), the anterior part of the Me (MeA) also receives a substantial olfactory input. In mice (Kang *et al.*, 2009), but not in rats (Martínez-Marcos, 2009), the posterodorsal part of the Me (MePD) has also been shown to receive a direct olfactory input (Fig. 7.5(C) and (D)). Attending to embryological, anatomical, and functional data, the medial amygdala (Me) is a very complex structure (Choi *et al.*, 2005). Thus, although the Me has traditionally been considered a pure striatal derivative (Swanson and Petrovich, 1998), recent evidence suggests that its cells arise from multiple sources including the ventral pallium, the striatum and the preoptic-entopeduncular histogenetic territory, and maybe parts of the hypothalamic neuroepithelium (Garcia-Lopez *et al.*, 2008; Medina *et al.*, 2004).

The MeA begins at the level of the NLOT, with which it limits laterally. More caudally, it is adjacent to the BAOT and the ACo. The inner part of the MeA limits with the BMA (Fig. 7.1(E) and (F)). Although the MeA lacks a clear lamination, the afferents arising from the main and accessory olfactory bulbs show a laminar pattern, the olfactory ones occupying a superficial location relative to the (thicker) vomeronasal input (Fig. 7.5(C)) (Kang *et al.*, 2009; Pro-Sistiaga *et al.*, 2007). As can be appreciated in Fig. 7.3(C), the MeA displays a weak subpial immunostaining for calretinin, whereas the immunoreactivity for neuropilin-2 extends from the ventral surface of the BAOT to deep layers of the MeA (Fig. 7.4(B)).

Regarding the MeP, several anatomical and functional evidences indicate that it is a heterogeneous structure in which ventral and dorsal divisions can be distinguished. The posterior ventral division (MePV) is located just medial to the ACo rostrally and PMCo caudally (Fig. 7.2(A) and (B)). The posterior dorsal division (MePD) seems to be continuous with the dorsal aspect of the MeA and extends dorsally adjacent to the basomedial nucleus of the amygdala and the intra-amygdaloid portion of the BST (BSTIA; Fig. 7.2(A) and (B)). The MePD and MePV can be differentiated with a number of genetic markers which reveal also differential embryological origins and functions of each subdivision (Choi *et al.*, 2005).

The vomeronasal system seems to be composed of at least two subsystems that can be traced into the medial extended amygdala (Martínez-Marcos and Halpern, 1999b). In the vomeronasal organ, neurons expressing V1R and V2R receptors are segregated and project in a nonoverlapping manner to the anterior and posterior divisions of the AOB, respectively (Jia and Halpern, 1996). Although both the anterior and posterior divisions of the AOB project to layer Ia of the Me, the deep cell layers of the MeAV (Mohedano-Moriano *et al.*, 2007), MeAD, and MePV (Martínez-Marcos and Halpern, 1999b) receive an exclusive input from the posterior AOB. As we have seen, this contrasts with the BSTMPM, which receives an exclusive input from the anterior AOB. These data indicate that, in spite of a massive overlap of the projections of both divisions of the AOB in layer I of the Me, the deep layers of the MeA and of the MePV receive information from V2R-expressing vomeronasal neurons, whereas the BSTMPM receives vomeronasal information only by V1R-expressing neurons.

2. Bed nucleus of the accessory olfactory tract

The BAOT is composed of cells associated to the axons of the accessory olfactory tract, and thus can be considered the vomeronasal equivalent of the NLOT. It is a small and round group of compacted cells located immediately posterior to the NLOT, medial to the ACo, and lateral to the MeA. In the BAOT, like in the rest of the vomeronasal amygdala, the vomeronasal input coincides with a dense immunoreactivity for calretinin (Fig. 7.3(C)) and neuropilin-2 (Fig. 7.4(B)). In addition to this input from the AOB, it has been recently demonstrated that the cells in the BAOT also receive synapses from axons originating in the MOB, thus revealing that the BAOT also processes olfactory information (Pro-Sistiaga *et al.*, 2007).

3. Anterior amygdaloid area

The anterior amygdaloid area is the rostral-most structure of the amygdala, where it is adjacent to the subcortical basal forebrain. The ventral (superficial) portion of the anterior amygdala (AAV) is usually considered an olfactory structure since it receives direct afferents from the MOB (Kevetter and Winans, 1981). However, recent experimental works using sensitive tracing techniques have demonstrated that the dorsal (deep) portion of the anterior amygdala (AAD) also receives direct projections from the AOB (Mohedano-Moriano *et al.*, 2007).

The AAV is medial to the NLOT, caudal to the caudal Tu, and rostral to the MeA (Fig. 7.1(C) and (D)). At rostral levels, the AAV is superficial to the AAD, magnocellular preoptic nucleus, and nucleus of the horizontal limb of the diagonal band. Caudally, it is superficial to the substantia innominata. In contrast, the AAD is deep to the LOT and ACo, laterally adjacent to the substantia innominata (SI) and medial to the Pir and the ventral endopiriform nucleus. It extends caudally until the anterior basomedial nucleus of the amygdala (Fig. 7.1(C)). The pallial or subpallial nature of the AAD is not clear yet (see Martínez-García *et al.*, 2007). However, recent data of the expression of genetic markers (Tole *et al.*, 2005) indicate that the AAD might be a subpallial derivative, as it is targeted by Pax6-expressing cells arising from the dorsal lateral ganglionic eminence. In line with this, the AAD shows some large acetylcholinesterase reactive cells that apparently correspond to displaced neurons of the basal cholinergic cells group (De Olmos *et al.*, 2004).

III. Functional Anatomy of the Chemosensory Amygdala

A. Olfactory amygdala

In contrast to other nuclei of the cortical amygdala, which are targeted by olfactory and vomeronasal inputs (ACo, NLOT, and CxA), the posterolateral cortical nucleus of the amygdala (PLCo) only receives inputs from the MOB. Its connectivity in the rat is well described. It is reciprocally connected with the rest of the olfactory cortex (Luskin and Price, 1983), including the APir and endopiriform nucleus (Behan and Haberly, 1999), and shows feedback projections to the MOB. It also projects to the vomeronasal amygdala (Canteras *et al.*, 1992), including the PMCo (Majak and Pitkänen, 2003), Me, and distinct subdivisions of the BST (Dong *et al.*, 2001) and receives afferents from the vomeronasal cortex (PMCo; Kemppainen *et al.*, 2002). In addition, the PLCo projects to the central extended amygdala (CeA and BSTLP) (Canteras *et al.*, 1992; Dong *et al.*, 2001), a projection that extends further rostrally to reach other ventral striatal regions such as the nucleus accumbens, the Tu, and the Calleja islands (Ubeda-Bañon *et al.*, 2007). In addition, the PLCo gives rise to important projections to the hippocampal formation (CA3, CA1, and ventral subiculum), as well as to intra-amygdaloid projections targeting the lateral nucleus (Majak and Pitkänen, 2003).

Therefore, the PLCo seems directly involved in the processing of olfactory stimuli through its interconnections with the MOBs and the different parts of the olfactory cortex. In addition, its direct and indirect (through the entorhinal cortex) projections to the hippocampal formation suggest that it plays an important role in the generation of olfactory memories or to engrave olfactory stimuli on episodic memories (Fig. 7.6). Moreover, through its direct projections to the lateral amygdala the PLCo might allow association of odors to stimuli of other modalities for emotional learning related to odors (e.g., odor fear conditioning).

As discussed above, also the PLCo gives rise to connections to the ventral striatum, classically considered as the main reward center in the brain (Fig. 7.6). These projections are very interesting from a functional point of view since they may be involved in processing the rewarding properties of odors with intrinsic biological relevance (chemical signals) or odors that become secondary rewarding stimuli when associated with other natural rewards, as has been shown for the case of sexual activity (Kippin *et al.*, 2003) or sexual pheromones (Martínez-Ricós *et al.*, 2007).

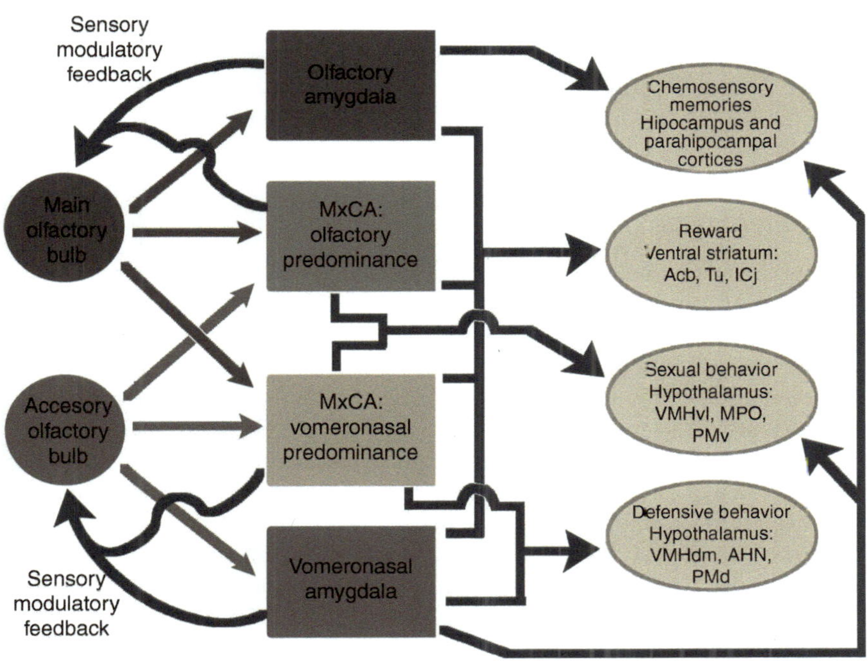

Figure 7.6 Schematic representation of the main inputs and outputs of the chemosensory structures of the amygdala, indicating the principal role that olfactory and vomeronasal information may be playing in different behavioral responses known to be influence by chemical signals. For abbreviations, see list. (See Color Insert.)

The APir was traditionally considered as a rostroventral extension of the LEnt (Krettek and Price, 1977) and, in fact, they share several anatomical features. Thus, like the LEnt, the APir is part of the olfactory cortex, *senso lato*, and it is interconnected with the remaining areas of the olfactory cortex (including part of the entorhinal cortex). However, recent hodological studies reveal specific patterns of efferent and afferent connections of the APir (Santiago and Shammah-Lagnado, 2005; Shammah-Lagnado and Santiago, 1999). The APir receive important thalamic afferents from gustatory and visceroceptive midline nuclei, as well as direct gustatory/visceroceptive afferents from the parabrachial nucleus. In addition, in contrast to the entorhinal cortex but similar to the PLCo, the APir projects massively to the central amygdala (Jolkkonen *et al.*, 2001; McDonald *et al.*, 1999) and the medial ventral striatum (Brog *et al.*, 1993; Shammah-Lagnado and Santiago, 1999).

This convergence of gustatory, interoceptive, and olfactory stimuli makes the APir a central node for mediating emotional responses to feeding or specific food items. Appetitive responses might be mediated by the APir projections to the ventral striatum whereas aversive responses would course through its output to the central extended amygdala.

Finally, there is a remarkable projection from the APir to the CA1 layer of the hippocampus. This pathway does not use the perforant path, possibly one of the main differences between the pattern of connectivity of the APir and the LEnt (Jolkkonen *et al.*, 2001). This direct projection may allow the APir to influence the formation of olfactory memories in relation, for instance, to food recognition (Fig. 7.6).

B. Vomeronasal amygdala

Among the structures considered strictly vomeronasal, the only structure with cortical characteristics and pallial origin (Medina *et al.*, 2004) is the PMCo, which, therefore, could be considered as the primary vomeronasal cortex.

The connectivity of the PMCo has been studied in the rat (Canteras *et al.*, 1992; Kemppainen *et al.*, 2002) and recently also in the sheep (Meurisse *et al.*, 2009). Among the main projections of the PMCo described in the rat, it is worth mentioning a massive glutamatergic projection to the granular layer of the AOB, which provides a feedback loop at the sensory level and modulates the pheromone signal processing (Fan and Luo, 2009; Martínez-Marcos and Halpern, 1999a). This feedback projection from the primary sensory cortex to the bulb recalls the olfactory system, further supporting the view of the PMCo as the primary vomeronasal cortex (Fig. 7.6).

Like the primary olfactory cortex, the PMCo is also interconnected with the remaining secondary vomeronasal nuclei (Me, BAOT, BST, contralateral PMCo). In addition, the PMCo is also interconnected with parts of the olfactory cortex (PLCo, Pir, LEnt, DEN), thus becoming a primary vomeronasal cortex that receives also tertiary olfactory inputs. This stresses the high degree of convergence between olfactory and vomeronasal stimuli, thus virtually refuting, from the anatomical point of view, the classical view of the "dual olfactory hypothesis."

In addition to the interconnections with other chemosensory centers of the cerebral hemispheres, the PMCo is also connected reciprocally with the hippocampal formation, in particular with the subiculum and CA3 layer of hippocampus (Canteras *et al.*, 1992; Kemppainen *et al.*, 2002). These interconnections of the PMCo and hippocampus suggest a possible involvement of vomeronasal stimuli in the generation of spatial maps and spatial learning, although functional evidence of this hypothesis is lacking.

The only major target of the PMCo that does not originate feedback projections to it is the ventral striatum. Specifically, the PMCo projects to the Tu and anteromedial ICj (Ubeda-Bañon *et al.*, 2008). This projection has been suggested to be involved in the neural processing of the reinforcing properties of sexual pheromones (Lanuza *et al.*, 2008; Fig. 7.6). As previously described, the PLCo also projects over the ventral striatum, and both projections seem to overlap significantly (compare Ubeda-Bañon *et al.*, 2007, 2008), although the projection from PLCo seems to terminate in a posterolateral portion of the ventral striatum as compared with the input from the PMCo (Martínez-Marcos, 2009).

Very few studies have tackled the behavioral or functional role of the PMCo. Romero *et al.* (1990) reported that lesions of the PMCo of female rats resulted in a decreased androtropism, for example, a decrease in the time that female rats spent in the proximity of a caged intact male as compared to a castrated male. However, a more recent study on the effects of lesions of the PMCo in sexual behavior of golden hamsters (Maras and Petrulis, 2008) reported no alterations of the preference for the urine of a conspecific of the opposite sex, but showed a mild alteration in copulatory behavior. It has to be taken into account that attraction in hamsters seems to be due to volatile pheromonal compounds in urine, likely detected by the olfactory system (O'Connell and Meredith, 1984). Consequently, in hamsters the PMCo might play a minor role in the reinforcing or attractive value of conspecifics' urine. However, the electrolytic lesions may have also affected the amygdalo-hippocampal transition area overlying the PMCo. At least in rats, this structure sends projections to hypothalamic centers related with sexual behavior (Canteras *et al.*, 1992). Further anatomical and functional studies in other species are therefore needed to clarify the function of this nucleus.

The BSTMPM and the adjoining subnuclei of the bed nucleus of the posterior part of the medial BST show specific patterns of connections with the hypothalamus and brainstem that have been well studied in the rat (Dong and Swanson, 2004; Dong *et al.*, 2001). These patterns of connections suggest that the posterior division of the BST, including the BSTMPM targeted by direct afferents from the AOB, is involved in defensive and reproductive behavioral responses that at least in mice are very likely mediated by vomeronasal stimuli (Leypold *et al.*, 2002; Stowers *et al.*, 2002). This nucleus has been reported to receive inputs exclusively from V1R vomeronasal receptors through connections from the anterior AOB (Mohedano-Moriano *et al.*, 2007). Functionally, it has been reported that low molecular weight constituents of male urine activating the anterior AOB mediate the pregnancy block effect and convey information about the identity of the mating male (Peele *et al.*, 2003), thus suggesting a detection through V1R vomeronasal receptors. In contrast, the major urinary proteins (MUPs) involved in intermale aggression in mice are known to be detected by V2R receptors (Chamero *et al.*, 2007). This renders further support to the view, put forward by Mohedano-Moriano *et al.* (2008) that pathways arising from V1R- and V2R-expressing vomeronasal neurons are segregated up to the hypothalamus. Differential activation of these two pathways by different pheromones would result in activation of different sets of hypothalamic nuclei resulting in facilitation of sexual or agonistic behaviors or in defined neuroendocrine responses (Fig. 7.6).

C. Mixed chemosensory amygdala

Among the structures of the MxCA with olfactory predominance, the ACo of the amygdala is best characterized. Based on anatomical data, two roles for the ACo have been suggested. Besides the direct inputs from the main and accessory olfactory bulbs, the afferents to the ACo from parts of the olfactory cortex (Luskin and Price, 1983) and from vomeronasal structures like the MeP and PMCo point to this nucleus as a site of convergence of different chemosensory inputs. However, the ACo not only projects to vomeronasal structures but also to hypothalamic centers involved in sexual behavior, like the medial preoptic nucleus or the ventromedial hypothalamic nucleus. For this reason, the ACo may be considered as an important center for the integration of olfactory and vomeronasal information involved in sexual behavior (Petrovich *et al.*, 1996).

Second, the ACo is connected with the BMA (Petrovich *et al.*, 1996), both receive convergent olfactory (Scalia and Winans, 1975) and gustatory (Bernard *et al.*, 1993) inputs, and both project to thalamic and hypothalamic centers related to taste. Therefore, the ACo and the BMA have been postulated to be part of a functional circuit involved in feeding behavior and, more specifically, in olfactory–gustatory integration (Petrovich *et al.*, 1996).

In contrast, functional data on the NLOT are fragmentary (De Olmos *et al.*, 2004), so that functional considerations are mainly based on a few studies analyzing specifically the connectivity of the nucleus in the rat (Santiago and Shammah-Lagnado, 2004). According to these studies (Haberly and Price, 1978; Luskin and Price, 1983), the NLOT is interconnected with most of the cortical olfactory structures, including the MOB, the anterior olfactory nucleus, and Pir. Afferents to the NLOT also originate in other regions of the cortical and subcortical telencephalon. Thus, the strong reactivity for acetylcholinesterase histochemistry seems related to afferents from the SI (Hecker and Mesulam, 1994). Moreover, the ventral subiculum (Canteras and Swanson, 1992) and LEnt (McDonald and Mascagni, 1997) also show important projections to the NLOT.

Concerning its projections, besides its connections with other olfactory cortical structures, the NLOT shows remarkably strong bilateral efferents to the basolateral nucleus of the amygdala (arising in its layer III cells) and to the ventral striatum, specifically to the Tu and ICj (arising in layer II cells). This distinct pattern of connections of layers II and III likely reflect the different embryological origin of the cells of both layers (Remedios *et al.*, 2007). In addition, the basolateral amygdala and the ventral striatum are both part of the reward circuitry of the brain (Baxter and Murray, 2002), thus suggesting a role of the NLOT in reward processing of chemosensory stimuli (Fig. 7.6).

Finally, to the best of our knowledge there is an almost complete lack of anatomical and functional data about the corticoamygdaloid transition area.

Concerning the MxCA with vomeronasal predominance, the Me is a very complex nucleus usually divided, as explained above, into anterior and posterior divisions (Gomez and Newman, 1992; Usunoff *et al.*, 2009), often further subdivided in dorsal and ventral subnuclei (Canteras *et al.*, 1995). This division fits the pattern of expression of genes of the Lhx family. Thus, the anterior (MeA, with dorsal and ventral divisions, MeAD, and MeAD) part of the Me expresses Lhx5. Within the MeP, this gene family also renders distinct expression patterns, as the MePD expresses Lhx6, whereas MePV is positive for Lhx9 (Choi *et al.*, 2005). These differential patterns of gene expression are related to the heterogeneous origin of the cells of the subnuclei of the Me, as analyzed in detail by Garcia-Lopez *et al.* (2008) in the mouse.

In addition, the divisions delineated by the expression of Lhx genes in the Me seem related to the different functions played by its subnuclei. Thus, the MePD (and also the BSTMPM) seems involved mainly in reproductive behaviors, whereas MePV is activated by the expression of defensive behaviors (Choi *et al.*, 2005). Both subnuclei would elicit these behavioral responses through direct pathways to different hypothalamic centers (Fig. 7.6). The functional neuroanatomy of the MeA is less studied. There is evidence in hamsters suggesting that a strong interaction of the MeAD and MePD is necessary for the attraction to possible mates (Maras and Petrulis, 2009).

Regarding the bed nucleus of the accessory tract, anatomical data are fragmentary and functional data controversial. Probably due to its small size and "hidden" position, there is not much information regarding the connectivity of this nucleus, although there is evidence of a profuse connectivity of the BAOT with the rest of the amygdaloid vomeronasal structures, including a centrifugal projection to the AOB (Martínez-Marcos and Halpern, 1999a). Also specific projections from V2R receptors through the posterior AOB to the deep aspect of the BAOT have been described in rats

(Mohedano-Moriano *et al.*, 2007), which suggest a possible role of this nucleus in behaviors driven by proteins secreted by the extraorbital lacrimal gland (Kimoto *et al.*, 2005), MUPs involved in intermale aggression (Chamero *et al.*, 2007) or nonvolatile ligands associated to the major histocompatibility complex (Brennan and Kendrick, 2006) including attraction and individual recognition, which are very important for adaptive sociosexual interactions. Electrolytic lesions of the BAOT in rats apparently increase maternal behavior in both males (Izquierdo *et al.*, 1992) and virgin females (Del Cerro *et al.*, 1991). However, the possible involvement of fibers of the accessory olfactory tract in the electrolytic lesions in these studies (thus interrupting the vomeronasal innervation of the rest of vomeronasal amygdaloid structures) should be taken into account to interpret these results.

In the same vein, part of the anterior amygdaloid area, namely the AAD, receives differential inputs from V2R receptors through the posterior AOB (Mohedano-Moriano *et al.*, 2007) and sends specific inputs to the hypothalamus (Mohedano-Moriano *et al.*, 2008). This pathway may also be involved in the response to molecules detected by this type of receptors (Brennan and Kendrick, 2006; Chamero *et al.*, 2007; Kimoto *et al.*, 2005), although there is no experimental evidence in support of this hypothesis.

IV. Evolutionary Relevance of the Chemosensory Amygdala

Anatomically, the chemosensory amygdala is well described in several species of amphibians, reptiles, and mammals (Lanuza and Halpern, 1997; Martínez-García *et al.*, 2007; Martínez-Marcos *et al.*, 1999; Moreno and Gonzalez, 2006; Pitkanen, 2000). In nonhuman primates, there are relatively few studies analyzing the cytoarchitecture, connectivity, and function of this set of nuclei. In humans, there are a few data on cytoarchitecture, and functional data come from patients undergoing brain infarction and functional imaging studies of volunteer subjects (Amaral *et al.*, 1992; Price, 1987, 1990), the connectivity being ignored. Therefore, the identity and boundaries of the different chemosensory centers of the amygdala of primates (particularly humans) are imprecisely determined.

Nevertheless, it is quite clear that rodents and primates must show important differences. The former are considered macrosmatic species, in which the olfactory and vomeronasal senses are the predominant sensory systems for numerous relevant biological functions (e.g., Brennan and Zufall, 2006; Del Cerro, 1998; Martínez-Ricós *et al.*, 2008), while most primates (specially humans) are considered microsmatic species, in which the chemical senses are less important for basic biological functions (e.g., mate choice), while other sensory modalities (e.g., vision) play a more important role (Krupp, 2008; Roney, 2003; Roney and Simmons, 2008). The functional relevance of the olfactory and vomeronasal systems in different taxa correlates with the development of the chemosensory amygdala (Martínez-García *et al.*, 2007) and, therefore, it is a significant feature to be taken into account when comparing the organization of the amygdala of rodents and primates.

Among primates, there are two big subdivisions from taxonomic and evolutionary points of view: the New World Monkeys (Platirrhine) such as the marmoset and the Old World Monkeys (Catarrhine) including macaques and humans. In New World monkeys, a functional vomeronasal system has been described with a vomeronasal organ present in adult animals. In Old World monkeys, however, the vomeronasal system appears to be vestigial in fetuses and absent or nonfunctional in adults (Maier, 1997; Martínez-Marcos, 2001; Smith *et al.*, 2001). Although some authors claim that the vomeronasal organ is recognizable in adults, there is no evidence of vomeronasal nerve or AOB in humans (the issue of the vomeronasal amygdala in humans is discussed below). "Pheromonal" functions in humans are under debate and, if they exist, could be mediated by the olfactory system (Brennan and Zufall, 2006; Meredith, 2001).

In the course of evolution, a key phenomenon for this divergence was the development of a multicolor vision. This trait is not only useful for arboreal species of primates to differentiate between the fruits and foliage, but also allows the development of new sexual communication systems. For example, the tonality of the anogenital skin in the sexual receptivity period in baboon females (Zhang and Webb, 2003). This change of evolutionary strategy could lead to a decrease of pheromonal importance in primates (Zhang and Webb, 2003).

As discussed above, there are few data regarding connectivity of the olfactory bulbs in primates. To our knowledge, studies in new world monkeys are limited to the projections of the MOB (Liebetanz *et al.*, 2002) with similar results to those of old world primates (Carmichael *et al.*, 1994; Turner *et al.*, 1978), thus leaving unidentified the vomeronasal amygdala of primates. This makes delimiting the chemosensory structures of the primate amygdala a very difficult task and leads to controversies about the true identity of the medial amygdala described in the human brain (Mai *et al.*, 2008). It is unknown, for instance, whether the vomeronasal inputs have been substituted by olfactory ones or have simply disappeared.

To discuss the hypothesis of a reduction of the size of the chemosensory amygdala associated with the development of color vision, we can take advantage of similar, better documented evolutionary modifications, as it is in the case of the LEnt.

The LEnt is a six-layered structure receiving a direct olfactory input. In rodents, virtually 100% of the LEnt can be considered as olfactory recipient (Insausti *et al.*, 2002) probably playing a role in the formation of olfactory memories (Ferry *et al.*, 2006) via the perforant path to the hippocampus (Steward, 1967). In macaques, about 15% of LEnt is olfactory recipient, and the olfactory input is likely to be even more reduced in humans (Insausti *et al.*, 2002). This reduction in the olfactory input is accompanied by a remarkable increase of inputs of other sensory modalities (mainly visual) or multimodal inputs.

A similar process may have happened in the case of the chemosensory amygdala. We hypothesize that in primates the importance of emotional processing of chemosensory stimuli has been reduced, although it is possible that this information keeps playing a very important role in some behaviors like breast-feeding (Varendi and Porter, 2001), maternal behavior, or even in the reproductive mate choice (Ober *et al.*, 1997). In contrast, other stimuli (visual) may have gained weight in amygdaloid processing and might play a key role for biologically relevant processes such as individual recognition and mate choice, which in rodents seem to be mainly chemosensory.

In the human species, the existence of true pheromones has been questioned many times (in part given the difficulty to design experiments that can test innate responses). As we have discussed before, humans lack a functional vomeronasal system and, therefore, in the case that human pheromones exist, they should be olfactory stimuli (very likely volatile molecules). To check this possibility, several studies have investigated the existence in humans of genes coding for vomeronasal receptors (Giorgi *et al.*, 2000), as well as the expression of those genes in the vomeronasal organ or in the olfactory epithelium (Kouros-Mehr *et al.*, 2001). Also, it has been tested whether in the human olfactory epithelium there are other kinds of receptors able to detect pheromonal signals, as it happens in rodents (Hagino-Yamagishi, 2008). These studies have shown that the human genome possesses a few genes coding for vomeronasal receptors type V1R, which express functional receptors when transfected into HeLa/Olf cells, and respond with cAMP as second messenger when exposed to different chemosensory stimulus (Shirokova *et al.*, 2008). Remarkably, studies demonstrating the functionality of those receptors *in vivo* are lacking.

These results indicate, as suggested above, that if pheromonal substances exist in humans, they would be detected via the olfactory system. According to this possibility, several studies have demonstrated the existence of volatile substances with pheromonal characteristics (Schaal *et al.*, 2003) in other mammalian species. This opens the possibility of the existence of volatile substances of similar characteristics in human beings (Schaal *et al.*, 2009), although this hypothesis has yet to be proved.

The existence of amygdaloid structures in primates (including humans) with anatomical (and maybe functional) characteristics similar to those in the rodent chemosensory amygdala opens the possibility of an amygdaloid processing of such stimuli. This would include emotional tagging of stimuli as attractive/reinforcing or aversive. This possibility is supported by functional magnetic resonance studies in humans in which different odors supposed to be innately attractive or aversive produced different activation patterns in the amygdala and were used as unconditioned stimuli to elicit conditioned emotional responses to neutral faces (Gottfried *et al.*, 2002). This emotional learning involved activation of the posterior amygdala (putative chemosensory amygdala). These data integrate the chemosensory amygdala within the global perspective of the amygdala as the center of the brain emotional processing. Further, they suggest that in humans there is a chemosensory amygdala able to recognize innately attractive or aversive olfactory stimulus and use them for the generation of learned (emotional) behavioral responses to conspecifics.

V. Conclusions and Future Directions

This chapter summarizes a new vision of the chemosensory amygdala that would include the olfactory, the vomeronasal, and the MxCA (where olfactory and vomeronasal inputs would converge). The chemosensory amygdala is included anatomically and functionally within the general scheme of the amygdaloid complex as a center for emotional processing. Evolutionary changes undergone by the chemosensory amygdala are discussed including changes occurred in primates and humans.

Acknowledgments

This study has been supported by the Spanish Ministry of Education and Science-FEDER (BFU2007-67912-C02-01/BFI to FMG and BFU2007-62290/BFI to AMM) and the Autonomous Government of Castilla-La Mancha (PCC08-0064 to AMM and EL).

References

Allison, A. (1953). The structure of the olfactory bulb and its relationship to the olfactory pathways in the rabbit and the rat. *J. Comp. Neurol.* **98,** 309–353.

Amaral, D. G., Price, J. L., Pitkanen, A., and Carmichael, T. (1992). Anatomical organization of the primate amygdala complex. *In* "The Amygdala," (J. Aggleton, Ed.), 1st edn., pp. 1–67. Wiley-Liss, New York.

Baxi, K. N., Dorries, K. M., and Eisthen, H. L. (2006). Is the vomeronasal system really specialized for detecting pheromones? *Trends Neurosci.* **29,** 1–7.

Baxter, M. G., and Murray, E. A. (2002). The amygdala and reward. *Nat. Rev. Neurosci.* **3,** 563–573.

Behan, M., and Haberly, L. B. (1999). Intrinsic and efferent connections of the endopiriform nucleus in rat. *J. Comp. Neurol.* **408,** 532–548.

Bernard, J. F., Alden, M., and Besson, J. M. (1993). The organization of the efferent projections from the pontine parabrachial area to the amygdaloid complex: A *Phaseolus vulgaris* leucoagglutinin (PHA-L) study in the rat. *J. Comp. Neurol.* **329,** 201–229.

Brennan, P. A., and Kendrick, K. M. (2006). Mammalian social odours: Attraction and individual recognition. *Philos. Trans. R. Soc. Lond. B Biol. Sci.* **361,** 2061–2078.

Brennan, P. A., and Zufall, F. (2006). Pheromonal communication in vertebrates. *Nature* **444,** 308–315.

Brog, J. S., Salyapongse, A., Deutch, A. Y., and Zahm, D. S. (1993). The patterns of afferent innervation of the core and shell in the "accumbens" part of the rat ventral striatum: Immunohistochemical detection of retrogradely transported fluoro-gold. *J. Comp. Neurol.* **338,** 255–278.

Bruce, H. M., and Parrott, D. M. (1960). Role of olfactory sense in pregnancy block by strange males. *Science* **131,** 1526.

Canteras, N. S., and Swanson, L. W. (1992). Projections of the ventral subiculum to the amygdala, septum, and hypothalamus: A PHAL anterograde tract-tracing study in the rat. *J. Comp. Neurol.* **324,** 180–194.

Canteras, N. S., Simerly, R. B., and Swanson, L. W. (1992). Connections of the posterior nucleus of the amygdala. *J. Comp. Neurol.* **324,** 143–179.

Canteras, N. S., Simerly, R. B., and Swanson, L. W. (1995). Organization of projections from the medial nucleus of the amygdala: A PHAL study in the rat. *J. Comp. Neurol.* **360,** 213–245.

Carmichael, S. T., Clugnet, M. C., and Price, J. L. (1994). Central olfactory connections in the macaque monkey. *J. Comp. Neurol.* **346,** 403–434.

Chamero, P., Marton, T. F., Logan, D. W., Flanagan, K., Cruz, J. R., Saghatelian, A., Cravatt, B. F., and Stowers, L. (2007). Identification of protein pheromones that promote aggressive behaviour. *Nature* **450,** 899–902.

Choi, G. B., Dong, H. W., Murphy, A. J., Valenzuela, D. M., Yancopoulos, G. D., Swanson, L. W., and Anderson, D. J. (2005). Lhx6 delineates a pathway mediating innate reproductive behaviors from the amygdala to the hypothalamus. *Neuron* **46,** 647–660.

De Olmos, J. S., Beltramino, C. A., and Alheid, G. (2004). Amygdala and extended amygdala of the rat: A cytoarchitectonical, fibroarchitectonical and chemoarchitectonical survey. *In* "The Rat Nervous System," (G. Paxinos, Ed.), 4th edn. Elsevier, San Diego.

Del Cerro, M. C. (1998). Role of the vomeronasal input in maternal behavior. *Psychoneuroendocrinology* **23,** 905–926.

Del Cerro, M. C., Izquierdo, M. A., Collado, P., Segovia, S., and Guillamón, A. (1991). Bilateral lesions of the bed nucleus of the accessory olfactory tract facilitate maternal behavior in virgin female rats. *Physiol. Behav.* **50,** 67–71.

Dong, H. W., and Swanson, L. W. (2004). Projections from bed nuclei of the stria terminalis, posterior division: Implications for cerebral hemisphere regulation of defensive and reproductive behaviors. *J. Comp. Neurol.* **471,** 396–433.

Dong, H. W., Petrovich, G. D., and Swanson, L. W. (2001). Topography of projections from amygdala to bed nuclei of the stria terminalis. *Brain Res. Brain Res. Rev.* **38,** 192–246.

Fan, S., and Luo, M. (2009). The organization of feedback projections in a pathway important for processing pheromonal signals. *Neuroscience* **161,** 489–500.

Ferry, B., Ferreira, G., Traissard, N., and Majchrzak, M. (2006). Selective involvement of the lateral entorhinal cortex in the control of the olfactory memory trace during conditioned odor aversion in the rat. *Behav. Neurosci.* **120,** 1180–1186.

Fink, R. P., and Heimer, L. (1967). Two methods for selective silver impregnation of degenerating axons and their synaptic endings in the central nervous system. *Brain Res.* **4,** 369–374.

Garcia-Lopez, M., Abellan, A., Legaz, I., Rubenstein, J. L., Puelles, L., and Medina, L. (2008). Histogenetic compartments of the mouse centromedial and extended amygdala based on gene expression patterns during development. *J. Comp. Neurol.* **506,** 46–74.

Giorgi, D., Friedman, C., Trask, B. J., and Rouquier, S. (2000). Characterization of nonfunctional V1R-like pheromone receptor sequences in human. *Genome Res.* **10,** 1979–1985.

Gomez, D. M., and Newman, S. W. (1992). Differential projections of the anterior and posterior regions of the medial amygdaloid nucleus in the Syrian hamster. *J. Comp. Neurol.* **317,** 195–218.

Gottfried, J. A., O'Doherty, J., and Dolan, R. J. (2002). Appetitive and aversive olfactory learning in humans studied using event-related functional magnetic resonance imaging. *J. Neurosci.* **22,** 10829–10837.

Haberly, L. B., and Price, J. L. (1978). Association and commissural fiber systems of the olfactory cortex of the rat. *J. Comp. Neurol.* **178,** 711–740.

Hagino-Yamagishi, K. (2008). Diverse systems for pheromone perception: Multiple receptor families in two olfactory systems. *Zool. Sci.* **25,** 1179–1189.

Halpern, M., and Martínez-Marcos, A. (2003). Structure and function of the vomeronasal system: An update. *Prog. Neurobiol.* **70,** 245–318.

Hecker, S., and Mesulam, M. M. (1994). Two types of cholinergic projections to the rat amygdala. *Neuroscience* **60,** 383–397.

Insausti, R., Marcos, P., Arroyo-Jiménez, M. M., Blaizot, X., and Martínez-Marcos, A. (2002). Comparative aspects of the olfactory portion of the entorhinal cortex and its projection to the hippocampus in rodents, nonhuman primates, and the human brain. *Brain Res. Bull.* **57,** 557–560.

Izquierdo, M. A., Collado, P., Segovia, S., Guillamón, A., and del Cerro, M. C. (1992). Maternal behavior induced in male rats by bilateral lesions of the bed nucleus of the accessory olfactory tract. *Physiol. Behav.* **52,** 707–712.

Jia, C., and Halpern, M. (1996). Subclasses of vomeronasal receptor neurons: Differential expression of G proteins ($G_{i\alpha 2}$ and $G_{o\alpha}$) and segregated projections to the accessory olfactory bulb. *Brain Res.* **719,** 117–128.

Johnston, J. B. (1923). Further contribution to the study of the evolution of the forebrain. *J. Comp. Neurol.* **35,** 337–481.

Jolkkonen, E., Miettinen, R., and Pitkänen, A. (2001). Projections from the amygdalo-piriform transition area to the amygdaloid complex: A PHA-l study in rat. *J. Comp. Neurol.* **432,** 440–465.

Kang, N., Baum, M. J., and Cherry, J. A. (2009). A direct main olfactory bulb projection to the 'vomeronasal' amygdala in female mice selectively responds to volatile pheromones from males. *Eur. J. Neurosci.* **29,** 624–634.

Karlson, P., and Luscher, M. (1959). Pheromones': A new term for a class of biologically active substances. *Nature* **183,** 55–56.

Kemppainen, S., and Pitkanen, A. (2000). Distribution of parvalbumin, calretinin, and calbindin-D(28 k) immunoreactivity in the rat amygdaloid complex and colocalization with gamma-aminobutyric acid. *J. Comp. Neurol.* **426,** 441–467.

Kemppainen, S., Jolkkonen, E., and Pitkanen, A. (2002). Projections from the posterior cortical nucleus of the amygdala to the hippocampal formation and parahippocampal region in rat. *Hippocampus* **12,** 735–755.

Kevetter, G. A., and Winans, S. S. (1981). Connections of the corticomedial amygdala in the golden hamster. II. Efferents of the "olfactory amygdala". *J. Comp. Neurol.* **197,** 99–111.

Kimoto, H., Haga, S., Sato, K., and Touhara, K. (2005). Sex-specific peptides from exocrine glands stimulate mouse vomeronasal sensory neurons. *Nature* **437,** 898–901.

Kippin, T. E., Cain, S. W., and Pfaus, J. G. (2003). Estrous odors and sexually conditioned neutral odors activate separate neural pathways in the male rat. *Neuroscience* **117,** 971–979.

Kouros-Mehr, H., Pintchovski, S., Melnyk, J., Chen, Y. J., Friedman, C., Trask, B., and Shizuya, H. (2001). Identification of non-functional human VNO receptor genes provides evidence for vestigiality of the human VNO. *Chem. Senses* **26,** 1167–1174.

Krettek, J. E., and Price, J. L. (1977). Projections from the amygdaloid complex and adjacent olfactory structures to the entorhinal cortex and to the subiculum in the rat and cat. *J. Comp. Neurol.* **172,** 723–752.

Krupp, D. B. (2008). Through evolution's eyes: Extracting mate preferences by linking visual attention to adaptive design. *Arch. Sex. Behav.* **37,** 57–63.

Lanuza, E., and Halpern, M. (1997). Afferent and efferent connections of the nucleus sphericus in the snake *Thamnophis sirtalis*: Convergence of olfactory and vomeronasal information in the lateral cortex and the amygdala. *J. Comp. Neurol.* **385,** 627–640.

Lanuza, E., Novejarque, A., Martínez-Ricós, J., Martínez-Hernández, J., Agustín-Pavón, C., and Martínez-García, F. (2008). Sexual pheromones and the evolution of the reward system of the brain: The chemosensory function of the amygdala. *Brain Res. Bull.* **75,** 460–466.

LeDoux, J. E. (2000). Emotion circuits in the brain. *Annu. Rev. Neurosci.* **23,** 155–184.

Leypold, B. G., Yu, C. R., Leinders-Zufall, T., Kim, M. M., Zufall, F., and Axel, R. (2002). Altered sexual and social behaviors in trp2 mutant mice. *Proc. Natl. Acad. Sci. USA* **99,** 6376–6381.

Liebetanz, D., Nitsche, M. A., Fromm, C., and Reyher, C. K. (2002). Central olfactory connections in the microsmatic marmoset monkey (*Callithrix jacchus*). *Cells Tissues Organs* **172,** 53–69.

Lin, W., Arellano, J., Slotnick, B., and Restrepo, D. (2004). Odors detected by mice deficient in cyclic nucleotide-gated channel subunit A2 stimulate the main olfactory system. *J. Neurosci.* **24,** 3703–3710.

Luskin, M. B., and Price, J. L. (1983). The topographic organization of associational fibers of the olfactory system in the rat, including centrifugal fibers to the olfactory bulb. *J. Comp. Neurol.* **216,** 264–291.

Mai, J. K., Paxinos, G., and Voss, T. (2008). Atlas of the Human Brain. Elsevier, New York.

Maier, W. (1997). The nasopalatine duct and the nasal floor cartilages in catarrhine primates. *Z. Morphol. Anthropol.* **81,** 289–300.

Majak, K., and Pitkänen, A. (2003). Projections from the periamygdaloid cortex to the amygdaloid complex, the hippocampal formation, and the parahippocampal region: A PHA-L study in the rat. *Hippocampus* **13,** 922–942.

Maras, P. M., and Petrulis, A. (2008). The posteromedial cortical amygdala regulates copulatory behavior, but not sexual odor preference, in the male Syrian hamster (*Mesocricetus auratus*). *Neuroscience* **156,** 425–435.

Maras, P. M., and Petrulis, A. (2009). Lesions that functionally disconnect the anterior and posterodorsal sub-regions of the medial amygdala eliminate opposite-sex odor preference in male Syrian hamsters (*Mesocricetus auratus*). *Neuroscience* **165,** 1052–1062.

Martínez-García, F., Novejarque, A., and Lanuza, E. (2007). Evolution of the Amygdala in Vertebrates. *In* "Evolution of Nervous Systems," (J. H. Kaas, Ed.), Vol. 2, pp. 255–334. Academic Press, Oxford.

Martínez-García, F., Novejarque, A., and Lanuza, E. (2008). Two interconnected functional systems in the amygdala of amniote vertebrates. *Brain Res. Bull.* **75,** 206–213.

Martínez-García, F., Martínez-Ricós, J., Agustín-Pavón, C., Martínez-Hernández, J., Novejarque, A., and Lanuza, E. (2009). Refining the dual olfactory hypothesis: Pheromone reward and odour experience. *Behav. Brain Res.* **200,** 277–286.

Martínez-Marcos, A. (2001). Controversies on the human vomeronasal system. *Eur. J. Anat.* **5,** 47–53.

Martínez-Marcos, A. (2009). On the organization of olfactory and vomeronasal cortices. *Prog. Neurobiol.* **87,** 21–30.

Martínez-Marcos, A., and Halpern, M. (1999a). Differential centrifugal afferents to the anterior and posterior accessory olfactory bulb. *NeuroReport* **10,** 2011–2015.

Martínez-Marcos, A., and Halpern, M. (1999b). Differential projections from the anterior and posterior divisions of the accessory olfactory bulb to the medial amygdala in the opossum, *Monodelphis domestica. Eur. J. Neurosci.* **11,** 3789–3799.

Martínez-Marcos, A., Lanuza, E., and Halpern, M. (1999). Organization of the ophidian amygdala: Chemosensory pathways to the hypothalamus. *J. Comp. Neurol.* **412,** 51–68.

Martínez-Ricós, J., Agustín-Pavón, C., Lanuza, E., and Martínez-García, F. (2007). Intraspecific communication through chemical signals in female mice: Reinforcing properties of involatile male sexual pheromones. *Chem. Senses* **32,** 139–148.

Martínez-Ricós, J., Agustín-Pavón, C., Lanuza, E., and Martínez-García, F. (2008). Role of the vomeronasal system in intersexual attraction in female mice. *Neuroscience* **153,** 383–395.

McDonald, A. J., and Mascagni, F. (1997). Projections of the lateral entorhinal cortex to the amygdala: A *Phaseolus vulgaris* leucoagglutinin study in the rat. *Neuroscience* **77,** 445–459.

McDonald, A. J., Shammah-Lagnado, S. J., Shi, C., and Davis, M. (1999). Cortical afferents to the extended amygdala. *Ann. NY Acad. Sci.* **877,** 309–338.

Medina, L., Legaz, I., González, G., De Castro, F., Rubenstein, J. L., and Puelles, L. (2004). Expression of Dbx1, Neurogenin 2, Semaphorin 5A, Cadherin 8, and Emx1 distinguish ventral and lateral pallial histogenetic divisions in the developing mouse claustroamygdaloid complex. *J. Comp. Neurol.* **474,** 504–523.

Meredith, M. (2001). Human vomeronasal organ function: A critical review of best and worst cases. *Chem. Senses* **26,** 433–445.

Meredith, M., and O'Connell, R. J. (1979). Efferent control of stimulus access to the hamster vomeronasal organ. *J. Physiol.* **286,** 301–316.

Meurisse, M., Chaillou, E., and Lévy, F. (2009). Afferent and efferent connections of the cortical and medial nuclei of the amygdala in sheep. *J. Chem. Neuroanat.* **37,** 87–97.

Mohedano-Moriano, A., Pro-Sistiaga, P., Ubeda-Bañón, I., Crespo, C., Insausti, R., and Martínez-Marcos, A. (2007). Segregated pathways to the vomeronasal amygdala: Differential projections from the anterior and posterior divisions of the accessory olfactory bulb. *Eur. J. Neurosci.* **25,** 2065–2080.

Mohedano-Moriano, A., Pro-Sistiaga, P., Ubeda-Bañon, I., de la Rosa-Prieto, C., Saiz-Sanchez, D., and Martínez-Marcos, A. (2008). V1R and V2R segregated vomeronasal pathways to the hypothalamus. *NeuroReport* **19,** 1623–1626.

Moreno, N., and Gonzalez, A. (2006). The common organization of the amygdaloid complex in tetrapods: New concepts based on developmental, hodological and neurochemical data in anuran amphibians. *Prog. Neurobiol.* **78,** 61–90.

Negus, V. E. (1956). The organ of Jacobson. *J. Anat.* **90,** 515–590.

Newman, S. W. (1999). The medial extended amygdala in male reproductive behavior. A node in the mammalian social behavior network. *Ann. NY Acad. Sci.* **877,** 242–257.

Ober, C., Weitkamp, L. R., Cox, N., Dytch, H., Kostyu, D., and Elias, S. (1997). HLA and mate choice in humans. *Am. J. Hum. Genet.* **61,** 497–504.

O'Connell, R. J., and Meredith, M. (1984). Effects of volatile and nonvolatile chemical signals on male sex behaviors mediated by the main and accessory olfactory systems. *Behav. Neurosci.* **98,** 1083–1093.

Ottersen, O. P. (1980). Afferent connections to the amygdaloid complex of the rat and cat: II. Afferents from the hypothalamus and the basal telencephalon. *J. Comp. Neurol.* **194,** 267–289.

Paxinos, G., and Franklin, K. B. J. (2001). The Mouse Brain in Stereotaxic Coordinates. Elsevier, San Diego.

Paxinos, G., Kus, L., Ashwell, K. W. S., and Watson, C. (1999). Chemoarchitectonic Atlas of the Rat Forebrain. Academic Press, London.

Peele, P., Salazar, I., Mimmack, M., Keverne, E. B., and Brennan, P. A. (2003). Low molecular weight constituents of male mouse urine mediate the pregnancy block effect and convey information about the identity of the mating male. *Eur. J. Neurosci.* **18,** 622–628.

Petrovich, G. D., Risold, P. Y., and Swanson, L. W. (1996). Organization of projections from the basomedial nucleus of the amygdala: A PHAL study in the rat. *J. Comp. Neurol.* **374,** 387–420.

Pitkanen, A. (2000). Connectivity of the rat amygdaloid complex. *In* "The Amygdala. A functional Analysis," (J. P. Aggleton, Ed.), 2nd edn., pp. 31–115. Oxford University Press, Oxford.

Pitkanen, A., Savander, V., and Ledoux, J. E. (1997). Organization of intra-amygdaloid circuitries in the rat: An emerging framework for understanding functions of the amygdala. *Trends Neurosci.* **20,** 517–523.

Powers, J. B., and Winans, S. S. (1975). Vomeronasal organ: Critical role in mediating sexual behavior of the male hamster. *Science* **187,** 961–963.

Price, J. L. (1987). The central olfactory and accessory olfactory systems. *In* "Neurobiology of Taste and Smell," (T. E. Finger and W. L. Silver, Eds.), pp. 179–203. John Wiley & Sons, New York.

Price, J. L. (1990). Olfactory system. *In* "The Human Nervous System," (G. Paxinos, Ed.), pp. 979–998. Academic Press, San Diego.

Pro-Sistiaga, P., Mohedano-Moriano, A., Ubeda-Bañon, I., Arroyo-Jimenez, M. M., Marcos, P., Artacho-Pérula, E., Crespo, C., Insausti, R., and Martínez-Marcos, A. (2007). Convergence of olfactory and vomeronasal projections in the rat basal telencephalon. *J. Comp. Neurol.* **504,** 346–362.

Pro-Sistiaga, P., Mohedano-Moriano, A., Ubeda-Bañon, I., de la Rosa-Prieto, C., Saiz-Sanchez, D., and Martínez-Marcos, A. (2008). Projections of olfactory bulbs to the olfactory and vomeronasal cortices. *NeuroReport* **19,** 1541–1544.

Raisman, G. (1972). An experimental study of the projection of the amygdala to the accessory olfactory bulb and its relationship to the concept of a dual olfactory system. *Exp. Brain Res.* **14,** 395–408.

Real, M. A., Heredia, R., Labrador, M. C., Dávila, J. C., and Guirado, S. (2009). Expression of somatostatin and neuropeptide Y in the embryonic, postnatal, and adult mouse amygdalar complex. *J. Comp. Neurol.* **513,** 335–348.

Remedios, R., Huilgol, D., Saha, B., Hari, P., Bhatnagar, L., Kowalczyk, T., Hevner, R. F., Suda, Y., Aizawa, S., Ohshima, T., Stoykova, A., and Tole, S. (2007). A stream of cells migrating from the caudal telencephalon reveals a link between the amygdala and neocortex. *Nat. Neurosci.* **10,** 1141–1150.

Restrepo, D., Arellano, J., Oliva, A. M., Schaefer, M. L., and Lin, W. (2004). Emerging views on the distinct but related roles of the main and accessory olfactory systems in responsiveness to chemosensory signals in mice. *Horm. Behav.* **46,** 247–256.

Romero, P. R., Beltramino, C. A., and Carrer, H. F. (1990). Participation of the olfactory system in the control of approach behavior of the female rat to the male. *Physiol. Behav.* **47,** 685–690.

Roney, J. R. (2003). Effects of visual exposure to the opposite sex: Cognitive aspects of mate attraction in human males. *Pers. Soc. Psychol. Bull.* **29,** 393–404.

Roney, J. R., and Simmons, Z. L. (2008). Women's estradiol predicts preference for facial cues of men's testosterone. *Horm. Behav.* **53,** 14–19.

Santiago, A. C., and Shammah-Lagnado, S. J. (2004). Efferent connections of the nucleus of the lateral olfactory tract in the rat. *J. Comp. Neurol.* **471,** 314–332.

Santiago, A. C., and Shammah-Lagnado, S. J. (2005). Afferent connections of the amygdalopiriform transition area in the rat. *J. Comp. Neurol.* **489,** 349–371.

Scalia, F., and Winans, S. S. (1975). The differential projections of the olfactory bulb and accessory olfactory bulb in mammals. *J. Comp. Neurol.* **161,** 31–55.

Schaal, B., Coureaud, G., Langlois, D., Giniès, C., Sémon, E., and Perrier, G. (2003). Chemical and behavioural characterization of the rabbit mammary pheromone. *Nature* **424,** 68–72.

Schaal, B., Coureaud, G., Doucet, S., Delaunay-El Allam, M., Moncomble, A. S., Montigny, D., Patris, B., and Holley, A. (2009). Mammary olfactory signalisation in females and odor processing in neonates: Ways evolved by rabbits and humans. *Behav. Brain Res.* **200,** 346–358.

Shammah-Lagnado, S. J., and Santiago, A. C. (1999). Projections of the amygdalopiriform transition area (APir). A PHA-L study in the rat. *Ann. NY Acad. Sci.* **877,** 655–660.

Shipley, M. T., Ennis, M., and Puche, A. C. (2004). Olfactory system. *In* "The Rat Nervous System," (G. Paxinos, Ed.), pp. 923–964. Elsevier Academic Press, San Diego.

Shirokova, E., Raguse, J. D., Meyerhof, W., and Krautwurst, D. (2008). The human vomeronasal type-1 receptor family—Detection of volatiles and cAMP signaling in HeLa/Olf cells. *FASEB J.* **22,** 1416–1425.

Smith, T. D., Siegel, M. I., and Bhatnagar, K. P. (2001). Reappraisal of the vomeronasal system of catarrhine primates: Ontogeny, morphology, functionality, and persisting questions. *Anat. Rec.* **265,** 176–192.

Steward, O. (1967). Topographic organization of the projections from the entorhinal area to the hippocampal formation of the rat. *J. Comp. Neurol.* **167,** 285–314.

Stowers, L., Holy, T. E., Meister, M., Dulac, C., and Koentges, G. (2002). Loss of sex discrimination and male–male aggression in mice deficient for TRP2. *Science* **295,** 1493–1500.

Swanson, L. W. (2004). Brain Maps: Structure of the Rat Brain. Elsevier, San Diego.

Swanson, L. W., and Petrovich, G. D. (1998). What is the amygdala? *Trends Neurosci.* **21,** 323–331.

Tole, S., Remedios, R., Saha, B., and Stoykova, A. (2005). Selective requirement of Pax6, but not Emx2, in the specification and development of several nuclei of the amygdaloid complex. *J. Neurosci.* **25,** 2753–2760.

Trinh, K., and Storm, D. R. (2004). Detection of odorants through the main olfactory epithelium and vomeronasal organ of mice. *Nutr. Rev.* **62,** S189–S192.

Turner, B. H., Gupta, K. C., and Mishkin, M. (1978). The locus and cytoarchitecture of the projection areas of the olfactory bulb in *Macaca mulatta*. *J. Comp. Neurol.* **177,** 381–396.

Ubeda-Bañon, I., Novejarque, A., Mohedano-Moriano, A., Pro-Sistiaga, P., de la Rosa-Prieto, C., Insausti, R., Martínez-García, F., Lanuza, E., and Martínez-Marcos, A. (2007). Projections from the posterolateral olfactory amygdala to the ventral striatum: Neural basis for reinforcing properties of chemical stimuli. *BMC Neurosci.* **8,** 103.

Ubeda-Bañon, I., Novejarque, A., Mohedano-Moriano, A., Pro-Sistiaga, P., Insausti, R., Martínez-García, F., Lanuza, E., and Martínez-Marcos, A. (2008). Vomeronasal inputs to the rodent ventral striatum. *Brain Res. Bull.* **75,** 467–473.

Usunoff, K. G., Schmitt, O., Itzev, D. E., Haas, S. J., Lazarov, N. E., Rolfs, A., and Wree, A. (2009). Efferent projections of the anterior and posterodorsal regions of the medial nucleus of the amygdala in the mouse. *Cells Tissues Organs* **190,** 256–285.

Vandenbergh, J. G. (1967). Effect of the presence of a male on the sexual maturation of female mice. *Endocrinology* **81,** 345–349.

Varendi, H., and Porter, R. H. (2001). Breast odour as the only maternal stimulus elicits crawling towards the odour source. *Acta Paediatr.* **90,** 372–375.

von Campenhausen, H., and Mori, K. (2000). Convergence of segregated pheromonal pathways from the accessory olfactory bulb to the cortex in the mouse. *Eur. J. Neurosci.* **12,** 33–46.

Whitten, W. K. (1956). Modification of the oestrous cycle of the mouse by external stimuli associated with the male. *J. Endocrinol.* **13,** 399–404.

Winans, S. S., and Scalia, F. (1970). Amygdaloid nucleus: New afferent input from the vomeronasal organ. *Science* **170,** 330–332.

Wouterlood, F. G., and Hrtig, W. (1995). Calretinin-immunoreactivity in mitral cells of the rat olfactory bulb. *Brain Res.* **682,** 93–100.

Wyatt, T. D. (2003). Pheromones and Animal Behaviour: Communication by Smell and Taste. Cambridge University Press, Cambridge.

Xu, F., Schaefer, M., Kida, I., Schafer, J., Liu, N., Rothman, D. L., Hyder, F., Restrepo, D., and Shepherd, G. M. (2005). Simultaneous activation of mouse main and accessory olfactory bulbs by odors or pheromones. *J. Comp. Neurol.* **489,** 491–500.

Zhang, J., and Webb, D. M. (2003). Evolutionary deterioration of the vomeronasal pheromone transduction pathway in catarrhine primates. *Proc. Natl. Acad. Sci. USA* **100,** 8337–8341.

Zufall, F., and Leinders-Zufall, T. (2007). Mammalian pheromone sensing. *Curr. Opin. Neurobiol.* **17,** 483–489.

CHAPTER EIGHT

TRPC Channels in Pheromone Sensing

Kirill Kiselyov,* Damian B. van Rossum,†,‡ *and* Randen L. Patterson†,‡

Contents

Abstract

Pheromone recognition relies on an amplification cascade that is triggered by pheromone binding to G protein-coupled receptors (GPCR). The first step in translation of GPCR activation by pheromones in the vomeronasal organ and main olfactory epithelium (MOE) into a cellular response is the activation of a transient receptor potential (TRP) family member, TRPC2 [Zufall, F., Ukhanov, K., Lucas, P., Liman, E. R., and Leinders-Zufall, T. (2005). Neurobiology of TRPC2: From gene to behavior. *Pflugers Arch.* **451**, 61–71; Yildirim, E., and Birnbaumer, L. (2007). TRPC2: Molecular biology and functional importance. *Handb. Exp. Pharmacol.* 53–75]. The members of the canonical (TRPC) family of TRP channels mediate membrane permeability, specifically, Ca^{2+} influx into the cytoplasm in response to activation of GPCR and tyrosine kinase receptors by hormones, neurotransmitters, and growth factors [Nilius, B. (2007). TRP channels in disease. *Biochim. Biophys. Acta* **1772**, 805–812; Venkatachalam, K., and Montell, C. (2007). TRP channels. *Annu. Rev. Biochem.* **76**, 387–417]. Mechanisms of their activation have been the focus of intense interest during the last decade. The data obtained from studies of TRPC2 have resulted in a better understanding of ion channel physiology and led to novel paradigms in modern cell biology

* Department of Biological Sciences, University of Pittsburgh, Pittsburgh, Pennsylvania, USA
† Department of Biology, The Pennsylvania State University, University Park, Pennsylvania, USA
‡ Center for Computational Proteomics, The Pennsylvania State University, University Park, Pennsylvania, USA

Vitamins and Hormones, Volume 83
ISSN 0083-6729, DOI: 10.1016/S0083-6729(10)83008-0

[Lucas, P., Ukhanov, K., Leinders-Zufall, T., and Zufall, F. (2003). A diacylglycerol-gated cation channel in vomeronasal neuron dendrites is impaired in TRPC2 mutant mice: Mechanism of pheromone transduction. *Neuron* **40,** 551–561; Stowers, L., Holy, T. E., Meister, M., Dulac, C., and Koentges, G. (2002). Loss of sex discrimination and male–male aggression in mice deficient for TRP2. *Science* **295,** 1493–1500; Leypold, B. G., Yu, C. R., Leinders-Zufall, T., Kim, M. M., Zufall, F., and Axel, R. (2002). Altered sexual and social behaviors in trp2 mutant mice. *Proc. Natl. Acad. Sci. USA* **99,** 6376–6381]. Although TRPC2 activation by pheromones presents one of the most straightforward examples of physiological function of TRPC channels, the molecular aspects of its activation are not well understood (Yildirim, E., and Birnbaumer, L. (2007). TRPC2: Molecular biology and functional importance. *Handb. Exp. Pharmacol.* 53–75). It is natural to expect that better understanding of TRPC2 activation mechanisms will lead to breakthroughs in understanding ion channel activation mechanisms, as well as applied behavioral pharmacology. The present review is focused on the current knowledge of TRPC2 physiology with a specific focus on TRPC activation mechanisms.

I. Pheromone Sensing Circuits

In the vomeronasal organ (VNO) and main olfactory epithelium (MOE), pheromone sensing relies on amplification cascades that are initiated by pheromone binding to G protein-coupled receptors (GPCR) and driven by G proteins (Yildirim and Birnbaumer, 2007; Zufall *et al.*, 2005). It appears that different components of the pheromone signal complex activate specific G protein cascades, which probably expands the repertoire of pheromone-driven behavior by enabling context-specific response modification.

The pheromone detection cascade starts with activation of GPCR and ends with cell depolarization induced by opening of TRPC2, a nonselective cation channel that belongs to the strikingly versatile transient receptor potential (TRP) channel family (Venkatachalam and Montell, 2007). The depolarization leads to generation of action potential and firing the neurons reporting to the specialized regions of the olfactory bulb. Corollary to the diminished role of pheromones in human behavior, and the loss of the VNO, TRPC2 is a pseudogene in humans and thus the exploration of TRPC function in pheromone recognition has focused on mice as a model system (Vannier *et al.*, 1999).

The mode of TRPC activation by pheromones emphasizes the versatility and modular organization of GPCR-dependent signaling cascade. Mouse VNO appears to contain at least two populations of pheromone-receptive neurons that differ in the composition of their prevailing signaling circuits and in their sensitivity to the specific components of the pheromone complex. Signal amplification/transduction in these populations relies on predominant expression of Gαi2 and Gαo heterotrimeric G proteins (Dulac and Torello, 2003; Mombaerts, 2004). Neurons from the apical part of the VNO are enriched in Gαi2 and express high levels of the putative pheromone sensor V1R, a GPCR with unknown functional involvement (Dulac and Torello, 2003; Mombaerts, 2004). Neurons from the basal part of the VNO organ display high levels of Gαo (Dulac and Torello, 2003; Mombaerts, 2004). The latter appears to drive amplification cascades triggered by V2R pheromone receptor that mediate the effects of major urinary protein complex, an aggression pheromone in mice (Stowers *et al.*, 2002). The functional link between V2R, Gαo, and TRPC2 activation has not been established. Instead, it has been inferred, based on the fact that impairing the receptor-TRPC2 axis by knockout of TRPC2 or by the suppression of GPCR function has similar cellular and behavioral manifestations (Hasen and Gammie, 2009; Stowers *et al.*, 2002). Although V1R, V2R, and TRPC2 functions are required in pheromone sensing (Yildirim and Birnbaumer, 2007; Zufall *et al.*, 2005), and TRPC2 can be activated by lipids in several physiological assays (Lucas *et al.*, 2003), the mechanistic details of signal translation between pheromone-sensing GPCR and TRPC2 are not well understood. Thus, investigating the intermediate steps between pheromone GPCR activation and TRPC2 gating deserve further investigation.

Numerous excellent reviews provide comprehensive analysis of behavioral and anatomical determinants of pheromone response, including behavioral analysis of TRPC2 knockout (KO) mice (Kato and Touhara, 2009; Touhara, 2007; Venkatachalam and Montell, 2007; Yildirim and Birnbaumer, 2007; Zufall *et al.*, 2005). These aspects of pheromone sensation will be only cursorily discussed in the present. Instead, we will focus on the possible mechanisms and unanswered questions in TRPC2 activation by pheromones.

II. TRPC2 and Pheromone Sensing

The core body of information establishing TRPC2 as an essential component of pheromone sensing signaling pathways comes from two lines of evidence obtained using TRPC2 KO mice: behavioral studies and physiological assays on isolated neurons from VNO. In male TRPC2 KO mice, male-on-male aggression as well as sexual behavior associated with pheromone-sensing (such as exclusively male-on-female mounting and pelvic thrusts) was nonexistent (Stowers *et al.*, 2002). Instead, the "typical" sexual behavior extended to the members of the same gender. TRPC2 KO in female mice had similar effects—the female mice stopped responding to male urine and displayed mounting and pelvic thrusts toward both male and female mice (Leypold *et al.*, 2002). These data are congruent with the behavioral characteristics of mice deficient in other components of VNO machinery or with destroyed VNO and thus they clearly warrant the conclusion that TRPC2 plays a key role in pheromone sensing.

At the ultrastructural level, TRPC2 is found in the VNO and is specifically enriched in the microvilla of the pheromone-reporting neurons (Menco *et al.*, 2001). It colocalizes with V1R, V2R, Gαi2, and Gαo, all implicated for pheromone sensing, further supporting TRPC2 role in pheromone recognition.

Electrophysiological recording from dissociated VNO from TRPC2 KO mice report dramatic loss of the currents normally associated with pheromone application (Stowers *et al.*, 2002). Although the fact that some pheromone-induced current remains in such neurons suggests that another channels also plays a role in pheromone sensing, it is clear that the majority of pheromone-induced neuronal current is provided by TRPC2 (Kelliher *et al.*, 2006).

The evidence above unequivocally places TRPC2 at the core of the pheromone-sensing machinery in mice. TRPC2 is one of the few TRPC channels with a concretely assigned biological function and it is perhaps the only TRP channel that has a specific behavioral role. It is clear that delineating its activation and regulation mechanisms will teach us a great deal about ion channels and about the integrative function of cells and signaling circuits. That fact that so little is known about this channel's function also promises a great deal of exciting developments in several fields of modern biomedical science.

III. TRPC Activation Mechanisms

A. TRPC2 domain architecture

TRPC2 is placed within the TRPC family due to its sequence similarity to the other TRPC channels. TRPC family members, TRPC1 and TRPC3-7 are ubiquitously expressed ion channels that, similar to other members of the TRP superfamily contain six transmembrane domains with a putative pore residing between the fifth and sixth domains (Venkatachalam and Montell, 2007). The varying length of the N- and C-termini of TRPCs accommodates a variety of functional domains including ankyrin repeats, calmodulin-binding sites, phosphorylation sites and sites of interaction with other molecules such as Homer, Orai, STIM1, Junctate, IP_3 receptor (IP_3R) and perhaps more (Kiselyov and Patterson, 2009; Ko *et al.*, 2009a).

All TRPC channels also have a TRP-box domain and a TRP_2 domain, both of which are present in most TRP channels including the founding member, the *Drosophila* photoreceptor TRP channel. The possible role of these domains in channel gating will be described later.

Although many commonalities exist between TRPC channels, the domain architecture of TRPC2 is quite distinct from all other TRPCs. For example, TRPC2 has two isoforms of very different lengths (long = 1264 amino acid (a.a.), short = 890 a.a.) (Yildirim *et al.*, 2003), while other TRPC isoforms vary at most by 100 a.a. In the N-terminus of the long TRPC2, NCBI Conserved Domain Database (CDD) predicts a sugar-binding domain (XRCC1) in its extreme N-terminus with high probability (Fig. 8.1A). In addition, the TRP_2 domain in TRPC2 is ~100 a.a. N-terminal to the first putative transmembrane helix, whereas the TRP_2 domain is ~150 a.a. N-terminal to the channel domain in all other TRPCs (Fig. 8.1B). At the amino acid level, the TRPC2 TRP_2 domain has some distinct substitutions when compared to the other TRPCs (Fig. 8.1B). For example, Y568 in TRPC2 is the only TRPC with an aromatic a.a. at this position. Further, L575 in TRPC2 corresponds to an arginine that is conserved in all other TRPCs. This leucine lies between two serine residues that are important for TRPC lipid-binding (van Rossum *et al.*, 2008). R587, A594, and A599 in TRPC2 are also distinct from the other TRPCs which contain a proline, serine/threonine, and threonine at these positions, respectively. It is tantalizing to consider that Y568 may be a site for tyrosine phosphorylation, and that A594 and A599 may be sites for PKA/PKG/PKC phosphorylation in the other TRPCs, but have been removed from TRPC2.

Due to the lack of domain architecture information available for TRPC2, we modeled TRPC2 for transmembrane domains, ankyrin repeats, peripheral lipid-binding, and calmodulin-binding, using Ada-BLAST (Hong *et al.*, 2009a,b; Ko *et al.*, 2009a). As shown in Figs. 8.1C and 8.2A, we observe signals for all of these functional and structural features. The predicted regions for each of these features are presented in Fig. 8.2B. We see many similarities, as well as some distinct differences when these results are compared to other TRPC channels. For instance, our results predict that TRPC2 has only three ankyrin repeats, unlike the rest of the TRPC channels in mice which appear to have four. Further, we observe that TRPC2 has a "hydrophobic inner-shell" domain (Mio *et al.*, 2007) just N-terminal to the transmembrane domains which we observe in all TRPC channels (Ko *et al.*, 2008, 2009a). Similar to TRPC3, 6, and 7, we also see three peripheral lipid-binding signals: one in the N-terminus of the channel, the TRP_2 domain, and the C-terminus of the channel, all of which have been experimentally validated for diacylglycerol (DAG)-sensitive TRPCs (Kwon *et al.*, 2007; van Rossum *et al.*, 2005, 2008). Our models predict two additional lipid-binding domains in the N-terminus of TRPC1, 4, and 5, suggesting a key difference between these two subclades of TRPCs (data

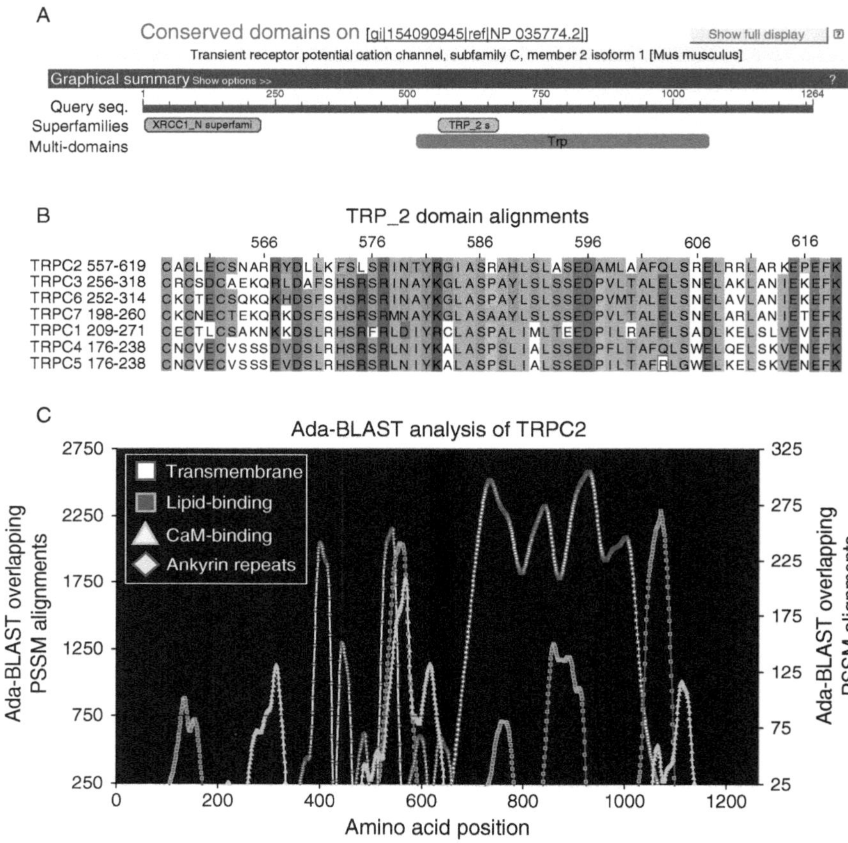

Figure 8.1 TRPC2 domain organization: (A) Graphical output of the domain architecture of mouse TRPC2 (NP_035774.2) as measured by NCBI CDD (default settings) (Marchler-Bauer *et al.*, 2005). (B) Multiple sequence alignment of the TRP_2 domain in mouse TRPC sequences. Numbering is per the mouse TRPC2 sequence. (C) Ada-Blast domain architecture predictions for transmembrane helices, ankyrin repeats, calmodulin-binding, and peripheral lipid-binding domains (*left axis*—transmembrane, *right axis*—calmodulin, peripheral lipid, ankyrin, *arbitrary units*) as per (Hong *et al.*, 2009a; Ko *et al.*, 2008, 2009b). All sequences, position-specific scoring matrices, and scripts used are available upon request. (See Color Insert.)

not shown). All TRPC channels also have a lipid-binding signal in the TRP-box domain just C-terminal to the sixth transmembrane. Indeed, the TRP-box has been demonstrated to bind phospholipids in TRPM4 (Nilius *et al.*, 2006). Our results also predict that TRPC2 may have up to seven calmodulin-binding domains. Interestingly, with the exception of the two most N-terminal predictions, these calmodulin-binding domains occur within peripheral lipid-binding predictions, as occurs in other DAG-sensitive

A

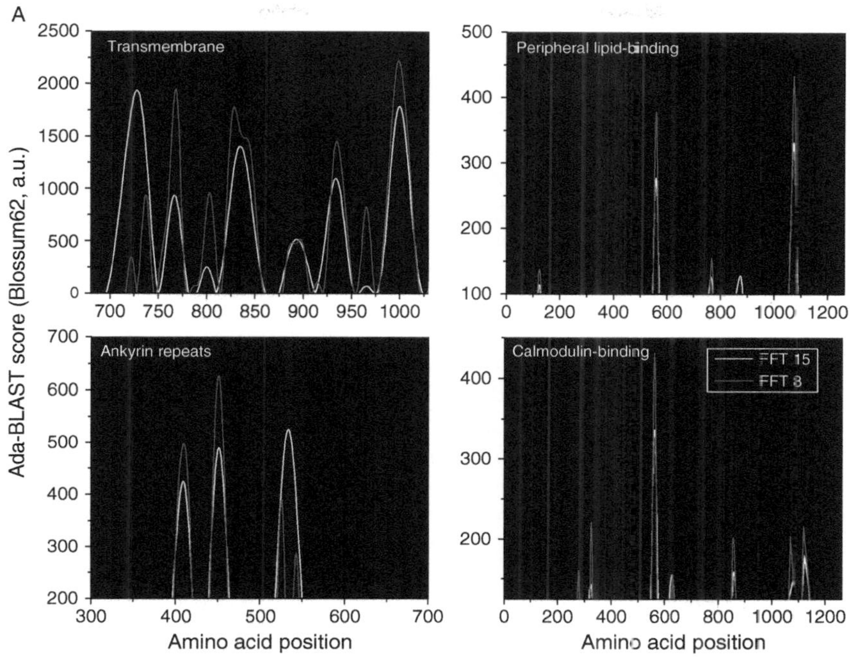

B

Putative domain architecture

	a.a.		a.a.		a.a.		a.a.
Inner shell	714–746	PLB1	95–152	ANK1	390–426	CBD1	260–298
TM1	748–779	PLB2	523–627	ANK2	431–171	CBD2	298–348
TM2	791–814	PLB3	840–896	ANK3	516–551	CBD3	545–580
TM3	815–847	PLB4	1040–1108			CBD4	598–648
TM4	880–908					CBD5	839–887
TM5	922–953					CBD6	1054–1088
Pore	956–974					CBD7	1093–1165
TM6	980–1019						

Figure 8.2 High resolution functional mapping: (A) Ada-BLAST positional data (generated as per (Hong *et al.*, 2009)) from Fig. 8.1C was subjected to Fourier-transformation curve fitting at two window sizes (red = 8 points, white = 15 points, origin 7.5). Following the data was base-line corrected (local minimum to local minimum). (B) Table depicting the boundaries for the measurements obtained in (A). (See Color Insert.)

TRPCs. A complete model on the inhibition of TRPC activity by calmodulin binding to and interrupting lipid-binding is provided in Ko *et al.* (2009a). Briefly, we propose that calmodulin-binding and phosphorylation of lipid-binding domains in TRPC channels disrupt the N- and C-termini of the channel binding to the plasma membrane (PM); thus, inactivating the channel and preparing the channel for endocytosis.

B. TRPC2 activation mechanisms

All TRPCs are activated as a result of the breakdown of the minor PM lipid PIP_2 by phospholipase C (PLC) (Kiselyov and Patterson, 2009; Venkatachalam and Montell, 2007). PLCβ is activated downstream of GPCR that activate the Gαq/11 subtype of heterotrimeric G proteins, while PLCγ is downstream of receptor tyrosine kinase receptors (e.g., growth factor receptors). Both types of PLC hydrolyze PIP_2 and yield two second messengers with drastically different properties and functions: IP_3 and DAG. IP_3 induces the release of Ca^{2+} ions stored in the endoplasmic reticulum (ER) into cytoplasm by opening the IP_3R, a ligand-gated ion channel that resides in the ER membrane. The resulting spike in cytoplasmic Ca^{2+} concentration affects a multitude of Ca^{2+}-dependent processes. Prolonged Ca^{2+} release from the ER triggers Ca^{2+} influx across the PM through the store-operated channels (SOC) (Putney, 2009).

With regards to the activation mechanisms, the TRPC family can be divided into two groups, on the basis of their sensitivity to DAG (Hofmann *et al.*, 1999). It has been demonstrated in several experimental systems, including excised patches, that DAG can activate TRPC2, TRPC3, TRPC6, and TRPC7, while only fragmentary reports exist on DAG-activation of TRPC1, TRPC4, and TRPC5 (Kiselyov and Patterson, 2009; Venkatachalam and Montell, 2007). Instead, there are numerous reports on activation of the latter channels by receptor stimulation as well as passive IP_3-dependent depletion of ER Ca^{2+} stores. In the case of TRPC3, its gating by store depletion has also been documented (Kim *et al.*, 2006; Kiselyov *et al.*, 1998; Worley *et al.*, 2007a; Yuan *et al.*, 2007). However, it appears that TRPC3 activation by store depletion depends on its interaction with other proteins such as Homer, Orai, and STIM1. Whether this activation mechanism is universal or specific to discrete cell-types has yet to be fully evaluated. Activation of recombinant TRPC2 by DAG has been demonstrated using several techniques including the excised patch (Lucas *et al.*, 2003), and thus, at present, the consensus is that these channels are somehow gated by DAG.

The apparent activation of TRPCs by DAG has just begun to be explored at the structural level. The simplest interpretation of the DAG effect on TRPC involved its direct gating of these channels, in line with the ligand-gated channel paradigm. However, two observations suggest that this picture may not be complete. First, when used at concentrations typical for TRPC activation in the recombinant protocols, DAG and its analogs cause destabilization of PM in several experimental systems. This membrane destabilization has been demonstrated to cause rapid vesicle insertion in both neurons and nonexcitable cells (Kiselyov and Patterson, 2009; Rigoni *et al.*, 2005; van Rossum *et al.*, 2008). Second, but no less important, it appears that all DAG-sensitive TRPC channels are regulated by their delivery to the PM. It has been shown that TRPC3 and TRPC6 expression on the PM is greatly increased following DAG application or receptor stimulation (Cayouette *et al.*, 2004; Singh *et al.*, 2004; van Rossum *et al.*, 2008). Such an effect has not been shown for the DAG-insensitive TRPC channels (van Rossum *et al.*, 2008).

Our recent report directly shows correlation between the TRP sensitivity to DAG and ability to be mobilized to the PM following stimulation. A comparative amino acid analysis of the "DAG sensitive" and "DAG insensitive" TRPCs suggested specific amino acid sequences within the TRP_2 domain of TRPC channels whose presence in the given TRPC member correlated with the previously published evidence of sensitivity of this channel to DAG. Our computational efforts using GDDA-BLAST predicted that the TRP_2 domain contains lipid binding and trafficking activity (Ko *et al.*, 2008). Point-mutations of the TRP_2 domain severely affected the DAG activation of TRPC3 and virtually abolished their insertion into the PM in response to stimulation (van Rossum *et al.*, 2008). However, it is important to note that other than insertion in the PM, these mutations do not alter vesicle movement or docking as the difference between WT and TRP_2 mutant TRPC3 cannot be discerned even with electron microscopy; biochemical and photobleaching techniques were employed to determine the changes in PM insertion (van Rossum *et al.*, 2008). Moreover, this result suggests that TRPC3 controls the fusion of other proteins contained in TRPC3-positive vesicles (i.e., if TRPC3 is not entering the membrane, how could other proteins contained in the same vesicle enter?). We hypothesize that TRP channels in general may be part of the SNARE complex for TRP-positive vesicles as this phenomenon has also been observed for TRPM7 (Ko *et al.*, 2009a; Krapivinsky *et al.*, 2006). Based on these data it was concluded that TRP_2 is a necessary requirement for TRPC mobilization to the PM in response to DAG and, perhaps, the entire phenomenon of TRPC activation by DAG.

Endogenous TRPC2 can be activated by DAG, suggesting that it is indeed a physiological signal (Lucas *et al.*, 2003; Stowers *et al.*, 2002). Thus, it is important to consider the source of DAG during stimulation of cells with pheromones. Neither Gαi2 nor Gαo has been directly implicated in PLC activation and it is unclear how (or whether) they provide the DAG necessary for the response of these channels in response to pheromone stimulation. It is possible that Gαi2 and Gαo effectors modulate TRPC2 activity without affecting DAG production. A couple of models can be made for DAG-dependent TRPC2 activation. The "insertion" model permits a situation when TRPC2 channels are preactivated in the delivery vesicles. In this model, upon insertion, TRPC2 is active until inactivated by an unknown mechanism (Ko *et al.*, 2009a). As calmodulin binding, phosphorylation, and endocytosis are negative regulators of all other DAG-sensitive TRPC channels, homology suggests that this is also the case for TRPC2 (Kiselyov and Patterson, 2009; Venkatachalam and Montell, 2007). There may also be other activators of TRPC2 that can increase channel activity after membrane insertion, although these have yet to be identified. A second model would be that TRPC2 basally present in the PM is first activated by receptor stimulation via an unknown mechanism. This activity from basal PM TRPC2 would then facilitate additional recruitment of active/activatable TRPC2 to the PM. Determining whether all newly inserted TRPC2 channels are constitutively active under physiological conditions would go far to elucidating the TRPC2 activation mechanism. Further investigations into the gating of this channel clearly promise exciting new developments and, perhaps, new paradigms in ion channel physiology.

In addition to DAG, all members of TRPC family are regulated by covalent modification (e.g., phosphorylation) and some respond to the ER Ca^{2+} store depletion (Kiselyov and Patterson, 2009; Venkatachalam and Montell, 2007). The latter topic will be discussed later. No information on TRPC2 modulation by covalent modification is available at this moment. However, it should be noted that regulation of TRPC2 by covalent modification is likely to be important for pheromone sensing as all other TRPC channels have been shown to be negatively regulated by either PKC or PKG phosphorylation (Chen *et al.*, 2009; Kwan *et al.*, 2004, 2006; Takahashi *et al.*, 2008; Venkatachalam *et al.*, 2003). Further, TRP channels are also regulated by nitrosylation (Yoshida *et al.*, 2006); thus, the number of covalent modifications that regulate TRPC2 are likely numerous and complex.

C. Regulation of TRPC activity by interaction with other proteins

The above-mentioned context dependent gating of TRPC channels by store depletion is perhaps the most interesting aspect of TRPC regulation. The available data point to a unique situation where a channel's gating behavior is a function of a dynamically controlled environment. A number of channels are regulated by subunits (e.g., voltage-gated sodium channels, voltage-gated potassium channels, etc.) but there are few examples when that channel's protein interaction environment is dynamic. This section will focus on proteins that interact with TRPC and whose expression and localization has been shown to be, or can be, dynamic.

Homer is a family of proteins that were initially cloned as immediate early gene products whose expression profile changes during long-term potentiation (Brakeman *et al.*, 1997; Xiao *et al.*, 1998). This family of proteins is coded in humans by three genes, each yielding isoforms due to alternative splicing (Fagni *et al.*, 2002; Worley *et al.*, 2007b; Xiao *et al.*, 2000). All isoforms contain EVH domains that mediate interaction of these proteins with proline-rich sequences in target proteins (Fagni *et al.*, 2002; Worley *et al.*, 2007b; Xiao *et al.*, 2000). The coiled-coil domains present in the long forms of Homers are responsible for Homer multimerization and formation of molecular complexes tethered by Homers. The first molecular complex shown to be tethered by Homers was the metabotropic glutamate receptor (mGluR)–IP_3R complex (Tu *et al.*, 1998). It was shown that expression of the short isoform of Homer that lacks coiled-coil domain and thus works as a dominant-negative, disengages mGluR–IP_3R complex, and retards the signal transduction between mGluR and IP_3R.

Several TRPC family members bear proline-rich sequences similar to those required for Homer binding. These sequences appear to mediate Homer binding to TRPC channels (Kim *et al.*, 2003, 2006; Yuan *et al.*, 2003). The Homer binding depends on proline-rich sequences in N- and C-termini of TRPC and has some specificity with regards to the type of TRPC involved in this interaction. Disruption of Homer binding by mutating the channel or by expressing the dominant-negative Homer drastically changed the gating mode of TRPC1 rendering the channel spontaneously active (Yuan *et al.*, 2003). The fact that the same treatment abolished TRPC1 interaction with IP_3R suggested that TRPC–IP_3R interaction is important for the TRPC gating. Delivery to the PM, complex assembly and gating of TRPC3 was altered as a result of interfering with Homer binding (Kim *et al.*, 2006). Taken together, these data suggest that Homer has an important role in tuning TRPC activity.

TRPC2 has the classic PXPF (PVPF) Homer-binding sequence in its N-terminal (a.a. 954–957 in the long isoform, a.a. 672–676 in the short form); no unconventional PSSP C-terminal Homer-binding sequence that has been implicated in TRPC1 interaction with Homer is present. Data do not exist for Homer gating of TRPC2. However, TRPC2 appears to bind Homer 1 and thus it is possible that Homers contribute to TRPC2 regulation (Yuan *et al.*, 2003). Future investigation will answer whether or not Homer is important for TRPC2 targeting and gating.

Other interesting candidates for regulation of TRPC2 activity are the recently characterized Orai and STIM1 proteins (Worley *et al.*, 2007a; Yuan *et al.*, 2007). STIM1 is a protein normally localized in the ER. Upon depletion of the ER Ca^{2+}, STIM1 translocates to the PM, where its interaction with Orai, a channel whose characteristics match the properties of the I_{CRAC}, the long-sought SOC in blood cells, and with TRPC mediates the gating of these channels by store depletion (Putney, 2009). Both STIM1 and Orai bind to TRPC2, yet the functional importance of such interaction is unclear (Worley *et al.*, 2007a).

IV. Perspectives: The "DAG Effect" and Beyond

TRPC2 channels undergo a context-specific activation mechanism that we are just beginning to uncover and understand. Progress in this direction should lead to a deeper understanding of sensory perception in general, as well as shed light on the structural/functional determinants of activity/regulation in the enigmatic canonical TRP family.

Research conducted over a decade has firmly established that TRPC2, 3, 6, and 7 can be discriminated/segregated from the other TRP channels by their sensitivity to DAG and DAG-derivatives (Hofmann *et al.*, 1999; Kiselyov and Patterson, 2009; van Rossum *et al.*, 2008; Venkatachalam and Montell, 2007). The "DAG effect" is nearly always defined by channel activity; however, recent progress has determined that channel activity is not the functional output for discriminating the "DAG effect." Take for example TRPC3, which is endogenously expressed in rat PC12 cells. Upon addition of OAG, no channel activity can be measured by fura-2AM, a calcium indicator dye, while cell surface biotinylation experiments of the same preparation show an OAG-dependent increase of TRPC3 in the PM (van Rossum *et al.*, 2008). Conversely, carbachol treatment results in both vesicle fusion and activity demonstrating the full orchestra of receptor-mediated events. TRPC2 is expressed in the testis but does not flux ions in response to DAG in this cell-type (Stamboulian *et al.*, 2005). Given the TRPC3 data, it is reasonable to consider that this could be a false negative and that TRPC2 may still be DAG-sensitive in the testes. Since surface expression defines the "DAG effect," not channel activity, it may also be possible that multiple channels, inside and outside of the TRP superfamily, have been erroneously excluded from the DAG-sensitive list.

The mode of regulation of the "DAG effect" is complex, involving a multitude of protein–protein and protein–lipid interactions. Integral to this cascade is the TRP_2 domain, mutation of which in TRPC3 blocks DAG-dependent channel insertion into the PM. Mutations in TRP_2 domain result in increased affinity for PM lipids and a correlated loss in DAG-dependent vesicle fusion (van Rossum *et al.*, 2008). These data support a model whereby TRPC1, 4, and 5 (which all have TRP_2 domains) are predicted to have higher affinity for PM lipids versus TRPC2, 3, 6, and 7. Biochemical tests of these predictions may reveal molecular mechanistic information for the differences between TRPC isoforms.

Whether this domain works in conjunction with another to fulfill the "DAG effect" is unknown. Nevertheless, the fact that the TRP_2 domain is fundamental to the vesicle fusion of its own channel is intriguing and suggests a model whereby DAG-sensitive TRPC channels can regulate the delivery of other cargo (i.e., SNARE-like). This model may provide a secondary function for TRPC channels when stimulated by DAG. Furthermore, this SNARE-like activity maybe an alternative explanation for TRPC channels and their permissive-positive effect on store-operated calcium entry. For example, TRPC2 expression enhances SOC and thus TRPC2 is store-linked (Jungnickel *et al.*, 2001; Vannier *et al.*, 1999); however, TRPC2 and its SNARE-like function in vesicles maybe promote surface expression of Orai or other positive regulators. Pore-dead TRPC2 mutants could be utilized to determine if TRPC2 activity is critical for this enhancement or if mutations in the TRP_2 domain could inhibit other store-linked proteins from PM expression. Alternatively, TRPC2 may fulfill an adaptor role and enrich positive regulators of SOC in signaling microdomains.

Future research is needed to flesh out the key players which modulate the signal relay between the pheromone receptor and TRPC2. TRPC2 is closely related to the other TRPC isoforms and can be seen, by evolutionary analysis, to share a common ancestor with the TRPC3/6/7 subclade (Yildirim and Birnbaumer, 2007). Therefore, known protein regulators/interactors (e.g., VAMP-2, PLCγ, BAP-135) of TRPC3, 6, and/or 7 are reasonable candidates for also regulating TRPC2. Recently, high throughput interaction studies of TRPC3 were published (Singh *et al.*, 2004). As well as providing proteins to test for their modulation of pheromone sensing, these data could also be exploited to construct a Boolean model for the putative TRPC2 "interactome" which may be useful to uncover subtle/counter-intuitive regulatory schemes.

TRP channels are polymodal in their activation and are responsive to a broad range of sensory signals such as temperature (hot and cold), osmolarity, pH, stretch, taste, and odorants to name a few (Kiselyov and Patterson, 2009; Venkatachalam and Montell, 2007). To date, fly TRP (photoreception) (Montell and Rubin, 1989), TRPC2 (Stowers *et al.*, 2002), and very recently TRPC5 (Blair *et al.*, 2009; Riccio *et al.*, 2009) are the only canonical TRP members associated with sensory perception. Despite this, there is some indirect evidence that supports a role for other TRPC channels in sensory pathways. For example, TRPC5 has been shown to be upregulated in response to acid, temperature, and stress (Holzer, 2009; Patterson RL, van Rossum DB, unpublished data). Therefore, TRPCs may modulate nociception pathways. In addition, recall that TRPC2 KO did not completely abolish SAG responsiveness; this may be compensated by other TRPCs expressed in the VNO (Kelliher *et al.*, 2006). Indeed, pheromone sensing in the VNO may be an ideal model system to study the functional role(s) of other TRPC channels. For example, domain substitution experiments between TRPC isoforms and TRPC2 could be conducted in this relatively straightforward system toward elucidating the molecular determinants that are either shared or distinctive. Taken together, there has never been a more fruitful time to synthesize many years of research and novel experimental support for molecular mechanisms of TRP channels in sensory perception.

ACKNOWLEDGMENTS

This work was supported by The National Science Foundation grant 428-15 691M (R. L. P., D. V. R., K. K.) and The National Institutes of Health HD058577 and ES016782 (K. K.) and GM087410 (R. L. P., D. V. R.). This work was also supported by the Searle Young

Investigators Award and start-up monies from Pennsylvania State University (R. L. P.), Funds from the Huck Life Science Institute's Center for Computational Proteomics (R. L. P. and D. V. R.) and a grant from the Pennsylvania Department of Health using Tobacco Settlement Funds to D. V. R. The Pennsylvania Department of Health specifically disclaims responsibility for any analyses, interpretations, or conclusions. We would also like to thank Drs. Bo. O. Rothe, Jim White, Kenji Cohan, Glenn M. Sharer, Sasha Kendall, and Berkeley Kendall for creative dialog.

REFERENCES

Blair, N. T., Kaczmarek, J. S., and Clapham, D. E. (2009). Intracellular calcium strongly potentiates agonist-activated TRPC5 channels. *J. Gen. Physiol.* **133,** 525–546.

Brakeman, P. R., Lanahan, A. A., O'Brien, R., Roche, K., Barnes, C. A., Huganir, R. L., and Worley, P. F. (1997). Homer: A protein that selectively binds metabotropic glutamate receptors. *Nature* **386,** 284–288.

Cayouette, S., Lussier, M. P., Mathieu, E. L., Bousquet, S. M., and Boulay, G. (2004). Exocytotic insertion of TRPC6 channel into the plasma membrane upon Gq protein-coupled receptor activation. *J. Biol. Chem.* **279,** 7241–7246.

Chen, J., Crossland, R. F., Noorani, M. M., and Marrelli, S. P. (2009). Inhibition of TRPC1/TRPC3 by PKG contributes to NO-mediated vasorelaxation. *Am. J. Physiol. Heart Circ. Physiol.* **297,** H417–H424.

Dulac, C., and Torello, A. T. (2003). Molecular detection of pheromone signals in mammals: From genes to behaviour. *Nat. Rev. Neurosci.* **4,** 551–562.

Fagni, L., Worley, P. F., and Ango, F. (2002). Homer as both a scaffold and transduction molecule. *Sci. STKE* re8.

Hasen, N. S., and Gammie, S. C. (2009). Trpc2 gene impacts on maternal aggression, accessory olfactory bulb anatomy and brain activity. *Genes Brain Behav.* **8,** 639–649.

Hofmann, T., Obukhov, A. G., Schaefer, M., Harteneck, C., Gudermann, T., and Schultz, G. (1999). Direct activation of human TRP6 and TRP3 channels by diacylglycerol. *Nature* **397,** 259–263.

Holzer, P. (2009). Acid-sensitive ion channels and receptors. *Handb. Exp. Pharmacol.* 283–332.

Hong, Y., Lee, D., Kang, J., van Rossum, D. B., and Patterson, R. L. (2009a). Adaptive BLASTing through the sequence dataspace: Theories on protein sequence embedding. *Phys. Arch.* arXiv:0911.0650v1, q-bio.Q, 1–21.

Hong, Y., Chalkia, D., Ko, K. D., Bhardwaj, G., Chang, G. S., van Rossum, D. B., and Patterson, R. L. (2009b). Phylogenetic profiles reveal structural and functional determinants of lipid-binding. *J. Proteomics Bioinform.* 139–149.

Jungnickel, M. K., Marrero, H., Birnbaumer, L., Lemos, J. R., and Florman, H. M. (2001). Trp2 regulates entry of Ca^{2+} into mouse sperm triggered by egg ZP3. *Nat. Cell Biol.* **3,** 499–502.

Kato, A., and Touhara, K. (2009). Mammalian olfactory receptors: Pharmacology, G protein coupling and desensitization. *Cell Mol. Life Sci.* **66,** 3743–3753.

Kelliher, K. R., Spehr, M., Li, X. H., Zufall, F., and Leinders-Zufall, T. (2006). Pheromonal recognition memory induced by TRPC2-independent vomeronasal sensing. *Eur. J. Neurosci.* **23,** 3385–3390.

Kim, S. J., Kim, Y. S., Yuan, J. P., Petralia, R. S., Worley, P. F., and Linden, D. J. (2003). Activation of the TRPC1 cation channel by metabotropic glutamate receptor mGluR1. *Nature* **426,** 285–291.

Kim, J. Y., Zeng, W., Kiselyov, K., Yuan, J. P., Dehoff, M. H., Mikoshiba, K., Worley, P. F., and Muallem, S. (2006). Homer 1 mediates store- and inositol 1, 4, 5-trisphosphate receptor-dependent translocation and retrieval of TRPC3 to the plasma membrane. *J. Biol. Chem.* **281,** 32540–32549.

Kiselyov, K., and Patterson, R. L. (2009). The integrative function of TRPC channels. *Front. Biosci.* **14,** 45–58.

Kiselyov, K. I., Xu, X., Mohayeva, G., Kuo, T., Pessah, I. N., Mignery, G. A., Zhu, X., Birnbaumer, L., and Muallem, S. (1998). Functional interaction between $InsP_3$ receptors and store-operated Htrp3 channels. *Nature* **396,** 478–482.

Ko, K. D., Hong, Y., Chang, G. S., Bhardwaj, G., van Rossum, D. B., and Patterson, R. L. (2008). Phylogenetic profiles as a unified framework for measuring protein structure, function and evolution. *Phys. Arch.* arXiv:0806.239, q-bio.Q.

Ko, K. D., Bhardwaj, G., Hong, Y., Chang, G. S., Kiselyov, K., van Rossum, D. B., and Patterson, R. L. (2009a). Phylogenetic profiles reveal structural/functional determinants of TRPC3 signal-sensing antennae. *Commun. Integr. Biol.* **2,** 133–137.

Ko, K. D., Hong, Y., Bhardwaj, G., Killick, T. M., van Rossum, D. B., and Patterson, R. L. (2009). Brainstorming through the sequence universe: Theories on the protein problem. *Phys. Arch.* arXiv:0911.0652v1, q-bio.QM, 1–21.

Krapivinsky, G., Mochida, S., Krapivinsky, L., Cibulsky, S. M., and Clapham, D. E. (2006). The TRPM7 ion channel functions in cholinergic synaptic vesicles and affects transmitter release. *Neuron* **52,** 485–496.

Kwan, H. Y., Huang, Y., and Yao, X. (2004). Regulation of canonical transient receptor potential isoform 3 (TRPC3) channel by protein kinase G. *Proc. Natl. Acad. Sci. USA* **101,** 2625–2630.

Kwan, H. Y., Huang, Y., and Yao, X. (2006). Protein kinase C can inhibit TRPC3 channels indirectly via stimulating protein kinase G. *J. Cell. Physiol.* **207,** 315–321.

Kwon, Y., Hofmann, T., and Montell, C. (2007). Integration of phosphoinositide- and calmodulin-mediated regulation of TRPC6. *Mol. Cell* **25,** 491–503.

Leypold, B. G., Yu, C. R., Leinders-Zufall, T., Kim, M. M., Zufall, F., and Axel, R. (2002). Altered sexual and social behaviors in trp2 mutant mice. *Proc. Natl. Acad. Sci. USA* **99,** 6376–6381.

Lucas, P., Ukhanov, K., Leinders-Zufall, T., and Zufall, F. (2003). A diacylglycerol-gated cation channel in vomeronasal neuron dendrites is impaired in TRPC2 mutant mice: Mechanism of pheromone transduction. *Neuron* **40,** 551–561.

Marchler-Bauer, A., Anderson, J. B., Cherukuri, P. F., Weese-Scott, C., Geer, L. Y., Gwadz, M., He, S., Hurwitz, D. I., Jackson, J. D., Ke, Z., *et al.* (2005). CDD: A conserved domain database for protein classification. *Nucleic Acids Res.* **33,** Database Issue: D192–D196.

Menco, B. P., Carr, V. M., Ezeh, P. I., Liman, E. R., and Yankova, M. P. (2001). Ultrastructural localization of G-proteins and the channel protein TRP2 to microvilli of rat vomeronasal receptor cells. *J. Comp. Neurol.* **438,** 468–489.

Mio, K., Ogura, T., Kiyonaka, S., Hiroaki, Y., Tanimura, Y., Fujiyoshi, Y., Mori, Y., and Sato, C. (2007). The TRPC3 channel has a large internal chamber surrounded by signal sensing antennas. *J. Mol. Biol.* **367,** 373–383.

Mombaerts, P. (2004). Genes and ligands for odorant, vomeronasal and taste receptors. *Nat. Rev. Neurosci.* **5,** 263–278.

Montell, C., and Rubin, G. M. (1989). Molecular characterization of the *Drosophila* trp locus: A putative integral membrane protein required for phototransduction. *Neuron* **2,** 1313–1323.

Nilius, B. (2007). TRP channels in disease. *Biochim. Biophys. Acta* **1772,** 805–812.

Nilius, B., Mahieu, F., Prenen, J., Janssens, A., Owsianik, G., Vennekens, R., and Voets, T. (2006). The Ca2+-activated cation channel TRPM4 is regulated by phosphatidylinositol 4, 5-biphosphate. *EMBO J.* **25,** 467–478.

Putney, J. W. (2009). Capacitative calcium entry: From concept to molecules. *Immunol. Rev.* **231,** 10–22.

Riccio, A., Li, Y., Moon, J., Kim, K. S., Smith, K. S., Rudolph, U., Gapon, S., Yao, G. L., Tsvetkov, E., Rodig, S. J., *et al.* (2009). Essential role for TRPC5 in amygdala function and fear-related behavior. *Cell* **137,** 761–772.

Rigoni, M., Caccin, P., Gschmeissner, S., Koster, G., Postle, A. D., Rossetto, O., Schiavo, G., and Montecucco, C. (2005). Equivalent effects of snake PLA2 neurotoxins and lysophospholipid–fatty acid mixtures. *Science* **310,** 1678–1680.

Singh, B. B., Lockwich, T. P., Bandyopadhyay, B. C., Liu, X., Bollimuntha, S., Brazer, S. C., Combs, C., Das, S., Leenders, A. G., Sheng, Z. H., *et al.* (2004). VAMP2-dependent exocytosis regulates plasma membrane insertion of TRPC3 channels and contributes to agonist-stimulated Ca^{2+} influx. *Mol. Cell* **15,** 635–646.

Stamboulian, S., Moutin, M. J., Treves, S., Pochon, N., Grunwald, D., Zorzato, F., De, W. M., Ronjat, M., and Arnoult, C. (2005). Junctate, an inositol 1, 4, 5-triphosphate receptor associated protein, is present in rodent sperm and binds TRPC2 and TRPC5 but not TRPC1 channels. *Dev. Biol.* **286,** 326–337.

Stowers, L., Holy, T. E., Meister, M., Dulac, C., and Koentges, G. (2002). Loss of sex discrimination and male-male aggression in mice deficient for TRP2. *Science* **295,** 1493–1500.

Takahashi, S., Lin, H., Geshi, N., Mori, Y., Kawarabayashi, Y., Takami, N., Mori, M. X., Honda, A., and Inoue, R. (2008). Nitric oxide-cGMP-protein kinase G pathway negatively regulates vascular transient receptor potential channel TRPC6. *J. Physiol.* **586,** 4209–4223.

Touhara, K. (2007). Molecular biology of peptide pheromone production and reception in mice. *Adv. Genet.* **59,** 147–171.

Tu, J. C., Xiao, B., Yuan, J. P., Lanahan, A. A., Leoffert, K., Li, M., Linden, D. J., and Worley, P. F. (1998). Homer binds a novel proline-rich motif and links group 1 metabotropic glutamate receptors with IP3 receptors. *Neuron* **21,** 717–726.

van Rossum, D. B., Patterson, R. L., Sharma, S., Barrow, R. K., Kornberg, M., Gill, D. L., and Snyder, S. H. (2005). Phospholipase Cgamma1 controls surface expression of TRPC3 through an intermolecular PH domain. *Nature* **434,** 99–104.

van Rossum, D. B., Oberdick, D., Rbaibi, Y., Bhardwaj, G., Barrow, R. K., Nikolaidis, N., Snyder, S. H., Kiselyov, K., and Patterson, R. L. (2008). TRP_2, a lipid/trafficking domain that mediates diacylglycerol-induced vesicle fusion. *J. Biol. Chem.* **283,** 34384–34392.

Vannier, B., Peyton, M., Boulay, G., Brown, D., Qin, N., Jiang, M., Zhu, X., and Birnbaumer, L. (1999). Mouse trp2, the homologue of the human trpc2 pseudogene, encodes mTrp2, a store depletion-activated capacitative Ca^{2+} entry channel. *Proc. Natl. Acad. Sci. USA* **96,** 2060–2064.

Venkatachalam, K., and Montell, C. (2007). TRP channels. *Annu. Rev. Biochem.* **76,** 387–417.

Venkatachalam, K., Zheng, F., and Gill, D. L. (2003). Regulation of canonical transient receptor potential (TRPC) channel function by diacylglycerol and protein kinase C. *J. Biol. Chem.* **278,** 29031–29040.

Worley, P. F., Zeng, W., Huang, G. N., Yuan, J. P., Kim, J. Y., Lee, M. G., and Muallem, S. (2007a). TRPC channels as STIM1-regulated store-operated channels. *Cell Calcium* **42,** 205–211.

Worley, P. F., Zeng, W., Huang, G., Kim, J. Y., Shin, D. M., Kim, M. S., Yuan, J. P., Kiselyov, K., and Muallem, S. (2007b). Homer proteins in Ca^{2+} signaling by excitable and non-excitable cells. *Cell Calcium* **42,** 363–371.

Xiao, B., Tu, J. C., Petralia, R. S., Yuan, J. P., Doan, A., Breder, C. D., Ruggiero, A., Lanahan, A. A., Wenthold, R. J., and Worley, P. F. (1998). Homer regulates the association of group 1 metabotropic glutamate receptors with multivalent complexes of homer-related, synaptic. *Neuron* **21,** 707–716.

Xiao, B., Tu, J. C., and Worley, P. F. (2000). Homer: A link between neural activity and glutamate receptor function. *Curr. Opin. Neurobiol.* **10,** 370–374.

Yildirim, E., and Birnbaumer, L. (2007). TRPC2: Molecular biology and functional importance. *Handb. Exp. Pharmacol.* 53–75.

Yildirim, E., Dietrich, A., and Birnbaumer, L. (2003). The mouse C-type transient receptor potential 2 (TRPC2) channel: Alternative splicing and calmodulin binding to its N terminus. *Proc. Natl. Acad. Sci. USA* **100,** 2220–2225.

Yoshida, T., Inoue, R., Morii, T., Takahashi, N., Yamamoto, S., Hara, Y., Tominaga, M., Shimizu, S., Sato, Y., and Mori, Y. (2006). Nitric oxide activates TRP channels by cysteine S-nitrosylation. *Nat. Chem. Biol.* **2,** 596–607.

Yuan, J. P., Kiselyov, K. I., Shin, D. M., Chen, J., Shcheynikov, N., Kang, H. S., Dehoff, M. H., Schwarz, M. K., Seeburg, P. H., Muallem, S., *et al.* (2003). Homer binds TRPC family channels and is required for gating of TRPC1 by IP_3-Receptors. *Cell* **114,** 777–789.

Yuan, J. P., Zeng, W., Huang, G. N., Worley, P. F., and Muallem, S. (2007). STIM1 heteromultimerizes TRPC channels to determine their function as store-operated channels. *Nat. Cell Biol.* **9,** 636–645.

Zufall, F., Ukhanov, K., Lucas, P., Liman, E. R., and Leinders-Zufall, T. (2005). Neurobiology of TRPC2: From gene to behavior. *Pflugers Arch.* **451,** 61–71.

CHAPTER NINE

Alarm Pheromones—Chemical Signaling in Response to Danger

François J. Verheggen,* Eric Haubruge,* *and* Mark C. Mescher†

Contents

Abstract

Many animals respond to the threat of predation by producing alarm signals that warn other individuals of the presence of danger or otherwise reduce the success of predators. While alarm signals may be visual or auditory as well as chemical, alarm pheromones are common, especially among insects and aquatic organisms. Plants too emit chemical signals in response to attack by insect herbivores that recruit the herbivores' natural enemies and can induce preparations for defense in neighboring plants (or other parts of the same plant). In this chapter, we discuss our current understanding of chemical alarm signaling in a variety of animal groups (including social and presocial insects, marine invertebrates, fish, and mammals) and in plants. We also briefly discuss the exploitation of alarm pheromones as foraging cues for natural enemies. We conclude with a brief discussion of the potential exploitation of alarm signaling to achieve the applied goal of managing pest species. © 2010 Elsevier Inc.

* Department of Functional and Evolutionary Entomology, Gembloux Agro-Bio Tech, Liege University, Gembloux, Belgium
† Department of Entomology, Center for Chemical Ecology, The Pennsylvania State University, University Park, Pennsylvania, USA

Vitamins and Hormones, Volume 83
ISSN 0083-6729, DOI: 10.1016/S0083-6729(10)83009-2

I. Introduction

In response to the approach of predators—or other rapid adverse changes in the immediate environment—many organisms emit alarm signals that can alert nearby individuals (conspecifics as well as others) of impending danger. Alarm signaling has frequently been viewed as an evolutionary puzzle because the fitness benefits to individuals receiving the signal are usually apparent while signaling often appears costly for signalers (e.g., Taylor *et al.*, 1990). Genuinely altruistic signaling can presumably evolve where the benefits preferentially fall on conspecifics with higher than average relatedness to the signaler (Sherman, 1977) as suggested by inclusive fitness theory (Hamilton, 1964). But alarm signaling may also directly benefit the fitness of the signaling individual itself, for example, if the antipredator or escape behaviors induced by the call reduce the probability of successful predation (Högstedt, 1983; Sherman, 1985) or attract the predator away from the signaling individual (Charnov and Krebs, 1974). Alarm calls may also have delayed benefits for the signaler, for example, by saving the lives of individuals who will reciprocate in the future (Trivers, 1971) or those of potential mates (Witkin and Fitkin, 1979) or other group members in circumstances where group living is beneficial (Smith, 1986).

Alarm signals frequently have visual and auditory components, especially in birds and mammals (e.g., Leavesley and Magrath, 2005; Seyfarth *et al.*, 1980; Sherman, 1977), but chemical alarm signals are also widespread (Wyatt, 2003). Chemical signals involved in communication with other conspecific individuals are called pheromones (from the Greek *pherein*, to transfer) and are thus distinguished from hormones (*hormon*, to excite) which mediate communication within an individual organism (Karlson and Lüscher, 1959). Most alarm pheromones likely have evolved from compounds originally having other functions. Specifically, it has been proposed that alarm pheromones may evolve either from chemicals involved in defense against predators or from compounds released upon injury (Wyatt, 2003). To the extent that these compounds serve as reliable cues to the presence of predators, potential receivers should evolve to detect them and respond in ways that enhance fitness. The acquisition of a true signaling function then entails further evolutionary elaboration of the cue specifically in response to selection acting on its role in communication (Maynard Smith and Harper, 2003).

A large literature addresses chemical identification of alarm pheromones and their impact on the behavior of nearby individuals. In order to conclude that particular compounds acts as an alarm pheromone, it is generally considered necessary to demonstrate that (i) the chemical(s) is released exclusively under exposure to hazard (e.g., predator attack), (ii) the signal is perceived by conspecifics, and (iii) it induces in the receiving individuals behavioral reactions similar to those induced when directly exposed to the same danger (Wyatt, 2003). The latter criteria is usually the most difficult to demonstrate, as it is not enough to demonstrate a modification in the behavior of the receiving individuals; the changes must clearly be appropriate responses to danger specific threat. Generally, adaptive responses to the reception of an alarm pheromone may be classified as evasive (e.g., receivers flee from the pheromone releaser) or aggressive (receivers move toward the signal and attack or harass the predator). Observed reactions can vary according to the concentration of pheromone released and also with prior experience of the receiver (Howse, 1998).

Alarm pheromones have documented in both vertebrate and nonvertebrate animals (Wyatt, 2003), and similar types of signaling seem to occur also in plants (Heil and Karban, 2010; Wittstock and Gershenzon, 2002). The chemical composition of alarm pheromones is highly variable: Table 9.1 presents a partial list of identified examples from animal systems. Alarm signals may be as simple as a single molecule (e.g., citral in mites, Kuwahara *et al.*, 1979), but can also be complicated chemical mixtures, whose activity is determined by their specific composition, the quantitative proportion of the different compounds, and the stereoisomerism of the dominating substances (Wadhams, 1990).

The remainder of this chapter reviews illustrative examples taken drawn from the tremendous diversity of alarm signaling systems that occur in presocial (aphids) and social (ants, termites, honeybees) insects, vertebrate animals, and plants.

II. Alarm Pheromones in Insects

Alarm pheromones appear to be the second most commonly produced class of chemical signals used by insects, after sex pheromones (Barbier, 1982). Alarm signaling has evolved in various Arthropod taxa in which the individuals are proximate enough to each other to rapidly communicate. Gregarious and social insects, including Hymenopterans and Hemipterans, have developed a diverse array of chemical compounds that function as releasers of alarm behavior (Table 9.1). Indeed, alarm pheromones appear to be highly adaptive for species in which individuals form aggregates that can exhibit a collective response to traumatic stimuli (Blum, 1985). In eusocial species, for example, they allow colony resources to be rapidly and efficiently deployed in response to specific threats. Insect alarm pheromones are usually short molecules of low molecular weight and simple structure (e.g., terpenoids or aliphatic ketones and esters). They are thus highly volatile and dissipate rapidly after emission as befits signals that operate over short time frames and at localized spatial scales (Payne, 1974). Various organs can be

Table 9.1 Some identified alarm pheromones in the animal kingdom

Animals	Principal compounds	Typical behavioral responses	Additional observations	References
Insects				
Hymenopterans				
Honeybees	Isopentyl acetate 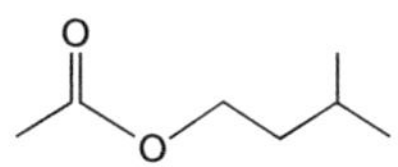 2-heptanone 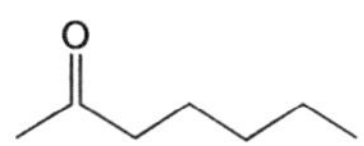	Recruitment and aggression	Over 20 active compounds have been identified in various bee species. Guarding workers release alarm pheromone in case of perturbation, which leads to the recruitment of nestmates and subsequent attack of the intruder.	Boch *et al.* (1962), Shearer and Boch (1965)
Ants	*n*-undecane 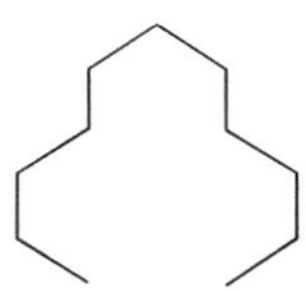 4-methyl-3-heptanone 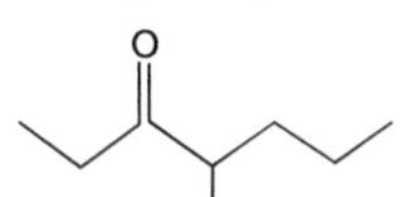	Fright reactions or recruitment and aggression	All Formicidae species produce and use an alarm pheromone whose secretion may induce escape behaviors or the recruitment of conspecifics and aggressive reactions.	Hughes et al. (2001), Stoeffler *et al.* (2007)

Homopterans				
Aphids	(E)-β-farnesene 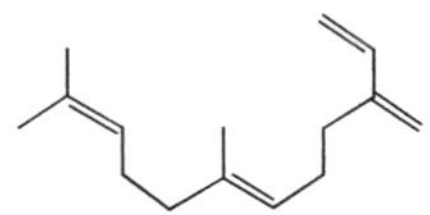 Germacrene A 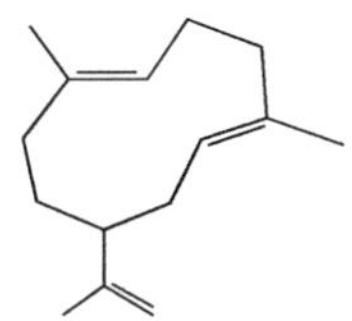	Fright reactions	(E)-β-farnesene is the only active component of the alarm pheromone of most Aphidinae species. Receiving individuals escape by running away from the emitter or falling off the plant.	Edwards *et al.* (1973), Bowers *et al.* (1977b)
Fish				
Ostariophysi	Hypoxanthine-3-N-oxide 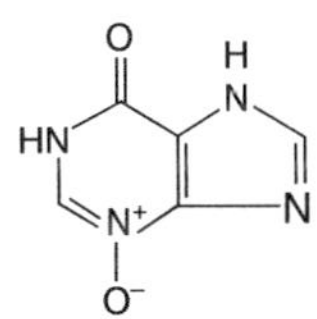	Fright reactions	Ostariophysan fish exhibit antipredator responses (increased shoaling and decreased area of movcmcnt) whcn exposed to compounds released from the damaged skin of other individuals. Exposure to low concentrations of hypoxanthine-3-*N*-oxide induces increase vigilance toward secondary (visual) risk-assessment cues.	Brown *et al.* (2004)

(*continued*)

Table 9.1 (*continued*)

Animals	Principal compounds	Typical behavioral responses	Additional observations	References
Cnidaria	Anthopleurine 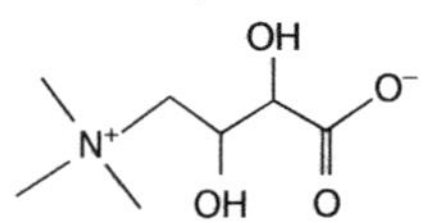	Fright reactions	Anthopleurine was the first reported cnidarian pheromone. The sea anemone *Anthopleura elegantissima*, releases anthopleurine from wounded tissues, inducing rapid withdrawal in nearby conspecifics.	Howe and Sheikh (1975)
Mites	Citral 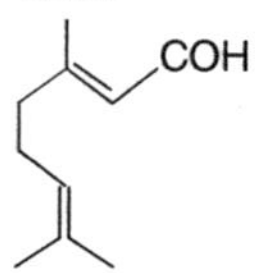	Fright reactions	Several families of mites produce citral as an alarm pheromone, whose perception induces avoidance behavior along with increased mobility.	Kuwahara *et al.* (1980)

involved in their production, including anal glands, mandibles, and stings. Although commonly comprising mixtures of several compounds, alarm pheromones tend to be less specialized than other types of pheromones, and few are species specific (Blum, 1985). This relative nonspecificity may be an advantage to species that are able to detect alarm signals of other insects sharing vulnerability to a common threat.

In noneusocial insects the effects of alarm pheromones are generally limited to causing dispersal. The response to alarm signals varies among eusocial species, but commonly involves attraction/recruitment of conspecific workers or soldiers and the adoption of aggressive postures. Below we discuss alarm signaling in aphids, ants, and honeybees.

A. Aphids

Because aphids are important agricultural pests throughout the world, their biology and behavior have been well studied. Aphid alarm signaling was first characterized in the 1970s. In response to predation and other disturbances, aphids secrete droplets from two cornicles situated on the upper surface of the abdomen near the tail that emit an odor repellent to conspecifics (Kislow and Edwards, 1972) (Fig. 9.1). This pheromone induces alate and apterous *Myzus persicae* (Hemiptera, Aphididae) to stop feeding and move away from the signaler or to drop from the host plant—waving their antennae before and during these aversive behaviors. Variation in response to alarm pheromone occurs both within and between species and correlates with to the relative risk of predation and the costs of escape (Pickett *et al.*, 1992).

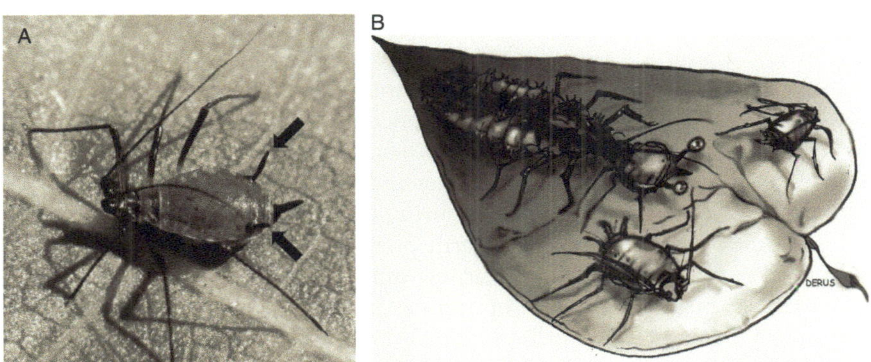

Figure 9.1 *Top*: In response to predation, aphids release an alarm pheromone from their cornicles that induces escape behavior in surrounding conspecifics. *Bottom*: The vetch aphid, *Megoura viciae* (Hemiptera, Aphididae), with arrows pointing to the alarm pheromone releasing organs (cornicles). The site of (E)-β-farnesene production remains unknown.

The active component of the liquid secreted from the cornicles of several economically important species of aphids was found to be a sesquiterpene ($C_{15}H_{24}$) named (E)-7,11-dimethyl-3-methylene-1,6,10-dodecatriene, or more commonly referred to as (E)-β-farnesene (Eβf) or *trans*-β-farnesene (Bowers *et al.*, 1972) (Table 9.1). This same compound was subsequently identified in many other aphid species including the green peach aphid *M. persicae* Sulzer (Edwards *et al.*, 1973; Wientjens *et al.*, 1973) and the pea aphid *Acyrthosiphon pisum* (Wohlers, 1981).

Germacrene A (Table 9.1), a biogenetic precursor of many sesquiterpenes, was later isolated from the alfalfa aphid and identified as an alarm pheromone (Bowers *et al.*, 1977b), though it appears to play this signaling role only within the genus *Therioaphis*. Pickett and Griffiths (1980) found *Megoura viciae* to synthesize additional monoterpenes, including α-pinene, β-pinene, and limonene, with (−)-α-pinene having the most significant alarm activity. (Z,E)-α-farnesene and (E,E)-α-farnesene were also reported in several aphid species (Gut and Van Oosten, 1985; Pickett and Griffiths, 1980), but did not show biological activity (Bowers *et al.*, 1977a).

Recently, Francis *et al.* (2005) characterized the volatile emissions of 23 aphid species and reported that Eβf was the only volatile chemical emitted in significant amounts by 16 of them. Eβf was a minor component of the volatile emissions of five other species. The remaining two species, *Euceraphis punctipennis* Zetterstedt and *Drepanosiphum platanoides* Schrank, did not release any Eβf, though other terpenes were isolated. In addition to the species examined by Francis *et al.* (2005), we have identified four additional aphid species that appear to produce Eβf as their only volatile chemical: *Rhopalosiphum maidis* Fitch, *Aphis glycines* Matsumura, *Aphis spiraecola* Pagenstecher, and *Brachycaudus persicae* Pesserini (Verheggen, unpublished data).

In *M. persicae*, the quantity and mode of action of the alarm pheromone was found to vary with morph and age of aphids (Gut and Van Oosten, 1985). The quantities of Eβf in aphids also increase in relation to increasing body weight (Byers, 2005), but its concentration declines exponentially with increasing body weight. In *A. pisum*, Verheggen *et al.* (2009) found that exposure to Eβf emitted by other individuals influences the levels of Eβf produced by immature aphids during development.

In addition to its role as an alarm pheromone in aphids, Eβf is also a common component of plant volatiles emissions—including both constitutive volatile blends (e.g., Agelopoulos *et al.*, 2000) and those induced by herbivore feeding (e.g., Turlings and Ton, 2006) or mechanical damage (e.g., Agelopoulos *et al.*, 1999). And Eβf is a constituent of various essential oils found in several plants family such as Asteraceae (Heuskin *et al.*, 2009; Reichling and Becker, 1978). It is thus tempting to speculate that Eβf production by plants functions to repel or habituate aphids or to otherwise interfere with alarm signaling, but there is currently little evidence that such effects occur (Petrescu *et al.*, 2001). Instead, it appears that the presence of other sesquiterpenes—like (−)-β-caryophyllene—in plant volatile blends allow aphids to distinguish the pure Eβf emitted by conspecifics from Eβf of plant origin (Dawson *et al.*, 1984). However, other terpenes like α-pinene or isothiocyanates have been reported to enhance the dispersal-inducing activity of Eβf, leading to an increased specificity of the alarm signal in some aphid species (Dawson *et al.*, 1987; Pickett and Griffiths, 1980). Interestingly, Eβf is present in trichomes of wild potato plants where its release under aphid infestation does appear to cause dispersal (Gibson and Pickett, 1983).

The behavioral effect of alarm pheromone on aphids varies across species and also with the amount of pheromone encountered by receiving individuals. Typical responses range from the cessation of feeding and removal of the stylet from host plant tissues to walking, jumping, or falling away from the source of emission (Braendle and Weisser, 2001; Chau and Mackauer, 1997; Clegg and Barlow, 1982; Edwards *et al.*, 1973; Losey and Denno, 1998; Montgomery and Nault, 1977a,b, 1978; Phelan *et al.*, 1976; Roitberg and Myers, 1978; Shah *et al.*, 1999; Wientjens *et al.*, 1973; Wohlers, 1980). In the sugarcane woolly aphid, *Ceratovacuna lanigera* Zehntner (Homoptera, Pemphigidae), the alarm pheromone reportedly elicited aggressive behavior from conspecifics (Arakaki, 1989). Eβf has also a repellent effect on the landing behavior of alate aphids, which can cause them to choose an alternative host plant (Lambers and Schepers, 1978; Phelan and Miller, 1982; Wohlers, 1982). Field experiments confirmed dispersal behavior of aphids subjected to their alarm pheromone in 41 species (Xiangyu *et al.*, 2002). Kunert *et al.* (2005) also found that Eβf exposure increased the production of winged individuals specialized for dispersal. Once Eβf concentrations decrease, aphids commonly reinfest host plants (Calabrese and Sorensen, 1978). Because the amounts of alarm pheromone emitted by an individual under natural conditions might be too low to warn all nearby conspecifics, two recent studies tested the hypothesis that aphids might amplify the alarm signal by emitting additional Eβf in response to the alarm signals of other individuals but found no evidence for such an effect (Hatano *et al.*, 2008; Verheggen *et al.*, 2008b).

In addition to serving as an alarm signal to conspecifics and other aphids, Eβf is exploited as a foraging cue by predators and parasitoids that feed on aphids. Details are presented in Section D.

B. Ants

The first published observation of an ant alarm pheromone was probably that of Goetsch (1934) who noted that crushed organs were capable of causing aggressive reactions in workers. Following this original observation, all Formicid species were subsequently found to produce and use an alarm pheromone (Hölldobler and Wilson, 1990), whose secretion may alert or recruit conspecifics and often stimulates aggressive reactions (Blum, 1985 and references therein). Although behavioral responses can differ drastically among ant species, alarm pheromones generally serve two distinct functions (Wilson and Regnier, 1971). The response to "aggressive alarms" is characterized by rapid movements oriented toward the emitter and by aggressive attitudes ranging from mandible and gaster movements to biting or stinging the antagonist (Fig. 9.2). Recruitment of more workers and intensified attacks on intruders are also observed. Responses to "panic alarms" entail escape, dispersion, and flight behaviors. Workers' displacement speed is increased, as well as the frequency of direction changes. The type of reaction was found to correlate with differences among species in the size and density of colonies, with species having larger and denser colonies being more prone to aggressive responses. For example, *Lasius fuliginosus* forms large subterranean colonies and the general response workers to the alarm pheromone, *n*-undecane (Table 9.1), entails running toward the pheromone source with mandibles opened (Stoeffler *et al.*, 2007). In contrast, workers of *Hypoponera opacior* and *Ponera pennsylvanica*, which have small colony sizes, drastically increase their mobility but do not run toward the emitter when exposed to the main constituent of their alarm pheromone, 2,5-dimethyl-3-isopentylpyrazine (Duffield *et al.*, 1976).

A variety of natural products and associated behaviors have been highlighted in the different formicid genera, with production sites including mandibular, pygidial, metapleural, and Dufour's glands. Ant alarm pheromones are usually aliphatic carbon chains shorter and more volatile than those characteristic of trail pheromones. These include ketones, alcohols, esters, aldehydes, alkylpyrazines, terpenes, short aliphatic hydrocarbons, and formic acid. As with aphid alarm signals, the alarm pheromones used by ants are thus well suited chemically for their role in mediating effective responses to threats that are highly localized in space in time. Different chemicals often

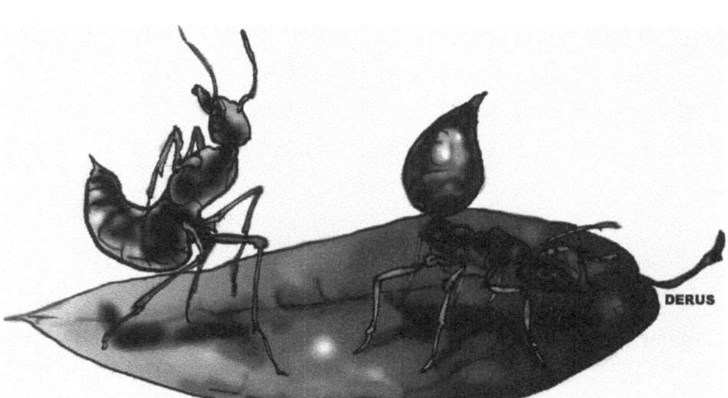

Figure 9.2 Two common alarm postures in Formicidae. Formicid ants respond to alarm pheromone with either aggressive or escape behaviors.

composed the alarm pheromone blend of a single ant species and these components can elicit different behaviors in receiving individuals. Moreover, because of differences in volatility, and perhaps also due to differences in the sensitivity of receiving individuals, the areas over which specific compounds induce active responses can also vary.

Minor workers of *Pheidole embolopyx* respond to encountering intruders of other species by secreting trail and alarm pheromones produced by the pygidial gland (Wilson and Hölldobler, 1985). In combination, these signals announce the presence of the enemy and lead to the recruitment of major workers who mount a sustained attack on the intruders.

The different components of the *Camponotus obscuripes* (Formicinae) alarm pheromone are produced in Dufour's gland and in the poison gland (Fujiwara-Tsujii *et al.*, 2006). The first gland contains a mixture of aliphatic carbon chains of which *n*-undecane represents 90%. Formic acid, a compound commonly used by ants for defense, trail marking, and recruitment, appears to be the only volatile chemical produced in the poison gland. In response to danger, *C. obscuripes* releases a mixture of these substances, each having a different volatility and function. Formic acid, perceived at longer distances, informs other colony members of the presence of a threat and helps them to locate the source of the emission. At shorter range, *n*-undecane and other associated saturated hydrocarbons induce aggression toward antagonists.

Among leaf cutting ants in the genus *Atta*, the mandibular gland secretions of most species contain mixtures of volatile, low-molecular-weight alcohols and ketones, which elicit the alarm response (Blum, 1968). The main volatile components of the mandibular glands of major workers are 4-methyl-3-heptanone (Table 9.1) and 2-heptanone (Hughes *et al.*, 2001), with the former being most active in eliciting alarm responses (Moser *et al.*, 1968). The latter chemical also occurs commonly in other ant genera (Feener *et al.*, 1996).

C. Honeybees

A vital role in honeybee colony defense is played by so-called guard bees, which patrol the nest entrance and represent the first line of defense. These guards are also specialized for the production of alarm pheromone which they release to recruit nestmates from the interior of the colony in case of danger (Boch *et al.*, 1962; Collins *et al.*, 1982). The perception of the pheromone increases workers movement and promotes aggression. Indeed, beekeepers are well acquainted with the banana-like odor released by stressed colonies, and with the fact that one bee sting is likely to be followed by others unless one rapidly moves away from the colony or uses smoke to sedate it. Although there is a striking variation in the intensity of their response (in docile colonies, only a few bees may respond while thousands of stinging individuals may attack in more aggressive colonies), only guarding workers produce the alarm pheromone (Alaux *et al.*, 2009; Vander Meer *et al.*, 1998).

The possibility that an alarm signal, of then unknown nature and origin, could act to alert honeybee workers was first suggested in the early 17th century (Butler, 1609, cited by Wilson, 1971). The signal was later proposed to be an odorant by Huber (1814), who noticed that presenting a honeybee worker's sting (attached to a forceps) to conspecifics changed their behavior from "quiet" to "aggressive." He concluded that "some odors incite honeybees to flee." It was later established that the honeybee alarm pheromone is produced in the mandibular as well as in the Koshewnikov gland associated with the sting apparatus (Boch *et al.*, 1962; Shearer and Boch, 1965)—though pheromone emission does not require that the sting be used.

Boch *et al.* (1962) first identified isopentyl acetate (previously called *iso*-amyl acetate) (Table 9.1) as a biologically active alarm pheromone associated with the sting (The use of smoke by beekeepers suppresses the activation of antennal receptors of isopentyl acetate, and therefore reduces nestmate recruitment.) (Visscher *et al.*, 1995). Subsequently, over 20 additional volatile aliphatic and aromatic active compounds of low molecular weight have been identified in the alarm pheromone blend (Hunt, 2007). In addition to isopentyl acetate, (Z)-11-eicosen-1-ol is thought to play an essential role (Boch *et al.*, 1962; Pickett *et al.*, 1982). Although both these compounds individually induce alarm responses in bee workers, when presented together they elicit behavioral responses comparable to the intact sting (Pickett *et al.*, 1982). Not all components of the pheromone blend in honeybees induce alarm behavior, some have other specialized functions including flight induction (e.g., benzyl acetate), and recruitment (e.g., 1-butanol, 1-octanol, hexyl acetate), while others play multiple roles (e.g., 1-hexanol, butyl acetate, isopentyl acetate, 2-nonanol) (Wager and Breed, 2000). Shearer and Boch (1965) reported alarm activity of 2-heptanone (Table 9.1) isolated from honeybee mandibular glands. With increasing age, the size of the gland and the amount of 2-heptanone increases (Vallet *et al.*, 1991). When filter paper treated with 2-heptanone is placed at the hive entrance, bees nearby become greatly agitated, assuming a characteristic aggressive posture and running toward the emission source in jerky circles or short zigzags. Contrary to longstanding expectations, the honeybee alarm pheromone blend does not seem to be implicated in target localization (Free, 1961; Wager and Breed, 2000).

D. Alarm pheromones used as kairomones by natural enemies

Semiochemicals provide a powerful way for organisms to communicate and coordinate their behaviors. But they also represent opportunities for other organisms to intercept and exploit such signals. Indeed, there are numerous

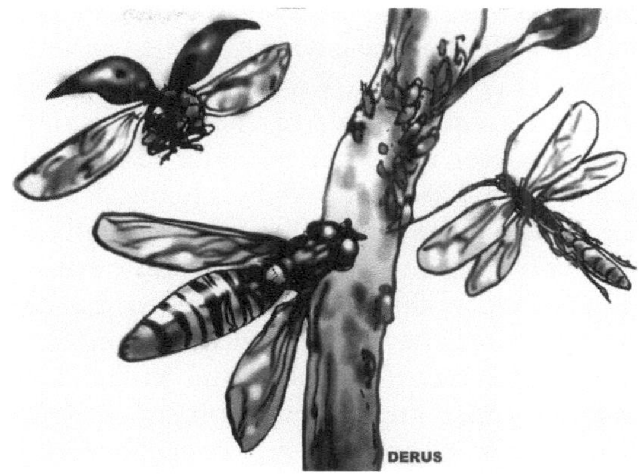

Figure 9.3 Like many natural enemies, aphid predators and parasitoids have evolved to perceive and exploit the alarm pheromones of their prey.

examples of natural enemies having learned or evolved to use the pheromones of their prey as foraging cues (Vet and Dicke, 1992).

For example, aphid natural enemies rely on semiochemicals, especially the aphid alarm pheromone, to locate aphid colonies (Fig. 9.3). Previous studies have demonstrated this phenomenon in lady beetles, *Coccinella* sp., *Adalia* sp., and *Harmonia* sp. (e.g., Francis *et al.*, 2004; Nakamuta, 1991; Verheggen *et al.*, 2007); hoverflies (e.g., Almohamad *et al.*, 2009; Verheggen *et al.*, 2008a, 2009); ground beetles (Kielty *et al.*, 1996); lacewings (Boo *et al.*, 1998; Zhu *et al.*, 1999); and parasitic wasp adults and larvae (Beale *et al.*, 2006).

Ant parasitoids also use alarm pheromone components to locate their specific hosts. Individuals of *Apocephalus paraponerae* (Diptera: Phoridae), which parasitizes workers of the giant tropical ant *Paraponera clavata* (Hymenoptera: Formicidae), locate fighting or injured workers of this host species by using 4-methyl-3-heptanone and 4-methyl-3-heptanol (Feener *et al.*, 1996). The cursorial spider *Habronestes bradleyi* (Araneae, Zodariidae), a specialist predator of the meat ant *Iridomyrmex purpureus*, likewise locates workers of its prey by using their alarm pheromone, which consists mainly of 6-methyl-5-hepten-2-one and is frequently released during territorial disputes among conspecifics (Allan *et al.*, 1996).

III. Alarm Pheromones in Marine Invertebrates

Alarm behaviors in aquatic invertebrates are also commonly mediated by chemical signals, and a growing number of aquatic organisms have been shown to display antipredator behavior in response to injury-released chemical cues from conspecifics, including mollusks (e.g., Spinella *et al.*, 1993), flatworms (e.g., Wisenden and Millard, 2001), annelids (e.g., Watson *et al.*, 2005), and echinoderms (e.g., Vadas and Elner, 2003).

The first report of a chemical alarm cue in a platyhelminth was the demonstration that predator avoidance behavior in a free-living flatworm, *Dugesia dorotocephala*, could be induced by chemical cues released from injured conspecifics (Wisenden and Millard, 2001). Despite their relatively simple nervous system, Planaria are apparently also capable of learned risk association, as following simultaneous exposure to the conspecific alarm signal and sunfish odor cues, they subsequently respond to the sunfish odor alone as an indicator of danger (Wisenden and Millard, 2001). Green sea urchins, *Lytechinus variegates*, employ a two-phased response to cues from damaged conspecifics entailing an initial rapid but ephemeral alarm response followed by a more sustained flight phase, which induces urchins to disperse (Vadas and Elner, 2003). Chemical alarm substances have also been documented in Gastropods. The snail *Littorina littorea*, common periwinkle, shows crawl-out responses (i.e., movement out of the water) in response to chemical stimuli from injured individuals (Jacobsen and Stabell, 1999). The first cnidarian pheromone to be documented was anthopleurine (Table 9.1), which is released from wounded tissues of the sea anemone *Anthopleura elegantissima*—for example, during attack by the nudibranch *Aeolidia papillosa*—and evokes rapid withdrawal in nearby conspecifics (Howe and Sheikh, 1975).

IV. Alarm Pheromones in Fish

Many fishes use alarm pheromones to warn conspecifics of potential threats in the surrounding environment (reviewed by Smith, 1992). The first suggestion that Ostariophysan fishes (the second largest superorder of fish) might exhibit a fright reaction in response to some signal from wounded conspecifics, and that this might reduce the receivers' vulnerability to subsequent predation, was made by von Frisch (1938). Pfeiffer (1963, 1977, 1978) subsequently documented alarm signaling in several Ostariophysan species. The secretion of the signals involves specialized epidermal cells that contain the alarm pheromone. When these cells are broken, as during predation events, this substance is released into the surrounding water (Fig. 9.4). Thus, senders cannot actively release their alarm substance (Smith, 1992), but the restricted context in which they are emitted reliably informs conspecifics of the presence of a predator. Fathead minnows (*Pimephales promelas*) and finescale dace (*Chrosomus neogaeus*) also exhibited significant antipredator responses (increased shoaling and decreased area of movement) when exposed to conspecific skin extract (Brown *et al.*,

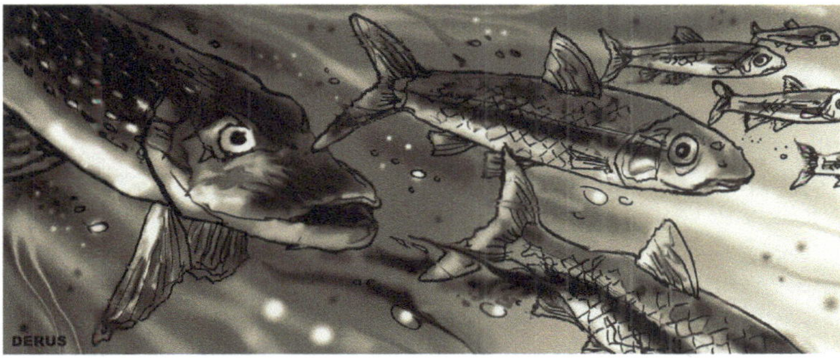

Figure 9.4 Ostariophysan fish species release an alarm signal when their skin is damaged, and receiving individuals exhibit fright reactions including increased shoaling and decreased area of movement.

2000). Similar reactions were observed in response to hypoxanthine-3-*N*-oxide (Table 9.1), one of several molecules thought to function as a chemical alarm signal in Ostariophysan species (Brown *et al.*, 2000). Complementary studies subsequently found that exposure to low concentrations of hypoxanthine-3-*N*-oxide may cause fish to increase vigilance toward secondary (i.e., visual) risk-assessment cues, leading to an increased alarm response in case of predator attack (Brown *et al.*, 2004). The fish fright reaction can also be detected visually by other nearby individuals leading to the rapid propagation of the alarm response through a group (Smith, 1992).

In the Percid fishes, physical injury also appears to be required for release of the active alarm pheromone component, and exposure to water that previously contained an injured individual leads to reduced movement ("freezing") and periods of inactivity in the receiver (Crane *et al.*, 2009). Fish alarm pheromones do not appear to be species specific, and usually induce equivalent alarm responses in other species (Smith, 1982). For example, the pumpkinseeds, *Lepomis gibbosus* (Acanthopterygii), exhibit antipredator responses when exposed to hypoxanthine-3-*N*-oxide, the putative Ostariophysan alarm pheromone (Golub *et al.*, 2005). This similarity of intra- and interspecific reactions in fishes, suggests corresponding similarities in signaling chemistry and reception mechanisms. This has led to some controversy as to whether alarm signals in fish should strictly be classed as pheromones or as allelochemicals (Burnard *et al.*, 2008).

V. Alarm Pheromones in Mammals

Mammals make wide use of pheromones to mark territories, attract mates, and coordinate group behavior. Chemical alarm signaling also occurs, but though many territorial and sexual pheromones have been identified in mammals, relatively little progress has been made in the chemical identification and functional analysis of mammal alarm pheromones (Hauser *et al.*, 2005). It is commonly thought that mammal alarm pheromones are volatile, and it is hypothesized that they may be low molecular weight compounds, such as fatty acids or steroids. The perception of these alarm signals seems to be mediated by an auxiliary olfactory sense organ called the vomeronasal organ (VON), or Jacobson's organ (Dulac and Axel, 1998).

Although, infochemicals appear to play a smaller role in communication between humans than in other mammals, the ability to produce and perceive pheromones has also been demonstrated in humans (McClintock, 1998). The existence of a human alarm pheromone has not been demonstrated, but it has been suggested that humans can detect differences between a neutral scent and a scent associated with frightened individuals (Ackerl *et al.*, 2002).

Chemical alarm signaling has been demonstrated in mice (Rottman and Snowdown, 1972). When exposed to the odor of a stressed conspecific, mice behaved aversively to the source of the odor, even though they responded positively to the sender's odor prior to the introduction of the stress. Stressed male Wistar rats release a volatile alarm pheromone, from the perianal region that elicits defensive and risk-assessment behavior in receiving individuals, characterized by hyperthermia, increased freezing, sniffing, and walking as well as a decreased resting behavior (Inagaki *et al.*, 2009; Kikusui *et al.*, 2001). So far, the chemical structure of this pheromone has not been elucidated.

Odor-induced fear responses have also been documented in cattle and shown to be at least partly mediated by olfactory cues in the urine of stressed individuals (Boissy *et al.*, 1998).

VI. Alarm Signals in Plants

Plants actively respond to damage induced by infesting arthropods by inducing direct defenses such as toxins and antifeedants (Gatehouse, 2002). But, they also typically release blends of volatile compounds from damaged tissues—as well as systemically—that appear to play a variety of signaling functions (Farmer, 2001). For example, these herbivore-induced plant volatiles can directly repel foraging herbivores, such as ovipositing butterflies and moths and host-seeking aphids (Dicke and Vet, 1999). Herbivore-induced volatiles also serve as key foraging cues for natural enemies of the feeding herbivores, including insect predators and parasitoids (e.g., Turlings *et al.*, 1998) and even for insectivorous birds (Mäntylä *et al.*, 2008). Moreover, these signals can convey complex and highly specific information about the status of emitting plants. For example, the highly specialized parasitoid wasp *Cotesia congregata* can consistently distinguish among volatile blends elicited by the feeding of two closely related caterpillar species and preferentially responds to the odors of plants infested by its host (De Moraes *et al.*, 1998).

There has been a longstanding debate about the extent to which damage-induce plant volatiles might also be important in signaling between neighboring plants (Farmer, 2001; Heil and Karban, 2010; Karban, 2008), but a number of recent studies suggests that these compounds play an important role in signaling between damaged and undamaged tissues of individual plants (e.g., Arimura *et al.*, 2000; Dolch and Tscharntke, 2000; Engelberth *et al.*, 2004; Karban and Maron, 2002; Karban *et al.*, 2003), and particularly in overcoming potential constraints on the internal (vascular) transmission of wound signals imposed by plants' modular architecture (Frost *et al.*, 2007; Heil and Silva Bueno, 2007; Karban *et al.*, 2006; Rodriguez-Saona *et al.*, 2009).

VII. Conclusion: Potential Applications of Alarm Pheromones

In addition to obviously intriguing questions about the evolution of alarm signaling within individuals species and differences in the way they function between taxa, understanding this class of semiochemical-mediated interactions also has potential for application to the management of pest species. Sex pheromones, mainly of Lepidopteran insects, have frequently been incorporated into management strategies (Copping, 2001). While few alarm pheromones have been employed in this context, some efforts have been made to incorporate them in push–pull strategies as behavior-manipulating stimuli to make the protected resource unattractive to the pest (Cook *et al.*, 2007). And honeybee alarm pheromone can be used to repel *Apis mellifera* from oilseed rape before insecticide applications (Free *et al.*, 1985).

A good deal of research has addressed the potential use of aphid alarm pheromone as a control mechanism. Following identification of the aphid alarm pheromone—Eβf in most species of Aphidinae—researchers began discussing the possibility of using this semiochemical to repel aphids (Bowers *et al.*, 1972), encouraged by the relative ease of extracting and purifying Eβf from plant material (Heuskin *et al.*, 2009). Early attempts to employ Eβf in the field were unsuccessful, however, as aphids recolonized host-plants very rapidly following exposure (Calabrese and Sorensen, 1978). Later, slow-release formulations of *Hemizygia petiolata* (Lamiaceae) containing high levels of Eβf were successfully employed to reduce pea aphid populations in field experiments (Bruce *et al.*, 2005). The increased aphid mobility induced by E*β*f exposition could also increase aphid exposure to insecticides and fungal control agents (Griffiths and Pickett, 1980). Similarly, application of farnesol and nerolidol, components of the two-spotted mite (*Tetranychus urticae*) alarm pheromone, increased mite mobility and subsequent exposure to coapplied acaricides, leading to enhanced control relative to the application of acaricides alone (Copping, 2001).

Studies on the role of E*β*f in interspecific interactions in natural systems also suggest its potential application to the control of aphid population mechanisms. As noted above, Gibson and Pickett (1983) demonstrated the ability of wild potatoes to repel aphids by naturally releasing E*β*f from their glandular trichomes. And work on the perception of the aphid alarm pheromone by predators highlights of its potential to increase aphid apparency to natural enemies (Almohamad *et al.*, 2008; Du *et al.*, 1998; Verheggen *et al.*, 2007, 2008a; Zhu *et al.*, 1999). Beale *et al.* (2006) exploited this potential by incorporating an E*β*f synthase gene into the genome of *Arabidopsis thaliana*, and demonstrated increased attraction of aphid parasitoids to the modified plants.

Because alarm pheromones can be attractants for certain organisms, they also have potential for use in baits or traps. Hughes et al. (2002) showed that an alarm pheromone produced by grass-cutting ants, 4-methyl-3-heptanone, has significant potential to improve the efficacy of baits used for the control of these insects, since individuals receiving the signal tend to move toward the source of emission.

Far fewer studies have addressed practical applications of non-insect alarm pheromones. However, alarm signals might well have applications in the control of aquatic pests. For example, the search for a method to decrease the decline of Britain's native white-clawed crayfish (*Austropotamobius pallipes*) caused by the presence of the induced signal crayfish (*Pacifastacus leniusculus*), originally from North America, has given rise to speculation that *P. leniusculus* pheromones (including sex, stress, and alarm pheromones) might improve the efficiency of existing baits (Stebbing *et al.*, 2003).

REFERENCES

Ackerl, K., Atzmueller, M., and Grammer, K. (2002). The scent of fear. *Neuroendocrinol. Lett.* **23,** 79–84.

Agelopoulos, N. G., Hooper, A. M., Maniar, S. P., Pickett, J. A., and Wadhams, L. J. (1999). A novel approach for isolation of volatile chemicals released by individual leaves of a plant in situ. *J. Chem. Ecol.* **25,** 1411–1425.

Agelopoulos, N. G., Chamberlain, K., and Pickett, J. A. (2000). Factors affecting volatile emissions of intact potato plants, *Solanum tuberosum*: Variability of quantities and stability of ratios. *J. Chem. Ecol.* **26,** 497–511.

Alaux, C., Sinha, S., Hasadsri, L., Hunt, G. J., Guzman-Novoa, E., DeGrandi-Hoffman, G., Uribe-Rubio, J. L., Southey, B. R., Rodriguez-Zas, S., and Robinson, G. E. (2009). Honey bee aggression supports a link between gene regulation and behavioral evolution. *PNAS* **106,** 15400–15405.

Allan, R. A., Elgar, M. A., and Capon, R. J. (1996). Exploitation of an ant chemical alarm signal by the zodariid spider *Habronestes bradleyi* Walckenaer. *Proc. Roy. Soc. B—Biol. Sci.* **263,** 69–73.

Almohamad, R., Verheggen, F. J., Francis, F., Lognay, G., and Haubruge, E. (2008). Emission of alarm pheromone by non-preyed aphid colonies. *J. Appl. Entomol.* **132,** 601–604.

Almohamad, R., Verheggen, F. J., and Haubruge, E. (2009). Searching and oviposition behavior of aphidophagous hoverflies (Diptera: Syrphidae): A review. *Biotechnol. Agron. Soc. Environ.* **13,** 467–481.

Arakaki, N. (1989). Alarm pheromone eliciting attack and escape responses in the sugar-cane woolly aphid, *Ceratovacuna-lanigera* (Homoptera, Pemphigidae). *J. Ethol.* **7,** 83–90.

Arimura, G.-I., Ozawa, R., Shimoda, T., Nishioka, T., Boland, W., and Takabayashi, J. (2000). Herbivory-induced volatiles elicit defence genes in lima bean leaves. *Nature* **406,** 512–515.

Barbier, M. (1982). Les phéromones. Aspects biochimiques et biologiques. Masson.

Beale, M. H., Birkett, M. A., Bruce, T. J. A., Chamberlain, K., Field, L. M., Huttly, A. K., Martin, J. L., Parker, R., Phillips, A. L., Pickett, J. A., Prosser, I. M., and Shewry, P. R. (2006). Aphid alarm pheromone produced by transgenic plants affects aphid and parasitoid behavior. *PNAS* **103,** 10509–10513.

Blum, M. S. (1968). Alarm pheromones. *Annu. Rev. Entomol.* **14,** 157–180.

Blum, M. S. (1985). Alarm pheromones. *In* "Comprehensive Insect physiology, Biochemistry and Pharmacology," (G. A. Kerkut and L. I. Gilbert, Eds.), pp. 193–224. Pergamon Press.

Boch, R., Shearer, D. A., and Stone, B. C. (1962). Identification of *iso*-amyl acetate as an active component in the sting pheromone of the honey bee. *Nature* **195,** 1018–1020.

Boissy, A., Terlouw, C., and Le Neindre, P. (1998). Presence of cues from stressed conspecifics increases reactivity to aversive events in cattle: Evidence for the existence of alarm substances in urine. *Physiol. Behav.* **63,** 489–495.

Boo, K. S., Chung, I. B., Han, K. S., Pickett, J. A., and Wadhams, L. J. (1998). Response of the lacewing *Chrysopa cognata* to pheromones of its aphid prey. *J. Chem. Ecol.* **24,** 631–643.

Bowers, W. S., Nault, L. R., Webb, R. E., and Dutky, S. R. (1972). Aphid alarm pheromone: Isolation, identification, synthesis. *Science* **177,** 1121–1122.

Bowers, W. S., Nishino, C., Montgomery, M. E., and Nault, L. R. (1977a). Structure–activity-relationships of analogs of aphid alarm pheromone, (E)-beta-farnesene. *J. Insect Physiol.* **23,** 697–701.

Bowers, W. S., Nishino, C., Montgomery, M. E., Nault, L. R., and Nielson, M. W. (1977b). Sesquiterpene progenitor, Germancrene A: An alarm pheromone in aphids. *Science* **196,** 680–681.

Braendle, C., and Weisser, W. W. (2001). Variation in escape behavior of red and green clones of the pea aphid. *J. Insect Behav.* **14,** 497–509.

Brown, G. E., Adrian, J. C., Smyth, E., Leet, H., and Brennan, S. (2000). Ostariophysan alarm pheromones: Laboratory and field tests of the functional significance of nitrogen oxides. *J. Chem. Ecol.* **26,** 139–154.

Brown, G. E., Poirier, J. F., and Adrian, J. C. (2004). Assessment of local predation risk: The role of subthreshold concentrations of chemical alarm cues. *Behav. Ecol.* **15,** 810–815.

Bruce, T. J. A., Birkett, M. A., Blande, J., Hooper, A. M., Martin, J. L., Khambay, B., Prosser, I., Smart, L. E., and Wadhams, L. J. (2005). Response of economically important aphids to components of *Hemizygia petiolata* essential oil. *Pest Manag. Sci.* **61,** 1115–1121.

Burnard, D., Gozlan, R. E., and Griffiths, S. W. (2008). The role of pheromones in freshwater fishes. *J. Fish Biol.* **73,** 1–16.
Byers, J. A. (2005). A cost of alarm pheromone production in cotton aphids, *Aphis gossypii*. *Naturwissenschaften* **92,** 69–72.
Calabrese, E. J., and Sorensen, A. J. (1978). Dispersal and recolonization by *Myzus persicae* following aphid alarm pheromone exposure. *Ann. Entomol. Soc. Am.* **71,** 181–182.
Charnov, E. L., and Krebs, J. R. (1974). The evolution of alarm calls, altruism or manipulation? *Am. Nat.* **109,** 107–112.
Chau, A., and Mackauer, M. (1997). Dropping of pea aphids from feeding site: A consequence of parasitism by the wasp, *Monoctonus paulensis*. *Entomol. Exp. Appl.* **83,** 247–252.
Clegg, J. M., and Barlow, C. A. (1982). Escape behavior of the pea aphid *Acyrthosiphon pisum* (Harris) in response to the alarm pheromone and vibration. *Can. J. Zool.* **60,** 2245–2252.
Collins, A. M., Rinderer, T. E., Harbo, J. R., and Bolten, A. B. (1982). Colony defense by Africanized and European honeybees. *Science* **218,** 72–74.
Cook, S. M., Khan, Z. R., and Pickett, J. A. (2007). The use of push-pull strategies in integrated pest managment. *Annu. Rev. Entomol.* **52,** 375–400.
Copping, L. G. (2001). The biopesticide manual. *British Crop Protection Council.*
Crane, A. L., Woods, D., and Mathis, A. (2009). Behavioural responses to alarm cues by free-ranging rainbow darters (*Etheostoma caeruleum*). *Behaviour* **146,** 1565–1572.
Dawson, G. W., Griffiths, D. C., Pickett, J. A., Smith, M. C., and Woodcock, C. M. (1984). Natural inhibition of the aphid alarm pheromone. *Entomol. Exp. Appl.* **36,** 197–199.
Dawson, G. W., Griffiths, D. C., Pickett, J. A., Wadhams, L. J., and Woodcock, C. M. (1987). Plant-derived synergists of alarm pheromone from turnip aphid, Lipaphis (Hyadaphis) erysimi (Homoptera, Aphididae). *J. Chem. Ecol.* **13,** 1663–1671.
De Moraes, C. M., Lewis, W. J., Paré, P. W., Alborn, H. T., and Tumlinson, J. H. (1998). Herbivore-infested plants selectively attract parasitoids. *Nature* **393,** 570–573.
Dicke, M., and Vet, L. E. M. (1999). Plant–carnivore interactions: Evolutionary and ecological consequences for plant, herbivore and carnivore. *In* "Herbivores: Between Plants and Predators," (H. Olff, V. K. Brown, and R. H. Drent, Eds.), pp. 483–520. Blackwell Science, Oxford.
Dolch, R., and Tscharntke, T. (2000). Defoliation of alders (*Alnus glutinosa*) affects herbivory by leaf beetles on undamaged neighbours. *Oecologia* **125,** 504–511.
Du, Y., Poppy, G. M., Powell, W., Pickett, J. A., Wadhams, L. J., and Woodcock, C. M. (1998). Identification of semiochemicals released during aphid feeding that attract parasitoid *Aphidius ervi*. *J. Chem. Ecol.* **24,** 1355–1368.
Duffield, R. M., Blum, M. S., and Wheeler, J. W. (1976). Alkylpyrazine alarm pheromones in primitive ants with small colonial units. *Comp. Biochem. Physiol. B* **54,** 439–440.
Dulac, C., and Axel, R. (1998). Expression of candidate pheromone receptor genes in vomeronasal neurons. *Chem. Senses* **23,** 467–475.
Edwards, L. J., Siddall, J. B., Dunham, L. L., Uden, P., and Kislow, C. J. (1973). Trans-beta-farnesene, alarm pheromone of the green peach aphid, *Myzus persicae* (Sulzer). *Nature* **241,** 126–127.
Engelberth, J., Alborn, H. T., Schmelz, E. A., and Tumlinson, J. H. (2004). Airborne signals prime plants against insect herbivore attack. *PNAS* **101,** 1781–1785.
Farmer, E. (2001). Surface-to-air signals. *Nature* **411,** 854–856.
Feener, D. H., Jacobs, L. F., and Schmidt, J. O. (1996). Specialized parasitoid attracted to a pheromone of ants. *Anim. Behav.* **51,** 61–66.
Francis, F., Lognay, G., and Haubruge, E. (2004). Olfactory responses to aphid and host plant volatile releases: E-B-Farnesene an effective kairomone for the predator *Adalia bipunctata*. *J. Chem. Ecol.* **30,** 741–755.
Francis, F., Vandermoten, S., Verheggen, F., Lognay, G., and Haubruge, E. (2005). Is the (E)-b-Farnesene only volatile terpenoid in aphids? *J. Appl. Entomol.* **129,** 6–11.

Free, J. B. (1961). The stimuli releasing the stinging response of honeybees. *Anim. Behav.* **9,** 193–196.

Free, J. B., Pickett, J. A., Ferguson, A. W., Simpkings, J. R., and Smith, M. C. (1985). Reppelling honeybees with alarm pheromones. *J. Agric. Sci.* **105,** 255–260.

Frost, C. J., Appel, H. M., Carlson, J. E., De Moraes, C. M., Mescher, M. C., and Schultz, J. C. (2007). Within-plant signaling by volatiles overcomes vascular constraints on systemic signaling and primes responses against herbivores. *Ecol. Lett.* **10,** 490–498.

Fujiwara-Tsujii, N., Yamagata, N., Takeda, T., Mizunami, M., and Yamaoka, R. (2006). Behavioral responses to the alarm pheromone of the ant *Camponotus obscuripes* (Hymenoptera: Formicidae). *Zool. Sci.* **23,** 353–358.

Gatehouse, J. A. (2002). Plant resistance toward insect herbivores: A dynamic interaction. *New Phytol.* **156,** 145–169.

Gibson, R. W., and Pickett, J. A. (1983). Wild potato repels aphids by release of aphid alarm pheromone. *Nature* **302,** 608–609.

Goetsch, W. (1934). Untersuchungen über di Zusammenarbeit im Ameisenstaat. *Zoomorphology* **28,** 319–401.

Golub, J. L., Vermette, V., and Brown, G. E. (2005). Response to conspecific and heterospecific alarm cues by pumpkinseeds in simple and complex habitats: Field verification of an ontogenetic shift. *J. Fish Biol.* **66,** 1073–1081.

Griffiths, D. C., and Pickett, J. A. (1980). A potential application of aphid alarm pheromones. *Entomol. Exp. Appl.* **27,** 199–201.

Gut, J., and Van Oosten, A. M. (1985). Functional-significance of the alarm pheromone composition in various morphs of the green peach aphid, *Myzus persicae*. *Entomol. Exp. Appl.* **37,** 199–204.

Hamilton, W. D. (1964). The genetical evolution of social behaviour. *J. Theor. Biol.* **7,** 1–16.

Hatano, E., Kunert, G., Bartram, S., Boland, W., Gershenzon, J., and Weisser, W. W. (2008). Do aphid colonies amplify their emission of alarm pheromone? *J. Chem. Ecol.* **34,** 1149–1152.

Hauser, R., Wiergowski, M., Marczak, M., Karaszewski, B., and Wodniak-Ochocinska, L. (2005). Alarm pheromones as an exponent of emotional state shortly before death—Science fiction or a new challenge? *Forensic Sci. Int.* **155,** 226–230.

Heil, M., and Karban, R. (2010). Explaining evolution of plant communication by airborne signals. *Trends Ecol. Evol.* **25,** 137–144.

Heil, M., and Silva Bueno, J. C. (2007). Within-plant signaling by volatiles leads to induction and priming of an indirect plant defense in nature. *PNAS* **104,** 5467–5472.

Heuskin, S., Godina, B., Leroy, P., Capella, Q., Wathelet, J. P., Verheggen, F., Haubruge, E., and Lognay, G. (2009). Fast gas chromatography characterisation of purified semiochemicals from essential oils of *Matricaria chamomilla* L. (Asteraceae) and *Nepeta cataria* L. (Lamiaceae). *J. Chromatogr. A* **1216,** 2768–2775.

Högstedt, G. (1983). Adaptation unto death: Function of fear screams. *Am. Nat.* **121,** 562–570.

Hölldobler, B., and Wilson, E. O. (1990). The Ants. Springer-Verlag, Berlin.

Howe, N. R., and Sheikh, Y. M. (1975). Anthopleurine: A sea anemone alarm pheromone. *Science* **189,** 386–388.

Howse, P. E. (1998). Pheromones and Behaviour. *In* "Insect Pheromones and their Use in Pest Management," (P. E. Howse, I. Stevens, and O. Jones, Eds.). Chapman and Hall.

Huber, F. (1814). Nouvelles observations sur les abeilles, 2nd Edt. Paris & Genève, Librairie Paschoud.

Hughes, W. O. H., Howse, P. E., and Goulson, D. (2001). Mandibular gland chemistry of grass-cutting ants: Species, caste, and colony variation. *J. Chem. Ecol.* **27,** 109–124.

Hughes, W. O. H., Howse, P. E., Vilela, E. F., Knapp, J. J., and Goulson, D. (2002). Field evaluation of potential of alarm pheromone compounds to enhance baits for control of grass-cutting ants (Hymenoptera: Formicidae). *J. Econ. Entomol.* **95,** 537–543.

Hunt, G. J. (2007). Flight and fight: A comparative view of the neurophysiology and genetics of honey bee defensive behavior. *J. Insect Physiol.* **53,** 399–410.

Inagaki, H., Nakamura, K., Kiyokawa, Y., Kikusui, T., Takeuchi, Y., and Mori, Y. (2009). The volatility of an alarm pheromone in male rats. *Physiol. Behav.* **96,** 749–752.

Jacobsen, H. P., and Stabell, O. B. (1999). Predator-induced alarm responses in the common periwinkle, *Littorina littorea*: Dependence on season, light conditions, and chemical labelling of predators. *Mar. Biol.* **134,** 551–557.

Karban, R. (2008). Plant behaviour and communication. *Ecol. Lett.* **11,** 727–739.

Karban, R., and Maron, J. (2002). The fitness consequences of interspecific eavesdropping between plants. *Ecol. Lett.* **83,** 1209–1213.

Karban, R., Maron, J., Felton, G. W., Ervin, G., and Eichenseer, H. (2003). Herbivore damage to sagebrush induces resistance in wild tobacco: Evidence for eavesdropping between plants. *Oikos* **100,** 325–332.

Karban, R., Shiojiri, K., Huntzinger, M., and McCall, A. C. (2006). Damage-induced resistance in sagebrush: Volatiles are key to intra- and interplant communication. *Ecology* **87,** 922–930.

Karlson, P., and Lüscher, M. (1959). 'Pheromones': A new term for a class of biologically active substances. *Nature* **4653,** 55–56.

Kielty, J. P., Allen-Williams, L. J., Underwood, N., and Eastwood, E. A. (1996). Behavioral responses of three species of ground beetle (Coleoptera: Carabidae) to olfactory cues associated with prey and habitat. *J. Insect Behav.* **9,** 237–250.

Kikusui, T., Takigami, S., Takeuchi, Y., and Mori, Y. (2001). Alarm pheromone enhances stress-induced hyperthermia in rats. *Physiol. Behav.* **72,** 45–50.

Kislow, C. J., and Edwards, L. J. (1972). Repellent odor in aphids. *Nature* **235,** 108–109.

Kunert, G., Otto, S., Röse, U. S. R., Gershenzon, J., and Weisser, W. W. (2005). Alarm pheromone mediates production of winged dispersal morphs in aphids. *Ecol. Lett.* **8,** 596–603.

Kuwahara, Y., Fukami, H., Ishii, S., Matsumoto, K., and Wada, Y. (1979). Pheromone study on acarid mites. II. Presence of the alarm pheromone in the mold mite, *Tyrophagus putrescentiae* (Schrank) (Acarina: Acaridae) and the site of its production. *Jpn. J. Sanit. Zool.* **30,** 309–314.

Kuwahara, Y., Matsumoto, K., and Wada, Y. (1980). Pheromone study on acarid mit IV. Citral: composition and function as an alarm pheromone and its secretory gland in four species of acarid mites. *Jpn. J. Sanit. Zool.* **31,** 73–80.

Lambers, D. H. R., and Schepers, A. (1978). Effect of trans-beta-farnesene, used as a repellant against landing aphid alatae in seed potato growing. *Potato Res.* **21,** 23–26.

Leavesley, A. J., and Magrath, R. D. (2005). Communicating about danger: Urgency alarm calling in a bird. *Anim. Behav.* **70,** 365–373.

Losey, J. E., and Denno, R. F. (1998). The escape response of pea aphids to foliar-foraging predators: Factors affecting dropping behaviour. *Ecol. Enomol.* **23,** 53–61.

Mäntylä, E., Alessio, G. A., Blande, J. D., Heijari, J., and Holopainen, J. K. (2008). From plants to birds: Higher avian predation rates in trees responding to insect herbivory. *PLoS ONE* **3,** e2832.

Maynard Smith, J., and Harper, D. (2003). Animal Signals Oxford University Press, Oxford.

McClintock, M. K. (1998). On the nature of mammalian and human pheromones. *In* "Olfaction and Taste Xii—An International Symposium," (C. Murphy, Ed.), Vol. 855, pp. 390–392. New York Acad Sciences, New York.

Montgomery, M. E., and Nault, L. R. (1977a). Aphid alarm pheromones—Dispersion of *Hyadaphis erysimi* and *Myzus persicae* (Hemiptera—Aphididae). *Ann. Entomol. Soc. Am.* **70,** 669–672.
Montgomery, M. E., and Nault, L. R. (1977b). Comparative response of aphids to alarm pheromone, (E)-beta-farnesene. *Entomol. Exp. Appl.* **22,** 236–242.
Montgomery, M. E., and Nault, L. R. (1978). Effects of age and wing polymorphism on sensitivity of *Myzus persicae* to alarm pheromone. *Ann. Entomol. Soc. Am.* **71,** 788–790.
Moser, J. C., Brownlee, R. C., and Silverstein, R. (1968). Alarm pheromone of the ant *Atta texana*. *J. Insect Physiol.* **14,** 529–535.
Nakamuta, K. (1991). Aphid alarm pheromone component, (E)-beta-farnesene, and local search by a predatory lady beetle, *Coccinella septempunctata* Bruckii mulsant (Coleoptera, Coccinellidae). *Appl. Entomol. Zool.* **26,** 1–7.
Payne, T. L. (1974). Pheromone perception. *In* "Pheromones," (M. C. Birch, Ed.). North-Holland Publishing Company.
Petrescu, A. S., Mondor, E. B., and Roitberg, B. D. (2001). Subversion of alarm communication: Do plants habituate aphids to their own alarm signals? *Can. J. Zool.* **79,** 737–740.
Pfeiffer, W. (1963). The fright reaction of North American fish. *Can. J. Zool.* **41,** 69–77.
Pfeiffer, W. (1977). The distribution of fright reaction and alarm substance cells in fishes. *Copeia* **00,** 653–665.
Pfeiffer, W. (1978). Heterocyclic compounds as releasers of the fright reaction in the giant danio *Danio malabaricus* (Jerdon) (Cyprinidae, Ostariophysi, Pisces). *J. Chem Ecol.* 665–673.
Phelan, P. L., and Miller, J. R. (1982). Post-landing behavior of alate *Myzus persicae* as altered by (E)-beta-farnesene and 3-carboxylic acids. *Entomol. Exp. Appl.* **32,** 46–53.
Phelan, P. L., Montgomery, M. E., and Nault, L. R. (1976). Orientation and locomotion of the apterous aphids dislodged from their hosts by alarm pheromone. *Ann. Entomol. Soc. Am.* **69,** 1153–1156.
Pickett, J. A., and Griffiths, D. C. (1980). Composition of aphid alarm pheromones. *J. Chem. Ecol.* **6,** 349–360.
Pickett, J. A., Williams, I. H., and Martin, A. P. (1982). (Z)-11-Eicosen-1-ol, an important new pheromonal component from the sting of the honeybee, *Apis mellifera* L. (Hymenoptera, Apidae). *J. Chem. Ecol.* **8,** 163–175.
Pickett, J. A., Wadhams, L. J., Woodcock, C. M., and Hardie, J. (1992). The chemical ecology of aphids. *Annu. Rev. Entomol.* **37,** 67–90.
Reichling, J., and Becker, H. (1978). Essential oil of Radix chamomillae (*Matricaria chamomilla* L.). *Z. Naturforsch. C* **33,** 589–591.
Rodriguez-Saona, C. R., Rodriguez-Saona, L. E., and Frost, C. J. (2009). Herbivore-induced volatiles in the perennial shrub, *Vaccinium corymbosum*, and their role in inter-branch signaling. *J. Chem. Ecol.* **35,** 163–175.
Roitberg, B. D., and Myers, J. H. (1978). Adaptation of alarm pheromone responses of pea aphid *Acyrthosiphon pisum* (Harris). *Can. J. Zool.* **56,** 103–108.
Rottman, S. J., and Snowdown, C. T. (1972). Demonstration and analysis of an alarm pheromone in mice. *J. Comp. Physiol. Psycol.* **81,** 483–490.
Seyfarth, R. M., Cheney, D. L., and Marler, P. (1980). Monkey responses to three different alarm calls: Evidence of predator classification and semantic communication. *Science* **210,** 801–803.
Shah, P. A., Pickett, J. A., and Vanderberg, J. D. (1999). Responses of Russian wheat aphid (Homoptera: Aphididae) to aphid alarm pheromone. *Environ. Entomol.* **28,** 983–985.
Shearer, D. A., and Boch, R. (1965). 2-Heptanone in the mandibular gland secretion of the honeybee. *Nature* **205,** 530.

Sherman, P. W. (1977). Nepotism and the evolution of alarm calls. *Science* **197,** 1246–1253.
Sherman, P. W. (1985). Alarm calls of Belding's ground squirrels to aerial predators: Nepotism or self-preservation? *Behav. Ecol. Sociobiol.* **17,** 313–323.
Smith, M. C. (1982). Reaction of *Percina nigrofasciata, Ammocrypta beani*, and *Etheostoma swaini* (Percidae, Pisces) to conspecific and intergeneric skin extracts. *Can. J. Zool.* **60,** 1067–1072.
Smith, R. J. F. (1986). Evolution of alarm signals; role of benefits derived from retaining group members of territorial neighbors. *Am. Nat.* **128,** 604–610.
Smith, R. J. F. (1992). Alarm signals in fishes. *Rev. Fish Biol.* **2,** 33–63.
Spinella, A., Alvarez, L. A., Passeggio, A., and Cimino, G. (1993). New 3-alkylpyridines from 3 mediterranean Cephalaspidean mollusks—Structure, ecological role and taxonomic relevance. *Tetrahedron* **49,** 1307–1314.
Stebbing, P. D., Watson, G. J., Bentley, M. G., Fraser, D., Jennings, R., Rushton, S. P., and Sibley, P. J. (2003). Reducing the threat: The potential use of pheromones to control invasive signal crayfish. *Bull. Fr. Peche Piscicult.* 219–224.
Stoeffler, M., Maier, T. S., Tolasch, T., and Steidle, J. L. M. (2007). Foreign-language skills in rove-beetles? Evidence for chemical mimicry of ant alarm pheromones in myrmecophilous Pella beetles (Coleoptera: Staphylinidae). *J. Chem. Ecol.* **33,** 1382–1392.
Taylor, R. J., Balph, D. F., and Balph, M. H. (1990). The evolution of alarm calling: A cost-benefit analysis. *Anim. Behav.* **39,** 860–868.
Trivers, R. L. (1971). The evolution of reciprocal altruism. *Q. Rev. Biol.* **46,** 35–57.
Turlings, T. C. J., and Ton, J. (2006). Exploiting scents of distress: The prospect of manipulating herbivore-induce plant odour to enhance the control of agricultural pests. *Curr. Opin. Plant Biol.* **9,** 421–427.
Turlings, T. C. J., Bernasconi, M., Bertossa, R., Bigler, F., Caloz, G., and Dorn, S. (1998). The induction of volatile emissions in maize by three herbivore species with different feeding habits: Possible consequences for their natural enemies. *Biol. Control* **11,** 122–129.
Vadas, R. L., and Elner, R. W. (2003). Responses to predation cues and food in two species of sympatric, tropical sea urchins. *Mar. Ecol.* **24,** 101–121.
Vallet, A., Cassier, P., and Lensky, Y. (1991). Ontogeny of the fine-structure of the mandibular glands of the honeybee (*Api mellifera* L) workers and the pheromonal activity of 2-heptanone. *J. Insect Physiol.* **37,** 789–804.
Vander Meer, R. K., Breed, M. D., Espelie, K. E., and Winston, M. L. (1998). Pheromone Communication in Social Insects Ants, Wasps, Bees, and Termites. Westview Press.
Verheggen, F. J., Fagel, Q., Heuskin, S., Lognay, G., Francis, F., and Haubruge, E. (2007). Electrophysiological and behavioral responses of the multicolored asian lady beetle, *Harmonia axyridis* pallas, to sesquiterpene semiochemicals. *J. Chem. Ecol.* **33,** 2148–2155.
Verheggen, F. J., Arnaud, L., Bartram, S., Gohy, M., and Haubruge, E. (2008a). Aphid and plant volatiles induce oviposition in an aphidophagous hoverfly. *J. Chem. Ecol.* **34,** 301–307.
Verheggen, F. J., Mescher, M. C., Haubruge, E., De Moraes, C. M., and Schwartzberg, E. G. (2008b). Emission of alarm pheromone in aphids: A non-contagious phenomenon. *J. Chem. Ecol.* **34,** 1146–1148.
Verheggen, F. J., Haubruge, E., De Moraes, C. M., and Mescher, M. C. (2009). Social enviroment influences aphid production of alarm pheromone. *Behav. Ecol.* **20,** 283–288.
Vet, L. E. M., and Dicke, M. (1992). Ecology of infochemical use by natural enemies in a tritrophic context. *Annu. Rev. Entomol.* **37,** 141–172.
Visscher, P. K., Vetter, R. S., and Robinson, G. E. (1995). Alarm pheromone perception in honey-bees is decreased by smoke (Hymenoptera, Apidae). *J. Insect Behav.* **8,** 11–18.
von Frisch, K. (1938). Zur psychologie des Fische-Schwarmes. *Naturwissenschaften* **26,** 601–606.

Wadhams, L. J. (1990). The use of coupled gas chromatography: Electrophysiological techniques in the identification of insect pheromones. *In* "Chromatography and Isolation of Insect Hormones and Pheromones," (A. R. McCaffery and A. R. Wilson, Eds.), pp. 289–298. Plenum, New York/London.

Wager, B. R., and Breed, M. D. (2000). Does honey bee sting alarm pheromone give orientation information to defensive bees? *Ann. Entomol. Soc. Am.* **93,** 1329–1332.

Watson, G. J., Hamilton, K. M., and Tuffnail, W. E. (2005). Chemical alarm signalling in the polychaete Nereis (Neanthes) virens (Sars) (Annelida: Polychaeta). *Anim. Behav.* **70,** 1125–1132.

Wientjens, W. H., Lakwijk, A. C., and Vanderma, T. (1973). Alarm pheromone of grain aphids. *Experientia* **29,** 658–660.

Wilson, E. O. (1971). The Insect Societies. Oxford University Press, London.

Wilson, E. O., and Hölldobler, B. (1985). Caste-specific techniques of defense in the polymorphic ant *Pheidole embolopyx* (Hymenoptera: Formicidae). *Insect. Soc.* **32,** 3–22.

Wilson, E. O., and Regnier, F. E. (1971). The evolution of the alarm-defense system in the formicine ants. *Am. Nat.* **105,** 279–289.

Wisenden, B. D., and Millard, M. C. (2001). Aquatic flatworms use chemical cues from injured conspecifics to assess predation risk and to associate risk with novel cues. *Anim. Behav.* **62,** 761–766.

Witkin, S. R., and Fitkin, M. S. (1979). Chickadee alarm calls: Does mate investment pay dividends? *Anim. Behav.* **27,** 1275–1276.

Wittstock, U., and Gershenzon, J. (2002). Constitutive plant toxins and their role in defense against herbivores and pathogens. *Curr. Opin. Plant Biol.* **5,** 300–3007.

Wohlers, P. (1980). Escape responses of pea aphids, *Acyrthosiphon pisum,* to alarm pheromones and additional stimuli. *Entomol. Exp. Appl.* **27,** 156–168.

Wohlers, P. (1981). Effect of the alarm pheromone (E)-beta-farnesene on dispersal behaviour of the pea aphid *Acyrthosiphon pisum. Entomol. Exp. Appl.* **29,** 117–124.

Wohlers, P. (1982). Effect of alarm pheromone (E)-beta-farnesene on aphid behavior during flight and after landing on plants. *Z. Angewandte Entomol.* **93,** 102–108.

Wyatt, T. D. (2003). Pheromones and Animal Behaviour. The Press Syndicate of the University of Cambridge, Oxford.

Xiangyu, J. G., Zhang, F., Fang, Y. L., Kan, W., Zhang, G. X., and Zhang, Z. N. (2002). Behavioural response of aphids to the alarm pheromone component (E)-beta-farnesene in the field. *Physiol. Entomol.* **27,** 307–311.

Zhu, J. W., Cossé, A. A., Obrycki, J. J., Boo, K. S., and Baker, T. C. (1999). Olfactory reactions of the twelve-spotted lady beetle, *Coleomegilla maculata* and the green lacewing, *Chrysoperla carnea* to semiochemicals released from their prey and host plant: Electroantennogram and behavioral responses. *J. Chem. Ecol.* **25,** 1163–1177.

CHAPTER TEN

Odorant-Binding Proteins in Insects

Jing-Jiang Zhou

Contents

Abstract

Our understanding of the molecular and biochemical mechanisms that mediate chemoreception in insects has been greatly improved after the discovery of olfactory and taste receptor proteins. However, after 50 years of the discovery of first insect sex pheromone from the silkmoth *Bombyx mori*, it is still unclear how hydrophobic compounds reach the dendrites of sensory neurons *in vivo* across aqueous space and interact with the sensory receptors. The presence of soluble polypeptides in high concentration in the lymph of chemosensilla still poses unanswered questions. More than two decades after their discovery and despite the wealth of structural and biochemical information available, the physiological function of odorant-binding proteins (OBPs) is not well understood. Here, I review the structural properties of different subclasses of insect OBPs and their binding to pheromones and other small ligands. Finally, I discuss current ideas and models on the role of such proteins in insect chemoreception. © 2010 Elsevier Inc.

I. Introduction

The perception of pheromone and other odorants occurs through a complex series of events, many aspects of which have been elucidated in recent years. Both invertebrates and vertebrates use their olfactory system to detect odorants. Chemical sensing is essential for feeding, mating, avoiding

Centre for Sustainable Pest and Disease Management, Insect Molecular Biology Group, Biological Chemistry Division, Rothamsted Research, Harpenden, UK

Vitamins and Hormones, Volume 83
ISSN 0083-6729, DOI: 10.1016/S0083-6729(10)83010-9

toxic substances, and withdrawing from hostile environments. For terrestrial animals, most odorants are air-born small hydrophobic molecules and need to be transported to reach olfactory receptors (ORs) through an aqueous medium (mucus in vertebrates and sensillum lymph in insects) which forms a hydrophilic barrier for the air-born odorants. Odorant-binding proteins (OBPs) are one class of olfactory proteins found in both vertebrates and insects, and thought to aid in capture and transport of odorants and pheromones to the receptors (Pelosi and Maida, 1990; Vogt *et al.*, 1985). OBPs are small, water-soluble, extracellular proteins that are located in the fluid surrounding the sensory dendrite. The need for odorant transport is unique for terrestrial animals, and in this regard OBPs represent a major evolutionary adaption of the olfactory system (Vogt *et al.*, 1991).

OBPs of vertebrates belong to the large superfamily of carrier proteins called lipocalins (Flower, 1996). They generally consist of chains of about 150 amino acids, and are mainly structured in β-sheet domains and fold in the typical β-barrel structure. In native conditions, they are usually present as homodimers. Each subunit presents a binding pocket located inside the barrel that can accommodate ligands of medium size (10–20 carbon atoms) and hydrophobic nature. In insects, OBPs can be divided into three subfamilies: pheromone-binding proteins (PBPs), general odorant-binding proteins (GOBPs) and antennal specific proteins (ASPs) or antennal-binding proteinx (ABPx). There is no homology between vertebrate OBPs and insect OBPs in amino acid sequence (Györgyi *et al.*, 1988) and three-dimensional structure (Sandler *et al.*, 2000; Zhou *et al.*, 2009). Vertebrate OBPs show a broad specificity toward odorants or the corresponding pheromones. Furthermore, the highest concentration of OBPs occurs in the lateral nasal gland rather than in the olfactory mucosa (Pevsner *et al.*, 1988), it is possible that these OBPs have no real role in olfaction. Insect OBPs are highly abundant (up to 10 mM) in the sensillum lymph of insect antennae (Klein, 1987; Vogt and Riddiford, 1981; Vogt *et al.*, 1989). One of the most extensively studied systems of chemical communication is that of pheromone detection of PBPs in Lepidopteran insects or moths. It is becoming increasingly clear that the insect PBPs show specific affinities to insect pheromone components and represent a family of proteins that have a specific role in sexual behavior. In addition, insect olfaction systems could serve as a model system for understanding the principles of animal olfaction and have attracted much attention since the identification of very specific olfactory pheromones (Kaissling *et al.*, 1978), the development of methods to record neural activity both extracellular (Boeckh and Boeckh, 1979) and intracellular (Hildebrand *et al.*, 1992), the detailed behavior studies to pheromones and analogs (Baker *et al.*, 1988) and the detailed morphological characterisation of olfactory organ, the antennae (O'Connell *et al.*, 1983). Another family of olfactory proteins were identified in locust and named as chemosensory proteins (CSPs) because they were found specifically expressed in chemosensory organs (Angeli *et al.*, 1999). This protein family has been reviewed in detail (Pelosi *et al.*, 1995, 2006). However, it is still arguable if they should be classified as a member of the OBP family. They share no similarity to OBPs and have completely different three-dimensional structures to OBPs. In this chapter, we focus on insect OBPs which have been intensively studied recently, in particularly on the PBPs of lepidopteran insects.

II. Diversity of Odorant-Binding Proteins

The first OBP of insects was discovered at the beginning of the 1980s in the giant moth *Antheraea polyphemus*. This protein, named PBP because it bound to radioactive pheromones, is 142 amino acids long with an isoelectric point of 4.7 (Vogt and Riddiford, 1981). At the same time, OBPs were found in cow (Pelosi *et al.*, 1981), later in rat (Pevsner *et al.*, 1986), frog (Lee *et al.*, 1987), human (Lacazette *et al.*, 2000), and bovine (Pevsner *et al.*, 1990). Meanwhile, additional insect OBPs were identified in the silkmoth *Bombyx mori* (Maida and Pelosi, 1989), the gypsy moth *Lymntria dispar* (Vogt *et al.*, 1989) and the turnip moth *Agrotis segetum* (Prestwich *et al.*, 1995). In these early biochemical studies, most sequences were partial as they were identified by determining N-terminal sequences using the tritium-labeled specific pheromones as a probe (Vogt *et al.*, 1991; Pelosi *et al.*, 2006). Full-length PBP cDNA sequences were identified and cloned first from the tobacco hawk moth *Manduca sexta* MsexPBP (Györgyi *et al.*, 1988), and then from the wild silkmoth *A. polyphemus* (Raming *et al.*, 1989), the Chinese oak silkmoth *Antheraea pernyi* (Raming *et al.*, 1990), and then many more. Another family of OBPs is the GOBPs. The GOBPs were defined based on their expression in both male and female antennae and their similarity to PBPs of Lepidopteran insects (Breer *et al.*, 1990) and further divided into GOBP1 and GOBP2 subfamilies (Vogt *et al.*, 1991). They are thought to interact with general odorants such as plant volatiles although this has not been experimentally demonstrated. A third family of proteins that are highly expressed in antennae have been identified and named as ABPs and ASPs (Krieger *et al.*, 1996).

Since the first OBPs were reported in the Lepidoptera, many papers have been published describing the proteins and associated genes in a wide range of insect species in the orders of Coleoptera (Nikonov *et al.*, 2002), Hymenoptera (Briand *et al.*, 2001), Diptera (Kim *et al.*, 1998), Orthoptera (Picone *et al.*, 2001), Dictyoptera (Riviere *et al.*, 2003), and Heteroptera (Vogt *et al.*, 1999). The recent availability of several insect genomes has allowed the identification of all the putative OBP genes in an insect genome. The most striking feature among all OBP sequences is six highly conserved cysteines with specific spacing between them (Breer *et al.*, 1990; Raming *et al.*, 1990). The number of amino acids between the second and third cysteines is always three; the number of amino acids between the fifth and sixth cysteines is always eight.

Such pattern in amino acid sequences has become a "signature" for insect OBPs. They are structurally important and form disulfide bridges to maintain the three-dimensional structures (Fig. 10.1; Sandler *et al.*, 2000; Tegoni *et al.*, 2004; Zhou *et al.*, 2009). This sequence motif has been used in OBP gene annotation from insect genomes. There are a large number of OBPs present within a variety of insect genomes (Pelosi *et al.*, 2006), and the identification of genes encoding OBPs has been mainly by means of bioinformatic approaches based on the characteristic features of the protein families (Hekmat-Scafe *et al.*, 2002; Li *et al.*, 2005; Liu *et al.*, 2009; Pelletier and Leal, 2009; Xu *et al.*, 2003; Zhou *et al.*, 2004a,b, 2006, 2008). These features include the six-cysteine signature, a size of 15–20 kDa, the α-helix pattern, the globular water-soluble nature, and the presence of a signal peptide. In the last few years, more than 400 OBPs have been isolated and cloned from more than 40 insect species, belonging to 10 different orders (Fig. 10.2). Among these, there are more than 150 OBPs from 34 species of 13 Lepidopteran families (Fig. 10.3). The large portion of these OBP genes has been identified from insect genome annotation projects, thus their involvement in olfaction remains to be demonstrated. However, these studies significantly enhanced the identification of more diverse OBPs in Dipteran insects and gave an insight into the evolution of OBPs as an abundant and rapidly evolving gene family through gene duplication (Vogt, 2002; Zhou *et al.*, 2008). So far, there is no report of any OBPs in

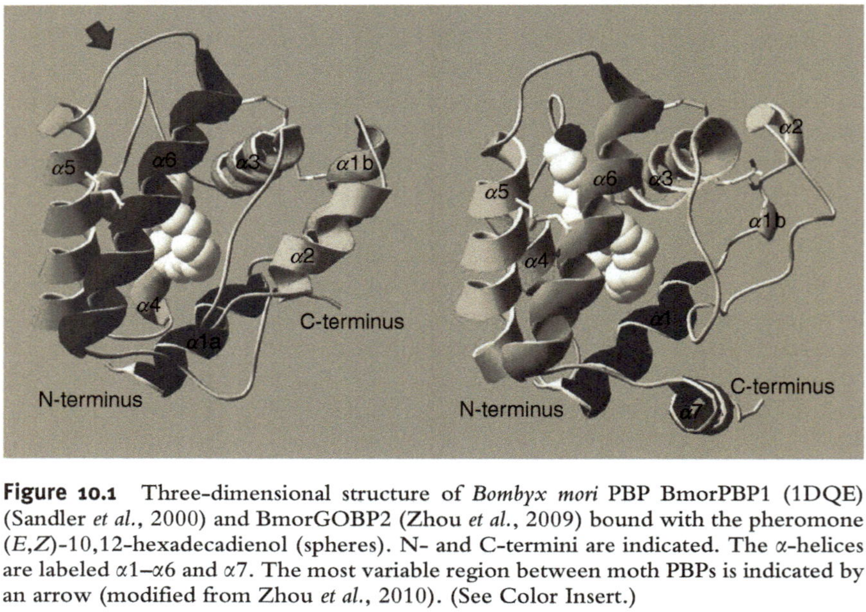

Figure 10.1 Three-dimensional structure of *Bombyx mori* PBP BmorPBP1 (1DQE) (Sandler *et al.*, 2000) and BmorGOBP2 (Zhou *et al.*, 2009) bound with the pheromone (*E*,*Z*)-10,12-hexadecadienol (spheres). N- and C-termini are indicated. The α-helices are labeled α1–α6 and α7. The most variable region between moth PBPs is indicated by an arrow (modified from Zhou *et al.*, 2010). (See Color Insert.)

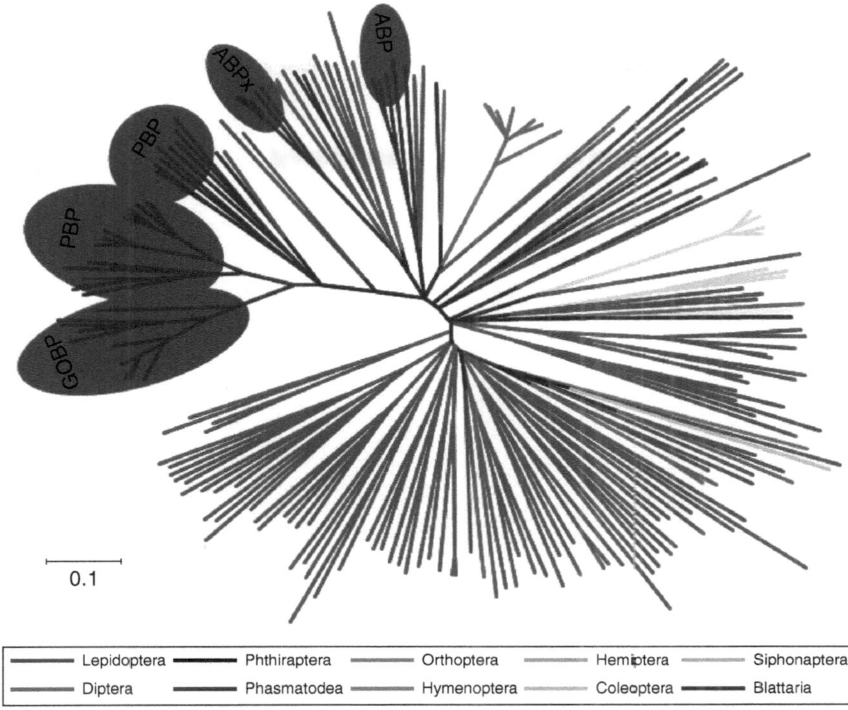

Figure 10.2 Cladograms of all OBPs of insects, whose sequences have been annotated. The mature amino acid sequences were aligned with ClustalW 8 with default gap-penalty parameters of gap opening 10 and extension 0.2. The cladograms were then constructed from these multiple alignments using MEGA4 software. The final unrooted consensus tree was generated with 1050 bootstrap trials using the neighbor-joining method and the p-distances model. The orders are color-coded (modified from Pelosi *et al.*, 2006). (See Color Insert.)

butterflies despite extensive study on their reproductive signaling (Nieberding *et al.*, 2008; Schneider and Seibt, 1969) and in any crustaceans.

While Lepidopteran OBPs represent a group of closely related proteins, they appear to be very divergent when compared with those of other insect Orders. Based on the OBP sequences of Dipteran species, where only the cysteine motif defines the relatedness while the rest of the sequences are very divergent, insect OBPs have been further grouped into: Classic OBPs (having typical six-cysteine signature and including PBPs, GOBPs, and ABPs), Dimer OBPs (having two six-cysteine signatures), Plus-C OBPs (having two additional conserved cysteines plus one proline), Minus-C OBPs (having lost two conserved cysteines), and Atypical OBPs (having 9–10 cysteines and a long C-terminus) (Hekmat-Scafe *et al.*, 2002; Xu *et al.*, 2003; Zhou *et al.*, 2004a,b).

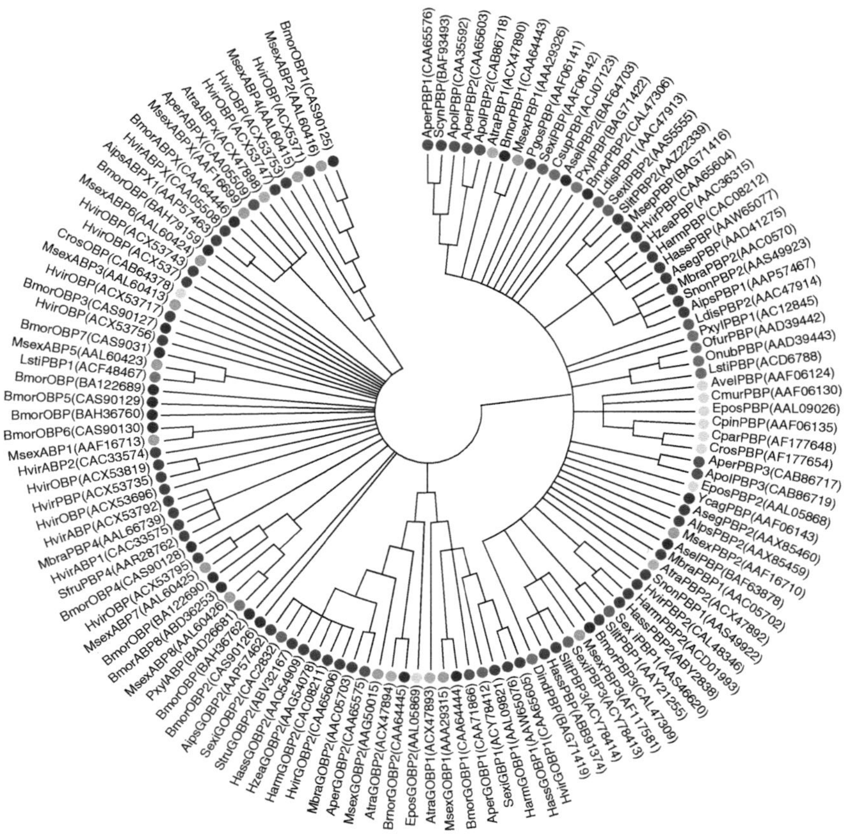

Figure 10.3 Sequence relatedness of Lepidopteran OBPs. The unrooted consensus tree was constructed from the multiple alignments using MEGA4 software, generated with 1500 bootstrap trials using the neighbor-joining method, 66 and presented with a cut off value of 65. The numbers are the bootstrap values calculated from 1500 replicates. For some OBP, names are presented as a three-letter code (first letter of genus followed by first two letters of species name) at the end of each line indicates the order, followed by the GenBank accession number in the parenthesis. The insect families are indicated by colored coded dots. Bmor, *Bombyx mori*; Lmad, *Leucophea madderae*; Mbra, *Mamestra brassicae*; Aper, *Antheraea pernyi*; Apol, *Antheraea polyphemus*; Msex, *Manduca sexta*; Hvir, *Heliothis virescens*; Avel, *Argyrotaenia velutinana*; Cros, *Ceratitis rosa*; Cpar, *Choristoneura parallela*; Cpin, *Choristoneura pinus*; Cmur, *Choristoneura murinana*; Epos, *Epiphyas postvittana*; Pgos, *Pectinophora gossypiella*; Ofur, *Ostrinia furnacalis*; Onub, *Ostrinia nubilalis*; Aips, *Agrotis ipsilon*; Aseg, *Agrotis segetum*; Hass, *Helicoverpa assulta*; Harm, *Helicoverpa armigera*; Hzea, *Heliothis zea*; Ldis, *Lymantria dispar*; Sexi, *Synanthedon exitiosa*; Ycag, *Yponomeuta cagnagellus*; Sfru, *Spodoptera frugiperda*; Pxyl, *Plutella xylostella*; Atra, *Amyelois transitella*.

In *Drosophila melanogaster* there are 61 genes (Hekmat-Scafe *et al.*, 2002; Zhou *et al.*, 2008). 49 encoding classical OBPs with the typical six-cysteine motif, while the remaining 12 exhibit specific characteristics in addition to this signature. It is worth noting that the 49 classical OBPs represent a family of divergent proteins, with the percentage of identical amino acids around 10–15%, reduced in some cases to as little as 4% (corresponding to the sole six-cysteine motif) and in only one case reaching the unusual value of 60%. The genome of *Anopheles gambiae* also contains a great number of genes encoding putative OBPs: 37 classical sequences and 35 with additional motifs (Biessmann *et al.*, 2002; Vogt *et al.*, 2002; Xu *et al.*, 2003; Zhou *et al.*, 2004a,b). The "Plus-C" OBPs were first reported both in *Drosophila* and *Anopheles* (Hekmat-Scafe, 2002; Zhou *et al.*, 2004a,b). Independent experimental work discovered and cloned a similar sequence in the cockroach *Leucophaea maderae* (Riviere *et al.*, 2003). Moreover, searching through the expressed sequence tag (EST) sequences deposited in the GenBank, members of Plus-C OBPs have been also found in the moths *M. sexta* and *B. mori*, thus suggesting that such polypeptides could also be present in other insect orders. Finally, the Atypical OBPs are a specific group of mosquito OBPs annotated from the genome of *A. gambiae*, *Aedes aegypti*, and *Culex quinquefascitus* (Pelletier and Leal, 2009; Xu *et al.*, 2003; Zhou *et al.*, 2008).

OBPs are generally divergent both across species of different genus and within the same species. There is a high conservation between species in a same genus (Zhou *et al.*, 2004a,b) and a certain degree of segregation of the sequences according to the Order (Pelosi *et al.*, 2006). However, sequences in some species of the same Order (e.g., in Hymenoptera), or even in the same species (e.g., *D. melanogaster* and *A. gambiae*), can be found in different branches of the phylogeny tree (Fig. 10.2). This indicates the existence of several subgroups of OBPs defined on the basis of sequence similarity. In the Order Hymenoptera, OBPs from 18 species of *Solenopsis* genus are clustered together, while the other OBPs are scattered in different branches. Another Order-specific cluster is formed by OBPs from 6 species of Coleoptera. On the other hand, the Dipteran OBPs are much more divergent. Lepidopteran OBPs are clearly a more specialised group of OBP family compared to OBPs from other orders with higher similarity between species. Furthermore, PBPs and GOBPs have clearly evolved along different lineages from the antennal proteins within Lepidopteran species (Figs. 10.2 and 10.3). They are derived from distinctly different though homologous genes, rather than from a common but alternatively processed transcript of a single gene (Krieger *et al.*, 1991). Figures 10.2 and 10.3 clearly show that Lepidopteran OBPs are grouped into three clusters: PBP, GOBP, and ABP, with the GOBPs further subdivided into two clusters: GOBP1 and GOBP2. PBPs of Lepidoptera are either specific to, or highly enriched in, the antennae of male moths and have been shown to bind the sex pheromones produced by females (Maida *et al.*, 2005; Steinbrecht, 1998;

Vogt and Riddiford, 1981). However, PBPs have also been found in the antennae of females and in male sensilla which are not pheromone-sensitive (Callahan *et al.*, 2000; Györgyi *et al.*, 1988; Krieger *et al.*, 1991, 1996, 1997; Picimbon and Gadenne, 2002; Vogt *et al.*, 1991, 2002). It has been proposed that they may bind other nonpheromone compounds. GOBPs are usually expressed equally in the antennae of both sexes and this is consistent with a proposed role in the detection of host volatiles, although this has not been demonstrated (Laue *et al.*, 1994; Steinbrecht, 1998; Vogt *et al.*, 1999). ABPs display limited sequence homology to PBPs and GOBPs but have the same sequence motif of the conserved cysteine residues as PBPs and GOBPs (Krieger *et al.*, 1996). No specific role has yet been proposed for them. However, one report showed the binding of BmorABPx and BmorGOBP2 of *B. mori* to sex pheromone components (Zhou *et al.*, 2009). Figure 10.3 also shows some family clusters of OBPs from different species, suggesting a common function of these clustered OBPs in the family. Most notably in *A. polyphemus* and *A. pernyi*, all three PBPs are very closely related. These two species share the same sex pheromone components. There is no report on the identification of GOBPs in *A. polyphemus* so as to compare them with GOBPs of *A. pernyi*. Figure 10.4 shows the sequence comparisons

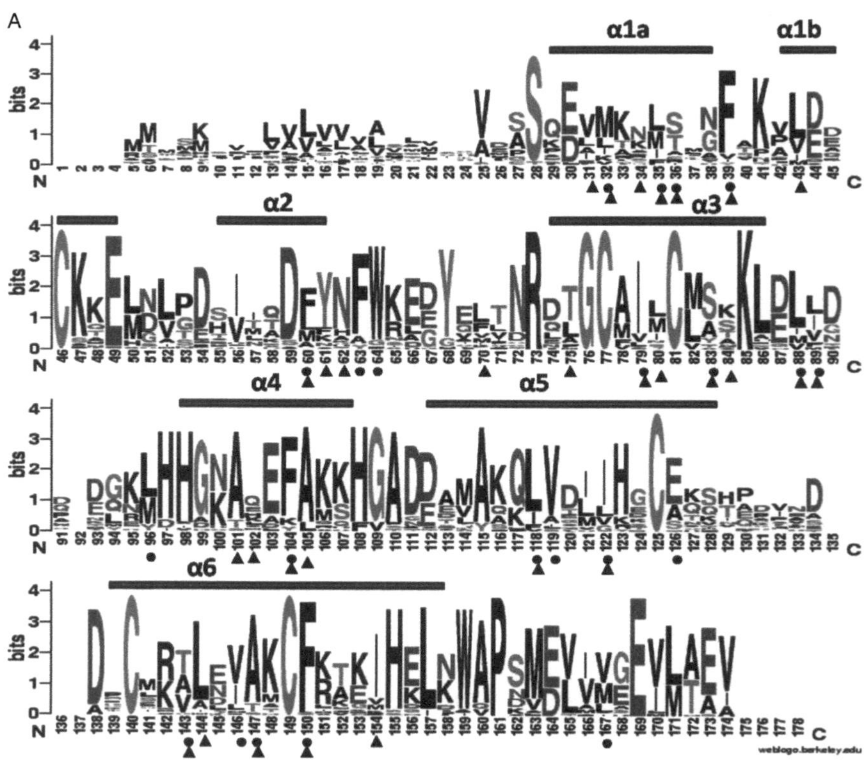

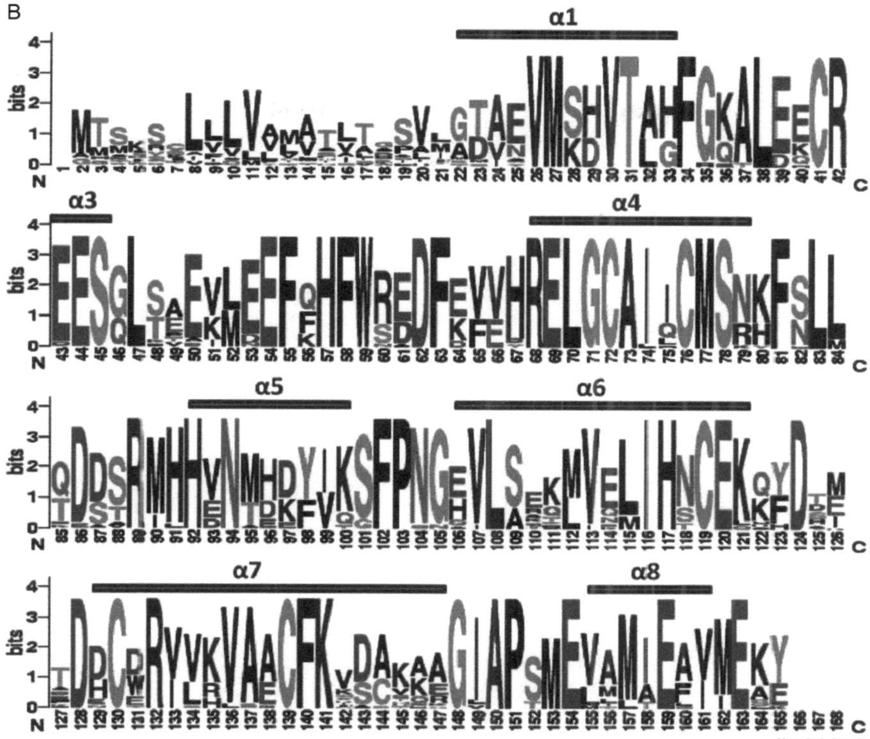

Figure 10.4 Alignment of Lepidopteran PBPs (A) and GOBPs (B) visualised with Weblogo (Crooks *et al.*, 2004). Each logo consists of stacks of symbols, one stack for each position in the sequence. The overall height of the stack indicates the sequence conservation at that position, while the height of symbols within the stack indicates the relative frequency of each amino or nucleic acid at that position. In general, a sequence logo provides a richer and more precise description of, for example, a binding site, than would a consensus sequence. Filled black dots and triangles indicate residues involved in the hydrophobic-binding pocket of BmorPBP1 (1DQE) (Sandler *et al.*, 2000) and ApolPBP (Mohanty *et al.*, 2004), respectively. Rectangle bars above weblogos indicate α-helix in the three-dimensional structure of BmorPBP1 (1DQE) (Sandler *et al.*, 2000) and BmorGOBP2 (Zhou *et al.*, 2009). (See Color Insert.)

between 32 PBPs from 13 Lepidopteran species and 20 GOBPs from the same species. Overall identity and similarity for the GOBPs is 31.0% and 87.5%, but only 3.9% identity and 69.1% similarity for the PBPs. In addition to the region of signal peptide sequences, the most diverse region in the PBP sequences is between α-helix 6 and α-helix 7, containing 10 amino acids at position 127–138 (Fig. 10.4A). This region is not part of the binding pocket (arrowed in Fig. 10.1) and is readily exposed for interaction with other molecules. Other highly divergent amino acid residues are at position 37 in α1a-helix, position 40 between α1a-helix and α1b-helix, position 57 in α2-helix, position 91 and 92 between α3-helix and α4-helix, and position 140 and 142 in α6-helix.

This divergence in PBP sequences is not affected by including extra 31 PBP sequences of other species for the comparison (data not shown). It is demonstrated that PBPs have very high solubility and a capacity of reversibly binding small molecules such as pheromones and odorants. The diversity of PBPs among different Lepidopteran species supports the previous assumption that PBPs function as a carrier for different pheromones among different insect species.

III. Pheromone and Ligand Binding

Reversible binding of pheromones and other odorants to insect OBPs has been demonstrated in several insect species (Table 10.1). The measured affinity constants (K_D) vary greatly. This may be due in some cases to the use of different techniques or experimental procedures. Most moth OBPs particularly PBPs bind hydrophobic alkyl (C14–C16) pheromones (Fig. 10.5), either an alkyl unsaturated alcohol like (*E*,*Z*)-10,12-hexadecadein-1-ol (E10, Z12-16OH or bombykol) of the silkmoth *B. mori*; an alkyl unsaturated aldehyde like (*Z*)-11-hexadecadein-1-al (Z11-16Ald) of the striped riceborer *Chilo suppressalis*; or an alkyl unsaturated acetate like (*E*,*Z*)-6,11-hexadecadienyl acetate (E6,Z11-16Ac) of *A. polyphemus* and *A. pernyi*. There are some variations on length of the carbon chain, side chains, and functional group. The characteristics that are important are the functional group, the position of unsaturations, and the location of the methyl end of the carbon chain. Figure 10.5 shows examples of some main components of insect sex pheromones. The sex pheromone of the fruit fly *D. melanogaster* is a C18 alkyl unsaturated acetate, (*Z*)-octadec-11-enyl acetate, or 11-*cis*-vaccenyl acetate.

Insect pheromones are usually blends of chemicals specific to a species. For example, in *B. mori*, the pheromone blend contains bombykol, (10*E*,12*E*)-hexadecadien-1-al (bombykal or E10, Z12-16Ald), and (10*E*,12*E*)-hexadecadien-1-ol (E10,E12-16OH) (Kaissling *et al.*, 1978). However, only bombykol is able to induce mating behavior at a physiological concentration while bombykal acts as an antagonist to bombykol (Butenandt *et al.*, 1961; Kaissling *et al.*, 1978). One important issue, related to the physiological function of OBPs, is whether these proteins can selectively bind and discriminate between the thousands of different semiochemicals presented to the olfactory repertoire. There is some evidence to support their selective binding, but the full understanding of the

Table 10.1 Binding of pheromones and odorants to OBPs of insects from different species

Species	Protein	Ligands	Method	K_D (μM)	References
Antheraea polyphemus	ApolPBP1	^{3}[H]-(*E*,*Z*)-6,11-C16-Ac	Native PAGE	–	Vogt and Riddiford (1981), Kaissling *et al.* (1985), Ziegelberger (1995), Maida *et al.* (2000, 2003)
A. polyphemus	ApolPBP1	^{3}[H]-(*E*,*Z*)-6,11-C16-DzAc	Photoaffinity	–	Prestwich (1993)
A. polyphemus	ApolPBP1	1-AMA + ligands	Fluorescence	0.5–1.4	Campanacci *et al.* (2001)
A. polyphemus	ApolPBPs	Pheromones	W Fluorescence	0.6–0.8	Leal *et al.* (2005a,b)
A. polyphemus	ApolPBPs	Pheromones	Extraction + GC/MS	–	Leal *et al.* (2005a,b)
A. polyphemus	ApolPBPs	Tritiated pheromones	Native PAGE	–	Maida *et al.* (2003)
Antheraea pernyi	AperPBPs	Tritiated pheromones	Native PAGE	–	Maida *et al.* (2003)
Bombyx mori	PBP	tritiated bombykol	Chromatography	–	Maida *et al.* (1993)
B. mori	PBP	Bombykol	W Fluorescence	1.1	Campanacci *et al.* (2001)
B. mori	PBP	Bombykol	Extraction + GC/MS	0.105	Leal *et al.* (2005a,b)
Lymantria dispar	PBP1,PBP2	Tritiated pheromones	Gel filtration	1.8–7.1	Plettner *et al.* (2000)
L. dispar	PBP1,PBP2	Pheromones and analogs	DNS-PBP and W Fluorescence	0.1–0.3	Honson *et al.* (2003)
Mamestra brassicae	MbraPBPs	Tritiated pheromones	Native PAGE	–	Maibeche-Coisne *et al.* (1997)
M. brassicae	MbraPBP1	1-AMA + ligands	Fluorescence	0.1–0.6	Campanacci *et al.* (2001)
Thaumatopoea pityocampa	PBP	^{3}[H]-(*Z*)-13-hexadecen-11-ynylDzAc	Photoaffinity	–	Feixas *et al.* (1995)

(*continued*)

Table 10.1 *(continued)*

Species	Protein	Ligands	Method	K_D (μM)	References
Manduca sexta	GOBP	General odorants	Photoaffinity	–	Feng and Prestwich (1997)
Apis melliphera	ASP1 (OBP)	Pheromones	Extraction	–	Danty *et al.* (1999)
A. melliphera	ASP1 (OBP)	9-Keto-2(*E*)-decenoic acid	W Fluorescence	0.07–0.06	Pesenti *et al.* (2008)
A. melliphera	ASP2 (OBP)	2-Heptanone, other ligands	Calorimetry, VOBA	0.14–0.45	Briand *et al.* (2001)
Drosophila melanogaster	LUSH (OBP)	1-NPN, ligands	Fluorescence	1.5 (1-NPN)	Zhou *et al.* (2004a,b)
Polistes dominulus	OBP-1	1-NPN, ligands	Fluorescence	2.1 (1-NPN)	Calvello *et al.* (2003)
Leucophaea maderae	PBP	ANS, ligands	Fluorescence	2.1 (ANS)	Riviere *et al.* (2003)
Acyrthosiphon pisum	OBP3	*E*-β-farnesene, analogs	Fluorescence	5.6 (1-NPN)	Qiao *et al.* (2009)

For explanation of the methods see text. Dissociation constants refer, where applicable, to the radioactive ligand or the fluorescent probe. 1-AMA: 1-aminoanthracence; ANS: 1-anilinonaphthalene-8-sulfonic acid; 1-NPN: *N*-phenyl-1-naphthylamine; DzAc: diazoacetate; DNS-PBP: dansylated PBP.

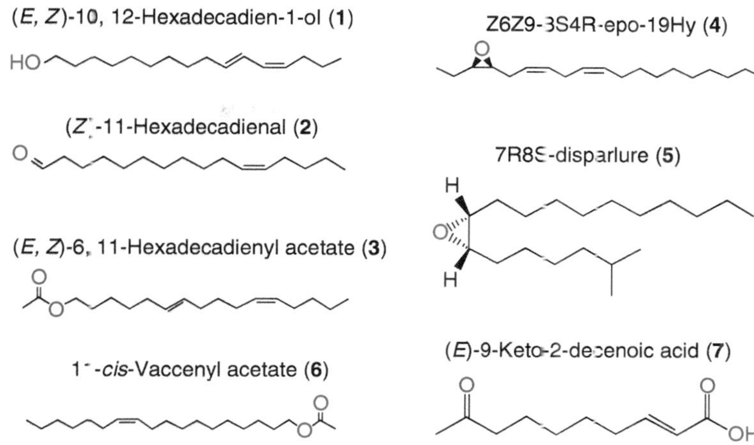

Figure 10.5 Structures of some main component of insect sex pheromones for the silkmoth *Bombyx mori* (1), the striped riceborer *Chilo suppressalis* (2), the Chinese oak silkmoth *Antheraea pernyi* (3), the Japanese giant looper *Ascotis selenaria cretacea* (4), the gypsy moth *Lymantria dispar* (5), the fruit fly *Drosophila melanogaster* (6), the honey bee *Apis mellifera* (7). (See Color Insert.)

discriminatory ability of OBPs remains elusive. Results from circular dichroism and spectroscopic experiments on the PBPs of *A. polyphemus* ApolPBPs are in favor of a fine specificity of the physiological ligand, which induces specific but limited conformational changes (Bette *et al.*, 2002; Mohl *et al.*, 2002). The OBP of the paper wasp *Polistes dominulus* exhibits a marked selective binding to oleoamide: both the *trans* isomer, elaidic amide, and the corresponding saturated compound, stearic amide, bind to the OBP with dissociation constants more than one order of magnitude higher than that of oleoamide (Calvello *et al.*, 2003). Different subfamilies of OBPs are found to associate with distinct classes of OR neurons. Thus, PBPs associate with pheromone-sensitive neurons, and GOBPs associate with general-odorant sensitive neurons (Vogt *et al.*, 1991) and are expressed by sensilla responding to plant odors (Laue *et al.*, 1994). Immunochemistry studies have proved that the PBP and GOBP indeed are present in different sensillum types in *A. polyphemus*, *A. pernyi*, *B. mori*, *D. melanogaster* (Shanbhag, *et al.*, 2001; Steinbrecht, 1998; Steinbrecht *et al.*, 1992, 1995). The results so far indicate a clear correlation in the numbers of receptor cell types, pheromone components, and PBPs within the same species in Lepidoptera.

The binding studies of PBPs demonstrated that the interactions between pheromones and PBPs are specific and selective (Du and Prestwich, 1995; Maida *et al.*, 1993). It was shown that each of three PBPs of *A. polyphemus* differentially bound the components of the acetate pheromone blend

(Maida *et al.*, 2003). The two PBPs of *A. pernyi* AperPBP1 and AperPBP2 were shown to exhibit opposite binding specificities for two pheromone component E6,11Z-16Ac and 4*E*,9*Z*-tetradecadienyl acetate (E4,9Z-14Ac) with K_D differing by a factor of 3.5–15 (Du and Prestwich, 1995). Dissociation constants in the micromolar range have also been measured with the two PBPs of *L. dispar* using tritium-labeled ligands and a binding assay in heterogeneous phase (Plettner *et al.*, 2000). In the same work, the authors also observed some selectivity of binding between the two enantiomers of the pheromone. However, in most of these early biochemistry studies, binding was measured after separation of the radioactive-labeled pheromone/protein mixture on a native electrophoresis gel. The prediction of the binding site sequences as Asp39-Lys58 for ApolPBPs was later shown to be incorrect by structural studies (Fig. 10.4A; Mohanty *et al.*, 2004). Furthermore, the three-dimensional structure of the BmorPBP1 revealed that photoactive compounds likely bind at the protein surface, not in the internal-binding site (Sandler *et al.*, 2000; Tegoni *et al.*, 2004). Most of the binding assays have now been performed with proteins expressed in heterologous systems. Several other modern techniques are employed to demonstrate the binding of OBPs to odorants and components of pheromone blends. These include X-ray crystallography, NMR structural characterisation, electrospraymass spectrometry (ESI-MS), and other biochemical methods such as fluorescence displacement (Campanacci *et al.*, 2001), intrinsic tryptophan quenching (Bette *et al.*, 2002), and a combination of the two (Zhou *et al.*, 2009). A "cold"-binding protocol was described for OBPs, that involves separation of the complex from free ligand by rapid ultrafiltration and evaluation of bound ligand following extraction using gas chromatography–mass spectrometry (GC–MS) analysis (Leal *et al.*, 2005a,b). This method has the advantage that it can be applied to mixtures of organic compounds, all incubated at the same time with the protein, allowing the identification of the best ligands in a single competitive experiment. Other protocols used to measure dissociation constants of ligands to insect OBPs involve calorimetry and VOBA (volatile odorant-binding assay) (Briand *et al.*, 2001). Recently, a two-phase-binding assay was used to measure the binding of *B. mori* OBPs BmorPBP1, BmorGOBP2, and BmorABPx in an equilibrium condition (Zhou *et al.*, 2009).

It has been shown that PBPs are able to bind several compounds besides the host-specific pheromone. In a fluorescent displacement-binding assay, the PBP of *M. sexta* MbraPBP1 binds all three components of the pheromone (*Z*)11-hexadecenol, (*Z*)11-hexadecenal, and (*Z*)11-hexadecenyl acetate with dissociation constants between 0.17 and 0.29 μM (Campanacci *et al.*, 2001). Fatty acids also bind well to MbraPBP1, especially palmitic acid, with a dissociation constant of 0.12 μM. The same study also reports that the PBP of *A. polyphemus*, ApolPBP1, binds the specific pheromone and a series of structurally related compounds. In this case, the components of the pheromonal blend E6,Z11-16Ald, E6,Z11-16Ac, and E4,Z9-14Ac display identical dissociation constants (0.50, 0.48, and 0.51 μM, respectively). Moreover, pheromones of other insect species, such as bombykol of *B. mori* and several fatty acids, also strongly bind to ApolPBP1 with similar affinities (K_D between 0.56 and 1.36 μM). The dissociation constant of the PBP of the cockroach *L. maderae* for a hydrophilic ligand, 3-hydroxy-butan-2-one has been estimated as 3.8 μM. It is noteworthy that a closely related compound, butane-2,3-diol, binds to the protein with comparable strength, while other components of the pheromone blend (3-methyl-2-butenoic acid and E-2-octenoic acid), as well as other organic compounds failed to show any measurable affinity (Riviere *et al.*, 2003). The *Drosophila* OBP LUSH failed to bind alcohols as well as a great number of volatiles known to elicit electrophysiological responses in the fly's antenna, but showed good affinity to a series of large aromatic compounds, including some phthalates (Zhou *et al.*, 2004a,b). The PBP of the silkmoth, *B. mori*, (BmorPBP1) was found to bind very strongly to nonpheromone compounds such as (10,12)-hexadeca-diyn-1-ol (Hooper *et al.*, 2009). In the case of the pea aphid, one OBP, ApisOBP3, specifically binds to the alarm pheromone (*E*)-*β*-farnesene and its corresponding alcohol farnesol and 3,7-dimethyloctyl acetate (Qiao *et al.*, 2009). All these results and additional data obtained with different OBPs indicate a rather broad specificity of binding, in contrast with the extremely high selectivity exhibited by insects in recognising their specific pheromones.

The difference in insect PBP primary sequences was correlated to structural differences of the sex pheromones (Prestwich *et al.*, 1995; Vogt *et al.*, 1991). This idea is further supported by the sequence comparison between PBPs and GOBPs (Fig. 10.4), and low values of identity (30–50%) between two PBPs of the gypsy moth *L. dispar*, whose pheromone, an internal epoxyde (7R,8S)-7,8-epoxy-2-methyloctadecane also called (+) disparlure (Bierl *et al.*, 1970), presents a structure markedly different from the 1-substituted linear chains of most Lepidopteran sex pheromones and is chemically unique pheromone within Lepidopteran species (Pelosi *et al.*, 2006). However, a detailed analysis with additional OBP sequences within PBP subfamily (Figs. 10.3 and 10.4) suggests that there is much higher identity between PBPs of different species and the difference in primary sequences may not be the only determinant of binding specificity. For example, the main sex pheromone component is Z11-16Ald and Z11-16Ac for the tobacco budworm *Heliothis virescens* and the cabbage moth *Mamestra brassicae*, respectively. The PBP of *L. dispar* LdisPBP1 has 60% identity to HvirPBP1 of *H. virescens*, and 58% identity to MbraPBP2 of *M. brassicae*, and LdisPBP2 shares 51% identity to HvirPBP2 and 49% to MbraPBP2. These values are calculated from full-length sequences, and the actual identity of the mature proteins will be higher. These identities are much higher than the overall identity of PBP (3.9%) and GOBP (31%) (Fig. 10.4). Another example is the PBPs (AselPBP1 and AselPBP2) of the Japanese giant looper *Ascotis selenaria cretacea* which also utilises a different pheromone Z6,Z9-3S4R-epo-19Hy from common alkyl pheromones of Lepidopteran insects. However, AselPBP2 shares 59% identity to SexiPBP2 of the peach tree borer *Synanthedon exitiosa* that uses Z3,Z13-18Ac. AselPBP1 shares 55% identity to SlitPBP1 of the oriental leafworm moth *Spodoptera litura* whose sex pheromone main component is Z9,E11-14Ac, and to AtraPBP2 of the orangeworm moth *Amyelois transitella* which uses Z11,Z13-16Ald as sex pheromone.

It seems that under competitive conditions PBPs may discriminate better between pheromone components. Using a cold-binding assay, Leal *et al.* (2005a,b) demonstrated a clear discriminatory binding of ApolPBP1 for the main pheromone component E6,Z11-16Ac over two other components E6,Z11-16Ald (fourfold) and E4,Z9-14Ac (twofold) only in the competitive assay. The selective and differential binding was shown in another competitive assay with E4,9Z-14Ac between PBPs of *A. polyphemus* and *A. pernyi* so that the PBP1 of both species showed preferential binding of E6,Z11-16Ac, and the PBP2 bound to E6,11Z-16Ald and the PBP3 preferentially bound to E4,9Z-14Ac (Maida *et al.*, 2003). The binding of LdisPBPs to the pheromone was enhanced in the presence of an antagonist (Honson *et al.*, 2003). For one PBP of the honey bee *Apis mellifera* AmelASP1, the specific binding for the main pheromone component (*E*)-9-keto-2-decenoic acid (9-ODA) was observed when AmelASP1 was crystallised in complex with the queen mandibular pheromone mixture containing more than three components (Pesenti *et al.*, 2008).

Several different OBPs in one species could be responsible for binding different pheromone components. One of them would function as a specific PBP and be able to activate pheromone-sensitive neuron; others would act as antagonist-binding proteins and be able to activate different neurons to prevent cross-species attraction or bind nonpheromone ligands for other functions. The analysis of signal peptide sequences indicated that multiple OBP classes may be coexpressed but independently processed within the same class of sensilla (Vogt *et al.*, 1991). Two species, for example, *B. mori* and *M. sexta*, utilise the same pheromone component, bombykal (Kaissling *et al.*, 1978) but in *B. mori* bombykal is an antagonist while in *M. sexta* bombykal is the main component of sex pheromone blend. BmorPBP1 was shown to bind bombykol and bombykal (Zhou *et al.*, 2009). BmorPBP1 and MsexPBP1 possess the highest similarity and could be bombykal-binding OBPs (Fig. 10.3). This could also mean that BmorPBP1 may bind bombykal and MsexPBP1 may bind bombykol to prevent cross-species mating. It is shown that the OBP of *A. gambiae* AgamOBP1 is also able to bind bombykol (Leal *et al.*, 2005a,b). Both PBPs of *A. polyphemus* ApolPBP1 and ApolPBP3 bind the tritium-labeled E6,11Z-16Ac not E6, Z11-16Ald. However, the PBPs in the related species *A. pernyi* AperPBP1 preferentially bind E6,11Z-16Ac and AperPBP2 bind E6,Z11-16Ald (Maida *et al.*, 2000). All PBPs from these two species strongly bind decylthio-1,1,1-trifluoropropa-mone (DTFP). This compound is an esterase inhibitor and inhibits the response of pheromone receptor cells (Pophof, 2004). Interestingly, ApolPBP1 was shown to bind the disparlure enantiomers of *L. dispar* (Plettner *et al.*, 2000) and sex pheromone bombykol of *B. mori* (Campanacci *et al.*, 2001). In a GC-based two phase-binding assay, where the protein was incubated with a mixture of bombykol and its four analogs, the GOBP of *B. mori* BmorGOBP2 displayed better discriminatory binding than BmorPBP1 between bombykol and bombykal although the BmorGOBP2 crystals can accommodate bombykol as well as its analogs without significant conformational change when it was individually complexed with these compounds (Zhou *et al.*, 2009).

The insect olfaction system is clearly capable of discrimination although each OBP exhibits a broad spectrum of binding. Such a system is at the same time specific and yet not limited in the number of potential ligands it can detect. On the other hand, a strong affinity of OBPs toward semiochemicals is not required when we consider that these proteins are highly concentrated up to 10 mM in the sensillar lymph (Klein, 1987; Vogt and Riddiford, 1981). In fact, with a protein concentration of 1 mM, even a dissociation constant of 10 mM is enough to keep 99% of the ligand bound to the protein (Pelosi *et al.*, 2006). The decision made by insects as how to respond to odor may rely on the olfactory messages (excitatory or inhibitory or both) delivered by OBPs at ORs and the interpretation of these messages at higher levels in the signaling transduction system. In addition to the high concentration in sensillar lymph, a large number of OBPs are present in insect genomes along with a large number of ORs (Table 10.2). Insect OBPs in combination with ORs have evolved to recognise at least a group of species-specific compounds and modulate insect behaviors in mating and host location.

It has been shown *in vitro* that OBPs can facilitate the passage of semiochemicals to the ORs, where the response of the insect to the chemical signal is initiated (Benton *et al.*, 2007; Grosse-Wilde *et al.*, 2006; Ha and Smith, 2006; Laughlin *et al.*, 2008; Syed *et al.*, 2006). In *B. mori*, the bombykol-responding and bombykal-responding neurons have been identified (Kaissling, 2009). Cells expressing BmorPBP1 are closely associated with the cells expressing BmorOR-1 and BmorOR-3 in the long sensilla (Grosse-Wilde *et al.*, 2006). Specific sensillar neurons, each sensitive to each of the sex pheromone components in *A. polyphemus* and *A. pernyi*, were also identified (Meng *et al.*, 1989). The OR of *A. polyphemus* ApolOR1-expressing cells are found to be surrounded by supporting cells coexpressing all three PBPs (Forstner *et al.*, 2009). ApolOR1 responds to all three pheromone components (E6,Z11-16Ac, E6,11Z-16Ald, and E4,Z9-14Ac) at nanomolar concentrations. However, at picomolar concentrations, the ApolOR1 cells respond only in the presence of ApolPBP2 and the pheromone E6,Z11-16Ald. Immunolocalisation studies of OBPs in *Drosophila* have shown a variety of different OBP combinations in morphologically

Table 10.2 OBPs and ORs identified from insect genomes

Species	*Drosophila melanogaster*	*Anopheles gambiae*	*Aedes aegypti*	*Bombyx mori*	*Acyrthosiphon pisum*	*Apis mellifera*	*Culex pipiens quinquefasciat us*	*Glossina morsitans morsitans*
OBP	61	72	64	45	15	21	53	20
	Hekmat-Scafe *et al.* (2002)	Xu *et al.* (2003)	Zhou *et al.* (2008)	Gong *et al.* (2009)	Zhou *et al.* (2010)	Forêt and Maleszka (2006)	Pelletier and Leal (2009)	Liu *et al.* (2009)
	Zhou *et al.* (2008)	Zhou *et al.* (2008)		Zhou *et al.* (2009)				
OR	62	79	131	41	79	170	n.a.	n.a.
	Robertson *et al.* (2003)	Hill *et al.* (2002)	Bohbot *et al.* (2007)	Wanner *et al.* (2007)	Smadja *et al.* (2009)	Robertson and Wanner (2006)		
	Gao and Chess (1999)	Fox *et al.* (2001)						

identical sensilla (Shanbhag *et al.*, 2001). In *L. dispar* antennae, there are two sensory neurons, one responding to (+)enantiomer of the pheromone and another to (−)enantiomer (Hansen, 1984). The sibling species *L. monacha* which coinhabit with *L. dispar* release this (−)enantiomer, which could be the sex pheromone for *L. monacha*. However in *D. melanogaster* and *L. dispar*, the cellular colocalisation of PBPs and ORs have not been demonstrated. More interestingly, the genome annotation of the waterflea *Daphnia pulex* found only gustatory receptors but no ORs (Peñalva-Arana *et al.*, 2009) and no OBPs (Zhou *et al.*, unpublished).

IV. Structure Aspects

Forty-seven three-dimensional structures of OBPs from seven species have been solved and deposited in the RCSB protein database (http://www.rcsb.org/pdb). Some of these are complexes with pheromone components and nonbiological compounds at different pHs, and some are site-directed mutants and dimeric forms. An excellent review provides most of the information available on such aspects (Tegoni *et al.*, 2004). All resolved OBP structures are very compact due to the presence of three interlocked disulfide bridges, and mainly fold into α-helical domains forming a conical shaped cavity for odorants (Fig. 10.1) despite the differences in their amino acid sequences. They include PBPs; BmorPBP1 of the silkmoth *B. mori*, ApolPBP of the giant moth *A. polyphemus*, LmadPBP of the cockroach *L. maderea* and AmelASP1 of the honey bee *A. mellifera*, the classic OBPs; LUSH of the fruit fly *D. melanogaster*, AgamOBP1 of the malaria mosquito *A. gambiae*, AaegOBP1 of the yellow fever mosquito *A. aegypti* and the GOBP; BmorGOBP2 of the silkmoth *B. mori*. Figure 10.1 shows two examples from *B. mori* OBPs BmorPBP1 and BmorGOBP2 complexed with the sex pheromone bombykol (Sandler *et al.*, 2000; Zhou *et al.*, 2009). The wall of the conical shape is formed by five helices (α1, α2, α4, α5, and α6) establishing a hydrophobic-binding cavity. The helices α3 is on top of the mouth of the conical shape with the edge formed by the loops between helices α1 and α2, α3, and α4, α5 and α6, which are the most divergent regions in the PBP sequences (Fig. 10.4A). The region between helices α3 and α4 is involved in the dimeric interaction between BmorPBP1 (Sandler *et al.*, 2000). The narrow end of the conical shape is formed by the loop between helices α4 and α5, the end of α6 and the end of C-terminus. In some insect OBPs the first and third α-helix is broken up into two or three smaller helices (α1a, α1b, α1c and α3a, α3b).

The C-termini of two Lepidopteran PBPs BmorPBP1 and ApolPBP form an α-helix and occupy the binding cavity at acid pH, this is thought to promote the release of the pheromone molecule from the binding cavity when the PBP/ligand complex reaches the ORs. At acidic pH, or in the absence of bombykol, the C-terminus of BmorPBP1 forms an α-helix and occupies the ligand-binding pocket (Damberger *et al.*, 2000; Horst *et al.*, 2001; Lee *et al.*, 2002). The complex BmorPBP1/bombykol undergoes a conformational change brought about by a reduction of pH near the ORs and releases bombykol (Lautenschlager *et al.*, 2005). The structure of the PBP ApolPBP of the giant moth *A. polyphemus*, was resolved as a complex with the specific pheromone at pH 6.3 using NMR spectroscopy (Mohanty *et al.*, 2004). At pH 4 and 5 the authors recorded an overall change of the spectrum, accompanied by loss of binding. A conformational change, similar to that observed for BmorPBP1, seems to also occur in this protein (Leal *et al.*, 2005a,b; Zubkov *et al.*, 2005). At pH 5.2, in fact, the ApolPBP exhibits a pH-induced structural change, where the protonation of His69, His70, and His95 in the binding pocket causes a reorientation of α-helices 1, 3, and 4, thus providing the driving force for the release of the pheromone molecule from the cavity. At this pH, binding of the pheromone is drastically reduced.

In other OBP structures, the C-termini partially occupy the binding cavity without forming an α-helix but they establish hydrogen bonds with amino acids in the cavity. The PBP LmadPBP of the cockroach *L. maderae* (Lartigue *et al.*, 2003) lacks the C-terminus common to Lepidopteran OBPs, being 19 residues shorter than *B. mori* PBP. Therefore, the formation of a seventh α-helix required for releasing the ligand out of the binding cavity cannot occur in this protein. Interestingly, components of the pheromonal blend of *L. maderae*, such as 3-hydroxy-butan-2-one, which bind the PBP with good affinity, are highly hydrophilic, unlike moth pheromones (Riviere *et al.*, 2003). Therefore, as the authors suggest, an active mechanism for releasing the ligand would not be needed in this case. The OBPs; LUSH, AgamOBP1, AaegOBP1 from Diptera and AmelASP1 from Hymenoptera, so called medium-chain PBPs, have a longer C-terminus than that of the LmadPBP but shorter than those of the PBPs of Lepidopteran species. The resolved structures of these OBPs show their C-terminus folds back into the core of the protein without forming an α-helix and the binding of ligands does not displace the C-terminus out of the binding cavity. There is no conformational change of LUSH associated with its acidic pH (Kruse *et al.*, 2003). The ligands are bound to AmelASP1 at acid pHs and released at neutral pH (Pesenti *et al.*, 2008). These observations are opposite to what is observed with other PBPs, such as those of *B. mori*, *A. polyphemus*, and *A. gambiae* (Horst *et al.*, 2001; Mohanty *et al.*, 2004). For both LUSH of *D. melanogaster* and AmelASP1 of *A. mellifera*, key amino acids were identified in determining pheromone release to OR by site-directed mutagenesis. The breaking of the salt-bridge between Lys87 and Asp118 of LUSH either by addition of ligand 11-*cis*-vaccenyl acetate or by mutation of Asp118 to Ala118 conferred activation of pheromone-sensitive neurons in a stimulation assay (Laughlin *et al.*, 2008), while for AmelASP1 hydrogen bonds established between Asp35 carboxylic side chain and the main chain N–H group and C=O group of Val118 of the C-terminus are shown to be critical for the pheromone binding and release (Pesenti *et al.*, 2009). The Asp35 of AmelASP1 is involved in forming a pH-induced and domain swapped asymmetric dimer in which the N-terminus of one monomer forms a parallel β-sheet with the C-terminus of another monomer after pH change from 5.5 to 7.0. This domain swapping favors the release of the pheromones at neutral pH and allows the dimer to accommodate more than one pheromone molecules (Pesenti *et al.*, 2009).

Finally, the structures of the mosquito OBPs; AgamOBP1 of *A. gambiae* and AaegOBP1 of *A. aegypti* present the common motif of the six α-helices, but with an additional interesting feature. The ligand-binding pocket has a tunnel-like structure running from one end of the protein to the other, thus potentially allowing a ligand to pass through the protein. Moreover, in the crystal structure, these OBPs are present as a dimer, with the binding pockets of the two units connected to make a continuous long tunnel (Leite *et al.*, 2009; Wogulis *et al.*, 2005). The C-termini of AgamOBP1 and AaegOBP1 fold back in the protein core and are locked by a double hydrogen/ionic bond between the carboxylic end of the last residue and two other amino acids at neutral pH. The authors proposed that acid pH would induce rupture of the ionic bond and lead to the expulsion of the C-terminus, leading to disruption of the binding site and allowing ligand release, thus sharing a similar mechanism of ligand expulsion triggered by the low pH near the axon membrane with Lepidopteran PBPs (Leite *et al.*, 2009; Wojtasek and Leal, 1999).

Three-dimensional crystal structures were solved for one member of the GOBP subfamily. The study showed that the C-termini of BmorGOBP2 form an α-helix at neutral pH and is not locked inside the binding cavity even in the absence of the sex pheromone (Fig. 10.1; Zhou *et al.*, 2009). The most significant differences between BmorGOBP2 and BmorPBP1 are at the C-terminus and in the second helix. The structures of BmorGOBP2 were also solved individually in the presence of the sex pheromone of *B. mori* bombykol and each of its analogs bombykal, (8*E*,10*Z*)-hexadecadien-1-ol, (10*E*)-hexadecen-12-yn-1-ol, (10*E*,12*Z*)-tetradecadien-1-ol. The structural differences between BmorGOBP2 complexes lie in the regions of amino acids 39–41, 62–66, 104–106, 123–128, and the C-terminus 139–141. These changes are of a similar size to those reported (Sandler *et al.*, 2000) as being responsible for the activation of the OBP LUSH of *D. melanogaster* (Laughlin *et al.*, 2008). However, inspection of all of the loops that differ in the BmorGOBP2 structures showed that they are involved in crystal contacts in one or both forms, so the conformational changes may not have physiological significance. In all structures, the ligand density is clearly directed toward Arg110 and the OH group is hydrogen-bonded to Arg110 not to Ser56 as in the BmorPBP1-bombykol complex

(Zhou *et al.*, 2009). It is proposed that the hydrogen bonds are involved in the discriminatory binding between bombykol and bombykal.

V. Function of OBPs

Although a pathway of signal transduction from the peripheral ORs to the areas of the central nervous system can explain how olfactory messages are translated into behavioral responses, the role of OBPs at the periphery of the olfactory system remains elusive. The discovery of membrane-bound ORs both in vertebrates and in insects and their functional expression in heterologous systems have shown that they can be directly activated by odorant and pheromone molecules. On the other hand, the very high concentration of OBPs as soluble proteins around olfactory dendrites and a large number of OBPs in insect genomes indicate important roles they may play. In fact, the great amount of energy involved in their synthesis and turnover cannot be justified without a great benefit for the individual or for the species. This is particularly true for insects, which often live on a very critical energy balance. The observations of rapid evolution and expansion in OBPs suggest they are involved in fast adaptation to changing environments. Several studies have confirmed their importance in mediating pheromone detection (Kaissling *et al.*, 1985) such as the immunohistochemical localisation of GOBPs and PBPs in separate sensilla (Laue *et al.*, 1994); the segregation of OBP types in *Drosophila* olfactory hairs (McKenna *et al.*, 1994; Pikielny *et al.*, 1994); the high turnover rate from mRNA to proteins (8×107 molecules/h/sensillum) (Vogt *et al.*, 1989); the different binding affinities for a variety of pheromone structures (Du and Prestwich, 1995; Leal *et al.*, 2005a,b; Pesenti *et al.*, 2008). Ultrastructural (Steinbrecht *et al.*, 1992, 1998), developmental (Vogt *et al.*, 1989), and electrophysiological studies (Laughlin *et al.*, 2008; van den Berg and Ziegelberger, 1991) have established the cellular locations for their olfaction functions. Recent studies have also proved that PBPs have an essential role in olfactory and pheromonal signal transduction (Benton *et al.*, 2006, 2007; Grosse-Wilde *et al.*, 2006; Pensenti *et al.*, 2009; Syed *et al.*, 2006). The molecular identification is performed by receptor sites on the antennal receptor neurons (Benton *et al.*, 2006, 2007). It is clear now that OBPs function as carriers to enhance the solubility of semiochemicals (pheromones and nonpheromones) and deliver them to membrane-bound ORs either on its own or in a complex with the OBP, or pass the pheromone to the sensory neuron membrane protein (SNMP), which then delivers it to the OR. Finally, the pheromone is degraded by special sensillar esterases (Ishida and Leal, 2008; Vogt *et al.*, 1985) (Fig. 10.6). The *B. mori* PBP1 BmorPBP1 and its binding to pheromone components have been the subject of intense study in recent years as a

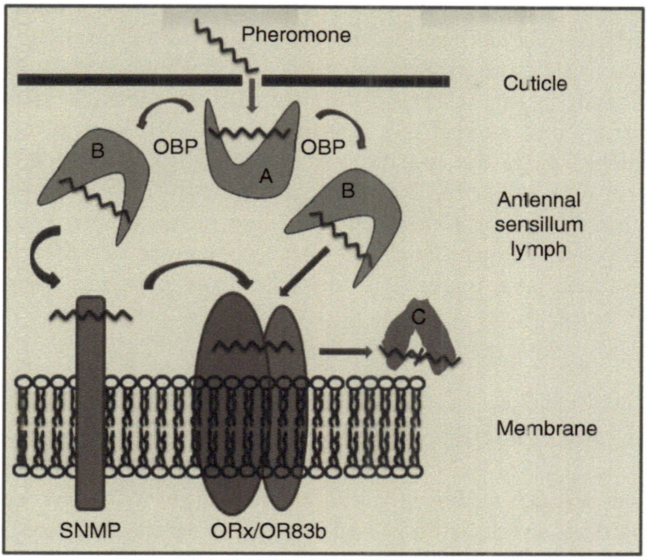

Figure 10.6 Pheromone transport by OBPs and possible signal transduction pathways to the olfactory receptor complex (modified from Benton *et al.*, 2007). (See Color Insert.)

model system for understanding the functions that OBPs may play in insect olfaction (Damberger *et al.*, 2000; Horst *et al.*, 2001; Leal *et al.*, 2005a,b; Lee *et al.*, 2002; Wojtasek and Leal, 1999). Coexpression of BmorPBP1 with BmorOR-1 in an "empty" neuron of *D. melanogaster* (Dobritsa *et al.*, 2003) increased sensitivity of the receptor to the sex pheromone component (10*E*,12*Z*)-hexadecadien-1-ol (bombykol) (Syed *et al.*, 2006). BmorPBP1 has also been shown to mediate a response to bombykol but not to another pheromone component bombykal in cultured HEK293 cells expressing BmorOR-1 (Grosse-Wilde *et al.*, 2006). Such functional evidence is lacking for OBPs of other insect species. Recent work on the *Drosophila* OBP LUSH revealed that it is required for the perception of the sex pheromone with deletion of the gene encoding LUSH suppressing electrophysiological and behavioral responses to the pheromone 11-*cis*-vaccenyl acetate (Ha and Smith, 2006). LUSH when bound to the pheromone makes a pheromone-specific conformational change that triggers the firing of pheromone-sensitive neurons (Laughlin *et al.*, 2008). Another two OBPs (Obp57d and Obp57e) were found to determine the differential behavior of two *Drosophila* species, *D. melanogaster* and *Drosophila sechellia*, to octanoic and hexanoic acids, which act as oviposition attractants for *D. sechellia*, but as repellents for other *Drosophila* species (Matsuo *et al.*, 2007).

Other roles have also proposed: (1) As a scavenger for removing the pheromones as well as foreign pheromones in order to maintain receptor activity (Kaissling, 1986; Pelosi and Maida, 1990); (2) As a filter to reduce the concentration of odorants when they become so high that long-term receptor desensitization could occur (Pelosi and Maida, 1990); (3) Electrophysiological recording on *A. polyphemus* and *B. mori* sensillae demonstrated that ApolPBPs and BmorPBPs contribute to OR activation, and this activation depends on the specific ternary association of a receptor, a PBP and a pheromone (Pophof, 2004). As a result, the role of these proteins seems to be that of an active receptor trigger rather than merely that of a passive transporter (Tegoni *et al.*, 2004); (4) Locations of OBPs in different parts of the insect also suggest different roles from olfaction and that of the antennal proteins.

VI. Conclusion

The structural studies provide some insight on how pheromone molecules are accommodated in and released from the hydrophobic cavity for seven OBPs (BmorPBP1, ApolPBP1, BmorGOBP2, AgamOBP1, AaegOBP1, LUSH, AmelASP1, LmadPBP1), but the exact mechanisms of odorant entry and release remain to be clarified for most insect OBPs. The precise role of OBPs in pheromone signaling remains unclear in most cases. Despite sharing a similar folding in three-dimensional structures, the insect OBP families exhibit structural diversities in the length, position, and angle of their α-helixes, in the length and path of their loops, and in the conformation of their C-termini. This diversity results in very different cavities, which vary in shape, position, and dimension of the solvent access, and in the nature of the amino acids that form their walls.

The pH-dependent mechanism of pheromone expulsion by the seventh helix proposed for BmorPBP1 is probably valid for PBPs of other moths that possess a long C-terminus, but is certainly not directly applicable to OBPs of other insect orders. For OBPs whose C-termini do not form α-helix in the binding cavity or form an α-helix but outside the binding cavity, there must be a different mechanism of pheromone or odor presentation to the OR.

Lepidopteran GOBPs and PBPs are highly conserved; this does not explain how various moth species utilise quite different habitats: *M. sexta* feed and deposit eggs only on tobacco plants; *B. mori* feed specifically on mulberry leaves; *L. dispar* live in deciduous forests throughout the northern hemisphere. The choice of habitats may be entirely determined at the level of the olfactory lobe. Furthermore, the binding of GOBPs to pheromone components suggests that they could be also PBPs and may serve as carriers for antagonists and scavengers for pheromone components in female insects (Zhou *et al.*, 2009) or act as PBPs. The evidence of OBP functions *in vivo* is still not sufficient, especially for the large number of divergent OBPs in Dipteran insects. Despite enormous effort, the binding specificity of OBPs is still unclear. The evidence of having one PBP binding specifically to one pheromone component remains elusive.

REFERENCES

Angeli, S., Ceron, F., Scaloni, A., Monti, M., Monteforti, G., Minnocci, A., Petacchi, R., and Pelosi, P. (1999). Purification, structural characterization, cloning and immunocytochemical localization of chemoreception proteins from *Schistocerca gregaria*. *Eur. J. Biochem.* **262,** 745–754.

Baker, T. C., Hansson, B. S., Löfstedt, C., and Löfqvist, J. (1988). Adaptation of antennal neurons in moths is associated with cessation of pheromone-mediated upwind flight. *Proc. Natl. Acad. Sci. USA* **85**(24), 9826–9830.

Benton, R., Sachse, S., Michnick, S. W., and Vosshall, L. B. (2006). A typical membrane topology and heteromeric function of *Drosophila* odorant receptors *in vivo*. *PLoS Biol.* **4**(2), e20.

Benton, R., Vannice, K. S., and Vosshall, L. B. (2007). An essential role for a CD36-related receptor in pheromone detection in *Drosophila*. *Nature* **450,** 289–293.

Bette, S., Breer, H., and Krieger, J. (2002). Probing a pheromone binding protein of the silkmoth *Antheraea polyphemus* by endogenous tryptophan fluorescence. *Insect Biochem. Mol. Biol.* **32,** 241–246.

Bierl, B. A., Beroza, M., and Collier, C. W. (1970). Potent sex attractant of the gypsy moth: Its isolation, identification, and synthesis. *Science* **170**(953), 87–89.

Biessmann, H., Walter, M. F., Dimitratos, S., and Woods, D. (2002). Isolation of cDNA clones encoding putative odourant binding proteins from the antennae of the malaria-transmitting mosquito, *Anopheles gambiae*. *Insect Mol. Biol.* **11**(2), 123–132.

Boeckh, J., and Boeckh, V. (1979). Threshold and odor specificity of pheromone-sensitive neurons in the deutocerebrum of *Antheraea pernyi* and *A. polyphemus* (Saturnidae). *J. Comp. Physiol.* **132,** 235–242.

Bohbot, J., Pitts, R. J., Kwon, H.-W., Rützler, M., Robertson, H. M., and Zwiebel, L. J. (2007). Molecular characterization of the *Aedes aegypti* odorant receptor gene family. *Insect Mol. Biol.* **16,** 525–537.

Breer, H., Boekhoff, I., and Tareilus, E. (1990). Rapid kinetics of second messenger formation in olfactory transduction. *Nature* **345**(6270), 65–68.

Briand, L., Nespoulous, C., Huet, J. C., Takahashi, M., and Pernollet, J. C. (2001). Ligand binding and physico-chemical properties of ASP2, a recombinant odorant-binding protein from honeybee (*Apis mellifera* L.). *Eur. J. Biochem.* **268,** 752–760.

Butenandt, A., Beckmann, R., and Stamm, D. (1961). Über den Sexuallockstoff des Seidenspinners. II. Konstitution und Konfiguration des Bombykols. *Z. Physiol. Chem.* **324,** 84–87.

Callahan, F. E., Vogt, R. G., Tucker, M. L., Dickens, J. C., and Mattoo, A. K. (2000). High level expression of "male specific" pheromone binding proteins (PBPs) in the antennae of female noctuiid moths. *Insect Biochem. Mol. Biol.* **30,** 507–514.

Calvello, M., Guerra, N., Brandazza, A., D'Ambrosio, C., Scaloni, A., Dani, F. R., Turillazzi, S., and Pelosi, P. (2003). Soluble proteins of chemical communication in the social wasp *Polistes dominulus*. *Cell. Mol. Life Sci.* **60,** 1933–1943.

Campanacci, V., Krieger, J., Bette, S., Sturgis, J. N., Lartigue, A., Cambillau, C., Breer, H., and Tegoni, M. (2001). Revisiting the specificity of *Mamestra brassicae* and *Antheraea*

polyphemus pheromone-binding proteins with a fluorescence binding assay. *J. Biol. Chem.* **276,** 20078–20084.
Crooks, G. E., Hon, G., Chandonia, J. M., and Brenner, S. E. (2004). WebLogo: A sequence logo generator. *Genome Res.* **14,** 1188–1190.
Damberger, F., Nikonova, L., Horst, R., Peng, G., Leal, W. S., and Wüthrich, K. (2000). NMR characterization of a pH-dependent equilibrium between two folded solution conformations of the pheromone-binding protein from *Bombyx mori*. *Protein Sci.* **9,** 1038–1041.
Danty, E., Briand, L., Michard-Vanhee, C., Perez, V., Arnold, G., Gaudemer, O., Huet, D., Huet, J. C., Ouali, C., Masson, C., and Pernollet, J. C. (1999). Cloning and expression of a queen pheromone-binding protein in the honeybee: An olfactory specific, developmentally regulated protein. *J. Neurosci.* **19,** 7468–7475.
Dobritsa, A. A., van der Goes van Naters, W., Warr, C. G., Steinbrecht, R. A., and Carlson, J. R. (2003). Integrating the molecular and cellular basis of odor coding in the *Drosophila antenna*. *Neuron* **37,** 827–841.
Du, G., and Prestwich, G. D. (1995). Protein structure encodes the ligand binding specificity in pheromone binding proteins. *Biochemistry* **34**(27), 8726–8732.
Feixas, J., Prestwich, G. D., and Guerrero, A. (1995). Ligand specificity of pheromone-binding proteins of the processionary moth. *Eur. J. Biochem.* **234,** 521–526.
Feng, L., and Prestwich, G. D. (1997). Expression and characterization of a lepidopteran general odorant binding protein. *Insect Biochem. Mol. Biol.* **27,** 405–412.
Flower, D. R. (1996). The lipocalin protein family: Structure and function. *Biochem. J.* **318,** 1–14.
Forêt, S., and Maleszka, R. (2006). Function and evolution of a gene family encoding odorant binding-like proteins in a social insect, the honey bee (*Apis mellifera*). *Genome Res.* **16,** 1404–1413.
Forstner, M., Breer, H., and Krieger, J. (2009). A receptor and binding protein interplay in the detection of a distinct pheromone component in the silkmoth *Antheraea polyphemus*. *Int. J. Biol. Sci.* **5**(7), 745–757.
Fox, A. N., Pitts, R. J., Robertson, H. M., Carlson, J. R., and Zwiebel, L. J. (2001). Candidate odorant receptors from the malaria vector mosquito *Anopheles gambiae* and evidence of down-regulation in response to blood feeding. *Proc. Natl. Acad. Sci. USA* **98,** 14693–14697.
Gao, Q., and Chess, A. (1999). Identification of candidate *Drosophila* olfactory receptors from genomic DNA sequence. *Genomics* **60,** 31–39.
Gong, D. P., Zhang, H. J., Zhao, P., Xia, Q. Y., and Xiang, Z. H. (2009). The odorant binding protein gene family from the genome of silkworm. *Bombyx mori*. *BMC Genomics.* **10,** 332.
Grosse-Wilde, E., Svatos, A., and Krieger, J. (2006). A pheromone-binding protein mediates the bombykol induced activation of a pheromone receptor in vitro. *Chem. Senses* **31,** 547–555.
Györgyi, T. K., Roby-Shemkovitz, A. J., and Lerner, M. R. (1988). Characterization and cDNA cloning of the pheromone-binding protein from the tobacco hornworm, *Manduca sexta*: A tissue-specific developmentally regulated protein. *Proc. Natl. Acad. Sci. USA* **85** (24), 9851–9855.
Ha, T. S., and Smith, D. P. (2006). A pheromone receptor mediates 11-*cis*-vaccenyl acetate-induced responses in *Drosophila*. *J. Neurosci.* **26**(34), 8727–8733.
Hansen, K. (1984). Discrimination and production of disparlure enantiomers by the gypsy moth and the nun moth. *Physiol. Entomol.* **9,** 9–18.
Hekmat-Scafe, D. S., Scafe, C. R., McKinney, A. J., and Tanouye, M. A. (2002). Genome-wide analysis of the odorant-binding protein gene family in *Drosophila melanogaster*. *Genome Res.* **12,** 1357–1369.

Hildebrand, J. G., Christensen, T. A., Harrow, I. D., Homberg, U., Matsumoto, S. G., and Waldrop, B. R. (1992). The roles of local interneurons in the processing of olfactory information in the antennal lobes of the moth *Manduca sexta*. *Acta Biol. Hung.* **43,** 167–174.

Hill, C. A., Fox, A. N., Pitts, R. J., Kent, L. B., Tan, P. L., Chrystal, M. A., Cravchik, A., Collins, F. H., Robertson, H. M., and Zwiebel, L. J. (2002). G protein-coupled receptors in *Anopheles gambiae*. *Science* **298**(5591), 176–178.

Honson, N., Johnson, M. A., Oliver, J. E., Prestwich, G. D., and Plettner, E. (2003). Structure-activity studies with pheromone-binding proteins of the gyspy moth, *Lymantria dispar*. *Chem. Senses* **28,** 479–489.

Hooper, A. M., Dufour, S., He, X., Muck, A., Zhou, J.-J., Almeida, R., Field, L. M., Svatos, A., and Pickett, J. A. (2009). High-throughput ESI-MS analysis of binding between the *Bombyx mori* pheromone-binding protein BmorPBP1, its pheromone components and some analogues. *Chem. Commun. (Camb.)* **14,** 5725–5727.

Horst, R., Damberger, F., Luginbühl, P., Güntert, P., Peng, G., Nikonova, L., *et al.* (2001). NMR structure reveals intramolecular regulation mechanism for pheromone binding and release. *Proc. Natl. Acad. Sci. USA* **98,** 14374–14379.

Ishida, Y., and Leal, W. S. (2008). Chiral discrimination of the Japanese beetle sex pheromone and a behavioral antagonist by a pheromone-degrading enzyme. *Proc. Natl. Acad. Sci. USA* **105,** 9076–9080.

Kaissling, K. E. (1986). Chemo-electrical transduction in insect olfactory receptors. *Annu. Rev. Neurosci.* **9,** 121–145.

Kaissling, K. E. (2009). Olfactory perireceptor and receptor events in moths: A kinetic model revised. *J. Comp. Physiol. A Neuroethol. Sens. Neural Behav. Physiol.* **195**(10), 895–922.

Kaissling, K. E., Kasang, G., Bestmann, H. J., Stransky, W., and Vostrowsky, O. (1978). A new pheromone of the silkworm moth *Bombyx mori*. *Naturwissenschaften* **65,** 382–384.

Kaissling, K.-E., Klein, U., De Kramer, J. J., Keil, T. A., Kanaujia, S., and Hemberger, J. (1985). Insect olfactory cells: Electrophysiological and biochemical studies. *In* "Molecular Basis of Nerve Activity," (J. P. Changeux, F. Hucho, A. Maelicke, and E. Neuman, Eds.), pp. 173–183. De Gruyter, Berlin.

Kim, M. S., Repp, A., and Smith, D. P. (1998). LUSH odorant-binding protein mediates chemosensory responses to alcohols in *Drosophila melanogaster*. *Genetics* **150,** 711–721.

Klein, U. (1987). Sensillum-lymph proteins from antennal olfactory hairs of the moth *Antheraea polyphemus* (Saturniidae). *J. Insect Biochem.* **17,** 1193–1204.

Krieger, J., Raming, K., and Breer, H. (1991). Cloning of genomic and complementary DNA encoding insect pheromone binding proteins: Evidence for microdiversity. *Biochim. Biophys. Acta* **1088,** 277–284.

Krieger, J., von Nickisch-Rosenegk, E., Mameli, M., Pelosi, P., and Breer, H. (1996). Binding proteins from the antennae of *Bombyx mori*. *Insect Biochem. Mol. Biol.* **26,** 297–307.

Krieger, J., Mameli, M., and Breer, H. (1997). Elements of the olfactory signaling pathways in insect antennae. *Invert. Neurosci.* **3,** 137–144.

Kruse, S. W., Zhao, R., Smith, D. P., and Jones, D. N. (2003). Structure of a specific alcohol-binding site defined by the odorant binding protein LUSH from *Drosophila melanogaster*. *Nat. Struct. Biol.* **10,** 694–700.

Lacazette, E., Gachon, A. M., and Pitiot, G. (2000). A novel human odorant-binding protein gene family resulting from genomic duplicons at 9q34: Differential expression in the oral and genital spheres. *Hum. Mol. Genet.* **9**(2), 289–301.

Lartigue, A., Gruez, A., Spinelli, S., Riviere, S., Brossut, R., Tegoni, M., and Cambillau, C. (2003). The crystal structure of a cockroach pheromone-binding protein suggests a new ligand binding and release mechanism. *J. Biol. Chem.* **278,** 30213–30218.

Laue, M., Steinbrecht, R. A., and Ziegelberger, G. (1994). Immunocytochemical localization of general odourant-binding protein in olfactory sensilla of the silkmoth *Antheraea polyphemus*. *Naturwissenschaften* **81,** 178–180.

Laughlin, J. D., Ha, T. S., Jones, D. N. M., and Smith, D. P. (2008). Activation of pheromone-sensitive neurons is mediated by conformational activation of pheromone-binding protein. *Cell* **133,** 1255–1265.

Lautenschlager, C., Leal, W. S., and Clardy, J. (2005). Coil-to-helix transition and ligand release of *Bombyx mori* pheromone-binding protein. *Biochem. Biophys. Res. Commun.* **335,** 1044–1050.

Leal, W. S., Chen, A. M., Ishida, Y., Chiang, V. P., Erickson, M. L., Morgan, T. I., and Tsuruda, J. M. (2005a). Kinetics and molecular properties of pheromone binding and release. *Proc. Natl. Acad. Sci. USA* **102,** 5386–5391.

Leal, W. S., Chen, A. M., and Erickson, M. L. (2005b). Selective and pH-dependent binding of a moth pheromone to a pheromone-binding protein. *J. Chem. Ecol.* **31,** 2493–2499.

Lee, K. H., Wells, R. G., and Reed, R. R. (1987). Isolation of an olfactory cDNA: Similarity to retinol-binding protein suggests a role in olfaction. *Science* **235,** 1053–1056.

Lee, D., Damberger, F. F., Peng, G., Horst, R., Güntert, P., Nikonova, L., *et al.* (2002). NMR structure of the unliganded *Bombyx mori* pheromone-binding protein at physiological pH. *FEBS Lett.* **531,** 314–318.

Leite, N. R., Krogh, R., Xu, W., Ishida, Y., Iulek, J., Leal, W. S., and Oliva, G. (2009). Structure of an odorant-binding protein from the mosquito *Aedes aegypti* suggests a binding pocket covered by a pH-sensitive "Lid". *PLoS ONE* **4,** e8006.

Li, Z., Pickett, J. A., Field, L. M., and Zhou, J.-J. (2005). Identification and expression profiling of putative odorant-binding proteins in the malaria mosquitoes, *Anopheles gambiae* and *Anopheles arabiensis*. *Arch. Insect Biochem. Physiol.* **58,** 175–189.

Liu, R., Lehane, S., He, X., Lehane, M., Hertz-Fowler, C., Berriman, M., Pickett, J. A., Field, L. M., and Zhou, J. J. (2009). Characterisations of odorant-binding proteins in the tsetse fly *Glossina morsitans morsitans*. *Cell Mol. Life Sci.* 2009 Dec 10. [Epub ahead of print].

Maibeche-Coisne, M., Sobrio, F., Delavnay, T., Lettere, M., Dubroca, J., Jacquin-Joly, E., and Nagnam-Le Meillour, P. (1997). Pheromone binding proteins of the moth *Mamestra brassicae*: Specificity of ligand binding. *Insect Biochem. Mol. Biol.* **27,** 213–221.

Maida, R., and Pelosi, P. (1989). Identification and partial purification of a pheromone-binding protein in *Bombyx mori*. *Ital. J. Biochem.* **38,** 211A–213A.

Maida, R., Steinbrecht, R. A., Ziegelberger, G., and Pelosi, P. (1993). The pheromone-binding protein of *Bombyx mori*: Purification, characterisation and immunocytochemical localisation. *Insect Biochem. Mol. Biol.* **23,** 243–253.

Maida, R., Krieger, J., Gebauer, T., Lange, U., and Ziegelberger, G. (2000). Three pheromone-binding proteins in olfactory sensilla of the two silkmoth species *Antheraea polyphemus* and *Antheraea pernyi*. *Eur. J. Biochem.* **267,** 2899–2908.

Maida, R., Ziegelberger, G., and Kaissling, K. E. (2003). Ligand binding to six recombinant pheromone-binding proteins of *Antheraea polyphemus* and *Antheraea pernyi*. *J. Comp. Physiol. [B]* **173,** 565–573.

Maida, R., Mameli, M., Müller, B., Krieger, J., and Steinbrecht, R. A. (2005). The expression pattern of four odorant-binding proteins in male and female silk moths, *Bombyx mori*. *J. Neurocytol.* **34,** 149–163.

Matsuo, T., Sugaya, S., Yasukawa, J., Aigaki, T., and Fuyama, Y. (2007). Odorant-binding proteins OBP57d and OBP57e affect taste perception and host–plant preference in *Drosophila sechellia*. *PLoS Biol.* **5,** e118.

McKenna, M. P., Hekmat-Scafe, D. S., Gaines, P., and Carlson, J. R. (1994). Putative *Drosophila* pheromone-binding proteins expressed in a subregion of the olfactory system. *J. Biol. Chem.* **269,** 16340–16347.
Meng, L. Z., Wu, C. H., Wicklein, M., Kaissling, K. E., and Bestmann, H. J. (1989). Number and sensitivity of three types of pheromone receptor cells in *Antheraea pernyi* and *A. polyphemus*. *J. Comp. Physiol. A* **165,** 139–146.
Mohanty, S., Zubkov, S., and Gronenborn, A. M. (2004). The solution NMR structure of *Antheraea polyphemus* PBP provides new insight into pheromone recognition by pheromone-binding proteins. *J. Mol. Biol.* **337,** 443–451.
Mohl, C., Breer, H., and Krieger, J. (2002). Species-specific pheromonal compounds induce distinct conformational changes of pheromone binding protein subtypes from *Antheraea polyphemus*. *Invert. Neurosci.* **4,** 165–174.
Nieberding, C. M., de Vos, H., Schneider, M. V., Lassance, J. M., Estramil, N., Andersson, J., Bång, J., Hedenström, E., Löfstedt, C., and Brakefield, P. M. (2008). The male sex pheromone of the butterfly *Bicyclus anynana*: Towards an evolutionary analysis. *PLoS ONE* **3**(7), e2751.
Nikonov, A. A., Peng, G., Tsurupa, G., and Leal, W. S. (2002). Unisex pheromone detectors and pheromone-binding proteins in scarab beetles. *Chem. Senses* **27,** 495–504.
O'Connell, R. J., Grant, A. J., Mayer, M. S., and Mankin, R. W. (1983). Morphological correlates of differences in pheromone sensitivity in insect sensilla. *Science* **220,** 1408–1410.
Pelletier, J., and Leal, W. S. (2009). Genome analysis and expression patterns of odorant-binding proteins from the southern house mosquito *Culex pipiens quinquefasciatus*. *PLoS ONE* **4,** e6237.
Pelosi, P., and Maida, R. (1990). Odorant binding proteins in vertebrates and insects: Similarities and possible common function. *Chem. Senses* **15,** 205–215.
Pelosi, P., Pisanelli, A. M., Baldaccini, N. E., and Gagliardo, A. (1981). Binding of [3H]-2-isobutyl-3-methoxypyrazine to cow olfactory mucosa. *Chem. Senses* **6,** 77–85.
Pelosi, P., Calvello, M., and Ban, L. (1995). Diversity of odorant-binding proteins and chemosensory proteins in insects. *Chem. Senses* **30**(Suppl. 1), i291–i292.
Pelosi, P., Zhou, J.-J., Ban, L. P., and Calvello, M. (2006). Soluble proteins in insect chemical communication. *Cell. Mol. Life Sci.* **63,** 1658–1676.
Peñalva-Arana, D. C., Lynch, M., and Robertson, H. M. (2009). The chemoreceptor genes of the waterflea *Daphnia pulex*: Many Grs but no Ors. *BMC Evol. Biol.* **9,** 79.
Pesenti, M. E., Spinelli, S., Bezirard, V., Briand, L., Pernollet, J. C., Tegoni, M., and Cambillau, C. (2008). Structural basis of the honey bee PBP pheromone and pH-induced conformational change. *J. Mol. Biol.* **380,** 158–169.
Pesenti, M. E., Spinelli, S., Bezirard, V., Briand, L., Pernollet, J. C., Campanacci, V., Tegoni, M., and Cambillau, C. (2009). Queen bee pheromone binding protein pH-induced domain swapping favors pheromone release. *J. Mol. Biol.* **390,** 981–990.
Pevsner, J., Sklar, P. B., and Snyder, S. H. (1986). Odorant-binding protein: Localization to nasal glands and secretions. *Proc. Natl. Acad. Sci. USA* **83,** 4942–4946.
Pevsner, J., Reed, R. R., Feinstein, P. G., and Snyder, S. H. (1988). Molecular cloning of odorant-binding protein: Member of a ligand carrier family. *Science* **241,** 336–339.
Pevsner, J., Hou, V., Snowman, A. M., and Snyder, S. H. (1990). Odorant-binding protein. Characterization of ligand binding. *J. Biol. Chem.* **265,** 6118–6125.
Picimbon, J. F., and Gadenne, C. (2002). Evolution of noctuid pheromone binding proteins: Identification of PBP in the black cutworm moth, *Agrotis ipsilon*. *Insect Biochem. Mol. Biol.* **32,** 839–846.
Picone, D., Crescenzi, O., Angeli, S., Marchese, S., Brandazza, A., Ferrara, L., Pelosi, P., and Scaloni, A. (2001). Bacterial expression and conformational analysis of a chemosensory protein from *Schistocerca gregaria*. *Eur. J. Biochem.* **268,** 4794–4801.

Pikielny, C. W., Hasan, G., Rouyer, F., and Rosbash, H. (1994). Members of a family of *Drosophila* putative odorant-binding proteins are expressed in different subsets of olfactory hairs. *Neuron* **12**(1), 35–49.

Plettner, E., Lazar, J., Prestwich, E. G., and Prestwich, G. D. (2000). Discrimination of pheromone enantiomers by two pheromone binding proteins from the gypsy moth *Lymantria dispar*. *Biochemistry* **39,** 8953–8962.

Pophof, B. (2004). Pheromone-binding proteins contribute to the activation of olfactory receptor neurons in the silkmoths *Antheraea polyphemus* and *Bombyx mori*. *Chem. Senses* **29,** 117–125.

Prestwich, G. D. (1993). Bacterial expression and photoaffinity labeling of a pheromone binding protein. *Protein Sci.* **2,** 420–428.

Prestwich, G. D., Du, G., and LaForest, S. (1995). How is pheromone specificity encoded in proteins? *Chem. Senses* **20,** 461–469.

Qiao, H., Tuccori, E., He, X., Gazzano, A., Field, L., Zhou, J.-J., and Pelosi, P. (2009). Discrimination of alarm pheromone (E)-beta-farnesene by aphid odorant-binding proteins. *Insect Biochem. Mol. Biol.* **39,** 414–419.

Raming, K., Krieger, J., and Breer, H. (1989). Molecular cloning of an insect pheromone-binding protein. *FEBS Lett.* **256,** 215–218.

Raming, K., Krieger, J., and Breer, H. (1990). Primary structure of a pheromone-binding protein from *Antheraea pernyi*: Homologies with other ligand-carrying proteins. *J. Comp. Physiol. [B]* **160,** 503–509.

Riviere, S., Lartigue, A., Quennedey, B., Campanacci, V., Farine, J. P., Tegoni, M., Cambillau, C., and Brossut, R. (2003). A pheromone-binding protein from the cockroach *Leucophaea maderae*: Cloning, expression and pheromone binding. *Biochem. J.* **371,** 573–579.

Robertson, H. M., and Wanner, K. W. (2006). The chemoreceptor superfamily in the honey bee, *Apis mellifera*: Expansion of the odorant, but not gustatory, receptor family. *Genome Res.* **16,** 1395–1403.

Robertson, H., Warr, C., and Carlson, J. (2003). Molecular evolution of the insect chemoreceptor gene superfamily in *Drosophila melanogaster*. *Proc. Natl. Acad. Sci. USA* **100,** 14537–14542.

Sandler, B. H., Nikonova, L., Leal, W. S., and Clardy, J. (2000). Sexual attraction in the silkworm moth: Structure of the pheromone-binding-protein-bombykol complex. *Chem. Biol.* **7,** 143–151.

Schneider, D., and Seibt, U. (1969). Sex pheromone of the queen bufferfly: Electroantennogram responses. *Science* **164,** 1173–1174.

Shanbhag, S. R., Hekmat-Scafe, D., Kim, M. S., Park, S. K., Carlson, J. R., Pikielny, C., Smith, D. P., and Steinbrecht, R. A. (2001). Expression mosaic of odorant-binding proteins in *Drosophila* olfactory organs. *Microsc. Res. Tech.* **55,** 297–306.

Smadja, C., Shi, P., Butlin, R. K., and Robertson, H. M. (2009). Large gene family expansions and adaptive evolution for odorant and gustatory receptors in the pea aphid, *Acyrthosiphon pisum*. *Mol. Biol. Evol.* **26,** 2073–2086.

Steinbrecht, R. A. (1998). Odorant-binding proteins: Expression and function. *Ann. NY Acad. Sci.* **30,** 323–332.

Steinbrecht, R. A., Ozaki, M., and Ziegelberger, G. (1992). Immunocytochemical localization of pheromone-binding protein in moth antennae. *Cell Tissue Res.* **282,** 203–217.

Steinbrecht, R. A., Laue, M., and Ziegelberger, G. (1995). Immunolocalization of pheromone-binding protein and general odorant-binding protein in olfactory sensilla of the silk moths *Antheraea* and *Bombyx*. *Cell Tissue Res.* **282,** 203–217.

Syed, Z., Ishida, Y., Taylor, K., Kimbrell, D. A., and Leal, W. S. (2006). Pheromone reception in fruit flies expressing a moth's odorant receptor. *Proc. Natl. Acad. Sci. USA* **103,** 16538–16543.

Tegoni, M., Campanacci, V., and Cambillau, C. (2004). Structural aspects of sexual attraction and chemical communication in insects. *Trends Biochem. Sci.* **29,** 257–264.

Van den Berg, M. J., and Ziegelberger, G. (1991). On the function of the pheromone binding protein in the olfactory hairs of *Antheraea polyphemus*. *J. Insect Physiol.* **37,** 79–85.

Vogt, R. G. (2002). Odorant binding protein homologues of the malaria mosquito *Anopheles gambiae*; Possible orthologues of the OS-E and OS-F OBPs of *Drosophila melanogaster*. *J. Chem. Ecol.* **28,** 2371–2376.

Vogt, R. G., and Riddiford, L. M. (1981). Pheromone binding and inactivation by moth antennae. *Nature* **293,** 161–163.

Vogt, R. G., Riddiford, L. M., and Prestwich, G. D. (1985). Kinetic properties of a sex pheromone-degrading enzyme: The sensillar esterase of *Antheraea polyphemus*. *Proc. Natl. Acad. Sci. USA* **82,** 8827–8831.

Vogt, R. G., Köehne, A. C., Dubnau, J. T., and Prestwich, G. D. (1989). Expression of pheromone binding proteins during antennal development in the gypsy moth *Lymantria dispar*. *J. Neurosci.* **9,** 3332–3346.

Vogt, R. G., Rybczynski, R., and Lerner, M. R. (1991). Molecular cloning and sequencing of general odorant-binding proteins GOBP1 and GOBP2 from the tobacco hawk moth *Manduca sexta*: Comparisons with other insect OBPs and their signal peptides. *J. Neurosci.* **11,** 2972–2984.

Vogt, R. G., Callahan, F. E., Rogers, M. E., and Dickens, J. C. (1999). Odorant binding protein diversity and distribution among the insect orders, as indicated by LAP, an OBP-related protein of the true bug *Lygus lineolaris* (Hemiptera, Heteroptera). *Chem Senses* **24,** 481–495.

Vogt, R. G., Rogers, M. E., Franco, M. D., and Sun, M. (2002). A comparative study of odorant binding protein genes: Differential expression of the PBP1-GOBP2 gene cluster in *Manduca sexta* (Lepidoptera) and the organization of OBP genes in *Drosophila melanogaster* (Diptera). *J. Exp. Biol.* **205,** 719–744.

Wanner, K. W., Anderson, A. R., Trowell, S. C., Theilmann, D. A., Robertson, H. M., and Newcomb, R. D. (2007). Female-biased expression of odourant receptor genes in the adult antennae of the silkworm, *Bombyx mori*. *Insect Mol. Biol.* **16,** 107–119.

Wogulis, M., Morgan, T., Ishida, Y., Leal, W. S., and Wilson, D. K. (2005). The crystal structure of an odorant binding protein from *Anopheles gambiae*: Evidence for a common ligand release mechanism. *Biochem. Biophys. Res. Commun.* **339,** 157–164.

Wojtasek, H., and Leal, W. S. (1999). Conformational change in the pheromone-binding protein from *Bombyx mori* induced by pH and by interaction with membranes. *J. Biol. Chem.* **274,** 30950–30956.

Xu, P. X., Zwiebel, L. J., and Smith, D. P. (2003). Identification of a distinct family of genes encoding atypical odorant-binding proteins in the malaria vector mosquito, *Anopheles gambiae*. *Insect Mol. Biol.* **12,** 549–560.

Zhou, J.-J., Zhang, G.-A., Huang, W., Birkett, M. A., Field, L. M., Pickett, J. A., and Pelosi, P. (2004a). Revisiting odorant-binding protein LUSH of *Drosophila melanogaster*: Evidence for odour recognition and discrimination. *FEBS Lett.* **558,** 23–26.

Zhou, J.-J., Huang, W., Zhang, G. A., Pickett, J. A., and Field, L. M. (2004b). "Plus-C" odorant-binding protein genes in two *Drosophila* species and the malaria mosquito *Anopheles gambiae*. *Gene* **327,** 117–129.

Zhou, J.-J., Kan, Y., Antoniw, J., Pickett, J. A., and Field, L. M. (2006). Genome and EST analyses and expression of a gene family with putative functions in insect chemoreception. *Chem. Senses* **31,** 453–465.

Zhou, J.-J., He, X. L., Pickett, J. A., and Field, L. M. (2008). Identification of odorant-binding proteins of the yellow fever mosquito *Aedes aegypti*, genome annotation and comparative analyses. *Insect Mol. Biol.* **17,** 147–163.

Zhou, J.-J., Robertson, G., He, X., Dufour, S., Hooper, A. M., Pickett, J. A., Keep, N. H., and Field, L. M. (2009). Characterisation of *Bombyx mori* Odorant-binding proteins reveals that a general odorant-binding protein discriminates between sex pheromone components. *J. Mol. Biol.* **389,** 529–545.
Zhou, J.-J., Field, L. M., and He, X. L. (2010). Insect odorant-binding proteins: Do they offer an alternative pest control strategy? *Outlooks Pest Manag.* **21**(1), 31–34.
Ziegelberger, G. (1995). Redox shift of the pheromone-binding protein in the silkmoth *Antheraea polyphemus*. *Eur. J. Biochem.* **232,** 706–711, 33.
Zubkov, S., Gronenborn, A. M., Byeon, I. J., and Mohanty, S. (2005). Structural consequences of the pH-induced conformational switch in *A. polyphemus* pheromone-binding protein: Mechanisms of ligand release. *J. Mol. Biol.* **354,** 1081–1090.

CHAPTER ELEVEN

Drosophila CheB proteins Involved in Gustatory Detection of Pheromones Are Related to a Human Neurodegeneration Factor

Claudio W. Pikielny

Contents

Abstract

The *Drosophila* CheBs proteins are expressed in a variety of sexually dimorphic subsets of taste hairs, some of which have been directly implicated in pheromone detection. Their remarkable collection of expression patterns suggests that CheBs have specialized roles in gustatory detection of pheromones. Indeed, mutations in the *CheB42a* gene specifically alter male response to female-specific cuticular hydrocarbons. Furthermore, CheBs belong to the large ML (MD-2-like) superfamily of lipid-binding proteins and share amino

Department of Genetics and Neuroscience Center, Dartmouth Medical School, Hanover, New Hampshire, USA

Vitamins and Hormones, Volume 83
ISSN 0083-6729, DOI: 10.1016/S0083-6729(10)83011-0

acids with an essential role in the function of human GM2-activator protein (GM2-AP), a protein whose absence results in neurodegeneration and death. As GM2-AP binds specifically to the GM2 ganglioside, we have proposed that CheB42a and other CheBs function by interacting directly with the lipid-like cuticular hydrocarbons of *Drosophila melanogaster* and modulating their detection by transmembrane receptors. Here I review the current knowledge of the CheB family and discuss possible models for their function.

I. Introduction

In most animal species, chemosensory detection of pheromones controls vital interactions between individuals such as mating and aggression (Touhara and Vosshall, 2009). One key property of a pheromone is the distance from the source at which it can be detected and affect the behavior of other individuals. Pheromones that are highly volatile can be detected at a long distance from the source, while detection of less volatile compounds requires direct contact with a chemosensory organ (Touhara, 2008; Wicker-Thomas, 2007). Many important insect pheromones are high molecular weight hydrocarbons with no functional group that display little if any volatility (Ferveur, 2005; Howard and Blomquist, 2005; Wicker-Thomas, 2007). For example, when the concentration of the mating pheromone of the house fly, (Z)-9-tricosene or muscalure, was measured for several days after spotting on the surface of a plant leaf, there was no detectable decrease (Witjes and Eltz, 2009).

In *Drosophila*, *cis*-vaccenyl acetate (cVA) is a male-specific volatile pheromone produced in the ejaculatory bulb that stimulates mating behavior in females, but when perceived by other males triggers aggression and inhibits courtship behavior. Recently, it has been shown that detection of cVA involves a specific pheromone-binding protein, LUSH, one or more specific olfactory receptor, and SNMP1 a CD36-related protein, as well as a sexually dimorphic olfactory circuit (Benton, 2007; Vosshall, 2008). However, most known pheromones in *Drosophila* are long-chain hydrocarbons with very low volatility that modulate courtship behavior and allow species discrimination (Ferveur, 2005; Billeter *et al.*, 2009), and are detected by gustatory organs (Boll and Noll, 2002; Bray and Amrein, 2003; Park *et al.*, 2006; Krstic *et al.*, 2009). More surprisingly, olfactory organs also detect these low volatility pheromones (Ejima *et al.*, 2005; Stockinger *et al.*, 2005; van der Goes van Naters and Carlson, 2007), albeit only within a range of a few millimeters (Gailey *et al.*, 1986). In this review, I will summarize our work on the *Drosophila* CheB protein family, and discuss the evidence that CheBs have a specialized role in gustatory detection of pheromones.

II. *Drosophila* CheBs Are Expressed in a Variety of Sex-Specific Subsets of Taste Hairs that May Be Specialized in Pheromone Detection

To discover molecules involved in gustatory detection of pheromones, we (Xu *et al.*, 2002) and others (Bray and Amrein, 2003) took advantage of the observation that the taste hairs on the front legs, but in no other part of the fly, are sexually dimorphic, both in numbers and in the pattern of their projections to the central nervous system (Possidente and Murphey, 1989). A subtractive cDNA cloning strategy (Xu *et al.*, 2002) led to the discovery of two genes that are specifically expressed in the front legs of males: CheA29a and CheB42a. Both CheA29a and CheB42a are part of small families of proteins encoded by the *Drosophila* genome, with 8 and 12 members, respectively (the nomenclature refers to Chemosensory protein families A and B, followed by the corresponding chromosomal band and a lower case letter to differentiate between related genes at the same locus). Systematic analyses of their expression patterns suggest that members of the CheB gene family are involved in gustatory perception of pheromones (Park *et al.*, 2006; Starostina *et al.*, 2009). Indeed, all 12 CheBs are expressed specifically in chemosensory organs, almost exclusively in gustatory organs; only two CheBs display detectable, but significantly lower expression in the antennae, the main olfactory organ (Table 11.1). Furthermore, expression of CheB42a, CheB93a, and CheB38c, which was examined at the cellular

Table 11.1 The 12 *Drosophila* CheBs are expressed in a variety of sexually dimorphic, gustatory-specific patterns

Group I	Group II
Specific expression in male front legs	Specific or preferential expression in wings of either sex
38a, 38b, 42a, 53a, 53b, 74a, 93b	38c (also in legs, except male front legs)
93a	42b (also in male antennae and front legs of males and females)
Expressed in distinct subset of male taste hairs from CheB42a	42c (also in front legs of both sexes)
Lower expression in male antennae	98 (wing-specific, higher in males than females)

Eight genes in group I are almost exclusively expressed in the front legs of males; one gene is also expressed at lower levels in male antennae. Expression at the cellular level of CheB42a and CheB93a is found in nonoverlapping subsets of taste hairs. Four genes in group II are each expressed in a unique pattern on taste hairs in other appendages (second and third pair of legs, wings). While genes in group II are all expressed in both males and females, expression of three of them is sexually dimorphic.

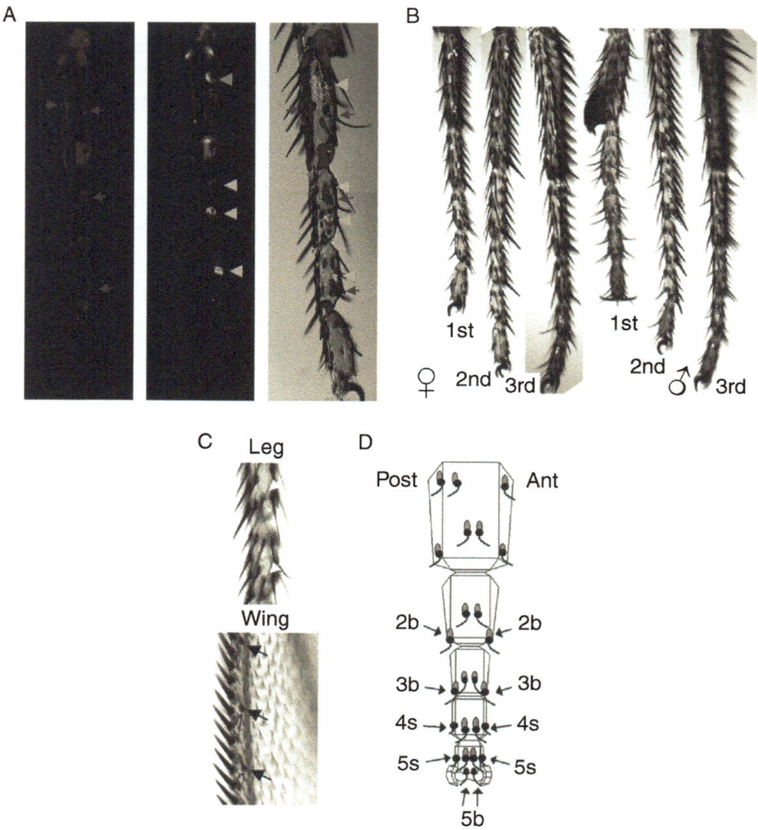

Figure 11.1 CheB42a, CheB93a, and CheB38c are expressed in three distinct, nonoverlapping, sexually dimorphic subsets of taste hairs. (A) Expression of CheB42a and CheB93a was analyzed by *in situ* hybridization. Expression of *CheB42a* (green) and *CheB93a* (red) occurs in two distinct subsets of taste hairs. Expression of CheB38c in the legs (B) and wings (C) is visualized through transgenic GFP expression using CheB42a regulatory sequences. (D) A schematic map indicates the position of all 21 gustatory sensilla on the tarsal segments of female front legs and the sites of GFP expression (green oval). Arrows indicate the position of the only five sensilla that respond to either sucrose, salt, or bitter compounds (Meunier *et al.*, 2000, 2003b). Modified from Starostina *et al.* (2009).

level, is associated with three distinct, nonoverlapping subsets of taste hairs on the legs and wings (Fig. 11.1). In addition to their gustatory specificity, expression of all but one of the 12 CheB genes is sexually dimorphic; seven are only expressed in the front legs of males, while four others display more complex patterns in both legs and wings (Table 11.1). To my knowledge, this is the only reported case in which the vast majority of genes in a family display strikingly sexually dimorphic expression outside of reproductive organs. Finally, while sharing their gustatory specificity and sexual dimorphism, expression of CheBs is remarkably varied, representing at least six distinct patterns, some of which overlap partially (Table 11.1).

Their sexually dimorphic expression in subsets of taste hairs suggests that CheBs may play a specific role in gustatory detection of pheromones. Indeed, none of the CheBs is detectably expressed in the gustatory hairs of the proboscis or internal taste organs which detect food components such as sugars, salt, and bitter compounds (Vosshall and Stocker, 2007). Furthermore, expression of the three CheB genes analyzed at the cellular level correlates almost perfectly with the taste hairs on front legs of both males and females that lack any detectable response to food chemicals (Fig. 11.1D) (Meunier *et al.*, 2000, 2003a; Starostina *et al.*, 2009). Finally, the 10 taste hairs on the front legs of males identified by expression of both CheB42a and Gr68a, a putative gustatory receptor for female pheromones, are indeed required for response to female cuticular hydrocarbons (Bray and Amrein, 2003; Park *et al.*, 2006). Therefore, expression of all genes in the CheB family may be restricted to taste hairs specialized in detecting pheromones.

III. CheB42a Is Required for Normal Response to Female-Specific Pheromones

One of the best-studied effects of *Drosophila* pheromones is the stimulation and modulation of mating behaviors through both olfactory and gustatory detection of pheromones (Villella and Hall, 2008). We therefore tested whether CheB42a is involved in male-specific gustatory detection of pheromones (Park *et al.*, 2006). Indeed, we found that while mutant males lacking CheB42a can perform most behaviors normally, they display a remarkably specific defect in their courtship behavior, progressing more rapidly than controls to attempted copulation, the final step in the sequence (Fig. 11.2). Using transgenes with and without a single nucleotide mutation in the initiator ATG of CheB42a, it was shown that this behavioral defect is due to the absence of the CheB42a protein (Fig. 11.2A and B). Does this abnormal behavior result from impaired chemosensory perception of cuticular hydrocarbons? To answer this question, we tested the response of mutant and control males to two different types of flies with altered hydrocarbon profiles. Indeed, *CheB42a* mutant males display the same increased zeal relative to controls in their attempt to copulate with males that emit female-specific pheromones as in the presence of normal females (Fig. 11.2D). In contrast, in the presence of females lacking cuticular hydrocarbons mutant males respond just like control males (Fig. 11.2C). Together, these experiments demonstrate that CheB42a is required for the normal response of males to female cuticular hydrocarbons.

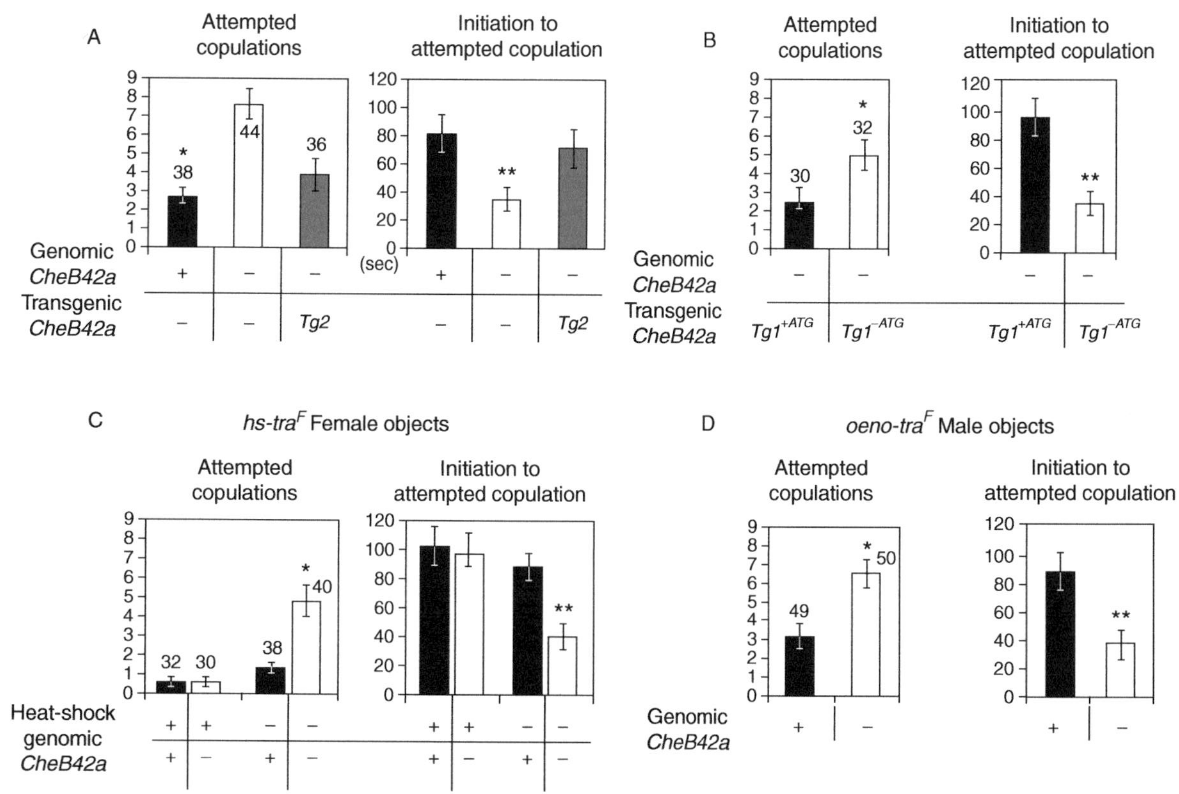

Figure 11.2 Female-specific cuticular hydrocarbons trigger earlier and more frequent copulation attempts from *CheB42a* mutant males. (A) Response of males to *w1118* virgin females was compared for control males (black bars), males homozygous for the $CheB42a^{\Delta 5\text{-}68}$ deletion of *CheB42a* (white bars), and $CheB42a^{\Delta 5\text{-}68}$ homozygous males that carry *Tg2*, a transgenic construct that encodes *CheB42a* but no other protein-

IV. CheBs Belong to the ML Superfamily of Lipid-Binding Proteins and Share Functionally Important Sequences with GM2-Activator Protein, an Essential Protein of Human Neurons

While simple BLAST searches failed to reveal any obvious relationship between CheBs and any other known protein (Xu *et al.*, 2002), extensive use of more sensitive approaches based on the presence of residues conserved among many different proteins revealed that CheBs are related to lipid-binding proteins of the ML family (MD2-like) (Starostina *et al.*, 2009) (Fig. 11.3). Sequence similarity among proteins in this family is very low, often undetectable by conventional BLAST searches (Inohara and Nunez, 2002). However, all ML proteins have very similar three-dimensional structures consisting of a single sheet of seven β-strands folding into a β-cup (Ichikawa *et al.*, 2005). Alignment of multiple ML proteins reveals a small number of conserved residues at fixed positions relative to this secondary structure, the most striking of which are four cysteine residues forming one disulfide bridge between β-strands 1 and 7, and another between β-strands 4 and 5 (Fig. 11.3B). Remarkably, CheBs share several blocks of conserved residues with human GM2-AP which are not present in other ML proteins with higher overall sequence similarity with GM2-AP (yellow and red blocks in Fig. 11.3A). The most conserved residues between CheBs and GM2-AP form motifs I and II, which coincide with key structural and functional elements of GM2-AP (Fig. 11.3C). Indeed, the three-dimensional structure of GM2-AP brings the two motifs into spatial proximity, allowing formation of a hydrogen bond (HB) between a lysine in motif I and a tyrosine in motif II,

coding gene (gray bars) (Lin *et al.*, 2005). $^{\star}p < 0.0000007$; $^{\star\star}p < 0.002$. (B) A single copy of alternative transgenes is the only genetic difference between the two types of males tested in this experiment which are heterozygous for *CheB42a*$^{\Delta 5\text{-}68}$ and *Δ5-22*, another deletion of the locus that removes not only *CheB42a* but also the neighboring *ppk25* gene (Lin *et al.*, 2005). Control males (black bars) carry *Tg1*$^{(+ATG)}$ (Lin *et al.*, 2005), a transgene that encodes both *CheB42a* and *ppk25*, while *Tg1*$^{(-ATG)}$ the transgene present in test males (white bars) is identical to $Tg_1^{(+ATG)}$, except for a point mutation that changes the initiating ATG of *CheB42a* to ATA resulting in the absence of detectable CheB42A protein (data not shown). $^{\star}p < 0.02$; $^{\star\star}p < 0.002$. (C) The response of *CheB42a*$^{\Delta 5\text{-}68}$ and control males was measured toward heat-shocked "*hs-traF*" females which carry the *hs-Gal4* and *UAS-traF* transgenes and lack cuticular hydrocarbons (Savarit *et al.*, 1999) or, as controls, genetically identical, nonheat-shocked *hs-traF* female siblings. $^{\star}p < 0.006$; $^{\star\star}p < 0.008$. (D) "*Oeno-traF*" males which carry the *oenocyte-Gal4* and *UAS-traF* transgenes and display female-specific hydrocarbon pheromones on their cuticles (Ferveur, 1997) were used as sexual objects for *CheB42a*$^{\Delta 5\text{-}68}$ and control males. $^{\star}p < 0.00038$; $^{\star\star}p < 0.00067$. Modified from Park *et al.* (2006).

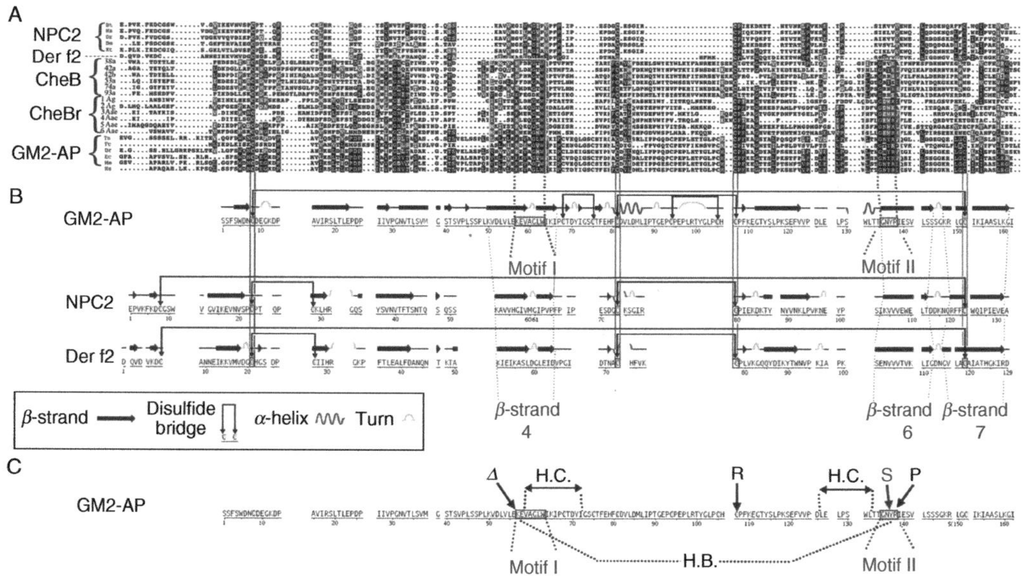

Figure 11.3 CheBs share key functional residues with human GM2-activator protein. (A) Alignment of six sequences from each of four groups: CheBs, CheBrs, proteins related to GM2-AP, and proteins related to NPC2, including the mite antigen Der f2. Three of the four cysteines involved in disulfide bonds in GM2-AP, NPC2, and Der f2 and the perfectly aligned cysteines in all other proteins in this alignment are boxed in purple. Residues present in human GM2-AP and conserved in at least 10 of the other 24 proteins in the alignment are shaded in black when identical, and green when similar. Sequence blocks found in CheBs, CheBrs, and GM2-APs, but not in NPC2 and Der f2, are boxed in yellow, and Motifs I and II, discussed in the text, are boxed in red. (B) The sequence alignment above was used to align the known secondary structures of Der f2 (Suzuki *et al.*, 2005), bovine NPC2 (Friedland *et al.*, 2003), and mouse GM2-AP (Wright *et al.*, 2000, 2003, 2004, 2005), obtained from the Protein Data Bank server at http://www.pdb.org/. Dotted lines indicate several secondary structure elements that are precisely aligned in the three proteins (the fourth, six, and seventh b-strands, and two turns, one interrupting β-strand 4, the other between β-strands 6 and 7). (C) Three known point mutations that inactivate human GM2-AP and result in Tay-Sachs disease, DK88,

and contributing to a hydrophobic cleft (HC) at the surface of the molecule (Wright *et al.*, 2005). This HC is thought to mediate the initial interaction of GM2-AP with GM2 present in the lysosomal membrane and act as a channel for transfer of the ganglioside to the internal pocket of GM2-AP. The functional importance of the conserved residues is reaffirmed by the observation that of the three mutations known to inactivate human GM2-AP, one deletes the conserved lysine in motif I and another changes the conserved arginine in motif II into a proline. The presence in CheBs of key functional residues of GM2-AP, particularly in view of the otherwise very low level of overall sequence similarity, suggests that CheBs share some functional properties with this human protein.

V. CheBs Likely Function as Gustatory-Specific Pheromone-Binding Proteins

Their inclusion in the ML family of lipid-binding proteins suggests that CheBs bind the lipid-like pheromones of *Drosophila* (Fig. 11.5) immediately before or after the latter are detected at the membrane of chemosensory neurons. One strong prediction of this hypothesis is that CheBs must be present in the inner lumen of taste hairs, the extracellular compartment where pheromones interact with putative receptors on the membrane of pheromone-sensing taste hairs (Fig. 11.4A; Shanbhag *et al.*, 2001). Expression of CheB42a occurs in thecogen cells, a specific type of non-neuronal cell (Park *et al.*, 2006). Thecogen cells are also called sheath cells because they wrap around the bodies of sensory neurons and border the lumen of internal taste hairs, into which they are thought to secrete soluble proteins. Indeed, the CheB42a protein can be detected in the lumen of pheromone-sensing hairs (Fig. 11.5B; Starostina *et al.*, 2009). Furthermore, double-staining with antibodies for PBPRP2, a protein of unknown function that is only secreted into the outer lumen (Shanbhag *et al.*, 2001), shows that CheB42a is only present in the inner lumen of pheromone-sensing hairs (Fig. 11.5C). These experiments show that CheB42a is indeed present

C138R, and R169P (Wright *et al.*, 2000), are indicated by black arrows. The synthetic Y137S mutation resulting in closure of the hydrophobic cleft and loss of ligand binding (Wright *et al.*, 2005) is shown by a red arrow. Two double-headed arrows indicate sequences that are nearby in space (Wright *et al.*, 2000), forming a hydrophobic cleft (HC) that interacts with ligands at the surface of the protein (Wright *et al.*, 2003, 2004, 2005). A hydrogen bond (HB) between K88 and Y137 is shown by a dotted line. The sequences of CheBs were reported previously (Xu *et al.*, 2002). References for the sequences in this alignment can be found in the original figure in Starostina *et al.* (2009). (See Color Insert.)

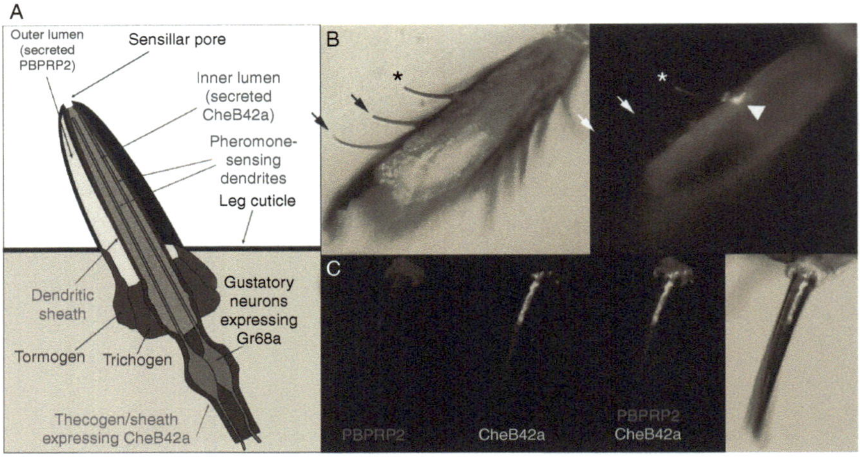

Figure 11.4 CheB42a is secreted into the extracellular compartment where pheromones are detected by gustatory neurons. (A) Cartoon showing the complex organization of a pheromone-sensing taste hair. (B) Paraffin section of a male front leg immunolabeled with anti-CheB42a (Xu *et al.*, 2002; Park *et al.*, 2006). One or more cells at the base of a taste hair (asterisk) and the corresponding hair shaft (arrowhead) are specifically labeled, while no labeling is associated with two other taste hairs (arrows) visible in this field. (C) Labeling with anti-CheB42a (green) and anti-PBPRP2 (red) (Park *et al.*, 2000) occur within the shaft of the same taste hair, but do not overlap. Modified from Starostina *et al.* (2009). (See Color Insert.)

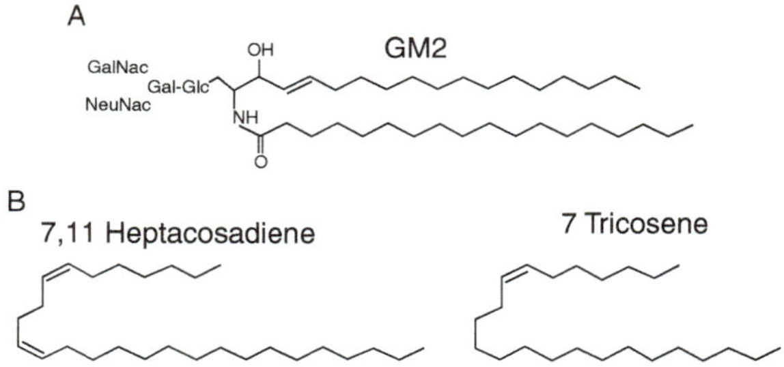

Figure 11.5 Courtship-activating pheromones of *Drosophila* are long-chain hydrocarbons resembling the aliphatic chains of GM2. The two major cuticular hydrocarbon pheromones of *Drosophila melanogaster*: (Z,Z)-7,11-heptacosadiene, and (Z)-7-tricosene (Ferveur, 2005) are shown above the GM2 glycolipid, the main ligand of GMAP (Wright *et al.*, 2003).

in the extracellular compartment where pheromone detection occurs, and support the possibility that CheBs represent a novel category of pheromone-binding protein with a specialized function in gustatory detection of contact pheromones.

VI. Models for the Function of CheBs in Gustatory Detection of Pheromones

What is the mechanism underlying the increased response of *CheB42a* mutant males to female-specific hydrocarbons, and more generally the function of CheBs in pheromone response? The current data is compatible with two opposing models (Fig. 11.6). In a first model, CheB42a decreases the stimulatory effect of female-specific cuticular hydrocarbons (Ferveur,

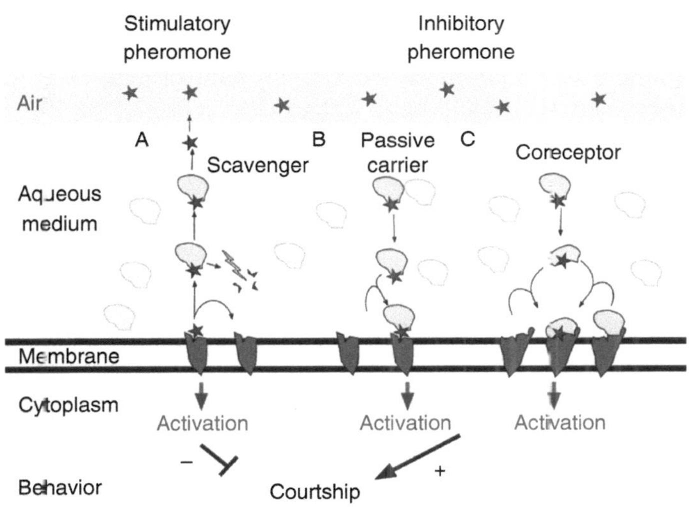

Figure 11.6 Models for CheB function. The following models for the function of CheB42a and other CheBs in detection of pheromones are based on the three general types of models that have been proposed for the function of pheromone-binding proteins and odorant-binding proteins (Kaissling, 2009; Pelosi *et al.*, 2006; Pevsner and Snyder, 1990; Stowers and Logan, 2008). (A) CheB42a may diminish or shorten the effect of a female pheromone that stimulates male courtship, either by facilitating its enzymatic inactivation or its diffusion back into the environment. Alternatively, CheB42a may be required for detection of an inhibitory pheromone. (B) CheB42a may be a passive carrier that facilitates the diffusion of its hydrophobic ligand through the aqueous phase between the air and the membrane of the chemosensory neuron. (C) By analogy with LUSH and MD2, CheB42a may function as coreceptor for an inhibitory pheromone.

2005). This possibility is supported by the expression of CheB42a in the same 10 taste hairs on male front legs that also express Gr68a, a gustatory receptor required for response to female-specific cuticular hydrocarbon pheromones (Bray and Amrein, 2003; Park *et al.*, 2006). One particularly attractive possibility is that CheB42a contributes to the turnover of female-specific pheromones inside the compartment where the latter are detected by the putative pheromone receptor Gr68a. Rapid turnover of pheromones by pheromone degrading enzymes within chemosensory organs is essential to prevent desensitization and to allow real-time monitoring of pheromone levels (Maibeche-Coisne *et al.*, 2004; Kaissling, 2009). In particular, the main house fly pheromone, Z(9)-tricosene, is enzymatically inactivated by oxydation into epoxyde and ketone derivatives (Ahmad *et al.*, 1987). Much in the same way that GM2-AP is required for hydrolysis of GM2 into GM1, CheB42a may therefore stimulate enzymatic inactivation of one of the female-specific dienes such as 7,11 heptacosadiene, that stimulate male courtship (Ferveur, 2005; Fig. 11.6A).

Alternatively, CheB42a may be required for detection of a hydrocarbon that inhibits male courtship behavior, such as 7-tricosene, which is produced by both males and females. Such a role would be analogous to that of several insect pheromone-binding proteins in detection of specific pheromones (Kaissling, 2009; Leal, 2005; Pelosi *et al.*, 2006). Pheromone-binding proteins and odorant-binding proteins, which are structurally unrelated to MLs, have long been proposed to act largely as passive carriers, facilitating diffusion of their hydrophobic ligands across the aqueous layer which covers the membranes of chemosensory neurons (Fig. 11.6B). By analogy, and consistent with GM2-AP's role as a cofactor for the Hexaminidase A enzyme (Kolter and Sandhoff, 2010), CheB42a may act as a passive carrier facilitating the interaction of inhibitory gustatory pheromones with their receptors. However, a recent series of elegant experiments have shown that an insect pheromone-binding protein, the *Drosophila* LUSH, plays a much more active role in olfactory detection of the volatile pheromone cVA (Laughlin *et al.*, 2008; Xu *et al.*, 2005). First, lack of LUSH not only disrupts cVA detection but also results in an increased baseline firing rate by cVA-detecting neurons, suggesting that LUSH itself interacts and regulates the activity of transmembrane receptors, even in the absence of cVA. Furthermore, cVA binding triggers a conformational change in LUSH, and a point mutation freezing LUSH in this active conformation results in cVA-independent activation of cVA-sensing neurons. Activation of transmembrane receptors therefore likely result from interactions with LUSH in an activated conformation triggered by cVA binding (Fig. 11.6C). Furthermore, the ML protein MD2 is an essential coreceptor in the detection of bacterial lipopolysaccharide by Toll-like receptor TLR4 (Jerala, 2007). CheBs could therefore play a similarly active role in detection of inhibitory gustatory pheromones.

VII. Conclusions and Future Directions

The *Drosophila* CheB protein family is unique among chemosensory families of proteins in the varied sexually dimorphic expression patterns displayed by its members, suggesting that it has a specialized role in gustatory detection of pheromones. Indeed, loss of the *CheB42a* gene results in abnormal male response to female pheromones. Furthermore, the conservation in CheBs of residues with critical roles for the function of human GM2-AP, suggests that related mechanisms are involved. Insights into the function of *Drosophila* CheBs should therefore illuminate our understanding of GM2-AP's role in neurodegeneration and vice versa.

ACKNOWLEDGMENTS

This work was supported by grants RO1DC04284 and R01DC007911 from the NIDCD to C. W. P., and through an award from the Biomedical Research Support Program for Medical Schools from the Howard Hughes Medical Institute to Dartmouth Medical School (76200-560801).

REFERENCES

Ahmad, S., Kirkland, K. E., and Blomquist, G. J. (1987). Evidence for a sex pheromone metabolizing cytochrome P-450 mono-oxygenase in the housefly. *Arch. Insect Biochem. Physiol.* **6,** 121–140.

Benton, R. (2007). Sensitivity and specificity in *Drosophila* pheromone perception. *Trends Neurosci.* **30,** 512–519.

Billeter, J. C., Atallah, J., Krupp, J. J., Millar, J. G., and Levine, J. D. (2009). Specialized cells tag sexual and species identity in *Drosophila melanogaster. Nature* **461,** 987–991.

Boll, W., and Noll, M. (2002). The *Drosophila* Pox neuro gene: Control of male courtship behavior and fertility as revealed by a complete dissection of all enhancers. *Development* **129,** 5667–5681.

Bray, S., and Amrein, H. (2003). A putative *Drosophila* pheromone receptor expressed in male-specific taste neurons is required for efficient courtship. *Neuron* **39,** 1019–1029.

Ejima, A., Smith, B. P., Lucas, C., Levine, J. D., and Griffith, L. C. (2005). Sequential learning of pheromonal cues modulates memory consolidation in trainer-specific associative courtship conditioning. *Curr. Biol.* **15,** 194–206.

Ferveur, J.-F. (1997). The pheromononal role of cuticular hydrocarbons in *Drosophila melanogaster. Bioessays* **19,** 353–358.

Ferveur, J. F (2005). Cuticular hydrocarbons: Their evolution and roles in *Drosophila* pheromonal communication. *Behav. Genet.* **35,** 279–295.

Friedland, N., Liou, H. L., Lobel, P., and Stock, A. M. (2003). Structure of a cholesterol-binding protein deficient in Niemann-Pick type C2 disease. *Proc. Natl. Acad. Sci. USA* **100,** 2512–2517.

Gailey, D., Lacaillade, R. C., and Hall, J. C. (1986). Chemosensory elements of courtship in normal and mutant, olfaction-deficient *Drosophila. Behav. Genet.* **16,** 375–405.

Howard, R. W., and Blomquist, G. J. (2005). Ecological, behavioral, and biochemical aspects of insect hydrocarbons. *Annu. Rev. Entomol.* **50,** 371–393.

Ichikawa, S., Takai, T., Inoue, T., Yuuki, T., Okumura, Y., Ogura, K., Inagaki, F., and Hatanaka, H. (2005). NMR study on the major mite allergen Der f 2: Its refined tertiary structure, epitopes for monoclonal antibodies and characteristics shared by ML protein group members. *J. Biochem. (Tokyo)* **137,** 255–263.

Inohara, N., and Nunez, G. (2002). ML — a conserved domain involved in innate immunity and lipid metabolism. *Trends Biochem. Sci.* **27,** 219–221.

Jerala, R. (2007). Structural biology of the LPS recognition. *Int. J. Med. Microbiol.* **297,** 353–363.

Kaissling, K. E. (2009). Olfactory perireceptor and receptor events in moths: A kinetic model revised. *J. Comp. Physiol. A Neuroethol. Sens. Neural Behav. Physiol* **195,** 895–922.

Kolter, T., and Sandhoff, K. (2010). Lysosomal degradation of membrane lipids. *FEBS Lett.* **584,** 1700–1712.

Krstic, D., Boll, W., and Noll, M. (2009). Sensory integration regulating male courtship behavior in *Drosophila. PLoS ONE* **4,** e4457.

Laughlin, J. D., Ha, T. S., Jones, D. N., and Smith, D. P. (2008). Activation of pheromone-sensitive neurons is mediated by conformational activation of pheromone-binding protein. *Cell* **133,** 1255–1265.

Leal, W. S. (2005). Pheromone Response. *In* "The Chemistry of Pheromones and Other Semiochemicals II," (S. Schulz, Ed.), Vol. 240, pp. 1–36. Springer, Berlin.

Lin, H., Mann, K. J., Starostina, E., Kinser, R. D., and Pikielny, C. W. (2005). A *Drosophila* DEG/ENaC channel subunit is required for male response to female pheromones. *Proc. Natl. Acad. Sci. USA* **102,** 12831–12836.

Maibeche-Coisne, M., Nikonov, A. A., Ishida, Y., Jacquin-Joly, E., and Leal, W. S. (2004). Pheromone anosmia in a scarab beetle induced by in vivo inhibition of a pheromone-degrading enzyme. *Proc. Natl. Acad. Sci. USA* **101,** 11459–11464.

Meunier, N., Ferveur, J. F., and Marion-Poll, F. (2000). Sex-specific non-pheromonal taste receptors in *Drosophila. Curr. Biol.* **10,** 1583–1586.

Meunier, N., Marion-Poll, F., Lansky, P., and Rospars, J. P. (2003a). Estimation of the individual firing frequencies of two neurons recorded with a single electrode. *Chem. Senses* **28,** 671–679.

Meunier, N., Marion-Poll, F., Rospars, J. P., and Tanimura, T. (2003b). Peripheral coding of bitter taste in *Drosophila. J. Neurobiol.* **56,** 139–152.

Park, S. K., Shanbhag, S. R., Wang, Q., Hasan, G., Steinbrecht, R. A., and Pikielny, C. W. (2000). Expression patterns of two putative odorant-binding proteins in the olfactory organs of *Drosophila melanogaster* have different implications for their functions. *Cell Tissue Res.* **300,** 181–192.

Park, S. K., Mann, K. J., Lin, H., Starostina, E., Kolski-Andreaco, A., and Pikielny, C. W. (2006). A *Drosophila* protein specific to pheromone-sensing gustatory hairs delays males' copulation attempts. *Curr. Biol.* **16,** 1154–1159.

Pelosi, P., Zhou, J. J., Ban, L. P., and Calvello, M. (2006). Soluble proteins in insect chemical communication. *Cell. Mol. Life Sci.* **63,** 1658–1676.

Pevsner, J., and Snyder, S. H. (1990). Odorant-binding protein: Odorant transport function in the vertebrate nasal epithelium. *Chem. Senses* **15,** 217–222.

Possidente, D. R., and Murphey, R. K. (1989). Genetic control of sexually dimorphic axon morphology in *Drosophila* sensory neurons. *Dev. Biol.* **132,** 448–457.

Savarit, F., Sureau, G., Cobb, M., and Ferveur, J.-F. (1999). Genetic Elimination of known pheromones reveals the fundamental basis of mating and isolation in *Drosophila. Proc. Nat. Acad. Sci. USA* **96,** 9015–9020.

Shanbhag, S. R., Park, S. K., Pikielny, C. W., and Steinbrecht, R. A. (2001). Gustatory organs of *Drosophila melanogaster*: Fine structure and expression of the putative odorant-binding protein PBPRP2. *Cell Tissue Res.* **304,** 423–437.

Starostina, E. Xu, A., Lin, H., and Pikielny, C. W. (2009). A *Drosophila* protein family implicated in pheromone perception is related to Tay-Sachs GM2-activator protein. *J. Biol. Chem.* **284,** 585–594.

Stockinger, P., Kvitsiani, D., Rotkopf, S., Tirian, L., and Dickson, B. J. (2005). Neural circuitry that governs *Drosophila* male courtship behavior. *Cell* **121,** 795–807

Stowers, L., and Logan, D. W. (2008). LUSH shapes up for a starring role in olfaction. *Cell* **133,** 1137–1139.

Suzuki, M., Tanaka, Y., Korematsu, S., Mikami, B., and Minato, N. (2005). Crystal structure and some properties of a major house dust mite allergen, Derf 2. *Biochem. Biophys. Res. Commun.* **339,** 679–686.

Touhara, K. (2008). Sexual communication via peptide and protein pheromones. *Curr. Opin. Pharmacol.*

Touhara, K., and Vosshall, L. B. (2009). Sensing odorants and pheromones with chemosensory receptors. *Annu. Rev. Physiol.* **71,** 307–332.

van der Goes van Naters, W., and Carlson, J. R. (2007). Receptors and neurons for fly odors in *Drosophila*. *Curr Biol.* **17,** 606–612.

Villella, A., and Hall, J. C. (2008). Neurogenetics of courtship and mating in *Drosophila*. *Adv. Genet.* **62,** 67–184.

Vosshall, L. B. (2008). Scent of a fly. *Neuron* **59,** 685–689.

Vosshall, L. B., and Stocker, R. F. (2007). Molecular architecture of smell and taste in *Drosophila. Annu. Rev. Neurosci.* **30,** 505–533.

Wicker-Thomas, C. (2007). Pheromonal communication involved in courtship behavior in Diptera. *J. Insect Physiol.* **53,** 1089–1100.

Witjes, S., and Eltz, T. (2009). Hydrocarbon footprints as a record of bumblebee flower visitation. *J. Chem. Ecol.*

Wright, C. S., Li, S. C., and Rastinejad, F. (2000). Crystal structure of human GM2-activator protein with a novel beta-cup topology. *J. Mol. Biol.* **304,** 411–422.

Wright, C. S., Zhao, Q., and Rastinejad, F. (2003). Structural analysis of lipid complexes of GM2-activator protein. *J. Mol. Biol.* **331,** 951–964.

Wright, C. S., Mi, L. Z., and Rastinejad, F. (2004). Evidence for lipid packaging in the crystal structure of the GM2-activator complex with platelet activating factor. *J. Mol. Biol.* **342,** 585–592.

Wright, C. S., Mi, L. Z., Lee, S., and Rastinejad, F. (2005). Crystal structure analysis of phosphatidylcholine-GM2-activator product complexes: Evidence for hydrolase activity. *Biochemistry* **44,** 13510–13521.

Xu, A., Park, S. K., D'Mello, S., Kim, E., Wang, Q., and Pikielny, C. W. (2002). Novel genes expressed in subsets of chemosensory sensilla on the front legs of male *Drosophila melanogaster*. *Cell Tissue Res.* **307,** 381–392.

Xu, P., Atkinson, R., Jones, D. N., and Smith, D. P. (2005). *Drosophila* OBP LUSH is required for activity of pheromone-sensitive neurons. *Neuron* **45,** 193–200.

CHAPTER TWELVE

Volatile Signals during Pregnancy

Stefano Vaglio

Contents

Abstract

Scents play a key role in mediating reproductive interactions in many vertebrates including mammals. Nowadays, several studies indicate that humans seem to use remarkably olfactory communication and are even able to produce and perceive pheromones. Furthermore, over the past several years, it became increasingly clear that pheromone-like chemical signals probably play a role in offspring identification and mother recognition. Recently developed technical procedures (solid-phase microextraction and dynamic headspace extraction) now allow investigators to characterize volatile compounds with high reliability. We analyzed the volatile compounds in sweat patch samples collected from the para-axillary and nipple–areola regions of women during pregnancy and after childbirth. We hypothesized that, at the time of birth and during the first weeks of life, the distinctive olfactory pattern of the para-axillary area is probably useful to newborn babies for recognizing and distinguishing their own mother, whereas the characteristic pattern of the nipple–areola region is probably useful as a guide to nourishment.

Laboratory of Anthropology, Department of Evolutionary Biology "Leo Pardi," University of Florence, Florence, Italy

Vitamins and Hormones, Volume 83
ISSN 0083-6729, DOI: 10.1016/S0083-6729(10)83012-2

I. Introduction

Scents play a significant role in mediating sexual behavior in many vertebrates, both in the recognition of opposite sex conspecifics and in assessing the suitability of different individuals as potential mates (Hurst, 2009). Moreover, in most mammalian species smell plays a fundamental role in response to chemical messengers related to different behaviors (Beauchamp *et al.*, 1976).

Within the overall olfactory communication, the so-called "individual odors", learned for recognition, do not seem to fit Karlson and Lüscher's definition of "pheromones" (Karlson and Lüscher, 1959). After years of debate, it seems clear that these variable odors are not pheromones whereas they are better referred to as "signature odors." But species-specific small molecules, which fit the classic pheromone definition, have now been identified for mammals. It appears clear that signature odors and pheromones can be mixed for effect (i.e., some mammals—including elephants and mice—present their small-molecule pheromones in the cleft of highly variable lipocalin proteins). Furthermore, pheromone signals can also be overlaid and improved with individual signature odors (Wyatt, 2009).

The importance of pheromones in intraspecies communication has long been known in insects, but several studies suggest that pheromones play an important role also in mammalian social behavior and, thus, in primates as well (Grammer *et al.*, 2005). Indeed pheromones affect reproductive behavior in many animal species: once released in the environment, through urine or glandular secretions, these volatile substances reach other individuals of the same species, signaling, for instance, mating availability and strengthening ties between mother and offspring, as well as regulating social relationships (Vaglio *et al.*, 2009).

In the past, the importance of human sense of smell has been underestimated. On the contrary, nowadays, several studies indicate that humans seem to use olfactory communication and are even able to produce and perceive certain pheromones which may play an important role in the behavioral and reproduction biology of humans (Hurst, 2009).

Actually in humans, the olfaction is a sensory modality of singular importance for the fine adjustment of early mother–infant interaction. While the precise role of maternal olfaction varies from one species to another, olfactory cues are in fact used in various aspects of parental care (Lévy *et al.*, 2004). Undoubtedly, infantile odors become strong stimuli allowing the normal development of maternal care and, moreover, provide a basis for individual recognition of the offspring in some species. Recognizable olfactory signatures reflect the product of particular genotype and, probably, are also influenced by the environment. Highly specialized neural mechanisms for processing of the infant signals have been developed. While there is no functional specificity of either the main or the accessory olfactory systems in the onset of maternal behavior among species, only the main olfactory system is implicated when individual odor discrimination of the young is required (Lévy and Keller, 2009).

It can be considered that the putative human pheromones are steroids present in the secretions of exocrine glands (Grammer *et al.*, 2005; Grosser *et al.*, 2000; Hauser *et al.*, 2005; Pause, 2004; Stern and Mc Clintock, 1998; Taylor, 1994). Estrogen derivatives are present in females (the so-called "copulins"—mixtures of aliphatic acids such as acetic, propionic, butyric, isovaleric, and isocaproic acid with estratetraenol), and androgen derivatives are present in males (androstenol, androstenone, and androstadienone). Furthermore, recent studies concerning the most volatile compounds of human sweat (Bernier *et al.*, 2000; Hauser *et al.*, 2005; Zeng *et al.*, 1991, 1996) have shown that the characteristic odor produced by the para-axillary region is due to the presence of volatile C6–C11 acids, the most abundant being *E*-3-methyl-2-hexenoic acid (*E*-3M2H).

II. Mother Recognition

In animal species, recognition between individuals is an essential requirement for any kind of further interaction. Recognition between mother and newborn is a fundamental behavioral interaction that is worthy of systematic investigation. The emotional relationship between a mother and her newborn begins with mutual recognition, which starts during gestation and continues through birth, augmented by body contact and lactation. Imprinting takes place through visual, auditory, and olfactory learning, which occurs very early during the so-called "critical period". Consequently, from the beginning of pregnancy, olfaction seems to represent a sort of Ariadne's thread that permits the infant to find its mother after birth (Vaglio *et al.*, 2009).

For newborn mammals, the mother's nipple region is of singular importance because it is the only source of necessary nutrients. Throughout the evolutionary history of our species, human infants, like other young mammals, have been entirely dependent upon milk delivered via the mother's nipples. Those babies who do not gain access to their mother's breasts, or who fail to suck adequately, would die shortly after birth. One would therefore expect that natural selection should have favored the evolution of mechanisms that make easy the establishment and maintenance of effective breast-feeding (Porter and Winberg, 1999).

It is now well established that the nutritional, immunological, and biochemical properties of breast milk promote health, growth, and development of the baby. Some of these factors may exert their influences only later in life. Furthermore, there are numerous claims of a positive association between breast-feeding and development of mother–infant bonding, as well as cognitive development (Atkinson *et al.*, 1990).

In addition to provide access to colostrums and milk, the nipple region is the source of chemical signals that appear to be uniquely salient for the newborn. Naturally occurring breast odors have been implicated in guiding the infant to the nipple, providing a basis for early individual recognition of the mother and influencing the behavioral state of the baby (Porter and Winberg, 1999).

A. Nonhuman mammals

Shortly after birth, young mammals have to locate, grasp, and begin to suck from a nipple of their mother. Thus, the nipple or breast is arguably the first "object" to which the newborn must direct appropriate behavioral responses in order to survive.

On this purpose, systematic studies have revealed that maternal odors play a critical role in eliciting nipple localization and sucking in the young of several species of mammals. For instance, in rat pups the initial nipple orientation is elicited by the odor of amniotic fluid and saliva that the mother spreads on her ventrum while grooming herself during birthing whereas, following the first successful feeding attempt, nipple localization and attachment are mediated by the odor of saliva that the pups themselves had previously deposited on their mother while sucking (Blass and Teicher, 1980). In contrast with the stimuli which control sucking by newborn rats, the olfactory signal that rabbit pups rely on to locate the nipples is produced and emitted at the mother's ventrum and is also found in the milk (Hudson and Distel, 1983). Like neonatal rabbits, newborn piglets also orient to odors emanating from their mother's nipple region (Morrow-Tesch and McGlone, 1990). Nipple localization poses a unique challenge for marsupials. After a short gestation period, the newborn crawls without assistance to the mother's pouch where it attaches itself to a nipple (Eisenberg, 1981): the infant is believed to make its way to the pouch by following an "odor trail" left by the mother that licks herself during delivery (Sharman and Calaby, 1964). Aside from the maternal odors which guide offspring directly to the nipple, lactating rodents emit chemical signals that function to keep their pups in the vicinity of the nest (Porter and Ruttle, 1975; Randall and Campbell, 1976; Schapiro and Salas, 1970). Under natural conditions, heightened ambulation in the absence of the maternal scent may facilitate pups relocation of the nest. Moreover, in several species of rodents, nursing mothers produce olfactory cues (so-called "maternal pheromones") which are uniquely attractive to their suckling young and elicit directional orientation to sites saturated with that odor (Breen and Leshner, 1977; Leon and Moltz, 1971; Porter *et al.*, 1978). On the other hand, a recent study about free-ranging domestic cats show that kittens respond from birth with efficient nipple-search behavior to inborn olfactory cues on the mother's ventrum and their emission is under hormonal control, but that kittens also quickly learn olfactory cues specific to their own mother and to their own particular nipples (Raihani *et al.*, 2009).

B. Humans

In humans, chemical cues from the breast region are particularly salient for newborn babies (Cernoch and Porter, 1985). Odors emanating from the breasts of lactating women appear to function as general attractants for babies, regardless of their feeding history and whether the source of the olfactory cues is the mother or an unfamiliar woman (Porter *et al.*, 1992).

Observations have documented the capability of human newborns to locate the nipple and initiate feeding without assistance (Widstrom *et al.*, 1987). Attractiveness of maternal breast odors in the biologically relevant context of breast-feeding is functionally analogous to the role of "nipple-search pheromone" in guiding young rabbits and piglets to the nipple. Although maternal odors may not be as critical for nipple localization in our own species, nonetheless they facilitate early breast-feeding attempts (Varendi *et al.*, 1997). In addition to helping to guide the infant directly to the nipple, maternal breast odors affect other aspects of neonatal behavior which increase the probability of successful nipple grasping and feeding (i.e., sucking movements and gross motor activity) (Russell, 1976).

Thus, maternal breast odors have been shown to elicit positive responses in newborn babies ranging in age from one hour to several weeks postpartum (Russell, 1976). Babies, including those who have had no prior breast-feeding experience, continue to be attracted to olfactory cues emanating from the breast of lactating females throughout the period of transition from colostrums to milk production. Moreover, each of these substances evokes directional head orientation by babies of the appropriate age (Marlier *et al.*, 1998).

The nipple/areola region is also supplied with a dense accumulation of skin glands which could contribute to the attractive chemical signal (Schaal and Porter, 1991; Stoddart, 1990). For example, ducts of sebaceous glands open directly on the tip of the nipple and are enlarged during lactation. Sebum production increases during the final trimester of pregnancy and remains elevated for several months after delivery in lactating mothers (Burton *et al.*, 1973). Likewise, the corpuscles of Montgomery located on the surface of the areola become more conspicuous during gestation and lactation. Excretions from these glands could themselves function as chemical signals or serve as odor fixatives that prolong the effectiveness of other attractive substances (Schaal and Porter, 1991; Stoddart, 1990). Diffusion of odor molecules may be enhanced by the relatively high surface temperature of the areola resulting from the rich supply of blood vessels in this region of the body (Mitz and Lalardrie, 1977).

Of course, natural secretions in addition to those already discussed might act as olfactory attractants for newborn babies. Maternal saliva has also been found to elicit investigative behavior in other mammalian species, including gerbils (Smith and Block, 1989), muck shrews (Stine and Dryden, 1977), and spiny mice (Porter *et al.*, 1990).

C. Fetal olfactory learning

Fetal olfactory learning has been documented in nonhuman mammals. For example, rat pups avoid odors which they had experienced in association with a noxious stimulus prior to birth (Smotherman, 1982). Aromatic substances in the mother's diet can taint the amniotic fluid and be detected by the fetus: young rats and rabbits whose mothers had eaten strongly flavored food while pregnant reacted more positively to these same dietary odors postnatally than did control pups (Hepper, 1988; Hudson and Altbacker, 1994). Data from experiments suggest that human fetuses might also be capable of perceiving odors and several authors have hypothesized that babies responsiveness to maternal breast odors may reflect exposure to similar cues prior to birth (i.e., continuity between the fetal olfactory environment and odors emitted in the nipple–areola region) (Schaal *et al.*, 1995; Varendi *et al.*, 1997).

Concerning humans, in support of the fetal olfactory learning hypothesis, newborn infants display clear behavioral attraction to the odor of amniotic fluid (Varendi *et al.*, 1996). Arguably, newborns are initially attracted to their own amniotic fluid because that odor is familiar (i.e., maintenance of a memory trace of their fetal olfactory environment). Moreover, while exposure to amniotic fluid is quickly eliminated after birth, breast-fed babies continue to have recurring close contact with cues emanating from the mother's nipple–areola region. Therefore, breast odors become increasingly familiar and attractive whereas amniotic fluid odor loses its positive hedonic value (Porter and Winberg, 1999).

Gas chromatography/mass spectrometry (GC-MS) analyses have identified similarities in the chemical profiles of volatile compounds from samples of human breast milk (collected 30 days postpartum) and amniotic fluid (Stafford and Horning, 1976). The overlapping odors of amniotic fluid and breast milk may account at least partially for newborn babies attraction to maternal breast odors. In effect, the odor of breast secretions may have a positive hedonic value because of its discernible resemblance to the "familiar" amniotic fluid odor. Despite such presumed similarity between amniotic fluid and breast odors, the scents are not functionally identical as evidenced by discriminative reactivity of babies to them (Varendi *et al.*, 1996, 1997).

III. Mother–Infant Interactions

Human chemical signals may also play a role in offspring identification. Odor cues from newborns are absolutely salient to their mothers (Kaitz *et al.*, 1987). Mothers are able to distinguish the odor of their own newborn baby from that of other newborns (Schaal *et al.*, 1980). Experiments also have demonstrated that adults can even recognize gender and individuality of nonrelated children (Chiarelli, 2001). Thus, body odors can provide humans with important information about the individual identity of their offspring (Doty, 1981; Olsson *et al.*, 2006; Porter and Moore, 1981; Porter *et al.*, 1983, 1985; Russell *et al.*, 1983).

On the other hand, children usually prefer parts of clothes which were in contact with the axilla and worn by their own mothers rather than clothes worn by other mothers (Schaal *et al.*, 1980). Therefore, as discussed above, chemical signals seem to have a fundamental role in the mechanism of mother–child identification (Porter *et al.*, 1983). Breast-feed versus bottle-feed infants show different reactions to maternal odors. Breast-feed infants are exposed to salient maternal odors and rapidly become familiarized with their mothers unique olfactory signature (Cernoch and Porter, 1985). Apparently, orientation to lactating-breast odors is an inborn adaptive response of newborns (Porter *et al.*, 1991).

Thus, it definitely seems an unavoidable conclusion that naturally occurring odors play an important role in mediating infant behavior (Vaglio, 2009).

A. Sociobiological remarks

As any other organism, humans are subject to invisible but potentially irresistible influences of metabolic materials on our muscle, motive and motor actions, both directly and indirectly (Morowitz, 2008; Srinivasan *et al.*, 2008). Obviously, mutual recognition among organisms is related to many aspects of the personal profile, both of metabolic-material biological similarity and morphologic-motor ecological familiarity (Lyon, 2006).

Mothers recognize the sounds of their own babies chortles and cries and may differentiate among their causes, from tiredness to hunger, from pain to scare. Yet mothers may pause for a moment to listen to cries from an unseen child which are similar enough to their own babies cries to require more attention before discounting and dismissing it as indeed being someone else's baby (Leavitt, 1998). Yet it is appreciated that the cry from any newborn can cause agitation and distress in any mother. Perhaps, this reflects the process of acquiring maternal memories: that is, at the time a mother has a newborn, she does not yet know her babies cry well enough to discriminate with certainty. Moreover, mothers of newborns are in states of hormonally heightened metabolic arousal and are thus readily responsive to both biologically and ecologically conditioned cues (Bath, 2000).

Immediacy of recognition of a simple similar-enough sound in a noisy place, such as a familiar name, is well enough known (the so-called "cocktail party syndrome"), even if that name was not in fact said, and so what was heard was only "similar enough" to seem "familiar enough." The connection among all aspects of recognition is surely not a set of discrete "signals" but, instead, a composition of several sorts of similarities and familiarities, including biochemical features. Probably these features serve to substantiate and sustain mutual recognition (Lier, 1988).

B. Functional significance of precocious olfactory interaction

Insights into the advantages of olfactory mediated early recognition of the mother, with respect to other sensory modalities, arise when one considers the ecology and natural history of our species. The reliance of infants on milk obtained by sucking at the mother's breast assures that they will have prolonged periods of exposure to the characteristic maternal odor beginning almost immediately after birth. Furthermore, the mother's olfactory signature will be experienced in conjunction with a combination of reinforcing stimuli (i.e., food, warmth, and tactile stimulation) which should further enhance learning of that chemical cue (Porter and Winberg, 1999).

Recognition of the mother's voice also develops very early (DeCasper and Fifer, 1980). There is evidence indicating that familiarization with the mother's voice may actually begin prior to birth (Fleming *et al.*, 1993), which could explain why young infants show plain indications that they recognize the voice of their mother but not those one of their father (DeCasper and Prescott, 1984). Mother's visual-facial features can likewise be used as a basis for early individual recognition (Bushnell *et al.*, 1989). Since the maternal odor signature is constantly emitted at the skin surface, olfactory recognition—in contrast with individual recognition mediated by vocal or visual cues—may occur regardless of lighting conditions or mother's clear behavioral state, providing that mother and infant are in close contact (Porter and Winberg, 1999).

Individual recognition is a necessary precursor for the development of an enduring social attachment. Olfactory recognition of the mother may play an important role in the initiation of the newborn's attachment to her; beginning shortly after birth, mothers and infants engage in a series of subtle reciprocal interactions, and mothers appear to be very sensitive to signals emitted by their baby (Lewis and Rosenblum, 1974). By conveying the impression that the mother can be distinguished from other individuals, infants may be able to exert some influence over her (Maurer and Salapatek, 1976; Robson and Moss, 1970).

C. Olfaction and maternal behavior

Olfactory cues have also been implicated as important mediating factors in the elicitation and maintenance of maternal behavior among terrestrial mammalian species. Several studies on domestic sheep (Lévy and Poindron, 1987; Lévy *et al.*, 1983) show the involved effects of odors associated with newborn young on the behavior of recently parturient mothers.

Human mothers, like recently parturient ewes, are capable of recognizing their offspring's characteristic odor shortly after birth (Porter *et al.*, 1983; Schaal *et al.*, 1980). An extended period of familiarization with the newborn is not necessary for mothers to develop the ability to recognize its odor (Kaitz *et al.*, 1987; Porter *et al.*, 1983; Russell *et al.*, 1983). Such early olfactory recognition of babies may be the result of rapid learning. Alternatively, because close genetic kin shares similar body odors (Hepper, 1988; Porter *et al.*, 1985), the mothers may have detected a resemblance between their newborn baby's scent and that one of other family members.

IV. Chemical Profile of Volatile Compounds During Pregnancy

In our recent study (Vaglio *et al.*, 2009), we hypothesized that women probably develop a volatile profile, through pregnancy and childbirth that enables identification of the mother by the newborn. The aim was to understand, through an analytical approach, how the volatile pattern of pregnant women changes during pregnancy and, consequently, to verify the effective role played by volatile chemical signals in the mechanism of mother–infant recognition.

We analyzed the chemical content of volatiles from sweat patch samples from the para-axillary and nipple–areola regions of women during pregnancy and after childbirth. Solid-phase microextraction (SPME) was used to extract the volatile compounds, which were then characterized and quantified by GC–MS (Fig. 12.1).

Results showed that during pregnancy women developed a distinctive pattern of five volatile compounds qualitatively common to the para-axillary and nipple–areola regions (1-dodecanol, 1-1′-oxybis octane, isocurcumenol, α-hexyl-cinnamic aldehyde, and isopropyl myristate) (Fig. 12.2).

Hypothetically, the differentiation of the olfactory pattern among pregnant women helps newborns to recognize their own mother and distinguish her from other individuals. At the time of birth and during the first weeks of life, the distinctive olfactory pattern of the para-axillary area might be useful to newborns to recognize and distinguish their mother, whereas the characteristic pattern of the nipple–areola region is probably useful as a guide to nourishment.

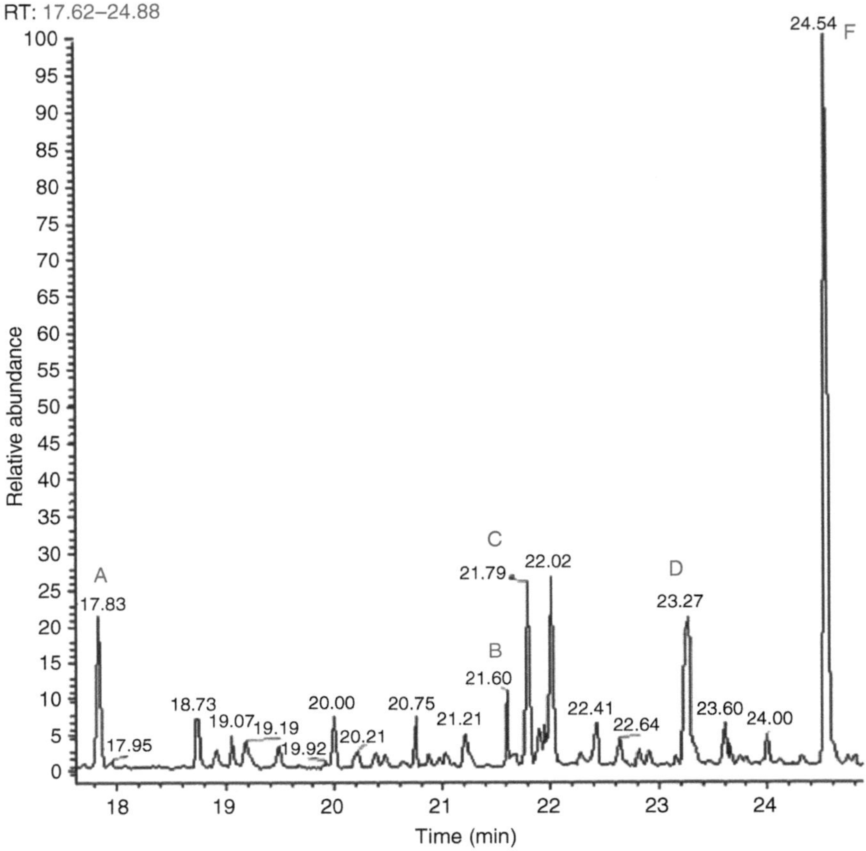

Figure 12.1 TIC profile of a nipple–areola sample during pregnancy. The range corresponds to the elution of the five frequently occurring compounds [(A) 1-dodecanol, RT 17.83 min; (B) 1-1′-oxybis octane, RT 21.60 min; (C) isocurcumenol, RT 21.79 min; (D) α-hexyl-cinnamic aldehyde, RT 23.27 min; (E) isopropyl myristate, RT 24.54 min]. It has been focused on the period between RT 17.60 min and 25.00 min that has been normalized. The unlabeled peaks are due to compounds present also in nonpregnant and nonlactating control or not common to all other samples. RT correspond to the following experimental conditions: the GC was equipped with a fused silica HP 5-MS capillary column (30 m × 0.25 mm crossbonded 5% phenyl–95% dimethylpolysiloxane, film thickness 0.50 μm); the injector and transfer line temperatures were maintained at 220°C and 250°C, respectively; injections were made in splitless mode with a constant flow of helium carrier gas of 1.1 ml/min; the oven temperature program, started at 40°C, was held for 3 min and then raised by 10°C/min to 100°C and in a second step by 5°C/min to the final temperature of 250°C.

V. Conclusions and Future Directions

In humans, as in other mammals, naturally occurring odors play an important role in the coordination of reciprocal mother–infant interactions

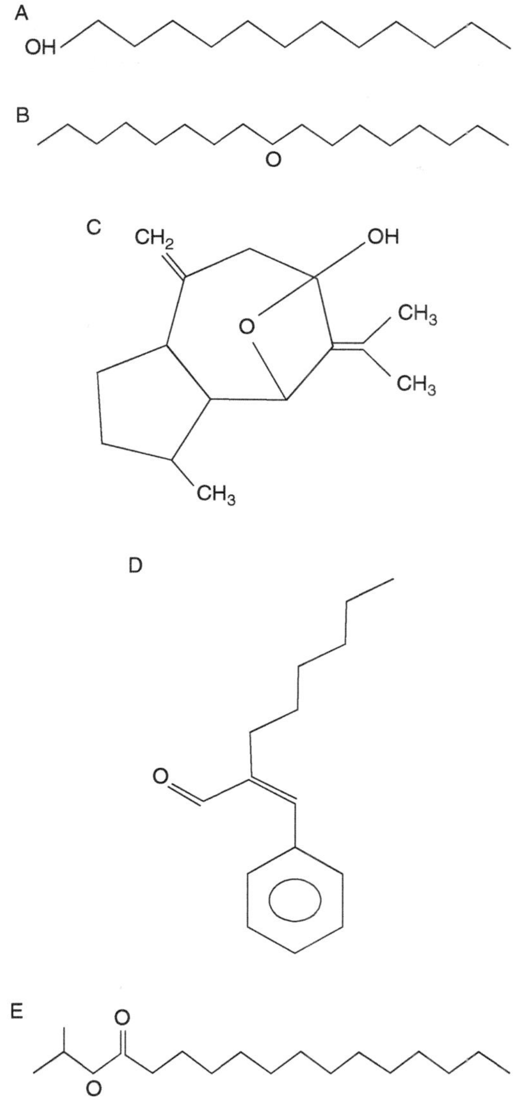

Figure 12.2 The five volatile compounds identified in sweat patch samples collected from the para-axillary and nipple–areola regions of women during pregnancy: (A) 1-dodecanol; (B) 1-1′-oxybis octane; (C) isocurcumenol; (D) α-hexyl-cinnamic aldehyde; and (E) isopropyl myristate.

during the early postpartum period. It is tentatively concluded that the olfactory cues emanating from the breasts of lactating mothers uniquely influence the behavior of newborn infants (Porter and Winberg, 1999).

Infants directional orientation to lactating females breast odors is clearly adaptive in that it helps them gain access to the nipple and thereby facilitates the intake of nutrients. The mother also benefits from this communication system, at least in a reproductive/genetic sense, since it contributes to the growth and survival of her offspring. On average, infants born of mothers who emit attractive breast odors should more readily establish effective feeding patterns than would establish the infants whose mothers fail to produce such chemical signals. Natural selection hence should favor the infants in the former category. Neonatal attraction to their nursing mother's breast odors therefore reflects the evolutionary history of our species as well as the prenatal/postnatal experience of individual infants (Porter and Winberg, 1999).

However, the nature of mother–infant interactions during breast-feeding and its preludes are still incompletely known. Since olfaction has been demonstrated to play a role in infants' sucking behavior, while its influence on maternal behavior in our species is not understood, it would be worthwhile to study this sensory modality in more detail.

The qualification of maternal breast odors as "pheromones" is just a semantic question (Beauchamp *et al.*, 1976). Anyhow, chemical signals originating from nursing mothers' nipple/areola region represent one of the best examples described to date of an olfactory cue that elicits specific behavioral responses in our species (i.e., facial orientation, rooting, and sucking activity by newborns).

The role of such attractive maternal odors in the mediation of early breast-feeding behavior by human infants appears to be similar to that of nipple-search pheromone as described in nonhuman mammals. In each instance, newborn babies overt reactivity to maternal breast odors contributes to successful nipple localization and milk ingestion. Thus, breast odors carry two functionally distinct categories of chemical signals: general attractants and individually olfactory signatures (Porter, 1991). As seen above, mothers can also be recognized by their axillary odors, which demonstrates that their olfactory signature is not localized solely in the breast region. It is likely, however, that babies first become acquainted with their mother's characteristic scent when sucking at her breast. Rapid learning of that salient phenotypic feature is triggered by neurophysiological and neurochemical activity occurring during the perinatal period.

So, thanks to several evidences, since many years it has been clear that the odor signals permit a correct development of mother–infant bond as well as cause the recognition of the mother by the infant at the time of birth. Consequently, it is reasonable to hypothesize that pregnant women develop a sort of specific odor profile during the overall period of pregnancy in order to be identified by the child after the birth. For this reason, it is very important to investigate, through analytical methods, the change of the profile of volatile compounds emitted by the skin of the pregnant women in the para-axillary and nipple–areola regions.

On this purpose, recent results show the effectiveness of the methodology used (Vaglio, 2009). Through the collection and analysis of the secretion released at the level of the para-axillary area and in the nipple areola region, it is possible to investigate the volatile compounds in a proper way. Up to now, these phenomena have often been investigated with inadequate methodologies and, as a consequence, the role of volatile compounds as regulators of mother–infant recognition has been underestimated. Moreover, recently developed technical instruments and procedures—as SPME, dynamic headspace extraction (DHS), and Maldi TOF/TOF—in addition to the classic ones—as GC–MS and liquid chromatography–mass spectrometry (LC–MS)—now allow investigators to characterize volatile and nonvolatile compounds with high reliability (Curran *et al.*, 2005).

Obviously, the study of the mechanism of mother–infant recognition is important not only for the acquisition of new knowledge concerning the emission of signal molecules essential for mother–child identification but also for its clear practical consequences. Indeed this information can be helpful for setting up the proper conditions to establish solid mother–child bonding. It can indicate the behavior during gestation and the initiation period of life of the newborn. Therefore, an understanding of the mechanisms of newborns recognition of their mother could have practical health implications (Vaglio, 2009).

ACKNOWLEDGMENTS

I thank the women who kindly participated in the research on which this material is based. I am deeply indebted to Susanna Pollastri for her editorial work on the chapter. Moreover, I would like to thank Leaf Lovejoy for useful suggestions. I also thank Professor Brunetto Chiarelli and Professor Giorgio Mello for their encouragement.

REFERENCES

Atkinson, S. A., Hanson, L. A., and Chandra, R. K. (1990). Human Lactation 4: Breastfeeding, Nutrition, Infection and Infant Growth in Developed and Emerging Countries Memorial University of Newfoundland, Arts Biomedical Publisher, St. John's, Terranova.

Bath, R. (2000). "Reading-your-baby lesson" for parents of excessively crying infants: The concept of "guided parent–infant training sessions". *Prax. Kinderpsychol. Kinderpsychiatr.* **49**(8), 537–549.

Beauchamp, G. K., Doty, R. L., Moulton, D. G., and Mugford, R. A. (1976). The pheromone concept in mammalian chemical communication: A brief critique. *In* "Mammalian Olfaction, Reproductive Processes and Behavior," (R. Doty, Ed.), pp. 143–160. Academic Press, New York, NY.

Bernier, U. R., Kline, D. L., Barnard, D. R., Schreck, C. E., and Yost, R. A. (2000). Analysis of human skin emanations by gas chromatography/mass spectrometry. *Anal. Chem.* **72**, 747–756.

Blass, E. M., and Teicher, M. H. (1980). First suckling response of the newborn albino rat: The roles of olfaction and amniotic fluid. *Science* **210,** 15–22.

Breen, M. F., and Leshner, A. I. (1977). Maternal pheromone: A demonstration of its existence in the mouse (*Mus musculus*). *Physiol. Behav.* **18,** 527–529.

Burton, J. L., Shuster, S., Cartlidge, M., Libman, L. J., and Martell, U. (1973). Lactation, sebum excretion and melanocyte-stimulating hormone. *Nature* **243,** 349–350.

Bushnell, I. W. R., Sai, F., and Mullin, J. T. (1989). Neonatal recognition of the mother's face. *Br. J. Dev. Psychol.* **7,** 3–15.

Cernoch, J. M., and Porter, R. H. (1985). Recognition of maternal axillary odors by infants. *Child Dev.* **56,** 1593–1598.

Chiarelli, B. (2001). Pheromonal communication and socialization. *In* "Evolutionary Anatomy of the Primate Cerebral Cortex," (D. Falk and K. R. Gibson, Eds.), pp. 165–176. Cambridge University Press, Cambridge, UK.

Curran, A. M., Rabin, S. I., Prada, P. A., and Furton, K. G. (2005). Comparison of the volatile organic compounds present in human odor using SPME-GC/MS. *J. Chem. Ecol.* **31,** 1607–1619.

DeCasper, A. J., and Fifer, W. P. (1980). Of human bonding: Newborns prefer their mothers' voices. *Science* **208,** 1174–1176.

DeCasper, A. J., and Prescott, P. A. (1984). Human newborns' perception of male voices: Preference, discrimination, and reinforcing value. *Dev. Psychobiol.* **17,** 481–491.

Doty, R. L. (1981). Olfactory communication in humans. *Chem. Senses* **6,** 351–376.

Eisenberg, J. F. (1981). The Mammalian Radiations. University of Chicago Press, Chicago, IL.

Fleming, A. S., Corter, C., Franks, P., Surbey, M., Schneider, B., and Steiner, M. (1993). Postpartum factors related to mother's attraction to newborn infant odors. *Dev. Psychobiol.* **26,** 115–132.

Grammer, K., Fink, B., and Neave, N. (2005). Human pheromones and sexual attraction. *Eur. J. Obstet. Gynecol. Reprod. Biol.* **118,** 135–142.

Grosser, B. I., Monti-Block, L., Jenings-White, C., and Berliner, D. L. (2000). Behavioral and electrophysiological effects of androstadienone. *Psychoneuroendocrinology* **25,** 289–299.

Hauser, R., Wiergowski, M., Gos, T., Marczak, M., Karaszewski, B., and Wodniak-Ochocinska, L. (2005). Alarm pheromones as an exponent of emotional state shortly before death. Science fiction or a new challenge? *Forensic Sci. Int.* **155,** 226–230.

Hepper, P. G. (1988). Adaptive fetal learning: Prenatal exposure to garlic affects postnatal preferences. *Anim. Behav.* **36,** 935–936.

Hudson, R., and Altbacker, V. (1994). Development of feeding and food preference in the European rabbit: Environmental and maturational determinants. *In* "Behavioral Aspects of Feeding," (B. G. Galef Jr., M. Mainardi, and P. Valsecchi, Eds.), pp. 125–145. Harwood, Chur, CH.

Hudson, R., and Distel, H. (1983). Nipple location by newborn rabbits: Behavioural evidence for pheromonal guidance. *Behaviour* **85,** 260–275.

Hurst, J. L. (2009). Female recognition and assessment of males through scent. *Behav. Brain Res.* **200**(2), 295–303.

Kaitz, M., Good, A., Rokem, A. M., and Eidelman, A. I. (1987). Mothers' recognition of their newborns by olfactory cues. *Dev. Psychobiol.* **20,** 587–591.

Karlson, P., and Lüscher, M. (1959). Pheromones: A new term for a class of biologically active substances. *Nature* **183,** 55–56.

Leavitt, L. A. (1998). Mothers' sensitivity to infant signals. *Pediatrics* **102**(5 Suppl. E), 1247–1249.

Leon, M., and Moltz, H. (1971). Maternal pheromone: Discrimination by pre-weanling albino rats. *Physiol. Behav.* **7,** 265–267.

Lévy, F., and Keller, M. (2009). Olfactory mediation of maternal behavior in selected mammalian species. *Behav. Brain Res.* **200**(2), 336–345.

Lévy, F., and Poindron, P. (1987). The importance of amniotic fluids for the establishment of maternal behaviour in experienced and inexperienced ewes. *Anim. Behav.* **35,** 1188–1192.
Lévy, F., Poindron, P., and Le Neindre, P. (1983). Attraction and repulsion by amniotic fluid and their olfactory control in the ewe around parturition. *Physiol. Behav.* **31,** 687–692.
Lévy, F., Keller, M., and Poindron, P. (2004). Olfactory regulation of maternal behavior in mammals. *Horm. Behav.* **46,** 284–302.
Lewis, M., and Rosenblum, L. A. (1974). The Effect of the Infant on its Caregiver. Wiley, New York, NY.
Lier, L. (1988). Mother–infant relationship in the first year of life. *Acta Paediatr. Scand.* **344,** 31–42.
Lyon, P. (2005). The biogenic approach to cognition. *Cogn. Process.* **7,** 11–29.
Marlier, L., Schaal, B., and Soussignan, R. (1998). Neonatal responsiveness to the odor of amniotic fluid and lacteal fluids: A test of perinatal chemosensory continuity. *Child Dev.* **69,** 611–623.
Maurer, D., and Salapatek, P. (1976). Developmental changes in the scanning of faces by young infants. *Child Dev.* **47,** 523–527.
Mitz, V., and Lalardrie, J. P. (1977). A propos de la vascularisation et de l'innervation sensitive du sein. *Senologia* **2,** 33–39.
Morowitz, H. J. (2008). Bacteriohopanetetrol and the sociology of science. *Complexity* **13** (5), 8–9.
Morrow-Tesch, J., and McGlone, J. J. (1990). Sensory systems and nipple attachment behavior in neonatal pigs. *Physiol. Behav.* **47,** 1–4.
Olsson, S. B., Barnard, J., and Turri, L. (2006). Olfaction and identification of unrelated individuals: Examination of the mysteries of human odor recognition. *J. Chem. Ecol.* **32,** 1635–1645.
Pause, B. M. (2004). Are androgen steroids acting as pheromones in humans? *Physiol. Behav.* **83,** 21–29.
Porter, R. H. (1991). Human reproduction and the mother–infant relationship: The role of odors. *In* "Smell and Taste in Health and Disease," (T. V. Getchell, R. L. Doty, L. M. Bartoshuk, and J. B. Snow Jr., Eds.), pp. 429–442. Raven Press, New York, NY.
Porter, R., and Moore, J. D. (1981). Human kin recognition by olfactory cues. *Physiol. Behav.* **27,** 493–495.
Porter, R. H., and Ruttle, K. (1975). The responses of one-day old *Acomys cahirinus* pups to naturally occurring chemical stimuli. *Z. Tierpsychol.* **38,** 154–162.
Porter, R. H., and Winberg, J. (1999). Unique salience of maternal breast odors for newborn infants. *Neurosci. Biobehav. Rev.* **23,** 439–449.
Porter, R. H., Doane, H. M., and Cavallaro, S. A. (1978). Temporal parameters of responsiveness to maternal pheromone in *Acomys cahirinus*. *Physiol. Behav.* **21,** 563–566.
Porter, R. H., Cernoch, J. M., and Mc Laughlin, F. J. (1983). Maternal recognition of neonates through olfactory cues. *Physiol. Behav.* **30,** 151–154.
Porter, R. H., Cernoch, J. M., and Baogh, R. D. (1985). Odour signatures and kin recognition. *Physiol. Behav.* **34,** 445–448.
Porter, R. H., McFadyen-Ketchum, S., and King, G. A. (1990). The influence of maternal labels on dietary preferences of spiny mouse weanlings. *Physiol. Behav.* **48,** 103–106.
Porter, R. H., Makin, J. W., Davis, L. D., and Christensen, K. M. (1991). An assessment of the salient olfactory environment of formula-fed infants. *Physiol. Behav.* **50**(5), 907–911.
Porter, R. H., Makin, J. W., Davis, L. B., and Christensen, K. M. (1992). Breast-fed infants respond to olfactory cues from their own mother and unfamiliar lactating females. *Infant Behav. Dev.* **15,** 85–93.
Raihani, G., Gonzàlez, D., Arteaga, L., and Hudson, R. (2009). Olfactory guidance of nipple attachment and suckling in kittens of the domestic cat: Inborn and learned responses. *Dev. Psychobiol.* **51**(8), 662–671.

Randall, P. K., and Campbell, B. A. (1976). Ontogeny of behavioral arousal in rats: Effect of maternal and sibling presence. *J. Comp. Physiol. Psychol.* **90,** 453–459.

Robson, K. S., and Moss, H. A. (1970). Patterns and determinants of maternal attachment. *J. Pediatr.* **77,** 976–985.

Russell, M. J. (1976). Human olfactory communication. *Nature* **260,** 520–522.

Russell, M. J., Mendelsson, T., and Peeke, H. (1983). Mother's identification of their infant's odors. *Ethol. Sociobiol.* **4,** 29–31.

Schaal, B., and Porter, R. H. (1991). "Microsmatic humans" revisited: The generation and perception of chemical signals. *In* Advances in the Study of Behavior, Vol. 20 pp. 135–199. Academic Press, New York, NY.

Schaal, B., Motagner, H., Hertling, E., Bolzoni, D., Moyse, R., and Quinchon, R. (1980). Les stimulations olfactives dans les relations entre l'enfant et la mere. *Reprod. Nutr. Dev.* **20,** 843–858.

Schaal, B., Marlier, L., and Soussignan, R. (1995). Responsiveness to the odour of amniotic fluid in the human neonate. *Biol. Neonate* **67,** 397–406.

Schapiro, S., and Salas, M. (1970). Behavioral response of infant rats to maternal odor. *Physiol. Behav.* **5,** 815–817.

Sharman, G., and Calaby, J. H. (1964). Reproductive behavior in the red kangaroo, *Megaleia rufa*, in captivity. *CSIRO Wildlife Res.* **9,** 58–85.

Smith, B. A., and Block, M. L. (1989). Preference of Mongolian gerbils for salivary cues: A developmental analysis. *Anim. Behav.* **39,** 512–521.

Smotherman, W. P. (1982). Odor aversion learning by the rat fetus. *Physiol. Behav.* **29,** 769–771.

Srinivasan, V., Morowitz, H. J., and Smith, E. (2008). Essential amino acids, from LUCA to LUCY. *Complexity* **13**(4), 8–9.

Stafford, M., and Horning, M. G. (1976). Profiles of volatile metabolites in body fluids. *J. Chromatogr.* **126,** 495–502.

Stern, K., and Mc Clintock, M. K. (1998). Regulation of ovulation by human pheromones. *Nature* **392,** 177–179.

Stine, C. J., and Dryden, G. L. (1977). Lip-licking behavior in captive musk shrews, *Suncus murinus*. *Behaviour* **62,** 298–313.

Stoddart, D. M. (1990). The Scented Ape. Cambridge University Press, Cambridge, UK.

Taylor, R. (1994). Brave new nose: Sniffing out human sexual chemistry. *J. Natl. Inst. Health Res.* **6,** 47–51.

Vaglio, S. (2009). Chemical communication and mother–infant recognition. *Comm. Integr. Biol.* **2**(3), 279–281.

Vaglio, S., Minicozzi, P., Bonometti, E., Mello, G., and Chiarelli, B. (2009). Volatile signals during pregnancy: A possible chemical basis for mother–infant recognition. *J. Chem. Ecol.* **35**(1), 131–139.

Varendi, H., Porter, R. H., and Winberg, J. (1996). Attractiveness of amniotic fluid odor: Evidence of prenatal olfactory learning. *Acta Paediatr.* **85,** 1223–1227.

Varendi, H., Porter, R. H., and Winberg, J. (1997). Natural odor preferences of newborns change over time. *Acta Paediatr.* **86,** 985–990.

Widstrom, A. M., Ransjo-Arvidson, A. B., Christensson, K., Matthiesen, A. S., Winberg, J., and Uvnas-Moberg, K. (1987). Gastric suction in healthy newborn infants. *Acta Paediatr. Scand.* **76,** 566–572.

Wyatt, T. D. (2009). Fifty years of pheromones. *Nature* **457,** 262–263.

Zeng, X. N., Leyden, J. J., Lawley, H. J., Sawano, K., Nohara, I., and Preti, G. (1991). Analysis of characteristic odors from human male axillae. *J. Chem. Ecol.* **17**(7), 1469–1492.

Zeng, X. N., Leyden, J. J., Spielman, A. I., and Preti, G. (1996). Analysis of characteristic human female axillary odors: Qualitative comparison to males. *J. Chem. Ecol.* **22**(2), 237–257.

CHAPTER THIRTEEN

Olfactory Sensitivity: Functioning in Schizophrenia and Implications for Understanding the Nature and Progression of Psychosis

Warrick J. Brewer* *and* Christos Pantelis†

Contents

* ORYGEN Youth Health Research Centre, Centre for Youth Mental Health, University of Melbourne, Victoria, Australia

† Melbourne Neuropsychiatry Centre, Department of Psychiatry, University of Melbourne, Victoria, Australia

Vitamins and Hormones, Volume 83
ISSN 0083-6729, DOI: 10.1016/S0083-6729(10)83013-4

Abstract

Prefrontal neural processes maturing during neurodevelopment parallel normal improvement in higher order olfactory processing (identification) from childhood. Hence, disorders of adolescence such as schizophrenia that implicate prefrontal regions are associated with olfactory identification deficits in the presence of relatively intact lower order olfactory processing capacity (sensation) and mediating neural processes (limbic system). Understanding the linear neural trajectory of olfactory processing can assist in detecting the location, nature, and extent of early compromise of circuitry implicated in neurodevelopmental disorders such as psychosis. More recently, relatively discreet odorant sensitivity problems in schizophrenia have been described and these appear related to secretion of malodorous compounds. These findings have significant implications for future genetic prediction of this disorder.

I. Introduction: Overview

While substantial research implicates early neurodevelopmental compromise in schizophrenia, overt symptoms of psychosis do not typically manifest until late adolescence. Furthermore, the mechanisms responsible for delay in symptom onset are not yet understood though they likely involve discordance in typical maturational processes due to a dynamic interaction between an early neurological compromise and developmental changes (McGlashan and Hoffman, 2000). Evidence of aberrant neurodevelopment in psychosis emphasises the importance of understanding this disorder in relation to normal maturational processes. In this context, we have previously identified early olfactory identification deficits prior to psychosis onset, where it appears that greater degree of deficit is likely predictive no so much of making a transition to psychosis, but of attracting a more significant diagnosis of schizophrenia (Brewer *et al.*, 2003). We argue that further understanding the role of olfactory processing during neuro-developmental disorders such as schizophrenia can play an important role in increasing our knowledge of risk factors leading to illness onset and progression (Brewer *et al.*, 2006).

Olfactory processing follows a largely linear trajectory, conveniently paralleling normal developmental trajectories of neural maturation; hence lower order olfactory detection and conscious sensation involve inferior neural mechanisms (epithelial layer, olfactory bulb, and entorhinal [limbic] cortex) that are maturing early in childhood. Olfactory identification, which relies upon the integrity of lower order sensitivity, is mediated by superior-prefrontal regions that are the site of significant maturation processes from adolescence to early adulthood. Olfactory identification is essentially the capacity to place conscious language around lower order limbic-system (emotional) excitation. Our research confirms that higher order olfactory identification deficits implicating prefrontal neural compromise occur largely in the context of the relatively intact lower order neural mechanisms that mediate olfactory sensitivity in chronic schizophrenia and in first-episode psychosis (Brewer *et al.*, 2001, 2007). However, while the nature of olfactory deficits in schizophrenia is well validated, understanding of the role of sensitivity is less understood.

In this chapter, we briefly describe the neural structures mediating detection, sensitivity to, and identification of odors. We summarise the relevant literature describing the status of these olfactory processes in schizophrenia, where findings suggest that olfactory identification deficits in schizophrenia occur largely in the context of relatively intact acuity. We then focus on a review of olfactory sensitivity in this disorder. This discussion occurs in the context of considering the staggered maturational trajectories of these aspects of lower and higher order olfactory function (detection/sensitivity and identification) and we suggest further research directions for understanding the nature and extent of the deficits observed in early-onset neurodevelopmental disorders.

II. Structural Organisation of Olfactory Function

Odor perception begins with stimulation of olfactory mucosa neurons in the olfactory epithelium located in the superior nasal cavity (Greer, 1991). Axons from these primary receptor neurons then innervate the ipsilateral olfactory bulbs. Subsequently, axons from second-order cells project to the piriform cortex of the temporal lobe, the ventral striatum and also to limbic-system structures including the entorhinal cortex and ventromedial hypothalamus (Eslinger *et al.*, 1982). Secondary projections from the primary recipient areas connect to the amygdala, hippocampus, and to the orbitofrontal cortex (OFC) both directly and indirectly through the dorsomedial thalamus. The indirect pathway is thought to be involved in the conscious recognition that an odor is present (Qureshy *et al.*, 2000).

Olfactory information may arrive directly at the prefrontal cortex, bypassing the influence of the reticular formation in the thalamus. Thus, with only two synapses between olfactory receptors and secondary cortical and subcortical areas (Eslinger *et al.*, 1982), the olfactory system provides the most direct environmental access to several structures implicated in schizophrenia (Moberg *et al.*, 2006).

A. Olfactory functioning: Terminology

Olfactory acuity (sensitivity) is defined as the ability to detect an odor. Threshold, a measure of acuity, refers to the lowest concentration of an odorant that an individual can identify, and varies enormously from person to person (Amoore, 1970). Hyposmia refers to a diminished sense of smell, and anosmia is total loss of the sense of smell when acuity is impaired.

Olfactory identification refers to the ability to recognise and name a common odor when presented with an odorant. As the peripheral olfactory nervous system must be functioning for perception of odor, an individual may fail to accurately identify an odor either due to deficits in acuity or in identification ability. In the presence of normal acuity, inability to identify common odors is termed olfactory agnosia (Kopala and Clark, 1990).

Varney (1988) stresses that in assessment of olfactory functioning, anosmia as an isolated symptom may be due to impaired peripheral innervation, fever, nasal obstruction, smoking, habituation, or the drying effects of medication. After accounting for such extraneous variables, impaired identification can be used to measure and localise more central pathology if sensory and cognitive parameters are clearly distinguished (Harrison and Pearson, 1989). The distinction between central rather than peripheral parameters may be related to identification of clinical subtypes such as negative symptom schizophrenia. Scientific interest in the association between schizophrenia and olfactory deficits has been enhanced by the development of a well standardised and clinically validated test of olfactory functioning—the University of Pennsylvania Smell Identification Test (UPSIT; Doty *et al.*, 1984). Norms for this task reflect increasing ability through childhood and adolescence until stabilised capacity in early adulthood. Hence, identification deficits in the presence of intact acuity likely reflect developmental arrest of prefrontal function, where increased degree of deficit is associated with lower age of onset of prefrontal compromise.

B. Olfactory identification is mediated by orbitofrontal processes

Olfactory identification represents a second-order olfactory function which is dependent on relatively intact functioning in the peripheral olfactory system. Therefore, given extraneous factors affecting acuity are accounted for, an inability to identify a smell in the presence of intact olfactory acuity can indicate compromise in central mechanisms—particularly the OFC.

The relatively discrete areas mediating olfactory identification ability have been examined by Zatorre *et al.* (1992) who found significant regional cerebral blood flow (rCBF) increases at the junction of the inferior frontal and temporal lobes bilaterally, corresponding to the piriform cortex, and unilaterally, in the right OFC. These findings were confirmed by Mozley *et al.* (1995) who found that during performance of olfactory identification tasks by patients with schizophrenia, abnormalities of rCBF were found in regions served by the lateral and intermediate branches of the olfactory tract, as well as the centrifugal fibers which originate in the ipsilateral brainstem and other structures important in olfactory feedback circuits. Thus, mean metabolism was lower in the superior frontal regions for patients who performed worse on the University of Pennsylvania Smell Identification Test (UPSIT: Doty *et al.*, 1984) and greater than mean metabolism was observed in the amygdala, thalamus, mamilliary bodies and pons, posterior corpus callosum, and midbrain. In a further Positron Emission Tomography (PET) study, Bertollo *et al.* (1996) demonstrated support for the finding of Zatorre *et al.* (1992) and demonstrated a significantly greater degree of hypometabolism in males with schizophrenia in the cortical area of the nondominant hemisphere that receives direct uncrossed olfactory projections. More recent findings implicate these same neural regions (Schneider *et al.*, 2007).

III. Olfactory Identification Deficits in Schizophrenia

Smell identification tests have been extensively employed in schizophrenia research as a measure of orbitofrontal functional integrity. Measured using the UPSIT, olfactory identification deficits are one of the most consistent observations in groups with chronic schizophrenia (Brewer *et al.*, 1996; Compton *et al.*, 2006; Malaspina and Coleman, 2003; Moberg *et al.*, 2006). There is also substantial evidence of olfactory identification deficits at psychosis onset (Brewer *et al.*, 2001; Good *et al.*, 2006; Moberg *et al.*, 1999; Seidman *et al.*, 1997), in ultrahigh risk groups who later develop psychosis (Brewer *et al.*, 2003) and in adolescents (11–17 years) with early-onset psychosis (Corcoran *et al.*, 2005). In addition, olfactory identification may serve as a genetic marker for psychosis (Kopala *et al.*, 2001). Twin and family studies have shown that olfactory identification ability of nonpsychotic family members and nonaffected twins is intermediate between their affected counterparts and controls (Compton *et al.*, 2006; Kopala *et al.*, 2001).

A. Implications of independent olfactory identification and sensitivity processes in schizophrenia

Kopala *et al.* (1990) reported identification deficits in the presence of intact acuity in schizophrenia. These authors used the literature by Potter and Butters (1980) and Jones-Gotman and Zatorre (1988) to account for their findings. Potter and Butters demonstrated a profound inability of patients with prefrontal lesions—specifically of the OFC, to distinguish odor qualities reliably, even when stimuli were highly discernible. These patients had known or suspected damage to the OFC and were not impaired in odor detection.

The only other condition identified where acuity and identification are dissociated is Korsakoff's amnestic syndrome. Here, the primary lesions are found in the dorsal-medial nucleus of the thalamus (Adams and Victor,

1985). Potter and Butters (1980) use their results to suggest a hierarchical organisation of olfactory processing passing from the mediodorsal nucleus of the thalamus to the temporal (entorhinal) lobe, and then to the lateral posterior OFC. This suggestion was based on the premise that their results supported evidence that prefrontal lesions produce more dramatic olfactory impairment than damage to the midline thalamus alone.

Jones-Gotman and Zatorre (1988) found that identification ability as measured by the UPSIT is significantly impaired following a unilateral excision in the temporal lobe or the OFC on either side, but not after a frontal lobe excision sparing the orbital cortex. Greater deficits were associated with OFC lesions than with lesions of the temporal area. Thresholds in both groups of lesioned patients were normal. Overall, it appears that if the orbital region is spared, identification ability is maintained, while if it is not, deficits in identification, but not acuity, are present. Projections to the dorsal thalamus and the frontal cortex are the major neocortical representations involved in odor discrimination, and thus involvement of either is inferred in identification deficits (Kopala and Clark, 1990).

IV. Olfactory Sensitivity Through Development

In contrast to the literature on identification ability, the available evidence suggests that children and young adults possess sensitivity comparable to that of persons in their thirties (Beauchamp and Pearson, 1991; Brewer and Pantelis, 2006; Schall *et al.*, 1998). However, methodological differences confound this evidence. For example, while Koelega (1994) found relative insensitivity of prepubescent children for 4–5 odorants compared to subjects aged 15 and 20 years, the musk-based steroidal odorants utilised are more likely to be detected postpuberty (see also Dorries *et al.*, 1989 who utilised androstenone). Such changes to sensitivity to some odors may be determined by hormonal or maturational changes. Strauss (1970) concluded that threshold detection ability for nonsteroidal substances increases progressively from age 8–10 through to adulthood (21–39 years). In contrast, the better controlled studies report no increase in sensitivity for nonsteroidal odorants (Cain *et al.*, 1995; Dorries *et al.*, 1989; Koelega and Koster, 1974; Larsson and Backman, 1997).

Difference in odor salience may affect sensitivity, which appears relevant to stage of development. For example, infants have higher levels of olfactory acuity for certain odorants (e.g., breast milk) rather than others (Beauchamp and Pearson, 1991; Koelega, 1994; Richman *et al.*, 1995; Schall, 1988). As indicated above, prepubescent children are as sensitive to nonsteroidal odors as adolescents and adults, while the ability to detect certain steroidal substances is only apparent postpubertally.

The nature of acuity deficits, the neural systems they implicate, and their effect on higher order identification ability are a possible confound, although for chronic schizophrenia patients, the literature suggests that identification deficits occur in the presence of relatively intact acuity for control odorants. This chapter now explores the history of acuity research in patients with psychosis and in normal controls, and outlines recent findings from the literature in people suffering from chronic schizophrenia.

A. Review of sensitivity literature in normal controls and in schizophrenia; Anosmia

The notion of olfactory processes operating independently in schizophrenia may have important implications for understanding the nature and role of the prefrontal cortex and associated limbic circuitry throughout the course of psychosis. Kopala's group has consistently found olfactory identification for *n*-butyl alcohol (NBA) or phenyl-ethyl alcohol (PEA) deficits occuring in the presence of intact acuity (Kopala *et al.*, 1989, 1992, 1998).

However, the literature describing olfactory acuity function in schizophrenia is less clear than that describing identification deficits. This may be due in part to some confusion in rationale that stems from literature in the early 1960s, where some research groups attempted to explore acuity for steroids in schizophrenia. More recently, Kopala's group for example has used tasks of acuity for more traditional *nonsteroidal* substances to demonstrate independence from identification ability. In addition, and as discussed below, the early steroid literature ignored an important finding that suggested that the acuity-for-steroids hypothesis was based upon a misleading premise. The following discussion argues that nonsteroidal substances should be utilised to investigate pure acuity performance rather than relying upon the use of steroidal-based compound.

B. Early odor research: Schizophrenia and abnormal sweat

Original interest in this subject was triggered by seeking to identify the odorous substance that clinicians believed might be secreted in the sweat of patients suffering from mental illness and followed a report by Smith and Sines (1960). These clinicians described a strange odor associated with the smell of sweat emitted from patients with hebephrenia. This odor appeared to be resistant to any amount of bathing and resembled a musky, stale urine smell. The authors suggested that identification of an odor that is unique in the apocrine sweat or in the sebaceous secretion of patients with schizophrenia might provide a clue to an "inborn error of metabolism. . ." (p. 74). These authors demonstrated that there was a readily identifiable scent found in the sweat of certain patients that could be distinguished from the usual smell of sweat. For example, anecdotal evidence from a psychiatrist, reported by Wiener (1966), suggested that the odor of schizophrenia "...had long been part of clinical diagnosis. (He)... remembered this from (his) state hospital days, and ...in analysis. (He could)... sometimes tell by the odour when an entering schizophrenic patient (was)...in crisis on a particular day-it really (was)...most reliable...p. 3165-6)". These observations apparently formed the impetus for Wiener's hypothesis of abnormal steroid secretion (Wiener, 1967). This hypothesis then triggered later research in acuity for steroids in schizophrenia (Bradley, 1984). Additional reports of the relationship apparently between this odor and acute crisis and its weakening during remission are still being made (Warrnambool Psychiatric Unit, personal communication).

In response to Smith and Sines' (1960) observation, Skinner *et al.* (1964) reported that the only abnormal bacterial organisms found in the axilliary area of such odorous patients was an excess of diptheroids. Skinner *et al.* (1964) suggested that this excess may be enhanced by the presence of the odorous substance or its precursor, or indeed, that the odorous substance may inhibit the growth of other organisms to produce a relative excess of diptheroids. Diptheroids are microorganisms resembling corynebacterium diptheriae (Professor Richard Brown, 1995, personal communication). Coryneform bacteria are able to act on steroid hormones to transform them to other steroids (Charney, 1966). However, Smith *et al.* (1969) then apparently isolated this odorous substance from the sweat of patients with schizophrenia using gas chromatography, mass spectrometry, and nuclear magnetic resonance spectroscopy. They reported its chemical structure as *trans*-3-methyl-2-hexenoic acid. This substance could not be related to bacteria formation, at least not "pseudomonas aeruginosa"—a common coryneform bacteria (Kloos and Musselwhite, 1975). The Smith *et al.* (1969) finding has been ignored in the literature focusing on steroid acuity in schizophrenia to date, and rather, reports of abnormal acuity in schizophrenia are based upon the misleading rationale that the abnormal odor secreted from patients' skin is predominately steroidal in nature. Further, results have been interpreted in this context to support the notion that acuity for steroids in these patients should be different to normals due to increased secretions in sweat. Acuity for hexanoic acid or its derivatives in humans has never been reported.

C. Early odor research: Schizophrenia and abnormal steroid secretion

A second strand of research emerged following the link made between abnormal steroid secretion and mental illness described above. Brooksbank and Pryse-Phillips (1964) demonstrated that psychiatric patients, particularly young males, had reduced adrostenol levels in their urine. These authors then demonstrated that the deficiency was found in patients with schizophrenia as distinct from other diagnostic categories.

The rationale for this research was based upon the extensive literature documenting endocrine abnormalities in mental illness (e.g., Bleuler, 1954; Reiss, 1958; Sands, 1957). The evidence suggested that not only was deficient gonadal secretion an outcome of mental illness, but that it was also a predisposing factor of a constitutional nature. Wiener (1966) had previously stated that the abnormal urinary secretion of metabolites in schizophrenia could profitably be viewed as signs of abnormal external chemical messengers (ECM; or pheromones). He went on to develop his hypothesis that there is a marked abnormal ECM system in schizophrenia (Wiener, 1967), where increased levels of steroids were found to be secreted in the blood, sweat, and urine. Liddell (1976) expanded this notion and demonstrated the utility of body odor as a diagnostic marker, particularly from substances secreted from the main apocrine glands in the axillae. Apocrine gland secretion is relatively odorless, but when left for several hours, bacteria decomposes the compound and liberates fatty acids. Development of axillary odor typically is associated with the coryneform bacteria which break down steroid hormones as described previously (Jackman, 1982; Jackman and Noble, 1983; Leydon *et al.*, 1981; Rennie *et al.*, 1991; Shehadeh and Kligman, 1963). The *normal* odor of sweat (particularly axillary sweat), urine, and breath is due to large quantities of butyric and hexanoic acids in the body (Liddell, 1976).

D. Steroid secretion and olfactory acuity for steroids in normals

The normal odor of the hexanoic acid derivative described above is similar to a stale urinous odor when it is exposed to moisture in the environment (personal observation). Its similarity to the steroidal odor of stale urine may explain in part why the focus of research in acuity in schizophrenia focused on acuity for steroids rather than on hexanoic acid *per se*. The urinous odor of steroids is confirmed from several sources. At least one of the common 16-unsaturated C-19 steroids possesses a smell varying between musk and urine that is secreted in normal males and in those with schizophrenia, usually from the metabolism of a precursor in the axillae by skin microorganisms (Bird and Gower, 1982). Five-α-androstenone has a urinous odor (Bird and Gower, 1982) and 5-α-androst-16-en-3-one (androstenol) is another steroid which possesses a urine-like musky odor, similar to testosterone (Kloek, 1961). This latter steroid occurs in the urine of normal men at three times the concentration than in women (Bird and Gower, 1982; Brooksbank, 1962; Claus and Alsing, 1976). Storage of this steroid also occurs in male fatty tissue, plasma, and in axillary sweat (Brooksbank *et al.*, 1974; Claus and Alsing, 1976; Gower and Bicknell, 1972; Gower *et al.*, 1985), and possibly in human skin (Berliner *et al.*, 1991).

The physiological function in humans of androstenol is unknown; however, when secreted in the saliva of the boar it acts as a releaser sex pheromone to elicit the characteristic immobilisation response of the oestrous sow to the advances of its mate (Melrose *et al.*, 1971). Androstenol (and androstenone) is a likely candidate as a pheromone in humans, although various other steroids can be detected at much higher concentrations (Brooksbank *et al.*, 1974).

Acuity for odors is decreased and is common in people following zinc depletion, associated with estrogen depletion in women. Furthermore, smell thresholds are significantly elevated during menstruation in females (Schneider, 1971). Acuity appears to be greater generally in women compared to males (Koelega and Koster, 1974; Stoddart, 1976; Wysocki and Gilbert, 1987), which appears to result from the higher potency of estrogens relative to androgens (Broverman *et al.*, 1968). Le Magnen (1952) hypothesised that sensitivity to urinoid odors is determined by sex hormones, where the presence of estrogens would improve sensitivity to these biological odors and the presence of androgens would lead to a low sensitivity. This hypothesis was supported by results from a study by Koelega and Koster (1974).

To complicate this picture, acuity for specific primary odors varies across individuals (Albone and Shirley, 1984; Clark and Ball, 1983) including the ability to detect androstenone and estrogen. Olfactory thresholds for 5-α-androstenones vary widely and reports on the percentage of the population that can detect this pheromone are varied (Albone and Shirley, 1984). Griffiths and Patterson (1970) showed that 8% of women and 44% of men are unable to smell androstenone while Beets and Theimer (1970) demonstrated, in contrast, that about 50% of men and women smell it normally while the remainder either cannot detect it at all, register a different sensation, or are inconsistent in their response. With some support for this finding, Amoore (1970) found that 50% of people cannot detect it at all, where there was apparently no difference according to sex, while Koelega and Koster (1974) observed that women are twice as sensitive to the compound as are men (Doty, 1977). However, Gower *et al.* (1985) reported that men may be no different to women in their acuity for this substance while anosmia did not differ greatly (9–20%). These authors found anosmia to the smell of 5-α-androst-16-en-3-α-ol was most marked in women (90%) rather than in men (45%).

Acuity for androstenone also differs significantly across geographic regions, where anosmia for this pheromone was most prevalent in the USA (33% M; 24% F) and lowest in Africa (22% M; 14% F). Men rate the smell of androstenone as being more pleasant than females rate it (Wysocki and Gilbert, 1987). Furthermore, the ability to detect this substance decreases with age beginning in the second decade of life while identification peaks through the sixth decade then declines. Intensity is usually rated as lower than for other primary odorants. Finally, subjects vary in their rating of androstenone as being "pleasant or unpleasant" (Van Toller *et al.*, 1983).

Hubert *et al.* (1980, 1981) suggest that little genetic variability is found within the normal range of olfactory acuity for non-steroidal substances; however, sensitivity to androstenone has a major genetic component (Wysocki and Beauchamp, 1984). Here, sensitivity may be conditioned in those who previously report that they cannot detect an odor (Wysocki *et al.*, 1989). Indeed, there may be three categories of human subjects: those truly anosmic, the inducible, and those who are constitutionally sensitive or have already experienced incidental induction. One explanation for these differences may be the formation of discrete receptors that can be induced in the epithelial layer, or alternatively exposure may affect changes in enzyme levels in the epithelial layers (Doty, 1977). Albone and Shirley (1984) suggest that secretions of steroids from the blood stream may enter the olfactory epithelium, thus altering the sensitivity to detection. These secretions are dependent upon hormone levels. Anosmia for 5-α-androstenone is probably the most common form of anosmia, which is of genetic origin (Wysocki and Beauchamp, 1984).

E. Acuity research in schizophrenia

It is likely that disturbance to the structure and function of peripheral and lower order mechanisms mediating olfactory processing in schizophrenia also contribute to reduction of sensitivity. Moberg *et al.* (2004) found smaller posterior nasal volumes in males with schizophrenia relative to comparison subjects, and suggested that this reflected early disruption in embryological development in males with schizophrenia. Moreover, these authors later reported physiological impairment in first-degree relatives of patients with schizophrenia, including left nostril detection impairments and reduced evoked response amplitudes (Turetsky *et al.*, 2008), that were comparable to those previously observed for schizophrenia patients. These authors then reported odor-specific hyposmia that was interpreted as implicating a disruption of cAMP mediated signal transduction in schizophrenia which was also found in unaffected first-degree relatives, thereby providing further evidence that these lower order dysfunctions are genetically mediated (Turetsky and Moberg, 2009a). However, these findings may involve a more complex explanation than the specific signal transduction mechanism cited (Serby, 2009; see also Turetsky and Moberg, 2009b). In a recent review, Turetsky *et al.* (2009a,b) report their findings that the normal relationship between olfactory bulb volume and odor detection threshold sensitivity found in normal controls was not found in patients with schizophrenia. This review also summarised the structural abnormalities of the olfactory cortex that implicate disruption to sensitivity. In addition, functional abnormalities of the olfactory cortex and epithelium have also been reported (see Turetsky *et al.*, 2009a,b).

F. Acuity for various odorants in schizophrenia

Bradley (1984) demonstrated that schizophrenic men had increased olfactory acuity for 16-androsten steroids than nonschizophrenic men. Her rationale was based upon the Brooksbank and Pryse-Phillips (1964) study discussed above demonstrating that abnormal secretion of steroids occurred in schizophrenia. It was expected that patients with reduced secretion would be more sensitive to those subjects with abnormal secretion who had habituated to the pheromonal odor.

While attempting to replicate the Bradley (1984) study, Isseroff *et al.* (1987) found that a large group of male and female patients with chronic schizophrenia had highly elevated thresholds for isoamyl-acetate (IA) in comparison to matched controls, which they attributed to the dehydration effects of neuroleptics. The study by Serby *et al.* (1990) discussed in the previous chapter supported this finding, where elevated olfactory thresholds for a musky odorant in males with schizophrenia were found. The odor of musk can be confused with steroidal compounds. However, these studies failed to account for the prevalence of androstenone agnosia in the general population of around 30% (Wysocki and Gilbert, 1987).

Geddes *et al.* (1991) were the first olfactory researchers to discriminate people with schizophrenia into positive and negative subtypes, with the aim of investigating possible associations with deficits in acuity. Their hypothesis was based on evidence demonstrating that removal of the temporal lobe increases odor detection thresholds without affecting odor recognition (Rausch and Serafetinides, 1975), and that the medial temporal lobe is implicated in schizophrenia (Trimble, 1987). The findings demonstrated that the negative symptom group had a significantly higher olfactory threshold than the positive group for a musk ketone, although neither group differed significantly from controls. These authors suggested these findings provided evidence for temporal lobe compromise in syndromal subgroups of schizophrenia, which is consistent with the notion of neuropsychological subtypes (Pantelis and Brewer, 1995, 1996; Pantelis *et al.*, 1992). Further support for this notion of subtyping was found by Brewer *et al.* (1996) who found that olfactory *identification* deficits were also related to increased levels of negative symptoms and, while identification ability was related to prefrontal and putative medial temporal function in controls, the identification deficit was related to prefrontal but not medial temporal function in patients with schizophrenia.

As noted previously, controlling for acuity levels is difficult, and in the Geddes *et al.* (1991) study, menstrual cycles which influence these levels significantly (Amoore, 1970) were not accounted for in the design. Moreover, specific use of odors that do not trigger a trigeminal nerve response such as phenyl-ethyl alcohol (PEA) is required in such research otherwise reported differences can be unnecessarily invalidated, or be erroneously attributed to threshold processing when it is a trigeminal response that is being reported.

Here, a response to apparently toxic stimuli such as isoamyl-acetate may still be reported by a subject due to reaction via the fifth cranial nerve in the presence of reduced sensitivity in the first cranial nerve (Martzke *et al.*, 1997). Furthermore, the use of inconsistent odorants across research groups is not helpful as acuity for individual substances varies considerably. Kopala's group has been consistent in this regard with their use of *n*-butyl alcohol or more recently, PEA. While it is conceded that accounting for the involvement of medial-temporal processes in acuity is difficult, utilisation of memory tasks known to index these areas (Jones-Gotman, 1991) could add weight to the evidence suggestive of compromise.

The notion of independent olfactory processes in schizophrenia should not be confused with the large literature documenting reduced global olfactory ability (acuity and identification) in patients with other psychopathologies. Identification deficits reported can often be secondary to acuity deficits in these reports and they are beyond the scope of this chapter. The only comparative study addressing this issue demonstrated that identification deficits in the presence of intact acuity were found to be peculiar to schizophrenia and not to patients with depression. Here, Gross-Isseroff *et al.* (1994) confirmed the study by Serby *et al.* (1990) demonstrating that acuity in depression was significantly reduced compared to controls. This reduction was apparently due to the introduction of antidepressant drug therapy.

The study by Kopala *et al.* (1998) discussed above confirmed the identification deficits in the presence of intact acuity for PEA and NBA in males with chronic schizophrenia. These findings were consistent with those from her 1989 and 1992 studies. However, in the 1998 study a subgroup of chronic patients suffering from polydipsia were found to suffer acuity deficits relative to nonpolydipsic/nomanetremic patients and normal controls which reflected a pattern of deficits similar to those found in more generalised organic pathology such as in Alzheimer's disease. The suggestion that there may be subgroups of patients with independent patterns of symptoms and related cognitive and/or olfactory function is consistent with the findings from Seidman *et al.* (1992, 1994), Geddes *et al.* (1991), and Brewer *et al.* (1996).

Research groups other than Kopala's have cited Wiener's hypothesis as a rationale for acuity assessment and consequently have incorporated steroids as odorants. The findings from these groups that acuity in schizophrenia is not intact, which is contrary to the conclusions by Kopala's group, can be seen to be less robust if trigeminal involvement is possible, or if the conclusions are based upon findings regarding acuity for steroids. The latter approach is problematic for two reasons as described above. First, steroid anosmia is not accounted for and, second, the rationale for assessment of steroids using Wiener's hypothesis is misleading. Wiener had made the false assumption that because the odor emanating from patients with schizophrenia was similar to a steroidal smell, coupled with emerging evidence of interruptions to steroid levels in similar patients, then their acuity for the same steroidal compound would be affected due to habituation effects. However, Smith *et al.* (1969) clarified this assumption when the odorant in question was identified as being a *nonsteroidal* hexanoic acid derivative. In addition, assessment of acuity with substances which have a similar odor to hexanoic acid (steroids or musk derivative) will most likely find raised thresholds due to habituation to the odor of hexanoic acid secreted in this patient group. These misleading assumptions confuse this area of research.

G. Hygiene naiveté in schizophrenia: Relationship to negative symptoms and olfactory deficits

A further strand to the focus in the literature emerged from the common observation of poor personal hygiene being apparent in patients with schizophrenia and that many of these patients are unaware of their malodorous state or of the effect of their body odor on others (Brewer *et al.*, 1996). Likely causes of poor personal hygiene have not been adequately explored, though Snowdon (1987) has suggested that poor hygiene reflects a more elemental disorder. For example, the deficits in olfactory function which have been identified in patients with schizophrenia and have been described previously may contribute to this lack of hygiene (Brewer *et al.*, 1996). As some patients with schizophrenia emit a peculiar odor from their sweat (Smith and Sines, 1960) as discussed previously, this problem may also contribute to their poor hygiene. Another possibility is that poor hygiene may be a secondary consequence of core negative symptoms, such as lack of motivation and apathy. Jackson (1987) identified a relationship between the negative symptoms of schizophrenia and social skills performance, which includes personal presentation and care, while only one study has found an association between negative symptoms and increased olfactory threshold (Geddes *et al.*, 1991). The only study to date to systematically examine the relationship between olfactory deficits, negative symptoms, and measures of social skills functioning was conducted by Brewer *et al.* (1996) who found that poor hygiene was found in those chronic patients with a greater degree of negative symptoms. In addition, degree of unpleasant odor was related to degree of negative symptoms and to deficits in olfactory identification. These patterns of results suggest that just as identification ability might be utilised as "component" challenges of circuitry implicated in the syndromes of schizophrenia, so might measures of acuity be utilised for similar purposes.

Harrison and Pearson (1989) have postulated that olfactory deficits in various neuropsychiatric conditions, including those discussed above concerning schizophrenia, implicate dysfunction of the central mechanisms mediating olfaction. However, some confusion remains in this vein of research if studies do not clearly discriminate between the abnormal steroid secretion hypothesis and difficulty in acuity for general substance *per se* as has been discussed. First, reports of "pure" olfactory acuity deficits *for the purposes of assessing acuity function specifically* in patients with schizophrenia should be the only relevant reports to add to the body of literature, and then, only if odorants that do not have a trigeminal component are utilised. Reports of acuity for steroids only confirm that there is a wide range of steroid anosmia in the population, and as such do not add anything to understanding of the process of acuity function *per se*. Furthermore, basing investigations of acuity for steroids upon Wiener's hypothesis is flawed and interpretation of findings as being relevant to the understanding of acuity should be ignored. A more appropriate direction for the steroidal acuity literature would be to investigate the subgroups of steroid anosmics in more detail, where the likely genetic component might direct researchers toward a more useful understanding of the neurobiology of schizophrenia. It is noteworthy that the larger proportion of studies in this area has concluded that acuity *per se* is impaired in schizophrenia while not accounting for subgroups of subjects who are anosmic to such substances.

Changes in acuity due to menstruation are a further complication in this research. In women, estradiol level is associated with their olfactory identification ability where lower estrogen level is associated with increased errors on the UPSIT (Kopala *et al.*, 1995). Therefore, it is important to examine men and women separately and to also monitor hormonal levels. In the absence of such invasive methodology, tracking the menstrual cycle provides a convenient and noninvasive method for studying estrogen fluctuations in humans (Hampson and Kimura, 1992).

In summary, the findings on acuity involving males and females with schizophrenia remain less clear than those for identification and therefore further investigation of patients with both first-episode and chronic schizophrenia is warranted. While it appears that independent medial temporal lobe involvement might be implicated in acuity processing, utilisation of substances that are less likely to trigger a trigeminal response is required and, further, it would be helpful if they are similar to those used in established research groups. In addition, use of odorants that have similar qualities to the odor of steroids are unhelpful, and findings from assessment of acuity for steroids should not be utilised to discount the findings of intact acuity in schizophrenia. Control of menstrual cycles is required when assessing female acuity. It is apparent that some acuity is required for unimpaired functioning of olfactory identification. Dissociation of these olfactory abilities may provide a framework for establishing the relative role of prefrontal relative to limbic neural circuitry in cognition.

We more recently examined the prevalence of acuity for pheromonal (steroidal) substances in a sample of patients with schizophrenia compared to patients with first-episode psychosis and normal controls. We aimed to extend the previous literature that has investigated chronic patient groups only. In addition, acuity for the odor found in schizophrenic sweat, and for a more traditional control substance was investigated in these same subject groups. The purpose of our aims was twofold. First, it was the first report of acuity for the substance identified by Smith *et al.* (1969) that was to be assessed. Second, utilising the more traditional control substance, we furthered Kopala's work in the chronic patient group to exploration of pure olfactory acuity at the outset of the illness. The relationship between acuity as a putative challenge of medial-temporal lobe function and identification as a probe of OFC function at stabilisation of the first episode of psychosis was examined. Finally, the presence of sex differences in acuity for schizophrenic sweat, pheromones, and for a control substance that does not trigger a trigeminal response was examined in all subject groups described above.

Our results confirmed that olfactory identification deficits that are present at early stabilisation of first onset psychosis occur in the presence of intact acuity for traditionally used substances (*n*-butyl alcohol; Brewer *et al.*, 2007). These results were important in demonstrating that, consistent with the appropriate literature, acuity *per se* appears to be intact at the outset of illness and remains relatively intact in patients who develop chronic illness. This contrasts with findings of increased threshold in the chronic patient group for HA, which has similar odorant properties to some musky steroidal compounds. In addition, while acuity was not related to identification ability in any group, the findings were consistent with previous reports of independent olfactory processing existing in patients with schizophrenia. These findings might also be utilised to suggest relatively intact functioning of limbic compared to prefrontal structures.

In addition, while acuity was not related to identification ability in any group in our 2007 study, the findings were consistent with previous reports of independent olfactory processing existing in patients with schizophrenia. These findings might also be utilised to suggest relatively intact functioning of limbic compared to prefrontal structures.

Our findings also supported the reports by Kopala *et al.* (1992, 1994a,b) and those by Wu *et al.* (1993) which suggested that olfactory identification deficits occur in patients with early psychosis and that they occur in the presence of intact acuity when nonsteroidal substances are utilised as test odorants (Kopala *et al.*, 1989, 1992, 1998). This pattern of dissociation supported the notion of a hierarchical organisation of olfactory processing passing from the dorsomedial nucleus of the thalamus to the temporal (entorhinal) lobe, and then to the posterior OFC (Jones-Gotman and Zatorre, 1988; Kopala and Clark, 1990; Potter and Butters, 1980).

In addition, our study was the first to have synthesised the HA derivative as the odorous compound described by Smith *et al.* (1969) that has been detected in the sweat of patients with chronic schizophrenia. It was also the first to report on acuity for this substance across the course of psychosis in comparison to controls. The presence of increased acuity threshold for this odor in the patients with chronic schizophrenia could not be explained by the effects of smoking, gender, premorbid IQ, phase of menstrual cycle, level of positive symptomatology, or compromise on tasks implicating medial temporal lobe function. The results suggested that steroidal anosmia limited the ability to detect HA in chronic patients in some way, as did higher doses of neuroleptic medication. Being neuroleptic naïve in the FE group did not result in improved acuity for HA. Further, acuity for HA was associated with the negative and disorganised symptoms of the illness. Increased emanation of this odor from the sweat of patients might be one explanation for elevated thresholds due to habituation. This is consistent with the findings of Brewer *et al.* (1996) demonstrating that increased body odor was associated with negative symptoms. These conclusions should be interpreted with caution; however, a role of elevated threshold for HA being indicative of poor prognosis may be suggested. Validation of this notion could only be gained by longitudinal investigation.

The odor of this compound that emanated from patients with chronic schizophrenia was first reported by Smith and Sines (1960) and may provide clues to compromise of metabolism. For example, these findings may implicate compromise of the tuberoinfundibular dopaminergic system, which originates in cell bodies of the arcuate nucleus of the hypothalamus and projects to the pituitary stalk. This system is important for prolactin regulation and may contribute to some other neuroendocrine abnormalities in schizophrenia (Kandel *et al.*, 1991). Further research is required to investigate the etiology of this abnormally high secretion of HA and, further, what relationship secretion levels have with positive symptoms. Anecdotal evidence suggests that exacerbated levels of this odor may precede relapse.

A related issue concerns the abnormal secretion of steroids in the body sweat of people with schizophrenia, which may smell similar to HA (Bird and Gower, 1982; Brooksbank and Pryse-Phillips, 1964; Kloek, 1961). Several studies have investigated acuity for steroids based upon the hypotheses by Wiener (1967), who suggested that abnormal pheromonal communication occurred in people with schizophrenia. Bradley (1984) tested the hypothesis that patients with schizophrenia would be abnormally conscious of pheromonal stimuli, even after accounting for the fact that males, who because of their own greater production of 16-androstenes, would be less sensitive to pheromonal odor than women. Bradley (1984) found that males with schizophrenia were more sensitive to steroids than normal male controls; however, these authors did not control for anosmia for steroid across the groups and for changes in acuity due to menstruation. They suggested reasonably, however, that increased acuity for male steroids was consistent with reduced levels of circulation of the same steroids, and that this might implicate compromise of gonadal function in some of the males who were assessed. The results from this current chapter suggest that anosmia for steroids is consistent between patient groups and normal controls. No gender differences were found, however the proportion of females to males across the groups was smaller than that in the Bradley (1984) study.

Isseroff *et al.* (1987) assessed acuity for isoamyl-acetate (IA) in people with schizophrenia compared to controls based upon a similar rationale to Bradley (1984). The authors also utilised a "hypersensitivity" argument that arose during the early 1960s to qualify the perceptual deficits in hallucinations and delusions, and suggested that patients with schizophrenia would be more sensitive to environmental stimuli. Results suggested that males with schizophrenia had elevated thresholds to IA in comparison to controls. No differences between the groups were found in acuity for androstenone, after controlling for steroid anosmia, and these authors concluded that the results from the Bradley (1984) study were achieved by chance due to the small number of subjects who were assessed. Isseroff *et al.* (1987) did not control for smoking, levels of symptoms, phase of menstrual cycle in the females, or dose of neuroleptic medication. However, they concluded that the most parsimonious explanation was the dehydration effects of neuroleptic medication. The more consistent literature by Kopala *et al.* (1989, 1992, 1998) demonstrates that olfactory acuity for a substance that is less likely to trigger a trigeminal response (NBA or PEA) is not affected by medication levels. The results we reported in the 2007 study support this finding.

Only two other exceptions to the findings of intact or increased acuity ability for odors in schizophrenia exist in the literature. Geddes *et al.* (1991) found increased olfactory thresholds for musk ketone in patients with schizophrenia who had more pronounced negative symptoms. These authors did not account for menstrual cycle phase or smoking. In addition, musk has a similar odor to some steroid compounds and steroid anosmia was not controlled for in this study. Results from Brewer *et al.* (2007) suggest that greater degree of negative symptoms is associated with reduced ability to detect HA, which is consistent with Geddes *et al.* (1991). Serby *et al.* (1990), using Geranoil as the acuity stimulus, observed elevated thresholds in their sample of 14 male patients with schizophrenia. This study did not account for medication or smoking effects, the sample is small, and the inconsistent use of substances other than NBA or PEA does not really assist the established progression of research in this area.

The findings of anosmia for steroid compounds in approximately one-third of subjects across the groups are consistent with previous reports in the literature (Gower *et al.*, 1985; Wysocki and Gilbert, 1987) and may be genetic in origin (Wysocki and Beauchamp, 1984). In addition, the ability to detect other individual odors requires intact specific genetic coding. Further research is required where an item analysis on the UPSIT in patients with psychosis may reveal, that patients may be anosmic for specific odors compared to controls. The gene marker for the ability to detect such odors could then be explored. Indeed, the ability to detect HA should be explored further in this context.

Use of HA had identified acuity deficits in patients with chronic schizophrenia, which may be related to neuroleptic medication dose. However, a similar effect would be expected in acuity ability for NBA if this was the case. No such effect was found in first-episode psychosis patients. The finding of a medication effect may be possibly linked to some relationship between neuroleptic dose and secretion of HA in sweat. For example, it is likely that this deficit may be related to habituation effects, where emanation of the odor of schizophrenia that occurs in a subgroup of patients, more particularly those with higher levels of negative symptoms (Brewer *et al.*, 1996) may desensitise their ability to detect the same odor compared to controls. This issue can only be adequately explored by investigating how neuroleptic medication disturbs hypothalamic processes in some way to lead to excess secretion of HA in sweat.

Although no direct evidence was available from serum estradiol data, the estrogen status of women could be inferred indirectly through the menstrual cycle information. Kopala *et al.* (1994a,b) reported that women with schizophrenia have lower peak serum estradiol levels than do control women, and that postmenopausal women with schizophrenia show deficits on UPSIT ability. In the current study, the findings of a significant difference in acuity for NBA between the women with highest estradiol level and those with a low level was found, where the former manifested an increased threshold score. These findings are consistent with previous research suggesting that smell thresholds are significantly elevated during menstruation (Koelega and Koster, 1974; Schneider, 1971).

V. Summary and Future Directions

Findings reported in Brewer et al (2007) were the first ever reported on acuity for HA in normal controls and in patients with psychosis and clarify the literature on acuity for steroids which has been based upon a misleading rationale since the early 1960s. This has implications for social skills training where the implication often is that some patients do not wash and that they have poor personal hygiene. If indeed they have some metabolic abnormality that results in increased secretion of HA, patients and carers need to be informed to avoid problems with stigma and false assumptions concerning selfcare.

Further research is required to determine the utility of such tasks to detect deficits in people who are at high risk for. To validate the usefulness of acuity as a probe of medial temporal regions, comparison of olfactory performance in patients with temporal lobe deficits to those with psychosis is required. This should determine whether deficits in acuity, and therefore identification, are present in temporal-lobe epilepsy patients and that these deficits occur in patterns that are dissociable from patterns found in patients with psychosis. Finally, exploration of the possible abnormal genetic marker associated with the detection of HA should be explored, along with an investigation into the process that triggers its abnormal level of secretion in the metabolism of patients with chronic schizophrenia.

ACKNOWLEDGMENTS

This research was supported by Program Grants from the NHMRC Australia (566529 and 350241). Associate Professor Brewer was supported by a Clinical Career Development Award from the NHMRC and the Colonial Foundation.

REFERENCES

Adams, R., and Victor, M. (1985). Principles of Neurology. McGraw Hill, New York.

Albone, E. S., and Shirley, S. G. (1984). Mammalian Semiochemistry. The Investigation of Chemical Signals Between Mammals. New York, John Wiley.

Amoore, J. E. (1970). Molecular Basis of Odor. Thomas, Illinois.

Beauchamp, G. K., and Pearson, P. (1991). Human development and taste. *Phsysiol. Behav.* **49,** 1009–1012.

Beets, M. G. J., and Theimer, T. (1970). Odours similarity between structurally unrelated odorants. *In* "Taste and Smell in Vertebrates," (G. E. W. Wolstenhome and J. Knights, Eds.). Churchill, London.

Berliner, D. L., Jennings-White, C., and Lavker, R. M. (1991). The human skin: Fragrances and pheromones. *J. Steroidal Biochem. Mol. Biol.* **39**(4B), 671–679.

Bertollo, D. N., Cowen, M. A., and Levy, A. V. (1996). Hypometabolism in olfactory cortical projection areas of male patients with schizophrenia: An initial positron emission tomography study. *Psychiatry Res.* **60,** 13–116.

Bird, S., and Gower, D. B. (1982). Axillary 5-alpha-androst-16-en-3-one, cholesterol and squalene in men: Preliminary evidence for 5-alpha-androst-16-en-3-one being a product of bacterial action. *J. Steroidal Biochem.* **17,** 517–522.

Bleuler, M. (1954). Endokrinologische Psychiatrie. Thieme, Stuttgart.

Bradley, E. A. (1984). Olfactory acuity to a pheromonal substance and psychotic illness. *Biol. Psychiatry* **19,** 899–905.

Brewer, W. J., Castle, D., and Pantelis, C. (2006). Olfaction and the Brain. Cambridge University Press, Melbourne.

Brewer, W. J., Edwards, J., Anderson, V., Robinson, T., and Pantelis, C. (1996). Neuropsychological, olfactory, and hygiene deficits in men with negative symptom schizophrenia. *Biol. Psychiatry* **40,** 1021–1031.

Brewer, W. J., Pantelis, C., Anderson, V., Velakoulis, D., Singh, B., Copolov, D. L., *et al.* (2001). Stability of olfactory identification deficits in neuroleptic-naive patients with first episode psychosis. *Am. J. Psychiatry* **158,** 107–115.

Brewer, W. J., Wood, S. J., McGorry, P. D., Francey, S. M., Phillips, L. J., Yung, A., *et al.* (2003). Impaired olfactory identification in individuals at ultra-high risk for psychosis who later develop schizophrenia. *Am. J. Psychiatry* **160,** 1790–1794.

Brewer, W. J., Pantelis, C., De Luca, C., and Wood, S. J. (2006). Olfactory processing and brain maturation. *In* "Olfaction and the Brain," (W. Brewer, D. Castle, and C. Pantelis, Eds.). Cambridge University Press, New York.

Brewer, W. J., Wood, S. J., Pantelis, C., Berger, G., Copolov, D. L., and McGorry, P. D. (2007). Olfactory sensitivity through the course of psychosis: Relationships to olfactory identification, symptomatology and the schizophrenia odour. *Psychiatry Res.* **149,** 97–104.

Brooksbank, B. W. L. (1962). Urinary excretion of androst-16-en-3-alpha-ol levels in normal subjects, and effects of treatment with trophic hormones. *J. Endocrinol.* **24,** 435–444.

Brooksbank, B. W. L., and Pryse-Phillips, W. (1964). Urinary alpha-16-androsten-3alpha-ol, 17-oxosteroids and mental illness. *BMJ* **20,** 1602–1606.

Brooksbank, B. W. L., Brown, R., and Gustafsson, J. A. (1974). The detection of 5-alpha-androst-16-en-3alpha-ol in human male axillary sweat. *Experientia* **30**(8), 864–865.

Broverman, D. M., Klaiber, E. L., Kobayahi, Y., and Vogel, W. (1968). Roles of activation and inhibition in sex differences in cognitive abilities. *Psychol. Rev.* **75,** 23–50.

Cain, W. S., Stevens, J. C., Nickou, C., *et al.* (1995). Life-span development of odor identification, learning and olfactory sensitivity. *Perception* **24,** 1457–1472.

Charney, W. (1966). Transformation of steroids by corynebacteriaceae. *J. Appl. Bacteriol.* **29,** 93–106.

Clark, T. O., and Ball, R. (1983). Sensitivities to five putative human pheromones in a population of young male service recruits. Mimeograph. From *Pharmabulletin* **80**, Health Commission of Victoria: Publisher.

Claus, R., and Alsing, W. (1976). Occurrence of 5-alpha-androst-16-en-3-one, a boar pheromone, in man and its relationship to testosterone. *J. Endocrinol.* **68,** 483–484.

Compton, M. T., McKenzie Mack, L., Esterberg, M. L., Bercu, Z., Kryda, A. D., Quintero, L., Weiss, P. S., and Walker, E. F. (2006). Associations between olfactory identification and verbal memory in patients with schizophrenia, first-degree relatives, and non-psychiatric controls. *Schizophr. Res.* **86**(1-3), 154–166, [Epub 2006 Jul 17].

Corcoran, C., Whitaker, A., Coleman, E., Fried, J., Feldman, J., Goudsmit, N., and Malaspina, D. (2005). Olfactory deficits, cognition and negative symptoms in early onset psychosis. *Schizophr. Res.* **80**(2-3), 283–293, [Epub 2005 Aug 26].

Dorries, K. M., Schmidt, H. J., Beauchamp, G. K., *et al.* (1989). Changes in sensitivity to the odor of androstenone during adolescence. *Dev. Psychobiol.* **22,** 423–425.

Doty, R. (1977). Chemical communication on sex and reproductive state in humans. *In* "Chemical Signals in Vertebrates," (D. Muller-Schwarze and M. M. Mozell, Eds.), Vol. 7, pp. 273–286. Plenum Press, New York.

Doty, R., Shaman, P., and Dann, W. (1984). Development of the University of Pennsylvania Smell Test: Standardised micro-encapsulated test of olfactory function. *Physiol. Behav.* **32,** 489–502.

Eslinger, P. J., Damasio, A. R., and Van Hoesen, G. W. (1982). Olfactory dysfunction in man: Anatomical and behavioral aspects. *Brain Cogn.* **1**(3), 259–285.

Geddes, J., Huws, R., and Pratt, P. (1991). Olfactory acuity in the positive and negative symptoms of schizophrenia. *Biol. Psychiatry* **29,** 774–778.

Good, K. P., Whitehorn, D., Rui, Q., Milliken, H., and Kopala, L. C. (2006). Olfactory identification deficits in first-episode psychosis may predict patients at risk for persistent negative and disorganized or cognitive symptoms. *Am. J. Psychiatry.* **163**(5), 932–933.

Gower, D. B., and Bicknell, D. C. (1972). Steroid excretion and biosynthesis, with special reference to 16-unsaturated C 19 steroids, in cases of testicular feminization and in a male pseudohermaphrodite. *Acta Endocrinol.* **70,** 567–581.

Gower, D. B., Bird, P. S., and House, F. R. (1985). Axillary 5-alpha-androst-16-en-3-one in men and women: Relationships with olfactory acuity to odorous 16-androstenes. *Experientia* **41,** 1134–1136.

Greer, F. R., Marshall, S., Cherry, J., and Suttie, J. W. (1991). Vitamin K status of lactating mothers, human milk, and breast-feeding infants. *Pediatrics.* **88**(4), 751–756.

Griffiths, N., and Patterson, R. (1970). Human olfactory responses to 5-alpha-androst-16-en-3-one: Principle component of boar taint. *J. Sci. Food Agric.* **21,** 4–6.

Gross-Isseroff, R., Luca-Haimovici, K., Sasson, Y., Kindler, S., and Zohar, J. (1994). Olfactory sensitivity in major depressive disorder and obsessive compulsive disorder. *Biol. Psychiatry* **53,** 798–802.

Hampson, E., and Kimura, D. (1992). Sex differences and hormonal influences on cognitive function in humans. *In* "Behavioral Endocrinology," (J. B. Becker, S. M. Breedlove, and D. Crews, Eds.). MIT Press.

Harrison, P. J., and Pearson, R. C. A. (1989). Olfaction and psychiatry. *Br. J. Psychiatry* **155,** 822–828.

Hubert, H. B., Fabsitz, R. R., Feinlab, M., and Brown, K. S. (1980).*Science* **208,** 608–609.

Hubert, H. B., Fabsitz, R. R., Brown, K. S., and Feinlab, M. (1981). *In* "Twin Research 3: Epidemiological and Clinical Studies," (L. Gedda, P. Parise, and W. E. Nance, Eds.), pp. 97–103. Liss, New York.

Isseroff, R. G., Stoler, M., Ophir, D., Lancet, D., and Sirota, P. (1987). Olfactory sensitivity to androstenone in schizophrenic patients. *Biol. Psychiatry* **22,** 922–925.

Jackman, P. J. H. (1982). Taxonomy of Aerobic Axillary Coryneforms Based on Electrophoretic Protein Patterns Unpublished PhD Thesis, University of London.

Jackman, P. J. H., and Noble, W. C. (1983). Normal axillary skin microflora in various populations. *Clin. Exp. Dermatol.* **8,** 259–268.

Jackson, H. J. (1987). Negative Symptoms and Social Skills Performance in Schizophrenia Unpublished Thesis for Master of Arts Degree, University of Melbourne, Victoria.

Jones-Gotman, M. (1991). Localisation of lesions by neuropsychological testing. *Epilepsia* **32**(Supp. 5), S41–S52.

Jones-Gotman, M., and Zatorre, R. J. (1988). Olfactory identification deficits in patients with focal cerebral excision. *Neuropsychologia* **26,** 387–400.

Kandel, E. R., Schwartz, J. H., and Jessell, T. M. (1991). Principles of Neural Science. 3rd edn. Elsevier, London.

Kloek, J. (1961). The smell of some steroid sex-hormones and their metabolites. *Psychiatry, Neurol. Neurochem.* **64,** 309–344.

Kloos, W. E., and Musselwhite, M. S. (1975). Distribution and persistence of staphylococcus and micrococcus species and other aerobic bacteria on human skin. *Appl. Microbiol.* **30,** 381–395.

Koelega, H. S. (1994). Prepubescent children may have specific deficits in olfactory sensitivity. *Percep. Motor Skills* **78,** 191–199.

Koelega, H. S., and Koster, E. P. (1974). Some experiments on sex differences in odor perception. *Ann. NY Acad. Sci.* **237,** 234–246.

Kopala, L., and Clark, C. (1990). Implications of olfactory agnosia for understanding sex differences in schizophrenia. *Schizophr. Bull.* **16,** 255–261.

Kopala, L., Clark, C., and Hurwitz, T. A. (1989). Sex differences in olfactory function in schizophrenia. *Am. J. Psychiatry* **146,** 1320–1322.

Kopala, L., Clark, C., and Hurwitz, T. (1992). Olfactory deficits in neuroleptic naive patients with schizophrenia. *Schizophr. Res.* **8,** 245–250.

Kopala, L. C., Good, K. P., and Honer, W. G. (1994a). Olfactory hallucinations and olfactory identification ability in patients with schizophrenia and other psychiatric disorders. *Schizophr. Res.* **12,** 205–211.

Kopala, L. C., Good, K. P., and Honer, W. G. (1994b). Olfactory identification ability in pre- and postmenopausal women with schizophrenia. *Biol. Psychiatry* **38,** 57–63.

Kopala, L. C., Good, K., Martzke, J., and Hurwitz, T. (1995). Olfactory deficits in schizophrenia are not a function of task complexity. *Schizophr. Res.* **17,** 195–199.

Kopala, L. C., Good, K. P., Koczapski, A. B., and Honer, W. G. (1998). Olfactory deficits in patients with schizophrenia and severe polydipsia. *Biol. Psychiatry* **43,** 497–502.

Kopala, L. C., Good, K. P., Morrison, K., Bassett, A. S., Alda, M., and Honer, W. G. (2001). Impaired olfactory identification in relatives of patients with familial schizophrenia. *Am. J. Psychiatry*. **158**(8), 1286–1290.

Larsson, M., and Backman, L. (1997). Age-related differences in episodic odour recognition: The role of access to specific odour names. *Memory* **5**(3), 361–378.

Le Magnen, J. (1952). Les phenomenes olfacto-sexuels chez le rat blanc. *Arch. Sci. Physiol. (Paris)* **6,** 295–332.

Leydon, J. J., McGinley, K. J., Holzle, E., Labows, J. N., and Kligman, A. M. (1981). The microbiology of the human axilla and its relationship to axillary odor. *J. Invest Dermatol.* **77,** 413–416.

Liddell, K. (1976). Smell as a diagnostic marker. *Postgrad. Med. J.* **52,** 136–138.

Malaspina, D., and Coleman, E. (2003). Olfaction and social drive in schizophrenia. *Arch. Gen. Psychiatry*. **60**(6), 578–584.

Martzke, J. S., Kopala, L. C., and Good, K. P. (1997). Olfactory dysfunction in neuropsychiatric disorders: Review and methodological considerations. *Biol. Psychiatry* **42,** 721–732.

McGlashan, T. H., and Hoffman, R. E. (2000). Schizophrenia as a disorder of developmentally reduced synaptic connectivity. *Arch. Gen. Psychiatry*. **57**(7), 637–648.

Melrose, D. R., Reed, H. C. B., and Patterson, R. L. S. (1971). Androgen steroids associated with boar odour as an aid to the detection of oestrus in pig artificial insemination. *Br. Vet. J.* **127,** 497–502.

Moberg, P. J., Agrin, R., Gur, R. E., Gur, R. C., Turetsky, B. I., and Doty, R. L. (1999). Olfactory dysfunction in schizophrenia: A qualitative and quantitative review. *Neuropsychopharmacol* **21,** 325–340.

Moberg, P. J., Arnold, S. E., Doty, R. L., Gur, R. E., Balderston, C. C., Roalf, D. R., Gur, R. C., Kohler, C. G., Kanes, S. J., Siegel, S. J., and Turetsky, B. I. (2006). Olfactory functioning in schizophrenia: Relationship to clinical, neuropsychological, and volumetric MRI measures. *J. Clin. Exp. Neuropsychol.* **28**(8), 1444–1461.

Moberg, P. J., Roalf, B. S., GUr, R. E., and Turetsky, B. I. (2004). Smaller nasal volumes as stigmata of aberrant neurodevelopment in schizophrenia. *Am. J. Psychiatry* **161,** 2314–2316.

Mozley, P. D., Stubbs, J. B., Kim, H. J., McElgin, W., Chumpradit, S., Kung, M. P., Romaniello, G., and Kung, H. F. (1995). Dosimetry of a D2/D3 dopamine receptor antagonist that can be used with PET or SPECT. *J. Nucl. Med.* **36**(7), 1322–1331.

Pantelis, C., and Brewer, W. J. (1995). Neuropsychological and olfactory dysfunction in schizophrenia: Relationship of frontal syndromes to syndromes of schizophrenia. *Schizophr. Res.* **17,** 35–45.

Pantelis, C., and Brewer, W. J. (1996). Neurocognitive and neurobehavioral patterns and the syndromes of schizophrenia: Role of frontal-subcortical networks. *In* "Schizophrenia: A Neuropsychological Perspective," (C. Pantelis, H. E. Nelson, and T. R. E. Barnes, Eds.), pp. 317–343. John Wiley & Sons, Chichester.

Pantelis, C., Barnes, T. R. E., and Nelson, H. E. (1992). Is the concept of frontal-subcortical dementia relevant to schizophrenia? *Br. J. Psychiatry* **160,** 442–450.

Potter, H., and Butters, N. (1980). An assessment of olfactory deficits in patients with damage to prefrontal cortex. *Neuropsychologia* **18,** 621–628.

Qureshy, A., Kawashima, R., Imran, M. B., Sugiura, M., Goto, R., Okada, K., Inoue, K., Itoh, M., Schormann, T., Zilles, K., and Fukuda, H. (2000). Functional mapping of human brain in olfactory processing: A PET study. *J. Neurophysiol.* **84**(3), 1656–1666.

Rausch, R., and Serafetinides, E. A. (1975). Specific alterations of olfactory function in humans with temporal lobe lesions. *Nature* **255,** 557–558.

Reiss, M. (1958). Psychoendocrinology. Grune and Stratton, New York.

Rennie, P. J., Gower, D. B., and Holland, K. T. (1991). In vitro and in vivo studies of human axillary odor and the cutaneous micro-flora. *Br. J. Dermatol.* **124,** 596–602.

Richman, R. A., Post, E. M., Sheehe, P. R., *et al.* (1995). Olfactory performance during childhood I. Development of an odourant identification test for children. *J. Pediatr.* **121,** 908–911.

Sands, D. E. (1957). *In* "Schizophrenia: Somatic Aspects," (D. Richter, Ed.), p. 77. Pergamon, London.

Schall, B. (1988). Olfaction in infants and children: Developmental and functional perspectives. *Chem. Senses* **13,** 145–190.

Schall, B., Marlier, L., and Soussignan, R. (1998). Olfactory function in the human fetus: Evidence from selective neonatal responsiveness to the odor of amniotic fluid. *Behav. Neurosci.* **112**(6), 1438–1449.

Schneider, F., Habel, U., Reske, M., Toni, I., Falkai, P., and Shah, J. (2007). Neural substrates of olfactory processing in schizophrenia patients and their healthy relatives. *Psychiatry Res.* **155,** 103–112.

Schneider, R. A. (1971). Newer insights into the role and modification of olfaction in man through clinical studies. *Ann. NY Acad. Sci.* **237,** 217–223.

Seidman, L. J., Talbot, N. L., Kalinowski, A. G., McCarley, R. W., Faraone, S. V., Kremen, W. S., Pepple, J. R., and Tsuang, M. T. (1992). Neuropsychological probes of fronto-limbic system dysfunction in schizophrenia: Olfactory identification and Wisconsin Card Sorting performance. *Schizophr. Res.* **6,** 55–65.

Seidman, L. J., Yurgelun-Todd, D., Kremen, W. S., Woods, B. T., Goldstein, J. M., Faraone, S. V., and Tsuang, M. T. (1994). Relationship of prefrontal and temporal lobe MRI measures to neuropsychological performance in chronic schizophrenia. *Biol. Psychiatry* **35,** 235–246.

Serby, M. (2009). Odor detection in schizophrenia: Alternative explanations. (Letter to the Editor). *Am. J. Psychiatry* **166,** 727.

Serby, M., Larson, P., and Kalkstein, D. (1990). Olfactory senses in psychoses. *Biol. Psychiatry* **28,** 829–830.

Shehadeh, N., and Kligman, A. M. (1963). The bacteria responsible for axillary odour. II. *J. Invest. Dermatol.* **41,** 3.

Skinner, K., Smith, K., and Rich, E. (1964). Bacteria and the "schizophrenic odor". *Arch. Gen. Psychiatry* 64, Abstracts.

Smith, K., and Sines, J. O. (1960). Demonstration of a peculiar odour in the sweat of schizophrenic patients. *Arch. Gen. Psychiatry* **2,** 184–188.

Smith, K., Thompson, G. F., and Koster, H. D. (1969). Sweat in schizophrenic patients: Identification of odorous substance. *Science* **166,** 398–399.

Snowdon, J. (1987). Uncleanliness among persons seen by community health workers. *Hosp. Commun. Psychiatry* **38**(5), 491–495.

Stoddart, D. M. (1976). Mammalian Odours and Pheromones. Camelot Press, Southampton.

Strauss, E. L. (1970). A study on olfactory acuity. *Ann. Otol. Rhinol. Laryngol.* **79**(1), 95–104.

Trimble, M. R. (1987). The neurology of schizophrenia. *Br. Med. Bull.* **43,** 616–633.

Turetsky, B. I., and Moberg, P. J. (2009a). An odor-specific threshold deficit implicates abnormal intracellular cyclic AMP signalling in schizophrenia. *Am. J. Psychiatry* **166,** 226–233.

Turetsky, B. I., and Moberg, P. J. (2009b). Letter to the Editor (Reply). *Am. J. Psychiatry* **166,** 728.

Turetsky, B. I., Kohler, C. G., Gur, R. E., and Moberg, P. J. (2008). Olfactory physiological impairment in first-degree relatives of schizophrenia patients. *Schizophr. Res.* **102,** 220–229.

Turetsky, B. I., Crutchley, P. C., Walker, J., Gur, R. E., and Moberg, P. J. (2009a). Depth of the olfactory sulcus: A marker of early embryonic disruption in schizophrenia? *Schizophr. Res.* **115,** 8–11.

Turetsky, B. I., Hahn, C., Borgmann-Winter, K., and Moberg, P. J. (2009b). Scents and nonsense: Olfactory dysfunction in schizophrenia. *Schizophr. Bull.* **35**(6), 1117–1131.

Van Toller, C., Kirk-Smith, M., Wood, N., Lombard, J., and Dodd, G. H. (1983). Skin conductance and subjective assessments associated with the odour of 5-alpha-androstanon-3-one. *Biol. Psychiatry* **16,** 85–107.

Varney, N. R. (1988). Prognostic significance of anosmia in patients with closed-head trauma. *J. Clin. Exp. Neuropsychol.* **10**(2), 250–254.

Wiener, H. (1966). External chemical messengers. I. Emission and reception in man. *NY State J. Med.* **Dec 15,** 3153–3171.

Wiener, H. (1967). External chemical messengers, II. Natural history of schizophrenia. *NY State J. Med.* **May 1,** 1144–1151.

Wu, J., Buschbaum, M. S., Moy, K., Denlea, N., Kesslak, P., Tseng, H., Plosnaj, D., Hetu, M., Potkin, S., Bracha, S., and Cotman, C. (1993). Olfactory memory in unmedicated schizophrenics. *Schizophr. Res.* **9,** 41–47.

Wysocki, C. J., and Beauchamp, G. K. (1984). Ability to smell androstenone is genetically determined. *Proc. Natl. Acad. Sci. USA* **81,** 4899–4902.

Wysocki, C. J., and Gilbert, A. N. (1987). National Geographic Smell Survey: The effects of age are heterogeneous. In Part 1. Characterisation of chemosensory changes in aging. *Ann. NY Acad. Sci.* 12–28.

Wysocki, C. J., Dorries, K, M., and Beauchamp, G. K. (1989). Ability to perceive androstenone can be acquired by ostensibly anosmic people. *P. Nat. Acad. Sci.* **86,** 7976–7978.

Zatorre, R. J., Jones-Gotman, M., Evans, A. C., and Meyer, E. (1992). Functional localisation and lateralisation of human olfactory cortex. *Nature* **360,** 339–340.

CHAPTER FOURTEEN

Olfactory Systems in Mate Recognition and Sexual Behavior

Matthieu Keller,[*,†,‡] Delphine Pillon,[*,†,‡] *and* Julie Bakker[§,¶,#]

Contents

Abstract

Olfactory signals play an important role so that breeding efforts are synchronized with appropriate social and environmental circumstances. In this context, the mammalian olfactory system is characterized by the existence of several olfactory subsystems that have evolved to process olfactory information. While the vomeronasal (or accessory) olfactory system is usually conceived as being involved in the processing of pheromonal signals due to its close connections

* INRA, UMR 85 Physiologie de la Reproduction et des Comportements, Nouzilly, France
† CNRS, UMR 6175, Nouzilly, France
‡ Université François Rabelais de Tours, Tours, France
§ Neuroendocrinologie du Comportement, GIGA-Neurosciences, University of Liège, Belgium
¶ Netherlands Institute for Neuroscience, Amsterdam, The Netherlands
# Medical Center, Vrije Universiteit, Amsterdam, The Netherlands

Vitamins and Hormones, Volume 83
ISSN 0083-6729, DOI: 10.1016/S0083-6729(10)83014-6

with the reproductive hypothalamus, the main olfactory system is, by contrast, considered as a general analyzer of volatile chemosignals, especially those that are used for the social identification of conspecifics. In fact, several recent sets of experiments suggest that both the main and accessory olfactory systems have the ability to process partly overlapping pheromonal chemosignals and that both systems converge at a downstream level of pheromonal processing. As a consequence, both systems have the ability to support complimentary aspects in mate discrimination and sexual behavior. However, the relative roles played by these systems and their interactions are at present still far from being understood.

I. Introduction

In order to maximize reproductive success, animals have evolved neural and endocrine mechanisms to coordinate breeding efforts with appropriate social and environmental circumstances. Among the social factors that influence mammalian reproductive function, olfaction is probably the most widespread and powerful. Indeed, chemical cues called pheromones are used to communicate species-specific information that modulates the reproductive behavior or physiology of the receiver individual. Pheromones have been shown to act as major regulators of all stages of reproductive behavior, including mating (Keller *et al.*, 2009), mother–young interactions at birth (Lévy and Keller, 2009; Lévy *et al.*, 2004), or sexual maturation (Vandenbergh, 1969). In the context of sexual behavior, pheromones are required to identify suitable mating partner or to trigger subsequent sexual motivation and copulatory behavior (Keller *et al.*, 2008).

In this review, we will refer to pheromones as chemosignals produced and released by individuals and processed by individuals of the same species and leading to short-term behavioral changes or more long-term physiological changes in the receiver individual (Karlson and Luscher, 1959). Although this rather simple definition is usually well accepted and shared, leading us to use the concept in a wide variety of contexts, readers should be aware that the concept is however controversial and that much more restrictive definitions can be sometimes used (Beauchamp *et al.*, 1976 or see reviews such as Brennan and Zufall, 2006 or Wyatt, 2003 for detailed analysis of current concepts and definitions related to pheromones). As a consequence, some of the examples depicted as being pheromonal effects may not always be shared by some investigators.

In addition, pheromones, as other olfactory chemosignals, are processed by the olfactory system. Interestingly, one of the specificity of the olfactory system, in comparison to other sensory systems, is the existence of various subsystems involved in the detection and processing of chemosignals

(Munger *et al.*, 2009; Tirindelli *et al.*, 2009). These olfactory subsystems have evolved so that they differ in their molecular/genetic basis, in their peripheral and central anatomy as well as in their function. However, these systems may also have complimentary roles in sustaining pheromone-dependent behaviors (for review please refer to Baum and Kelliher, 2009; Keller *et al.*, 2009; Kelliher, 2007). Therefore, an old-standing question in the field is to know the relative involvement of each of these subsystems in the control of pheromone-dependent behaviors. Among the various olfactory subsystems that have been identified so far, the main and the accessory (or vomeronasal) olfactory systems are probably the best characterized and even if a growing number of studies have shown the existence of other olfactory subsystems, namely the Gruenberg ganglion or the septal organ of Masera, little is currently known about their involvement in the control of reproductive behaviors (Munger *et al.*, 2009). As a consequence, this review will only concentrate on the relative roles of both main and accessory olfactory systems in mammalian mate discrimination and sexual behavior.

II. A Short Introduction to the Organization of the Accessory and Main Olfactory Subsystems

A. Architecture of the main olfactory system

In the main olfactory system (MOS), chemosignals are detected by olfactory receptors inserted into the plasma membrane of ciliated olfactory sensory neurons which are located in the main olfactory epithelium (MOE), lying at the end of the nasal cavity. Olfactory receptors are G protein–coupled seven transmembrane proteins encoded by approximately 1000 genes in rodents, thus forming the largest gene family in mammals (Buck and Axel, 1991). Beside olfactory receptors, another family of olfactory receptors, the trace amine associated-receptors, has been more recently identified in the MOE (Liberles and Buck, 2006). Readers interested in the genetic and molecular organization of olfactory detection and processing could refer to recent exhaustive reviews (Munger *et al.*, 2009; Tirindelli *et al.*, 2009).

MOE sensory neurons project their axons through the cribriform plate to the glomeruli of the main olfactory bulb (MOB), in which they make synapse with dendrites of mitral/tufted cells. In these MOB glomeruli, MOE sensory projections are precisely organized so that sensory neurons expressing a given odorant receptor send their axons to a few converging glomeruli with a fixed topographical localization (Buck, 2000). The mitral and tufted cells abutting these MOB glomeruli then transmit olfactory signals to various forebrain and limbic targets including the piriform or

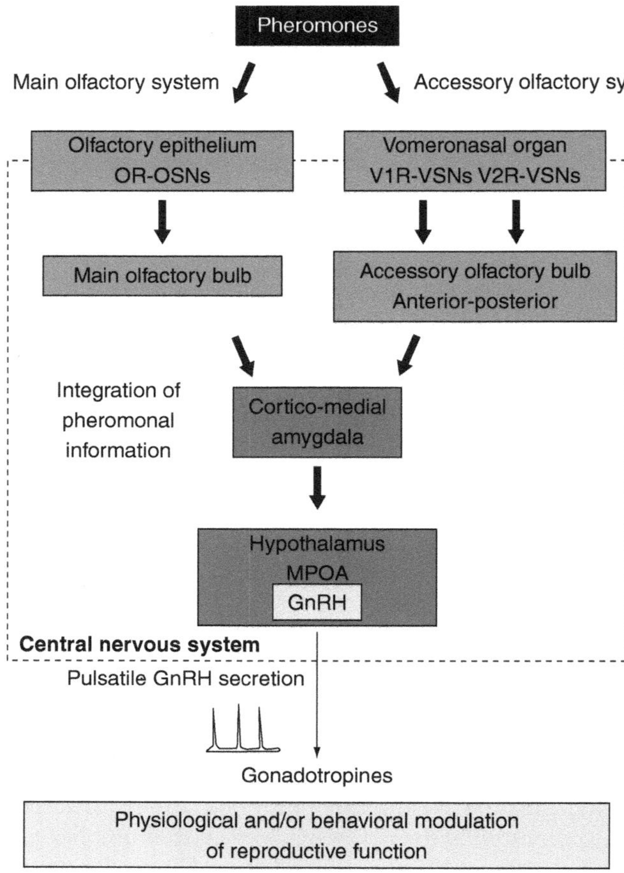

Figure 14.1 Schematic organization of mammalian main and accessory olfactory systems and their connections with the reproductive system at the level of GnRH neurons located in the reproductive hypothalamus.

the entorhinal cortices as well as the anterior cortical nucleus of the amygdala (Scalia and Winans, 1975, Fig. 14.1).

B. Neuroanatomical organization of the accessory olfactory system

The organization of the accessory olfactory system (AOS) differs widely, from a neuroanatomical perspective, in comparison to the one observed in the MOS. Indeed, the AOS is more closely related to the reproductive hypothalamus, thus being able to influence more long-term neuroendocrine or physiological changes. In this context, classical pheromonal effects mediated through the AOS include various examples impacting reproductive function such as modulation of puberty onset (Drickamer and Hoover, 1979; Vandenbergh, 1969), changes in estrus cyclicity (Whitten, 1956) or pregnancy block during the first stages of pregnancy (Brennan, 2009; Bruce, 1959).

In the AOS, the very first stage of pheromone detection takes place at the level of sensory neurons that are found in the vomeronasal organ (VNO; Fig. 14.1). The VNO is a sort of blind-ended tube that is running along the basis of the nasal septum and which opens via a narrow duct into the nasal cavity or into the mouth depending on species. Pheromones gain access to the lumen of the VNO by a vascular pumping mechanism activated once aroused animals investigate the olfactory source through direct physical contact (Meredith, 1994; Meredith and O'Connell, 1979). Once pheromones are pumped in the lumen of the VNO, pheromones then interact with vomeronasal receptors located on the membrane of VNO sensory neurons. These vomeronasal receptors have been classified in two distinct families: the vomeronasal type 1 (V1Rs) and type 2 (V2Rs) receptors (Munger *et al.*, 2009; Tirindelli *et al.*, 2009). The processing of pheromonal information through the vomeronasal system is obviously complex as it is segregated into two parallel streams. Indeed, both types of V1Rs- and V2Rs-sensory neurons are expressed in excluding regions of the VNO: while V1Rs-sensory neurons are expressed in the apical part of the VNO, near the lumen, V2Rs-sensory neurons are expressed in the more basal region (Brennan, 2004).

Such segregated organization between both streams of pheromonal information is conserved one step downstream at the level of the accessory olfactory bulb (AOB), where vomeronasal sensory neurons project their axons. Indeed, V1Rs-sensory neurons send projections exclusively to the rostral AOB, while V2Rs-sensory neurons project to its caudal part. This topographical segregation is thought to sustain functional differences as both AOB regions respond differentially to pheromonal stimuli in mice (Brennan *et al.*, 1999; Halem *et al.*, 2001). Finally, it has been shown that AOB mitral cells are only activated when mice contact various regions of the body of an anesthetized stimulus female, thus providing further support to the notion that the vomeronasal system is activated when animals investigate directly pheromonal source (Luo *et al.*, 2003).

When leaving the AOB, mitral cells project to the medial nucleus of the amygdala, where the pheromonal informations processed segregated so far (rostral versus caudal parts of the vomeronasal pathway) express some degree of convergence into partly overlapping projections (Von Campenhausen and Mori, 2000). Olfactory information reaches then various hypothalamic and limbic regions highly involved in the regulation of reproductive function and behavior. These regions include especially the bed nucleus of the stria terminalis (BnST), the medial preoptic area (MPOA), and the ventromedial hypothalamus (VMN; Scalia and Winans, 1975).

C. Main and accessory olfactory pathways impact partly overlapping neuroanatomical targets in limbic or hypothalamic structures

As exposed shortly above, both olfactory systems exhibit segregated detection and projection pathways at both peripheral (olfactory sensory neurons) and more central (olfactory bulbs) levels. However, a certain degree of convergence is observed between the two systems at the level of the cortical-medial amygdala (Gomez and Newman, 1992; Kevetter and Winans, 1981a,b; Meredith, 1991, 1998). Indeed, electrophysiological responses have been recorded in response to electrical stimulations of both the MOB and VNO at the single cell level (Licht and Meredith, 1987), thus suggesting that pheromonal signals mediated through both systems could interact and then impact the downstream network involved in the regulation of sexual behavior and including the BnST, MPOA, or VMN. In a reproductive context, another important site of cellular convergence of both olfactory systems is the gonadotropin-releasing hormone (GnRH) neurons that are found scattered in the MPOA. Indeed, it is widely accepted that the effects of pheromones on reproductive function are mainly mediated by GnRH neurons which represent the final output pathway of the neuronal network controlling fertility in all mammalian species. Several sets of experiments have now clearly demonstrated that both the vomeronasal and main olfactory subsystems project (at least indirectly) to GnRH neurons (Boehm *et al.*, 2005), and various experiments suggest that pheromonal signals processed through these systems have the potential to activate these neurons (Coquelin *et al.*, 1984; Meredith and Fewell, 2001; Pfeiffer and Johnston, 1994; Westberry and Meredith, 2003a,b).

III. Both MOS and AOS Are Functionally Involved in Pheromonal Processing

The vomeronasal system is usually considered as the main focus for pheromonal research due to its close connection with the reproductive hypothalamus and is therefore conceived to mediate the physiological and neuroendocrine changes induced by pheromones. For example, lesioning any level of the vomeronasal pathway has been consistently shown to disrupt pheromonal effects such as puberty acceleration or pregnancy block (Bellringer *et al.*, 1980; Lloyd-Thomas and Keverne, 1982; Lomas and Keverne, 1982). Using both *in vitro* electrophysiological and imaging methods, several groups have demonstrated that VNO sensory neurons can express very low threshold responses to various volatile pheromones (Del Punta *et al.*, 2002; Leinders-Zufall *et al.*, 2000). It is debatable whether these volatiles can have freely access to the VNO in the airstream and it is generally thought that they have to be transported into the VNO lumen, when the animals contact the pheromonal source, by carrier proteins belonging to the lipocalin family (Wysocki *et al.*, 1980). Some members of this family, including the major urinary proteins (MUPs; Hurst *et al.*, 2001) are now well characterized. Interestingly, these carrier proteins are also thought to serve by themselves for individual recognition, due to their high degree of polymorphism and their ability to stimulate the expression of the immediate early gene egr-1 in specific regions of the AOB (Brennan *et al.*, 1999; Hurst *et al.*, 2001). Other example of rather nonvolatile pheromonal signal processed by the vomeronasal system includes the male-specific exocrine gland-secreting peptide 1 which is secreted from the extraorbital lacrimal gland. This peptide is transferred through direct contact to the female VNO, where it stimulates V2R-expressing vomeronasal sensory neurons and elicits sex-specific electrophysiological response (Kimoto *et al.*, 2005). As a whole, these data suggest that the VNO has the ability to process a wide set of both volatile and peptide- or protein-related pheromonal chemosignals.

The case of the pregnancy block effect (also known as the Bruce effect) is a good example illustrating how pheromones detected by the AOS are able to induce long-term changes in the reproductive axis (Fig. 14.2). Indeed, the pregnancy block effects result from a neuroendocrine reflex triggered by the exposure of recently mated female mice to chemosignals from an unfamiliar male. The effect of male chemosignals on pregnancy is mediated by the suppression of prolactin release from the pituitary, due to increased dopamine release from neurons in the hypothalamic arcuate nucleus (Brennan, 2009). Prolactin is luteotrophic in mice, and thus reduction in prolactin blood levels results in failure of the corpora lutea. The consequent reduction in circulating progesterone levels prevents embryo implantation and thus terminates pregnancy and induces a return into estrus.

Beside the role of the AOS in pheromonal communication, it has also been known for a long time that the MOS has the ability to detect and process various pheromones. Indeed, the MOS is involved in the processing of volatile pheromonal signals related to social attraction and recognition, thus allowing animals to discriminate conspecifics according to their reproductive status. Indeed, urine consists of a mixture of distinct chemicals that vary, among others, according to the sex or physiology of the emitter (Andreolini *et al.*, 1987; Jemiolo *et al.*, 1989). For example, the volatile urinary compound (methylthio)-methanethiol (MTMT), that is present in male mice urine, activates a subset of mitral cells in the female MOB, and enhances female attractiveness of gonadectomized male urine when added to it (Lin *et al.*, 2005, Fig. 14.3). The MOS is also involved in the processing of the volatile steroid androstenone which is found in boar saliva and triggers tonic immobilization when detected by receptive sows (Dorries *et al.*, 1995, 1997).

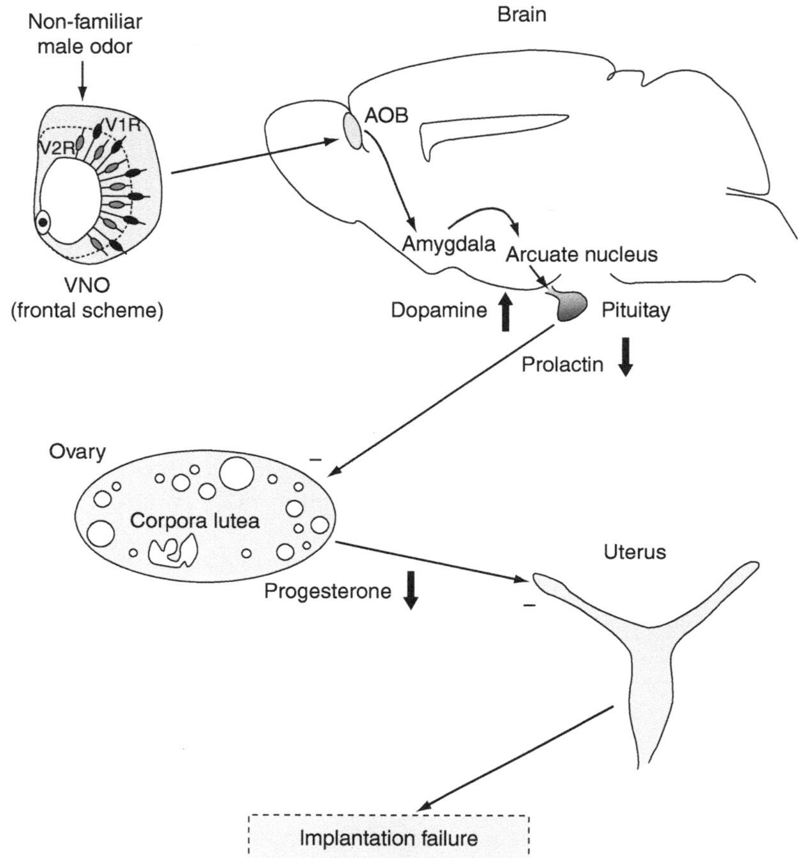

Figure 14.2 Schematic in the pregnancy block effect in mice. Exposure to the odor of an unfamiliar male triggers a neuroendocrine reflex leading to implantation failure. Unfamiliar male odor is processed by the vomeronasal organ, the accessory olfactory bulb, and finally the arcuate nucleus where it induces a decrease in prolactin secretion from the pituitary. The reduction in circulating prolactin results in failure of the corpora lutea and the consequent reduction in circulating progesterone levels prevents embryo implantation and thus terminates pregnancy and induces a return into estrus

This volatile chemosignal still produces its effect in sows having their VNO blocked, thus demonstrating that androstenone is detected and processed by the MOS. The MOS is also involved in the processing of male pheromones in the context of the male effect in sheep. This pheromonal effect is characterized by a reactivation of the whole gonadotropic axis in ewes exposed to ram pheromones during the seasonal period of anestrous (Cohen-Tannoudji *et al.*, 1989; Delgadillo *et al.*, 2009; Gelez and Fabre-Nys, 2004). In this example again, lesioning the AOS does not affect the LH and ovulatory

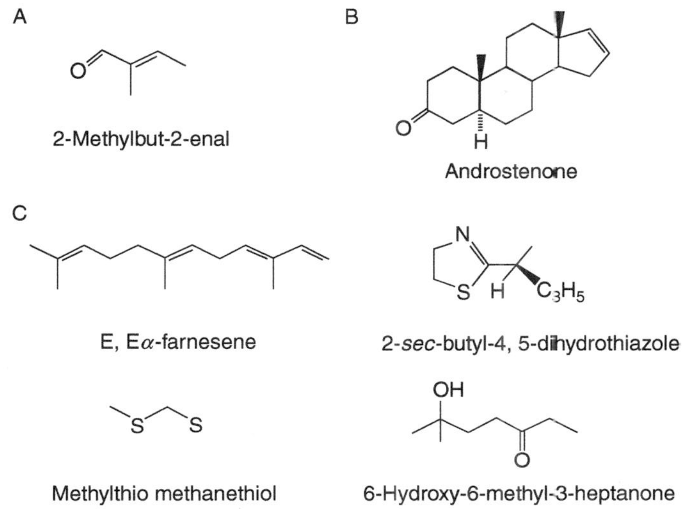

Figure 14.3 A few examples of mammalian pheromones involved in the control of mate recognition and sexual behavior. (A) 2-Methylbut-2-enal, the rabbit mammary pheromone that is released in the milk of the female rabbit and triggers the stereotyped nipple-search behavior. (B) Androstenone is released from the boar saliva and induces tonic immobility in receptive sow. (C) Some pheromones found in male mice urine and mediating various physiological or behavioral responses in the female, including mate discrimination or puberty acceleration.

responses of the ewe to the ram. Finally, quite convincing pheromonal effects have been demonstrated in humans who do not have a functional vomeronasal system (Meredith, 2001; Wysocki and Preti, 2004). Indeed, it has been demonstrated that exposing women to axillaries extracts from women in the follicular phase of their menstrual cycle shortens the length of the recipient's menstrual cycle (Stern and McClintock, 1998). Male and female axillaries stimulations have also been demonstrated to induce changes in LH pulses and mood in recipient women (Preti *et al.*, 2003; Shinohara *et al.*, 2001). Additionally, these kind of putative pheromonal signals only induce brain activation, revealed by functional brain imaging, in human with intact main olfactory function (Savic *et al.*, 2009). Finally, women can also differentiate and even show preference for the odor of male individuals with a dissimilar MHC genetic background (i.e., a different major histocompatibility complex; Jacob *et al.*, 2002), thus giving some support to the existence of an MOS-mediated pheromonal communication in human in a reproductive context.

As a whole, the view emerging from previous examples is that each olfactory system has the ability to process specific chemosignals. However, this functional dichotomy is only schematic because sensory neurons of both systems have the ability to detect partly overlapping sets of chemosignals and to process them in parallel. Indeed, calcium imaging studies performed on *in vitro* preparation of nasal tissue have shown that some sensory neurons respond to MHC-related peptides in both the VNO and the MOE (Spehr *et al.*, 2006a). The mechanisms underlying the detection of MHC peptides by VNO or MOE sensory neurons seem however to differ between both olfactory systems. Indeed, not only do thresholds of sensory neuron responses to MHC peptides differ in both VNO and MOE (Leinders-Zufall *et al.*, 2004; Spehr *et al.*, 2006b), but their detection also depends on distinct sets of transduction mechanisms. For example, the drug 2-aminoethoxydiphenylborate is able to inhibit local field potential to MHC peptides in the VNO but not in the MOE. Another example can be illustrated with the case of the volatile 2-heptanone; its detection appears to be dependent on the Trp2 (transient receptor potential cation 2 channel) gene in the VNO, while in the MOE, detection of 2-heptanone depends on the CNGA2 (Leypold *et al.*, 2002; Lin *et al.*, 2004), a channel that is only expressed in the MOE. At the behavioral level, the processing of these same olfactory signals is apparently not redundant as specific activation of each system leads obviously to different behavioral outputs. Thus, in the AOS, MHC-class I peptides signals have been shown to be used in the context of the Bruce effect (Leinders-Zufall *et al.*, 2004) while processing of MHC-class I peptides in the MOE supports social preferences (Spehr *et al.*, 2006b), thus demonstrating that MHC processing via the MOE does not replace vomeronasal inputs.

IV. Involvement of Both Olfactory Systems in the Control of Mate Discrimination and Sexual Behavior

Sexual behavior, as many socially motivated behaviors, can be divided into two phases: a motivational phase where pheromones allow partners to attract and identify each other (mate attraction and discrimination), which is followed by a sequence of interactions leading to copulation (consummatory sexual behavior). Attraction to as well as discrimination of the opposite-sex partner is usually thought to be dependent upon the main olfactory pathway as it is conceived as a general analyzer of the numerous volatile odors present in the environment, while the AOS is thought to control copulatory behavior due to its connections with the reproductive hypothalamus (Keverne, 2004). As we will see, this dichotomy is also rather schematic and both MOS and AOS can participate to the discrimination of a potential mate as well as the control of sexual behavior, depending on situations and/or species.

A. Pheromonal control of mate discrimination

The usual conception that attraction/discrimination toward the opposite sex involves the MOS is based on the observation that olfactory sexual discrimination can be achieved from a distance, on the basis of volatile olfactory cues only (as mentioned in part II, it is usually admitted that pheromones can gain access to the VNO only after direct physical investigation of the olfactory source). Such results have been repeatedly observed in different behavioral paradigms including habituation/dishabituation tests (Baum and Keverne, 2002; Pierman *et al.*, 2006), Y-maze preference tests (Keller *et al.*, 2006a,b; Pankevich *et al.*, 2006), or olfactometer studies based on go/no-go conditioning procedures (Keller *et al.*, 2009; Wesson *et al.*, 2006). In support to these results, it has been shown at the neurobiological level that stimulation with urinary volatiles or even with specific volatile urinary compounds such as MTMT, can induce clear MOB electrophysiological responses (Lin *et al.*, 2005). In addition, other experiments using mapping of immediate early genes expression showed that stimulation with urinary volatiles induced specific activation patterns at the level of the MOB glomerular cell layer (Martel and Baum, 2007; Martel *et al.*, 2007). Finally, the involvement of the MOS in mate discrimination has been confirmed by lesion of MOE function using intranasal application of zinc sulfate or intraperitonal injections of dichlobenil, both being chemicals destroying MOE sensory neurons without damaging the vomeronasal sensory neurons (Keller *et al.*, 2006a,b; Yoon *et al.*, 2005). MOS lesion abolished the usual preference for opposite-sex olfactory cues usually observed in both sexes when tested in a Y-maze. Interestingly, the effect of zinc sulfate lesioning was not only obtained when the animals were provided with volatile stimuli only, but also when direct contact with the olfactory source was provided, thus allowing the AOS potential access to both volatile and nonvolatile olfactory cues. This latter result suggests that volatiles detected and processed through the MOS are needed for the subsequent attraction of the animal toward deposit sources. This is in line with experiments performed in OMP-ntr mice, where the enzymatic activity of a nitroreductase enzyme is able to induce specific destruction of MOE sensory neurons and as a result disrupts the ability of female mice to localize male urinary deposit in the home cage (Ma *et al.*, 2002).

Complementary to the results described above, surgical ablation of the VNO is clearly ineffective in disrupting mate discrimination in both male and female mice (Keller *et al.*, 2006c; Pankevich *et al.*, 2004, 2006). Indeed, VNO-lesioned animals can perfectly discriminate body or urinary volatiles in a habituation/dishabituation test as well as express opposite-sex preference using volatile odors. Such a lack of VNO involvement in mate discrimination has also been shown in female ferrets where VNO lesion is ineffective in disrupting opposite-sex discrimination (Woodley *et al.*, 2004).

By contrast, blocking the nares of the animals produced deficits in both male and female ferrets (Kelliher and Baum, 2001). Other evidence comes from pig where VNO duct occlusion failed to disrupt female attraction toward the boar pheromone, androstenone (Dorries *et al.*, 1997). These results demonstrating the lack of a role for the VNO in mate discrimination have been confirmed by lesions performed downstream in the AOS, at the level of the AOB (Jakupovic *et al.*, 2008; Martinez-Ricos *et al.*, 2008).

Despite these convergent results, a role for the VNO in sex discrimination and mate recognition has been claimed by studies using Trp2-KO male mice (Leypold *et al.*, 2002; Stowers *et al.*, 2002). Deletion of Trp2 results in a large reduction of electrophysiological responses in VNO sensory neurons after exposure to urinary odorants and at the behavioral level, Trp2-KO male mice show indiscriminate attempts of mounts toward male and female stimulus subjects (Leypold *et al.*, 2002; Stowers *et al.*, 2002). Based on these data, the authors concluded that the VNO is needed for mate recognition. However, neither study measured olfactory sex discrimination directly, and therefore it remains questionable whether Trp2-KO males can discriminate between the sexes on the basis of pheromonal chemosignals. Fortunately, these results can be reconciled with previous findings because it has been shown that Trp2-KO mice still exhibit electrophysiological responses after MHC-class I peptides stimulation (Kelliher *et al.*, 2006). Furthermore, these mice show a pregnancy block effect when they are exposed to the odor of a strange male. These results suggest that Trp2 ablation is not equivalent to a total elimination of VNO function. Instead, it seems likely that some vomeronasal function is retained in Trp2-KO mice. It is also possible that developmental compensatory processes allow some recovery of vomeronasal function in these animals.

Finally, in contrast to the data presented so far, the rat appears as an exception because lesion of the AOS impacts attraction to opposite-sex odors quite extensively (Ichikawa, 1989; Romero *et al.*, 1990), therefore leading to extreme caution when extrapolating results from one species to another.

B. Pheromonal control of sexual behavior

1. Pheromonal control of male sexual behavior

The involvement of the MOS versus the AOS in the expression of sexual behavior is a subject of controversy. In the male, the involvement of VNO in copulatory behavior seems to vary greatly according to species. While in hamsters or prosimian primates (*Microcebus murinus*), surgical destruction of the VNO had quite important effects on male sexual behavior (Aujard, 1997; Powers and Winans, 1975), this seems not to be the case in male mice. Indeed, lesioning the VNO does not (Pankevich *et al.*, 2004) or only partly impact sexual behavior (Clancy *et al.*, 1984). As well, Trp2-KO male also demonstrate normal copulatory abilities (Stowers *et al.*, 2002), thus suggesting a role for the MOS (Keller *et al.*, 2006a). In support to this hypothesis, male mice sexual behavior has been shown to be more generally dependent on the MOS. Indeed, various studies, using either chemical lesions of the MOE with dichlobenil (Yoon *et al.*, 2005) or zinc sulfate (Keller *et al.*, 2006b) or using genetically engineered mice lacking CNGA2 (Mandiyan *et al.*, 2005) demonstrated a clear disruption of sexual behavior after destruction/inactivation of the MOE.

Interestingly, sexual experience is a factor allowing the integration of chemosignals originating from both MOS and AOS. Indeed, in hamsters, the control of male sexual behavior is varying according to previous sexual experience (Meredith, 1986; Pfeiffer and Johnston, 1994). In sexually naïve males, severe deficits in sexual behavior are observed in VNO-lesioned animals, thus showing that these inputs are needed for normal copulatory performance in these animals. By contrast, once animals have gained sexual experience, either main or vomeronasal inputs are sufficient for mating to occur. Only lesioning of both systems can impair copulation in these sexually experienced males. It has been suggested that the effect of olfactory deprivation on sexual behavior may be mediated by GnRH neurons. Indeed, GnRH cells receive olfactory information from both the MOS and the AOS. At the same time, an intracerebroventricular injection of GnRH is able to overcome the absence of VNO olfactory inputs in a way similar to that of sexual experience (Fernandez-Fewell and Meredith, 1994, 1995; Meredith, 1998; Meredith and Howard, 1992). Therefore, one hypothesis is that sexual experience modulates the relative functional efficiency of these MOB-to-GnRH neuron connections: these connections gaining functional efficiency only after a sufficient amount of sexual experience. In this context, female chemosensory cues are able to induce a higher Fos immunocytochemical labeling in the MPOA in sexually experienced than in inexperienced males. Compensation between both olfactory systems according sexual experience seems however not to be a general rule. For example, in male mice MOE lesion disrupts sexual behavior in both naïve and sexually experienced animals (Keller *et al.*, 2006b), suggesting that vomeronasal inputs are not able to sustain copulation by themselves in mice and underlying differences between species.

2. Pheromonal control of female sexual behavior

In the female, early studies (Edwards and Burge, 1973; Thompson and Edwards, 1972) suggested a role for the MOS in the display of female sexual receptivity, since destruction of the MOE by intranasal infusion with zinc sulfate attenuated lordosis behavior. In accordance with these results, recent experiments also confirmed that MOE zinc sulfate lesion reduced lordosis (Keller *et al.*, 2006a). An explanation for these effects is that deprivation of MOS sensory input may induce less activation of the centers regulating lordosis in the brain, for example the VMN, and as a consequence disrupts lordosis behavior. However, these effects of MOE lesions are clearly not as effective in disrupting lordosis as VNO lesions. Indeed, VNO lesions greatly abolished lordosis behavior in females of various species including rats (Rajendren *et al.*, 1990), mice (Keller *et al.*, 2006c), hamsters (Mackay-Sim and Rose, 1986), or voles (Curtis *et al.*, 2001). Intriguingly, studies on the role of the VNO in pregnancy block effect in mice showed that VNO ablation did not prevent female mice from becoming pregnant (Kelliher *et al.*, 2006; Lloyd-Thomas and Keverne,1982), suggesting that the VNO may not mediate female sexual receptivity in mice. However, both sets of data can be reconciled because it has been shown that the disruptive consequences of VNO lesions can be partly overcome over time and long-term exposure to the male. For example, the lordosis quotient of VNO-lesioned female rats increased after prolonged exposure to the male (Rajendren *et al.*, 1990), suggesting that some compensatory mechanisms can occur over time. The degree of sexual or olfactory sensory experience prior to VNO removal may also play a role in these compensatory mechanisms (Martínez-García *et al.,* 2009).

V. General Conclusions

In conclusion, we have reviewed the current conceptions of how the mammalian main and accessory olfactory subsystems interact to detect and process partially overlapping sets of pheromonal signals, giving rise to a model that involves parallel processing of the same molecules but through different mechanisms leading to specific behavioral outputs. Indeed, the most salient feature of this review is that there are no general rules that allow classification of the AOS more as a pheromone detector than the MOS. Consequently, both systems should be conceived as complementary rather than as separate pathways for mate discrimination and the stimulation of sexual motivation and behavior. Further experimentation will be needed to understand how chemosensory cues are integrated with hormonal and neuroendocrine factors to control courtship and mating behaviors, especially at the level of the hypothalamus. In addition, the reader must remind that most of the data reported in this manuscript refer to rodent literature. This is justified by the fact that the most recent advances in the field have been performed in these species and also according to the great importance of olfactory communication in these species, but this should lead to some caution when extrapolating to other species, as by definition pheromones are species-specific signals. Therefore, great heuristic value will be undoubtedly provided by comparative research in relation to species-specific evolutionary and ecological constraints.

ACKNOWLEDGMENTS

Matthieu Keller is a CNRS research associate (France). Delphine Pillon is associate professor at the University of Tours. Julie Bakker is an FNRS research associate. This work has been performed under the support of ANR 2009 CESA-006-02.

REFERENCES

Andreolini, F., Jemiolo, B., and Novotny, M. (1987). Dynamics of excretion of urinary chemosignals in the house mouse (*Mus musculus*) during the natural estrous cycle. *Experientia* **43,** 998–1002.

Aujard, F. (1997). Effect of vomeronasal organ removal on male socio-sexual responses to female in a prosimian primate (*Microcebus murinus*). *Physiol. Behav.* **6,** 1003–1008.

Baum, M. J., and Kelliher, K. R. (2009). Complementary roles of the main and accessory olfactory systems in mammalian mate recognition. *Annu. Rev. Physiol.* **71,** 141–160.

Baum, M. J., and Keverne, E. B. (2002). Sex difference in attraction thresholds for volatile odors from male and estrous female mouse urine. *Horm. Behav.* **41,** 213–219.

Beauchamp, G. K., Doty, R. L., Moulton, D. G., and Mugford, R. A. (1976). The pheromone conception mammalian chemical communication: A critique. *In* "Mammalian Olfaction, Reproductive Success and Behavior," (R. L. Doty, Ed.), pp. 144–160. New-York, Academic Press.

Bellringer, J. F., Pratt, H. P., and Keverne, E. B. (1980). Involvement of the vomeronasal organ and prolactin in pheromonal induction of delayed implantation in mice. *J. Reprod. Fertil.* **59,** 223–228.

Boehm, U., Zou, Z., and Buck, L. B. (2005). Feedback loops link odor and pheromone signaling with reproduction. *Cell* **123,** 683–695.

Brennan, P. A. (2004). The nose knows who's who: Chemosensory individuality and mate recognition in mice. *Horm. Behav.* **46,** 231–240.

Brennan, P. A. (2009). Outstanding issues surrounding vomeronasal mechanisms of pregnancy block and individual recognition in mice. *Behav. Brain Res.* **200,** 287–294.

Brennan, P. A., and Zufall, F. (2006). Pheromonal communication in vertebrates. *Nature* **444,** 308–315.

Brennan, P. A., Schellinck, H. M., and Keverne, E. B. (1999). Patterns of expression of the immediate-early gene egr-1 in the accessory olfactory bulb of female mice exposed to pheromonal constituents of male urine. *Neuroscience* **90,** 1463–1470.

Bruce, H. M. (1959). An exteroceptive block to pregnancy in the mouse. *Nature* **184,** 105.

Buck, L. B. (2000). The molecular architecture of odor and pheromone sensing in mammals. *Cell* **100,** 611–618.

Buck, L. B., and Axel, R. (1991). A novel multigene family may encode odorant receptors: A molecular basis for odor recognition. *Cell* **65,** 175–187.

Clancy, A. N., Coquelin, A., Macrides, F., Gorski, R. A., and Noble, E. P. (1984). Sexual behavior and aggression in male mice: Involvement of the vomeronasal system. *J. Neurosci.* **4,** 2222–2229.

Cohen-Tannoudji, J., Lavenet, C., Locatelli, A., Tillet, Y., and Signoret, J. P. (1989). Non involvement of the accessory olfactory system in the LH response of anoestrous ewes to male odour. *J. Reprod. Fertil.* **86,** 135–144.

Coquelin, A., Clancy, A. N., Macrides, F., Noble, E. P., and Gorski, R. A. (1984). Pheromonally induced release of luteinizing hormone in male mice: Involvement of the vomeronasal system. *J. Neurosci.* **4,** 2230–2236.

Curtis, J. T., Liu, Y., and Wang, Z. (2001). Lesions of the vomeronasal organ disrupt mating induced pair bonding in female prairie voles (*Microtus ochrogaster*). *Brain Res.* **901,** 167–174.

Del Punta, K., Puche, A., Adams, N. C., Rodriguez, I., and Mombaerts, P. (2002). A divergent pattern of sensory axonal projections is rendered convergent by second-order neurons in the accessory olfactory bulb. *Neuron* **35,** 1057–1066.

Delgadillo, J. A., Gelez, H., Ungerfeld, R., Hawken, P. A., and Martin, G. B. (2009). The 'male effect' in sheep and goats—Revisiting the dogmas. *Behav. Brain Res.* **200,** 304–314.

Dorries, K. M., Adkins-Regan, E., and Halpern, B. P. (1995). Olfactory sensitivity to the pheromone, androstenone, is sexually dimorphic in the pig. *Physiol. Behav.* **57,** 255–259.

Dorries, K. M., Adkins-Regan, E., and Halpern, B. P. (1997). Sensitivity and behavioral responses to the pheromone androstenone are not mediated by the vomeronasal organ in domestic pigs. *Brain Behav. Evol.* **49,** 53–62.

Drickamer, L. C., and Hoover, J. E. (1979). Effects of urine from pregnant and lactating female house mice on sexual maturation of juvenile females. *Dev. Psychobiol.* **12,** 545–551.

Edwards, D. A., and Burge, K. G. (1973). Olfactory control of the sexual behavior of male and female mice. *Physiol. Behav.* **11,** 867–872.

Fernandez-Fewell, G. D., and Meredith, M. (1994). c-Fos expression in vomeronasal pathways of mated or pheromone-stimulated male golden hamsters: Contributions from vomeronasal sensory input and expression related to mating performance. *J. Neurosci.* **14,** 3643–3654.

Fernandez-Fewell, G. D., and Meredith, M. (1995). Facilitation of mating behavior in male hamsters by LHRH and Ac LHRH 5-10: Interaction with the vomeronasal system. *Physiol. Behav.* **57,** 213–221.

Gelez, H., and Fabre-Nys, C. (2004). The "male effect" in sheep and goats: A review of the respective roles of the two olfactory systems. *Horm. Behav.* **46,** 257–271.

Gomez, D. M., and Newman, S. W. (1992). Differential projections of the anterior and posterior regions of the medial amygdaloid nucleus in the Syrian hamster. *J. Comp. Neurol.* **317,** 195–218.

Halem, H. A., Baum, M. J., and Cherry, J. A. (2001). Sex difference and steroid modulation of pheromone-induced immediate early genes in the two zones of the mouse accessory olfactory system. *J. Neurosci.* **21,** 2474–2480.

Hurst, J. L., Payne, C. E., Nevison, C. M., Marie, A. D., Humphries, R. E., Robertson, D. H., Cavaggioni, A., and Beynon, R. J. (2001). Individual recognition in mice mediated by major urinary proteins. *Nature* **414,** 631–634.

Ichikawa, M. (1989). Recovery of olfactory behavior following removal of accessory olfactory bulb in adult rat. *Brain Res.* **498,** 45–52.

Jacob, S., McClintock, M. K., Zelano, B., and Ober, C. (2002). Paternally inherited HLA alleles are associated with women's choice of male odor. *Nat. Genet.* **30,** 175–179.

Jakupovic, J., Kang, N., and Baum, M. J. (2008). Effect of bilateral accessory olfactory bulb lesions on volatile urinary odor discrimination and investigation as well as mating behavior in male mice. *Physiol. Behav.* **93,** 467–473.

Jemiolo, B., Andreolini, F., Xie, T. M., Wiesler, D., and Novotny, M. (1989). Puberty-affecting synthetic analogs of urinary chemosignals in the house mouse, *Mus domesticus*. *Physiol. Behav.* **46,** 293–298.

Karlson, P., and Luscher, M. (1959). 'Pheromones': A new term for a class of biologically active substances. *Nature* **183,** 55–56.

Keller, M., Douhard, Q., Baum, M. J., and Bakker, J. (2006a). Destruction of the main olfactory epithelium reduces female sexual behavior and olfactory investigation in female mice. *Chem. Senses* **31,** 315–323.

Keller, M., Douhard, Q., Baum, M. J., and Bakker, J. (2006b). Sexual experience does not compensate for the disruptive effects of zinc sulfate—Lesioning of the main olfactory epithelium on sexual behavior in male mice. *Chem. Senses* **31,** 753–762.

Keller, M., Pierman, S., Douhard, Q., Baum, M. J., and Bakker, J. (2006c). The vomeronasal organ is required for the expression of lordosis behaviour, but not sex discrimination in female mice. *Eur. J. Neurosci.* **23,** 521–530.

Keller, M., Baum, M. J., and Bakker, J. (2008). Olfactory control of sex-recognition and sexual behavior in mice. *In* "Chemical Signals in Vertebrates XI," (J. L. Hurst, R. J. Beynon, S. C. Roberts, and T. D. Wyatt, Eds.), pp. 241–250. Springer-Verlag, New York.

Keller, M., Baum, M. J., Brock, O., Brennan, P., and Bakker, J. (2009). The main and the accessory olfactory systems interact in the control of mate recognition and sexual behavior. *Behav. Brain Res.* **200,** 268–276.

Kelliher, K. R. (2007). The combined role of the main olfactory and vomeronasal systems in social communication in mammals. *Horm. Behav.* **52,** 561–570.

Kelliher, K. R., and Baum, M. J. (2001). Nares occlusion eliminates heterosexual partner selection without disrupting coitus in ferrets of both sexes. *J. Neurosci.* **21,** 5832–5840.

Kelliher, K. R., Spehr, M., Li, X. H., Zufall, F., and Leinders-Zufall, T. (2006). Pheromonal recognition memory induced by TRPC2-independent vomeronasal sensing. *Eur. J. Neurosci.* **23,** 3385–3390.

Keverne, E. B. (2004). Importance of olfactory and vomeronasal systems for male sexual function. *Physiol. Behav.* **83,** 177–187.

Kevetter, G. A., and Winans, S. S. (1981a). Connections of the corticomedial amygdala in the golden hamster. II. Efferents of the "olfactory amygdala". *J. Comp. Neurol.* **197,** 99–111.

Kevetter, G. A., and Winans, S. S. (1981b). Connections of the corticomedial amygdala in the golden hamster. I. Efferents of the "vomeronasal amygdala". *J. Comp. Neurol.* **197,** 81–98.

Kimoto, H., Haga, S., Sato, K., and Touhara, K. (2005). Sex-specific peptides from exocrine glands stimulate mouse vomeronasal sensory neurons. *Nature* **437,** 898–901.

Leinders-Zufall, T., Lane, A. P., Puche, A. C., Ma, W., Novotny, M. V., Shipley, M. T., and Zufall, F. (2000). Ultrasensitive pheromone detection by mammalian vomeronasal neurons. *Nature* **405,** 792–796.

Leinders-Zufall, T., Brennan, P., Widmayer, P., Chandramani, S. P., Maul-Pavicic, A., Jäger, M., Li, X. H., Breer, H., Zufall, F., and Boehm, T. (2004). MHC class I peptides as chemosensory signals in the vomeronasal organ. *Science* **306,** 1033–1037.

Lévy, F., and Keller, M. (2009). Olfactory mediation of maternal behaviour in selected mammalian species. *Behav. Brain Res.* **200,** 336–345.

Lévy, F., Keller, M., and Poindron, P. (2004). Olfactory regulation of maternal behavior in mammals. *Horm. Behav.* **46,** 284–302.

Leypold, B. G., Yu, C. R., Leinders-Zufall, T., Kim, M. M., Zufall F., and Axel, R. (2002). Altered sexual and social behaviors in trp2 mutant mice. *Proc. Natl. Acad. Sci. USA* **99,** 6376–6381.

Liberles, S. D., and Buck, L. B. (2006). A class of chemosensory receptors in the olfactory epithelium. *Nature* **42,** 645–650.

Licht, G., and Meredith, M. (1987). Convergence of main and accessory olfactory pathways onto single neurons in the hamster amygdala. *Exp. Brain Res.* **69,** 7–18.

Lin, W., Arellano, J., Slotnick, B., and Restrepo, D. (2004). Odors detected by mice deficient in cyclic nucleotide-gated channel subunit A2 stimulate the main olfactory system. *J. Neurosci.* **24,** 3703–3710.

Lin, D. Y., Zhang, S. Z., Block, E., and Katz, L. C. (2005). Encoding social signals in the mouse main olfactory bulb. *Nature* **434,** 470–477.

Lloyd-Thomas, A., and Keverne, E. B. (1982). Role of the brain and accessory olfactory system in the block to pregnancy in mice. *Neuroscience* **7,** 907–913.

Lomas, D. E., and Keverne, E. B. (1982). Role of the vomeronasal organ and prolactin in the acceleration of puberty in female mice. *J. Reprod. Fertil.* **66,** 101–107.

Luo, M., Fee, M. S., and Katz, L. C. (2003). Encoding pheromonal signals in the accessory olfactory bulb of behaving mice. *Science* **299,** 1196–1201.

Ma, D., Allen, N. D., Van Bergen, Y. C., Jones, C. M., Baum, M. J., Keverne, E. B., and Brennan, P. A. (2002). Selective ablation of olfactory receptor neurons without functional impairment of vomeronasal receptor neurons in OMP-ntr transgenic mice. *Eur. J. Neurosci.* **16,** 2317–2323.

Mackay-Sim, A., and Rose, J. D. (1986). Removal of the vomeronasal organ impairs lordosis in female hamsters: Effect is reversed by luteinising hormone-releasing hormone. *Neuroendocrinology* **42,** 489–493.

Mandiyan, V. S., Coats, J. K., and Shah, N. M. (2005). Deficits in sexual and aggressive behaviors in Cnga2 mutant mice. *Nat. Neurosci.* **8,** 1660–1662.

Martel, K. L., and Baum, M. J. (2007). Sexually dimorphic activation of the accessory, but not the main, olfactory bulb in mice by urinary volatiles. *Eur. J. Neurosci.* **26,** 463–475.

Martel, K. L., Keller, M., Douhard, Q., Bakker, J., and Baum, M. J. (2007). Comparison of odor induced glomerular activation in the main olfactory bulb of aromatase knock-out and wild type female mice. *Neurosci. Lett.* **421,** 101–105.

Martínez-García, F., Martínez-Ricós, J., Agustín-Pavón, C., Martínez-Hernández, J., Novejarque, A., and Lanuza, E. (2009). Refining the dual olfactory hypothesis: Pheromone reward and odour experience. *Behav. Brain Res.* **200,** 277–286.

Martinez-Ricos, J., Agustin-Pavon, C., Lanuza, E., and Martinez-Garcia, F. (2008). Role of the vomeronasal system in intersexual attraction in female mice. *Neuroscience* **153,** 383–395.

Meredith, M. (1986). Vomeronasal organ removal before sexual experience impairs male hamster mating behavior. *Physiol. Behav.* **36,** 737–743.

Meredith, M. (1991). Sensory processing in the main and accessory olfactory systems: Comparisons and contrasts. *J. Steroid Biochem. Mol. Biol.* **39,** 601–614.

Meredith, M. (1994). Chronic recording of vomeronasal pump activation in awake behaving hamsters. *Physiol. Behav.* **56,** 345–354.

Meredith, M. (1998). Vomeronasal, olfactory, hormonal convergence in the brain. Cooperation or coincidence? *Ann. NY Acad. Sci.* **855,** 349–361.

Meredith, M. (2001). Human vomeronasal organ function: a critical review of best and worst cases. *Chem. Senses* **26,** 433–445.

Meredith, M., and Fewell, G. (2001). Vomeronasal organ: Electrical stimulation activates Fos in mating pathways and in GnRH neurons. *Brain Res.* **922,** 87–94.

Meredith, M., and Howard, G. (1992). Intracerebroventricular LHRH relieves behavioral deficits due to vomeronasal organ removal. *Brain Res. Bull.* **29,** 75–79.

Meredith, M., and O'Connell, R. J. (1979). Efferent control of stimulus access to the hamster vomeronasal organ. *J. Physiol.* **286,** 301–316.

Munger, S. D., Leinders-Zufall, T., and Zufall, F. (2009). Subsystem organization of the mammalian sense of smell. *Annu. Rev. Physiol.* **71,** 115–140.

Pankevich, D. E., Baum, M. J., and Cherry, J. A. (2004). Olfactory sex discrimination persists, whereas the preference for urinary odorants from estrous females disappears in male mice after vomeronasal organ removal. *J. Neurosci.* **24,** 9451–9947.

Pankevich, D. E., Cherry, J. A., and Baum, M. J. (2006). Effect of vomeronasal organ removal from male mice on their preference for and neural Fos responses to female urinary odors. *Behav. Neurosci.* **120,** 925–936.

Pfeiffer, C. A., and Johnston, R. E. (1994). Hormonal and behavioral responses of male hamsters to females and female odors: Roles of olfaction, the vomeronasal system, and sexual experience. *Physiol. Behav.* **55,** 129–138.

Pierman, S., Douhard, Q., Balthazart, J., Baum, M. J., and Bakker, J. (2006). Attraction thresholds and sex discrimination of urinary odorants in male and female aromatase knockout (ArKO) mice. *Horm. Behav.* **49,** 96–104.

Powers, J. B., and Winans, S. S. (1975). Vomeronasal organ: Critical role in mediating sexual behavior of the male hamster. *Science* **187,** 961–963.

Preti, G., Wysocki, C. J., Barnhart, K. T., Sondheimer, S. J., and Leyden, J. J. (2003). Male axillary extracts contain pheromones that affect pulsatile secretion of luteinizing hormone and mood in women recipients. *Biol. Reprod.* **68,** 2107–2113.

Rajendren, G., Dudley, C. A., and Moss, R. L. (1990). Role of the vomeronasal organ in the male-induced enhancement of sexual receptivity in female rats. *Neuroendocrinology* **52,** 368–372.

Romero, P. R., Beltramino, C. A., and Carrer, H. F. (1990). Participation of the olfactory system in the control of approach behavior of the female rat to the male. *Physiol. Behav.* **47,** 685–690.

Savic, I., Hedén-Blomqvist, E., and Berglund, H. (2009). Pheromone signal transduction in humans: What can be learned from olfactory loss. *Hum. Brain Mapp.* **30,** 3057–3065.

Scalia, F., and Winans, S. S. (1975). The differential projections of the olfactory bulb and accessory olfactory bulb in mammals. *J. Comp. Neurol.* **161,** 31–55.

Shinohara, K., Morofushi, M., Funabashi, T., and Kimura, F. (2001). Axillary pheromones modulate pulsatile LH secretion in humans. *NeuroReport* **12,** 893–895.

Spehr, M., Spehr, J., Ukhanov, K., Kelliher, K. R., Leinders-Zufall, T., and Zufall, F. (2006a). Parallel processing of social signals by the mammalian main and accessory olfactory systems. *Cell. Mol. Life Sci.* **63,** 1476–1484.

Spehr, M., Kelliher, K. R., Li, X. H., Boehm, T., Leinders-Zufall, T., and Zufall, F. (2006b). Essential role of the main olfactory system in social recognition of major histocompatibility complex peptide ligands. *J. Neurosci.* **26,** 1961–1970.

Stern, K., and McClintock, M. K. (1998). Regulation of ovulation by human pheromones. *Nature* **392,** 177–179.

Stowers, L., Holy, T. E., Meister, M., Dulac, C., and Koentges, G. (2002). Loss of sex discrimination and male-male aggression in mice deficient for TRP2. *Science* **295,** 1493–1500.

Thompson, M. L., and Edwards, D. A. (1972). Olfactory bulb ablation and hormonally induced mating in spayed female mice. *Physiol. Behav.* **8,** 1141–1146.

Tirindelli, R., Dibattista, M., Pifferi, S., and Menini, A. (2009). From pheromones to behavior. *Physiol. Rev.* **89,** 921–956.

Vandenbergh, J. G. (1969). Male odor accelerates female sexual maturation in mice. *Endocrinology* **84,** 658–660.

Von Campenhausen, H., and Mori, K. (2000). Convergence of segregated pheromonal pathways from the accessory olfactory bulb to the cortex in the mouse. *Eur. J. Neurosci.* **12,** 33–46.

Wesson, D. W., Keller, M., Douhard, Q., Baum, M. J., and Bakker, J. (2006). Enhanced urinary odor discrimination in female aromatase knockout (ArKO) mice. *Horm. Behav.* **49,** 80–86.

Westberry, J., and Meredith, M. (2003a). The influence of chemosensory input and gonadotropin releasing hormone on mating behavior circuits in male hamsters. *Brain Res.* **974,** 1–16.

Westberry, J. M., and Meredith, M. (2003b). Pre-exposure to female chemosignals or intracerebral GnRH restores mating behavior in naive male hamsters with vomeronasal organ lesions. *Chem. Senses* **28,** 191–196.

Whitten, W. K. (1956). Modification of the oestrous cycle of the mouse by external stimuli associated with the male. *J. Endocrinol.* **13,** 399–404.
Woodley, S. K., Cloe, A. L., Waters, P., and Baum, M. J. (2004). Effects of vomeronasal organ removal on olfactory sex discrimination and odor preferences of female ferrets. *Chem. Senses* **29,** 659–669.
Wyatt, T. D. (2003). Pheromones and Animal Behaviour. Communication by Smell and Taste. Cambridge University Press, Cambridge, United-Kingdom.
Wysocki, C. J., Wellington, J. L., and Beauchamp, G. K. (1980). Access of urinary nonvolatiles to the mammalian vomeronasal organ. *Science* **207,** 781–783.
Wysocki, C. J., and Preti, G. (2004). Facts, fallacies, fears, and frustrations with human pheromones. *Anat. Rec. A Discov. Mol. Cell Evol. Biol.* **281,** 1201–1211.
Yoon, H., Enquist, L. W., and Dulac, C. (2005). Olfactory inputs to hypothalamic neurons controlling reproduction and fertility. *Cell* **123,** 669–682.

CHAPTER FIFTEEN

Communication by Olfactory Signals in Rabbits: Its Role in Reproduction

Angel I. Melo *and* Gabriela González-Mariscal

Contents

Abstract

Rabbits use a variety of olfactory signals to transmit information related with reproduction. Such cues are produced in skin glands (submandibular, anal, Harder's, lachrymal, preputial) and the mammary gland–nipple complex. Some signals are transmitted by active behaviors, for example, chin-marking, urination, and defecation, while others are transmitted passively (e.g., mammary pheromone (MP) and inguinal gland secretions). We show that sex steroids regulate: chinning frequency and the chin gland's size, weight and secretory activity in bucks and does by acting on specific brain regions or on the chin gland, respectively. The "mammary pheromone," identified in milk as 2-methyl-but-2-enal, is essential for guiding the pups to the nipples, but its origin (mammary gland, ventral skin, nipple) remains to be determined. Estradiol, progesterone, and prolactin regulate the emission of an olfactory cue that also triggers nipple-search behavior in the pups, but its chemical identity and relation with the MP are unclear.

Centro de Investigación en Reproducción Animal, CINVESTAV-Universidad Autónoma de Tlaxcala, Tlaxcala, Tlax., México

Vitamins and Hormones, Volume 83
ISSN 0083-6729, DOI: 10.1016/S0083-6729(10)83015-8

I. Introduction

Olfactory signals play a major role in regulating a variety of biological functions in mammals, among them, onset of puberty, synchronization of estrus, ovulation, identification of kin, mate choice, pregnancy block, and selectivity of nursing. Yet, despite their obvious importance, investigation of the specific signals involved in modulating any of the above processes has been rather patchy. For instance, the participation of olfactory cues in pregnancy block, identification of kin, and onset of puberty has been explored mainly in mice (Dluzen and Vandenbergh, 1992; Price and Vandenbergh, 1992). Ferrets have been the preferred species for studying the role of male scents in promoting pair formation and mating-induced ovulation (Bakker and Baum, 2000). Mate choice and estrus synchronization by pheromones have been documented largely in rats (McClintock, 1982; Schank and McClintock, 1997). Abundant research exists in sheep to support an association between specific olfactory signals from the lamb and the likelihood of nursing by the ewe (Poindron *et al.*, 2007). In these instances, a particular species has been selected mainly because the phenomenon under investigation is reliably expressed or is easy to measure in it. Rabbits, by contrast, have not been consistently used as a model in which to explore the modulation of a specific function by olfactory signals. Yet, as we illustrate in this review, there is abundant evidence showing that secretions from several body sources in male and female rabbits participate in regulating (or are associated with) specific aspects of reproduction, namely, mating, maternal behavior, nursing, and social hierarchy. We hope that putting together this information will bring insight into the ways by which olfactory and endocrine signals are integrated in the rabbit brain to control complex behaviors. We also trust that our work will encourage other investigators to use rabbits as a model for studying the participation of olfactory signals in reproductive phenomena that are common to all mammals.

II. Communication by Chemical Signals

A. Chin glands and their secretions

1. Histology, sexual dimorphism, and regulation by steroid hormones

Skin glands in mammals are classified into holocrine (e.g., sebaceous glands), and merocrine (e.g., sweat glands). The submandibular or chin gland of rabbits is a modified sweat gland (apocrine; Lyne *et al.*, 1964) developed from the external root sheath of the hair follicle and attached to it (Wales and Ebling, 1971). Chin glands enlarge at puberty (ca. 13 weeks of age) in both sexes, but at the onset of sexual maturity (ca. 24 weeks of age) their anatomy, histology, and biological function show a marked sexual dimorphism (Mykytowycz, 1965; Wales and Ebling, 1971). As adults, the chin glands are larger and heavier in males (458–1000 mg) than in females (156–242 mg) and their weight is correlated with body weight in males, though not in females. In addition, the chin glands of dominant males have twice the size and weight of those of subordinates (Mykytowycz, 1965; Mykytowycz and Dudzinski, 1966; Wales and Ebling, 1971). The submandibular gland comprises three groups of lobes: two deeply seated lateral ones and a central lobe located under the chin. The three lobes are a conglomerate of tubules lying in the subcutaneous tissue of the submandibular region and their excretory ducts open on the surface of the skin. Each tubule is lined with a columnar or cuboidal epithelium of secretory cells. Each lobe has tubules with three types of cells: type A (nonvacuolated), type B (vacuolated), and dark (Lyne *et al.*, 1964). The shape and size of these secretory cells depends on the functional state of the secretory cycles, that is, resting, synthesizing, or discharging (Kurosumi *et al.*, 1961; Mykytowycz, 1965). Male glands contain significantly less secretory acini/field and the diameter of acini is larger than in the female gland (Cerbón *et al.*, 1996). The size, histology, and secretory activity of chin glands largely depend on sexual hormones. Thus, gonadectomy reduces by almost three times the chin gland weight in males, though the opposite effect occurs in females (Mykytowycz, 1965). In addition, gonadectomy in males reduces the number of secretory cells and the size of tubules (Wales and Ebling, 1971) and increases the number of acini/field and reduces their diameter (Cerbón *et al.*, 1996). The administration of testosterone to castrated males restores the weight of the gland, but the coadministration with estradiol benzoate (EB) reverses the effects of testosterone. EB injected alone to intact males reduces gland weight and activity (Wales and Ebling, 1971). The secretory activity of the chin gland changes across the reproductive cycle as estrous females show a higher number of acini/field than do pregnant (days 20 and 29) and lactating (day 6) does (Cerbón *et al.*, 1996). These results further support a role of steroid hormones in the regulation of chin gland secretions and agree with the finding that the female submandibular gland contains receptors for estradiol and progesterone (Camacho-Arroyo *et al.*, 1999) and also for glucocorticoids (Hernández *et al.*, 1982).

2. Chemical composition of chin gland secretions

Thin-layer chromatography, electrophoresis (Goodrich and Mykytowycz, 1972), and gas-chromatography (Hayes *et al.*, 2001) have been used to identify the components of chin gland secretions. A variety of molecules have been detected, including, proteins, carbohydrates, hydrocarbons, non-glycerol esters, fatty acids, cholesterol, triglycerides, diglycerides, and monoglycerides (Goodrich and Mykytowycz, 1972) as well as aromatic compounds (naphthalene, benzaldehyde, ethyl benzene, acetophenone, 2,6-di-*tert*-butyl-*p*-cresol; Goodrich, 1983). Recently, Hayes *et al.* collected chin gland secretions from wild rabbits, either using "chinning poles" placed in the field (Hayes *et al.*, 2002a) or directly from the chin skin (Hayes *et al.*, 2002b). They identified 34 volatile components consisting mainly of aromatic and aliphatic hydrocarbons, alkyl-substituted benzene derivatives being the most common. From these, 2-phenoxyethanol was found in dominant but never in subordinate males (Hayes *et al.*, 2001, 2003). Although these authors did not find evidence that rabbits could distinguish between samples with or without 2-phenoxyethanol, they did determine that this substance acts as a fixative that prolongs the duration of the dominant male's scent-mark (Hayes *et al.*, 2003).

B. Chin-marking (chinning) in males and females

1. Ontogeny and sexual differences

In mammals, there are two ways for distributing skin gland secretions: passive and active marking (Mykytowycz, 1970). The former is accomplished through the mere presence of glands on the body, that is, animals do not have to deposit secretions actively on objects in the environment as odors emanate directly from the source. By contrast, in active marking, the secretions of skin glands are applied directly on objects in the surrounding area through a variety of scent-marking behaviors. Rabbits deposit submandibular gland secretions by rubbing their chin on objects such as grass blades, stones, bricks, stumps, the entrance to a burrow, the corner of a post, another rabbit (subordinate or juvenile), or on dung-hills (fecal pellets coated with secretions). Chin-marking is a stereotyped motor pattern that includes (a) the orientation of the animal's jaw against the object to be marked and (b) the performance of a forward head movement in which the rabbit rubs its chin against the object, leaving submandibular gland secretions behind (Fig. 15.1). Thus, the neck muscles, the visual perception of the object, and the tactile sensations

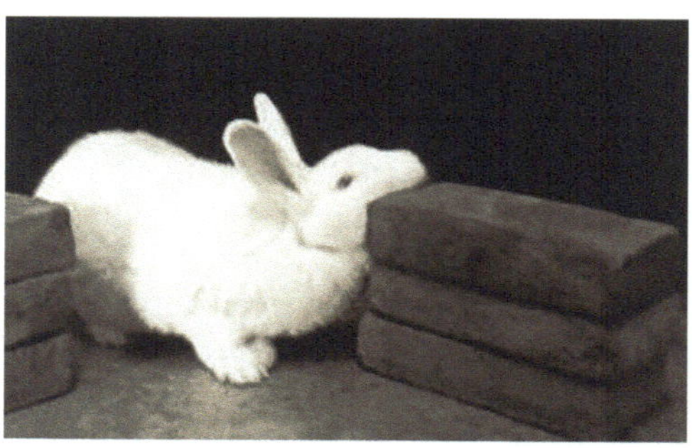

Figure 15.1 Rabbit chin-marking a brick pile placed inside the arena used to quantify this behavior in our laboratory.

perceived during chin-rubbing could contribute to modulate the execution of this form of scent-marking.

Chinning is displayed by all members of the colony, but its frequency is related to the age, sex, social status, and reproductive state of the individual. The onset of chinning is at 41 ± 16 days of age in females and 47 ± 13 days in males and at this time the frequency is higher in females than in males. Thereafter, chinning increases gradually but at a higher rate in males such that, by 100 days of age, a clear sexual dimorphism is established and males will continue to mark at a higher frequency than females throughout adulthood (González-Mariscal *et al.*, 1992; Fig. 15.2). The frequency of chinning is higher in dominant than in subordinate individuals, both in wild animals studied during the breeding season (Mykytowycz, 1962; Mykytowycz and Ward, 1971) and in domestic breeds kept under laboratory conditions (Arteaga *et al.*, 2008). Moreover, dominant males mate with almost all the females of the colony and they usually mark during sexual excitement (Myers and Poole, 1961).

2. Neuroendocrine regulation

Several lines of evidence have shown a correlation between chinning frequency and sexual receptivity in does. Thus, during estrus, when serum levels of estradiol are high and those of progesterone are low (Ramírez and Beyer, 1988) does show high scores of chinning (González-Mariscal *et al.*, 1990; Soares and Diamond, 1982) and sexual receptivity (Beyer and Rivaud, 1969; Stoufflet and Caillol, 1988). By contrast, low chinning scores

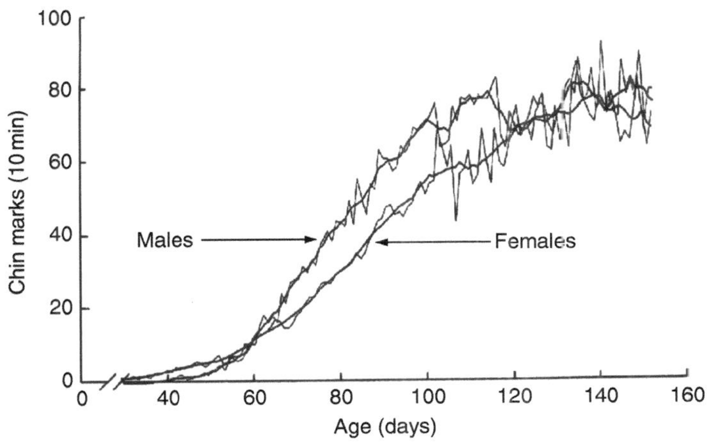

Figure 15.2 Ontogeny of chin-marking in male and female rabbits from 31 to 150 days of age. Dotted lines are original data (mean of means); solid lines are smoothed profiles of each curve. Reproduced from González-Mariscal *et al.* (1992) with the kind permission of Elsevier.

are observed during anestrus (Hudson *et al.*, 1994). Across pregnancy, when circulating levels of estradiol are low and those of progesterone are high, both chinning (González-Mariscal *et al.*, 1990, 1994b; Fig. 15.3) and sexual behavior (Beyer and Rivaud, 1969) are practically suppressed.

Similarly, ovariectomized (ovx) rabbits show practically no chinning or sexual behavior but the administration of EB restores both behaviors (Hudson *et al.*, 1990). The addition of progesterone to such EB-treated does inhibits both behaviors while its withdrawal allows the rapid restoration of scent-marking and sexual receptivity (Hudson *et al.*, 1990; Fig. 15.4).

A participation of the progesterone receptor (PR) in these effects is supported by the findings that (a) the administration of antiprogestins (RU486 or CDB 2914) to ovx rabbits given EB + progesterone attenuates

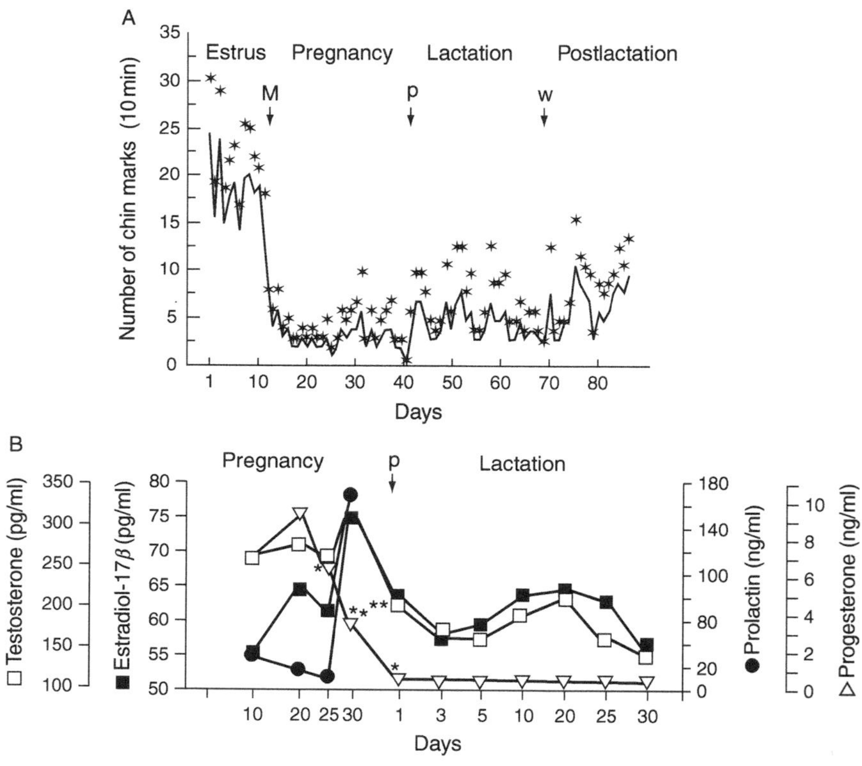

Figure 15.3 (A) Variations in the frequency of chinning across the doe's reproductive cycle (mean ± s.e.). M = mating; p = parturition; w = weaning. Reproduced from González-Mariscal *et al.* (1990), with the kind permission of Elsevier. (B) Variations in the serum concentration of estradiol, progesterone, testosterone, and prolactin observed across the doe's reproductive cycle. Reproduced from González-Mariscal *et al.* (1994b) with the kind permission of Elsevier.

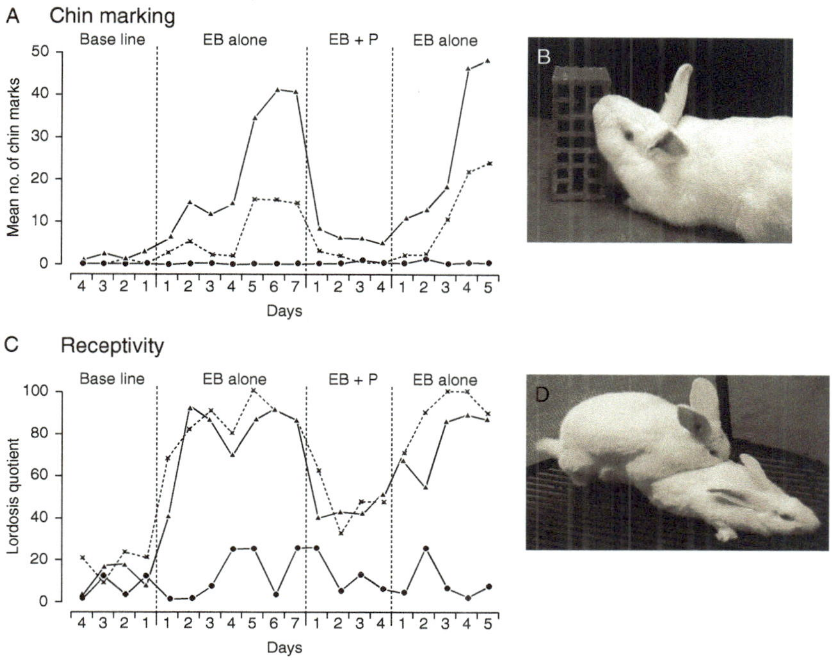

Figure 15.4 Effect of injecting ovx does with estradiol benzoate (EB; 1 μg/day, dotted lines, or 10 μg/day, solid line with triangles) or oil (solid line with circles), alone or combined with progesterone (P; 10 mg/day), on chinning (panels A, B) and sexual receptivity (panels C, D). Reproduced from Hudson *et al.* (1990) with the kind permission of Elsevier.

the inhibitory action of progesterone on chinning (Hoffman and González-Mariscal, 2006) and (b) chlormadinone acetate, a synthetic progestin with a higher potency than progesterone, reduces chinning frequency in ovx EB-treated does (Hoffman and González-Mariscal, 2007).

A correlation between chinning frequency and sexual behavior has also been documented in males. Thus, while intact bucks display high levels of both behaviors, castration eliminates or reduces them (Beyer *et al.*, 1980; González-Mariscal *et al.*, 1993). The administration of treatments that restore sexual behavior in castrated bucks also stimulate chinning, namely, testosterone propionate (TP) or the combination of low doses of EB plus 5α-dihydrotestosterone propionate (Beyer *et al.*, 1975, 1980; González-Mariscal *et al.*, 1993; McDonald *et al.*, 1970).

Chinning frequency is also regulated by inhibitory mechanisms that are independent of steroid hormones. Following mating, in females a drastic decrease in chinning (and ambulation in an open field) occurs and persists for 1 h. (González-Mariscal *et al.*, 1997). A transitory rise in chinning frequency is evident 12 h later but this behavior decreases thereafter and remains practically suppressed across pregnancy (González-Mariscal *et al.*, 1990). These immediate decreases in chinning frequency provoked by copulation cannot be attributed to progesterone as this hormone is released by the corpus luteum (derived from the ruptured follicles after mating-induced ovulation) approximately 40 h later (Ramírez and Beyer, 1988). Indeed, the antiprogestin RU486 does not prevent the immediate postmating inhibition of chinning in intact does (Hoffman and González-Mariscal, 2007). A similar chinning inhibitory mechanism, triggered by copulation, also operates in males. Following the display of a single ejaculation, scent-marking (but not ambulation in an open field) is drastically reduced for 1 h (González-Mariscal *et al.*, 1997). Yet, in contrast to females, chinning recovers by 2 h postcopula in bucks.

The neural substrate where steroid hormones act to stimulate chinning has been little studied. Based on the finding that the stimulation of sexual behavior by steroid hormones correlates with an increase in chinning frequency in both sexes, we implanted gonadectomized males and females with TP or EB, respectively, into brain areas known to regulate mating in rabbits. We found that bilateral implants of EB into the ventromedial hypothalamus (VMH) or the medial preoptic area (MPOA) reliably stimulated chinning in females (Fig. 15.5A). Most does implanted into the VMH and around half of the ones that received EB into the MPOA or diagonal band of Broca (DBB) showed lordosis. These data indicate that in female rabbits the VMH is an estrogen-sensitive brain area that stimulates both chinning and sexual behavior, while the MPOA seems to contain subpopulations of neurons involved in one or the other behavior (Melo *et al.*, 2008). Our results are consistent with the data from Palka and Sawyer (1966a,b) who found that estradiol or testosterone implants into the VMH and neighboring structures (e.g., ventrolateral part of the VMH, nucleus X, and ventral premammillary area) stimulated lordosis and support the hypothesis that chinning and sexual behavior are under the control of estrogens acting on common brain structures of the diencephalon. Indeed, high concentrations of estrogen receptor α-immunoreactive neurons are present in the hypothalamus and premammillary area of ovx does (Caba *et al.*, 2003).

In males, TP implants into the MPOA or DBB effectively stimulated chinning, but not sexual behavior. Implants into VMH did not stimulate any of the two behaviors (Melo *et al.*, 2008; Fig. 15.5B).

3. Sensory regulation

Chinning frequency is also regulated by the detection of odorants in the environment. For instance, male rabbits preferentially chin-mark objects previously marked by conspecifics over unmarked ones (Black-Cleworth

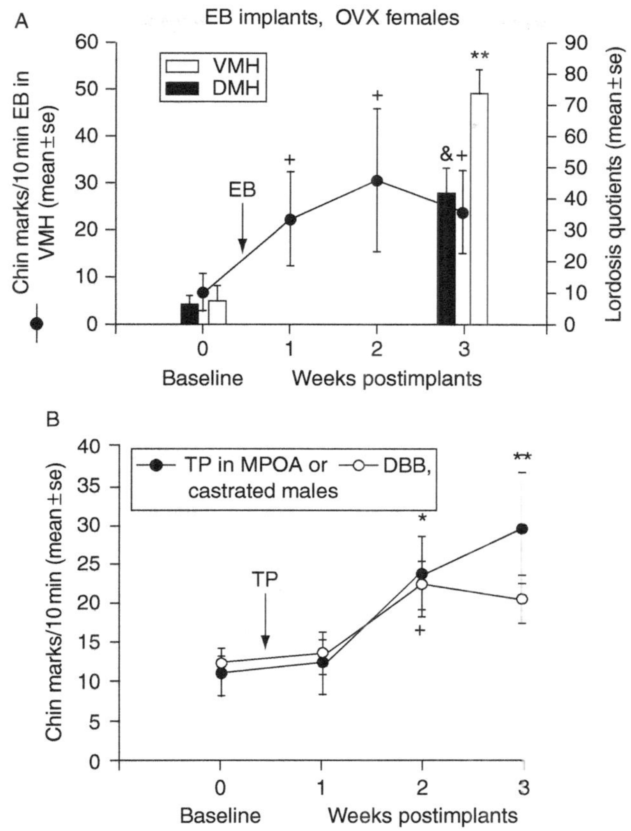

Figure 15.5 (A) Effect of implanting estradiol benzoate (EB) into the ventromedial (VMH) or dorsomedial (DMH) hypothalamus of ovx does on chinning and sexual receptivity. Scent-marking was stimulated only by implants in the VMH while lordosis was elicited from either implantation site. (B) Chinning frequency (but not sexual behavior) increased in castrated bucks following TP implants into the medial preoptic area (MPOA) or diagonal band of Broca (DBB). Reproduced from Melo *et al.* (2008) with the kind permission of Elsevier.

and Verberne, 1975). Females chin-mark more frequently the bricks previously marked by males than those marked by females, bricks marked by animals kept under long, rather than short, photoperiod and those marked with chin gland secretion rather than with donor's urine or with carrot or lemon juice (Hudson and Vodermayer, 1992). The olfactory perception of the animal's own deposited secretions also modulates chinning frequency: removal of the submandibular glands provoked, one month later, a significant reduction in scent-marking even in gonadally intact males (Chirino *et al.*, 1993).

The perception of male submandibular gland secretions allows females to discriminate between dominant (high chinning) and subordinate (low chinning) males: does spend more time near high-ranking individuals, chinning frequently around them (Reece-Engel, 1988). Chin-marking, in the context of an aggressive chase between two males, precedes and follows paw-scraping and is nearly always performed by the aggressor individual (Bell, 1980). This observation coincides with the recent finding that, in domestic male rabbits studied in a laboratory setting, a significant correlation exists between chinning frequency and the likelihood of winning a confrontation with another buck (Arteaga *et al.*, 2008).

The possibility that chinning frequency could also be modulated by the perception of the visual characteristics of the marked objects was initially suggested by Black-Cleworth and Verberne (1975). In a recent study, we varied the visual aspect and the texture of the objects placed for marking, as well as the location of the chinning arena, and we determined chinning frequency and ambulation in an open field across tests that lasted longer than usual (Hoffman *et al.*, 2010). Bricks with a rough surface elicited significantly more scent-marks than did polished onyx spheres but chinning and ambulation habituated with time and both behaviors were expressed at low levels by 30 min. High scent-marking scores were reinstated when (following a 5-min interval in which rabbits were removed from the arena) the original objects were replaced by visually different ones. Ambulation increased only when the arena was moved to a different location. Modifying the olfactory characteristics of the objects did not restimulate chinning or ambulation. These results indicate that both behaviors can be stimulated by the texture of objects or the visual characteristics of a new environment.

4. Biological significance

Despite being a conspicuous behavior, little is known about the significance of chin-marking in rabbit colonies. Wild rabbits organize themselves into social groups of 4–6 females and 1–2 males around a central warren, each with its own territory and a clearly established dominance hierarchy (Mykytowycz, 1962, 1965, 1968). They communicate with each other through chemical signals that include the secretions from the chin and inguinal glands as well as urine and fecal pellets coated with secretion from the anal glands. It has been proposed that the main functions of chinning are to establish and maintain social rank within the colony, to authenticate territoriality, and to enhance self-confidence (Mykytowycz, 1962, 1965; Mykytowycz *et al.*, 1976). Indeed, in wild rabbits, chin-marking is more frequent within their own territory than in a foreign area, and exposing animals in an arena to some components isolated from chin gland secretions significantly modifies their heart-rate (Goodrich, 1983). Moreover, as stated earlier, the frequency of chinning, the size and weight of the chin glands, and their secretory activity correlate positively with social rank and reproductive activity (Arteaga *et al.*, 2008; Bell, 1985; Black-Cleworth and Verberne, 1975; Mykytowycz, 1962, 1965; Mykytowycz and Dudzinski, 1966; Wales and Ebling, 1971). Although dominance hierarchies are more prominent in males than in females, to regulate access to limited resources, both sexes have a separate linear rank order (Holst *et al.*, 2002). The annual reproductive success of females is influenced to a large extent by their social rank, as evidenced by the higher fecundity and lower offspring mortality of high-ranking females (Holst *et al.*, 2002).

Another function proposed for chinning is to aid in mate selection. Under natural conditions, females must choose a buck to mate with and odors coming from the scent-marks could provide information about the quality of potential candidates, such as, social rank, health status, genotype, or ownership of territory (Reece-Engel, 1990). Although few studies have directly addressed these possibilities, our finding that mating drastically reduces chinning in bucks and does agrees with an important role of this behavior in the selection (and acquisition) of a sexual partner.

C. Chemical signals from the mammary gland

1. Nipple-search behavior in newborns

Mother rabbits nurse their young only once a day, inside the maternal nest; each nursing bout lasts around 3 min (González-Mariscal *et al.*, 1994b, 2007). These conditions demand that the pups, which are born altricial, with their eyelids closed, find the maternal nipples (in the darkness of an underground burrow) within a short period of time and suckle enough milk to sustain them for the next 24 h. Early work from Schley (1976) and Hudson and Distel (1983) provided behavioral evidence that an olfactory signal, emanating from the mother's belly, triggered in the pups a stereotyped behavior that guided them toward the maternal nipples and allowed them to suckle. The motor pattern provoked by the perception of such olfactory cue consists of rapid lateral and rostrocaudal head movements which are accompanied by slower motions of the frontal extremities; upon locating the nipple the young open their mouths and immediately grasp the nipple. The emission of this olfactory signal (originally termed "nipple-search pheromone," NSP) was quantified through a bioassay that counts the number of pups that find the maternal nipples within a few seconds and suckle them (Hudson and Distel, 1983). NSP is perceived by the main olfactory system of the pups as sectioning the lateral olfactory nerves prevents them from locating the maternal nipples (Hudson and Distel, 1986).

2. Hormonal regulation of NSP emission

As stated earlier, perception of the NSP from the mother's ventrum is critical for the young's survival during early lactation. Yet, this olfactory cue is also emitted by pregnant and, to a lesser extent, estrous does (Hudson and Distel, 1984). In the latter long photoperiods promote the emission of higher levels of NSP than do short ones (Hudson and Distel, 1990). This effect is mediated by melatonin (which is secreted during darkness; Brainard *et al.*, 1984; Reiter, 1993) because s.c. implants of minipumps that gradually release this hormone mimic the effects of short photoperiod in estrous does housed under long photoperiod conditions (Hudson *et al.*, 1994). Together, the above evidence suggested an important role of ovarian hormones in regulating the emission of NSP. To test this possibility we administered specific combinations of EB and progesterone to ovx does and found that, indeed, EB alone stimulated the emission of NSP, though to a lesser extent than when combined with progesterone (Hudson *et al.*, 1990). Moreover, withdrawal of progesterone (but continuation of EB) led to a decrease in the levels of NSP, which rose to maximal ones with daily injections of prolactin (González-Mariscal *et al.*, 1994a; Fig. 15.6). These results show that, across the doe rabbit's reproductive cycle (i.e., estrus, pregnancy, lactation) concomitant changes in ovarian and pituitary hormones regulate the emission of the NSP. At the same time, these findings question the significance of such olfactory cue during estrus and pregnancy, when suckling young are absent.

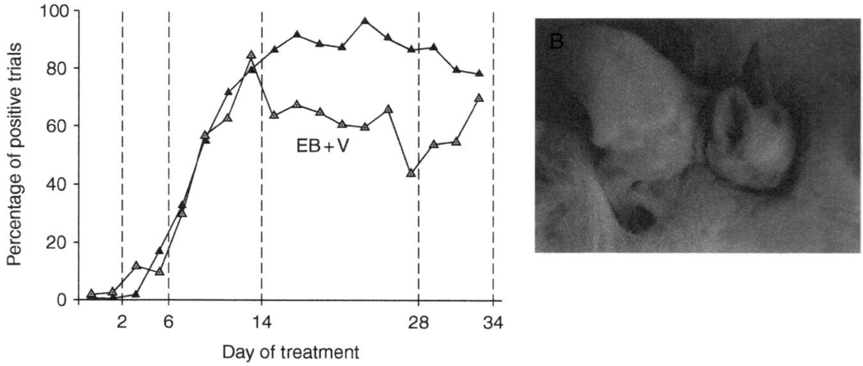

Figure 15.6 (A) Injections of estradiol benzoate (EB; 10 μg/day) plus progesterone (10 mg/day) stimulated nipple pheromone emission (NPE) in ovx does. Withdrawal of P followed by injections of prolactin (PRL) maintained maximal levels of NPE while injections of vehicle (V) did not. Modified from González-Mariscal *et al.* (1994a). (B) Bioassay, developed by Hudson and Distel (1983), used to quantify NPE. A female rabbit was held on its back, a pup was lightly held, placed on her belly, and allowed to search for nipples for 10 s. The proportion of pups that found a nipple and sucked it allowed us to determine the emission of "nipple pheromone."

3. The "mammary pheromone"

A volatile substance contained in milk, capable of triggering in the pups the same stereotyped behavioral responses they show when placed on a mother's belly, was identified by Schaal *et al.* (2003) as the compound 2-methyl-but-2-enal (2MB2) and termed "mammary pheromone" (MP). When synthetic MP was offered on a glass rod, rabbit pups showed the above-described rapid head movements characteristic of "nipple-search" behavior and grasped the rod carrying 2MB2. Moreover, MP was species-specific as neither hares nor kittens or rat pups showed these responses when exposed to 2MB2 while pups from several rabbit breeds invariably did (Schaal *et al.*, 2003). Interestingly, the percentage of rabbit pups that show the above behavioral responses varies with time of day and prandial state (Moncomble *et al.*, 2005).

4. Source(s) of mammary gland pheromone(s)

The identification of 2MB2 in milk prompted the investigation into the source(s) of this olfactory cue. While pups exposed to samples of milk ejected through the nipples responded effectively, milk taken directly from the alveoli of the mammary gland did not provoke this effect (Moncomble *et al.*, 2005). Moreover, behavioral responses were also lacking when the young were exposed to *tissue* derived from the mammary gland itself or from beneath the nipples. By using a different approach, we found that the surgical removal of the nipples before mating did not antagonize maternal behavior, as females willingly entered the nest box and positioned themselves over the litter. Yet, when pups were placed on the belly of such thelectomized mothers they did not show the rapid head movements associated with the perception of the NSP; rather, they performed a "swimming-like" behavior in which they slowly moved across the female's belly using their four extremities (González-Mariscal *et al.*, 2000). Taken together, the above results hint that the nipple may be a critical structure in which the olfactory cues that trigger nipple-search behavior in the pups are produced or modified.

III. Other Sources of Chemical Signals

In addition to the chin glands and the mammary gland–nipple complex, rabbits produce odoriferous substances in several other skin glands, namely, inguinal, anal, lachrymal, Harder's (located between the eyeball and the median corner of the orbit), and preputial (located around the entrance of the vagina; Martínez-Gómez *et al.*, 1997). In inguinal glands a regulation by steroid hormones, similar to that described for chin glands, has been reported (see above; Wales and Ebling, 1971). Harder's glands are larger in bucks than in does and their weight (as that of lachrymal glands) is largest during the breeding period. The activity of Harder's glands is correlated with social hierarchy as dominant rabbits (male and female) show histological evidence of more intense secretory function than subordinates. Gonadectomy decreases the size of both Harder's and lachrymal glands in males but provokes the opposite effect in females (Mykytowycz and Dudzinski, 1966). Anal glands do not show a sexual dimorphism in size but castration in males reduces their volume while the injection of testosterone reverses this effect (Coujard, 1947). The odor of anal gland secretions becomes stronger with increasing age, is more intense in bucks than in does, is reduced by castration, and is maximal during the breeding season (Hesterman and Mykytowycz, 1968).

The effect of the secretions from the above-described skin glands on the behavioral or physiological reactions of recipient conspecifics has been much less explored. To test whether inguinal gland secretions advertise sexual receptivity, stud males were exposed to the secretions from estrous or ovx does and their behavioral responses were recorded. No differences were found between the reactions elicited by these two stimuli, results suggesting that inguinal gland secretions do not communicate the female's reproductive state to the buck (Ordinola *et al.*, 1997). Another function for inguinal gland secretions has been proposed, namely, individual recognition. Mother rabbits confronted with their own progeny, smeared with the inguinal gland secretions of other females, sniffed and nudged them more than the unscented pups, and even chased and bit them (Mykytowycz and Goodrich, 1974).

In addition to the secretions produced by skin glands, urine contains signals that may convey information about the sex, age, social status, and individual identity of the depositing animal (for review, see Bell, 1980).

IV. Conclusions and Future Directions

This review has presented evidence that rabbits produce an abundance of olfactory signals, whose function is becoming apparent in specific cases. Notably, several experimental approaches have provided evidence on the neuroendocrine regulation of chin-marking. This behavior is tightly controlled, in both sexes, by gonadal steroids that act on specific nuclei of the diencephalon to stimulate chinning, alone or (in females) together with sexual receptivity. Although chinning is a stereotyped motor pattern, the perception of visual, tactile, or olfactory cues modulates its frequency of expression. This indicates that the stimulation of chinning most likely involves the activation of cortical and telencephalic neurons which, in turn, connect to and stimulate motoneurons in the brainstem and high spinal cord that control the jaw and neck movements characteristic of chinning. A common neural substrate with sexual receptivity seems to exist only at the level of the diencephalon as (from evidence in rodents) there is a separate lordosis-controlling system that involves axons descending to the brainstem, mesencephalic central gray, and spinal cord (Melo *et al.*, 2008; Fig. 15.7).

However, a powerful, immediate inhibition of chinning is exerted by mating in bucks and does. Exploring this phenomenon in the future, using the tools of pharmacology, will yield information on the neurotransmitters involved in the onset and offset of chin-marking. Additionally, as this behavior is steroid dependent, experiments that lesion brain regions containing estrogen receptors (in females) will enrich the information obtained

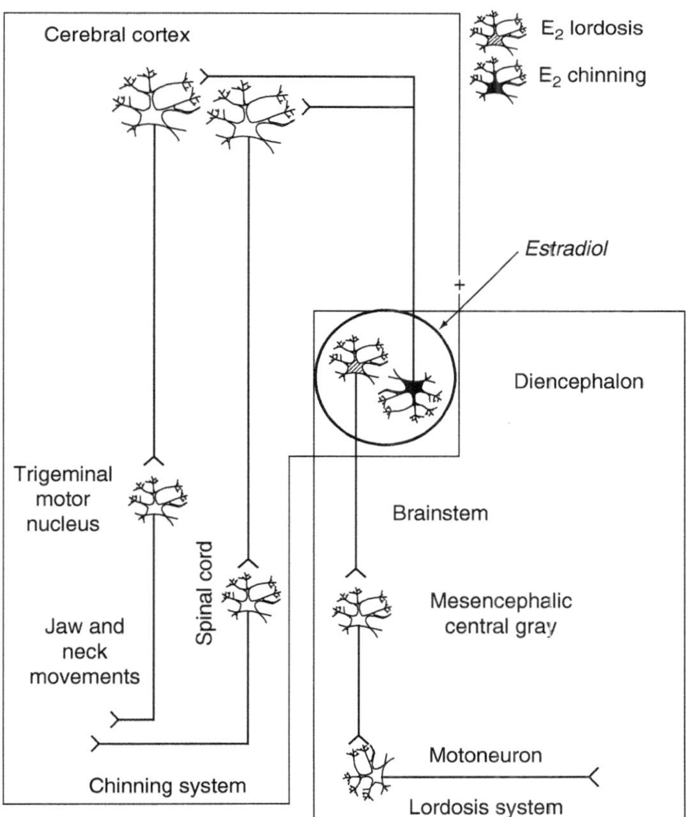

Figure 15.7 Diagram showing two neuronal estradiol-sensitive neuronal systems that could control the expression of chinning and sexual behavior in female rabbits. Reproduced from Melo *et al.* (2008) with the kind permission of Elsevier.

from the intracerebral implantation of EB. More work in males is needed in this regard, for example, nothing is known about the distribution of androgen receptors in the brain nor about the sites where TP implants can effectively stimulate sexual behavior.

The biological function of depositing a variety of odoriferous substances in the environment for the life of an individual has received relatively little attention in rabbits. Only a few experiments have documented the effect of the presence of a conspecific's scent-marks on the recipient's behavior (see Section IIA and B). The scanty evidence available suggests that chin-marks are associated with sexual behavior while inguinal gland secretions are related with individual identification. Yet, *all* skin glands investigated show the *same* response to sex steroids, in terms of effects of gonadectomy and hormonal replacement, a clear sexual dimorphism, and an increased gland size during the breeding season. This common response may indicate that gonadal steroids promote the production of "the adequate" scent-marks (by their action on the glands themselves) and also the *possibility* of engaging in scent-marking by acting on the neural substrate that regulates the motor aspects of this behavior. Finally, the *voluntary* choice to scent-mark (or not) would involve the complex evaluation by the animal of the signals (social, physical) in its environment. A final reflection concerning the biological meaning of scent-marks is how the olfactory cues of a given species can influence the population dynamics of a different one. Recently, Monclús *et al.* (2009) found that the distribution of foxes in central Spain was correlated with the distribution of rabbits, a finding indicating the complex evolution of mechanisms for detecting or emitting olfactory signals in predator and prey, respectively.

The olfactory cue emanating from the doe's nipples is the example for which a function has been more firmly established. The role of guiding the young to the mother's nipples is obviously essential for their survival. Yet, whether that is the sole role of the MP (or NSP) remains to be established. As recently discussed by Caba and González-Mariscal (2009), the anticipatory motor activity displayed by rabbit pups before nursing (Caba *et al.*, 2008; Hudson and Distel, 1982; Jilge, 1995) can be a consequence of the physiological response to milk intake, the perception of the NSP, or both. The demonstration that this cue is present in milk (Keil *et al.*, 1990), that its chemical identity has been determined (Schaal *et al.*, 2003), and that synthetic 2MB2 is readily available allows the performance of experiments in which potential additional roles of the MP can be explored. Determining the source of the MP and establishing whether it has the same chemical identity as the NSP are unsolved issues that demand using a multidisciplinary approach. Knowledge of the hormonal combinations that stimulate the emission of a cue that triggers the stereotyped nipple-search behavior in the pups (see Section IIC) should aid in this regard.

We conclude this review by emphasizing that the robust behavioral responses identified in rabbits, either in association with scent deposition or as a consequence of having perceived an olfactory cue, make them an ideal model for investigating major issues in neuroendocrinology, olfaction physiology, behavioral ecology, or psychobiology. Hopefully, interdisciplinary approaches will be used in future studies to address problems specific to those fields.

ACKNOWLEDGMENTS

The authors thank M.Sc. César G. Toriz González, Irene Ochoa, Carlos E. Aguilar, and Ma. de los Angeles Martínez for their help in preparation of figures.

REFERENCES

Arteaga, L., Bautista, A., Martínez-Gomez, M., Nicolás, L., and Hudson, R. (2008). Scent marking, dominance and serum testosterone levels in male domestic rabbits. *Physiol. Behav.* **94,** 510–515.

Bakker, J., and Baum, M. J. (2000). Neuroendocrine regulation of GnRH release in induced ovulators. *Front. Neuroendocrinol.* **21,** 220–262.

Bell, D. J. (1980). Social olfaction in lagomorphs. *Symp. Zool. Soc. Lond.* **45,** 141–164.

Bell, D. J. (1985). The rabbits and hares: Order lagomorpha. *In* "Social Odours in Mammalians," (R. E. Brown and D. W. MacDonald, Eds.), Vol. 2, pp. 507–530.

Beyer, C., and Rivaud, N. (1969). Sexual behavior in pregnant and lactating domestic rabbits. *Physiol. Behav.* **4,** 753–757.

Beyer, C., de la Torre, L., Larsson, K., and Pérez-Palacios, G. (1975). Synergistic actions of estrogen and androgen on the sexual behavior of the castrated male rabbit. *Horm. Behav.* **6,** 301–306.

Beyer, C., Velazquez, J., Larsson, K., and Contreras, J. L. (1980). Androgen regulation of the motor copulatory pattern in the male New Zealand White rabbit. *Horm. Behav.* **14,** 179–190.

Black-Cleworth, P., and Verberne, G. (1975). Scent-marking, dominance and flehmen behavior in domestic rabbits in an artificial laboratory territory. *Chem. Senses Flav.* **1,** 465–594.

Brainard, G. C., Matthews, S. A., Steger, R. W., Reiter, R. J., and Asch, R. (1984). Day: night variations of melatonin, 5-hydoxyindole acetic acid, serotonin, serotonin N-acetyltransferase, tryptophan, norepinephrine and dopamine in the rabbit pineal gland. *Life Sci.* **35,** 1615–1622.

Caba, M., and González-Mariscal, G. (2009). The rabbit pup, a natural model of nursing anticipatory activity. *Eur. J. Neurosci.* **30,** 1697–1706.

Caba, M., Beyer, C., González-Mariscal, G., and Morrell, J. I. (2003). Immunocytochemical detection of estrogen receptor-α in the female rabbit forebrain: Topography and regulation by estradiol. *Neuroendocrinology* **77,** 208–222.

Caba, M., Tovar, A., Silver, R., Morgado, E., Meza, E., Zavaleta, Y., and Juárez, C. (2008). Nature's food anticipatory experiment: Entrainment of locomotor behavior, suprachiasmatic and dorsomedial hypothalamic nuclei by suckling in rabbit pups. *Eur. J. Neurosci.* **27,** 432–443.

Camacho-Arroyo, I., Cerbón, M., Gamboa-Domínguez, A., González-Agüero, G., and González-Mariscal, G. (1999). Immunocytochemical detection of estrogen and progesterone receptors in the rabbit submandibular gland. *Comp. Biochem. Physiol. A Mol. Integr. Physiol.* **123,** 179–186.

Cerbón, M. A., Camacho-Arroyo, I., Gamboa-Domínguez, A., and González-Mariscal, G. (1996). The rabbit submandibular glads: Sexual dimorphism, effects of gonadectomy, and variations across the female reproductive cycle. *J. Comp. Physiol. A* **178,** 351–357.

Chirino, R., González-Mariscal, G., Carrillo, P., and Pacheco, P. (1993). Effect of removing the chin-marking behaviour in male rabbits of the New Zealand race. *Z. Sâugertierkunde.* **58,** 116–121.

Coujard, R. (1947). Étude des glandes odorantes du lapin et de leur influencement par les hormones sexuelles. *Rev. Can. Biol.* **6,** 3–25.

Dluzen, D., and Vandenbergh, J. G. (1992). Puberty acceleration in mice induced with a partially purified male urine extract: Effects on catecholamine release from the olfactory bulbs and hypothalamus. *Brain Res.* **585,** 367–371.

González-Mariscal, G., Melo, A. I., Zavala, A., and Beyer, C. (1990). Variations in chin-marking behavior of New Zealand female rabbits throughout the whole reproductive cycle. *Physiol. Behav.* **48,** 361–365.

González-Mariscal, G., Melo, A. I., Zavala, A., and Beyer, C. (1992). Chin-marking behavior in male and female New Zealand rabbits: Onset, development, and activation by steroids. *Physiol. Behav.* **52,** 889–893.

González-Mariscal, G., Melo, A. I., Zavala, A., Chirino, R., and Beyer, C. (1993). Sex steroid regulation of chin-marking behavior in male New Zealand rabbits. *Physiol. Behav.* **54,** 1035–1040.

González-Mariscal, G., Chirino, R., and Hudson, R. (1994a). Prolactin stimulates emission of nipple pheromone in ovariectomized New Zealand white rabbits. *Biol. Reprod.* **50,** 373–376.

González-Mariscal, G., Díaz-Sánchez, V., Melo, A. I., Beyer, C., and Rosenblatt, J. S. (1994b). Maternal behavior in New Zealand white rabbits: Quantification of somatic events, motor patterns and steroid plasma levels. *Physiol. Behav.* **55,** 1081–1089.

González-Mariscal, G., Albonetti, M. E., Cuamatzi, E., and Beyer, C. (1997). Transitory inhibition of scent-marking by copulation in male and female rabbits. *Anim. Behav.* **53,** 323–333.

González-Mariscal, G., Melo, A. I., Parlow, A. F., Beyer, C., and Rosenblatt, J. S. (2000). Pharmacological evidence that prolactin acts from late gestation to promote maternal behavior in rabbits. *J. Neuroendocrinol.* **12,** 983–992.

González-Mariscal, G., Mc Nitt, J. I., and Lukefahr, S. D. (2007). Maternal care of rabbits in the lab and on the farm: Endocrine regulation of behavior and productivity. *Horm. Behav.* **52,** 86–91.

Goodrich, B. S. (1983). Studies of the chemical composition of secretion from skin gland of the rabbis *Oryctolagus cuniculus* (L.). *In* "Chemical Signals in Vertebrates III," (R. M. Silverstein and D. Müller-Scwarze, Eds.), pp. 275–290. Plenum Publ. Corp., New York.

Goodrich, B. S., and Mykytowycz, R. (1972). Individual and sex differences in the chemical composition of pheromone-like substances from the skin glands of the rabbits *Oryctolagus cuniculus* (L.). *J. Mammal.* **53,** 540–548.

Hayes, R. A., Richardson, B. J., and Wyllie, S. G. (2001). Increased social dominance in male rabbits, *Oryctolagus cuniculus*, is associated with increased of 2-phenoxy ethanol from the chin gland. *In* "Chemical Signals in Vertebrates," (A. Marchlewska-Koj, J. J. Lepri, and D. Müller-Schwarze, Eds.), Vol. 9, pp. 335–342. Plenum/Kluwer Press, New York.

Hayes, R. A., Richardson, B. J., and Wyllie, S. G. (2002a). Semiochemicals and social signaling in the wild European rabbit in Australia: I. Scent profiles of chin gland secretion from the field. *J. Chem. Ecol.* **28,** 363–383.

Hayes, R. A., Richardson, B. J., Claus, S. C., and Wyllie, S. G. (2002b). Semiochemicals and social signaling in the wild European rabbit in Australia: II Variations in chemical composition of chin gland secretion across sampling sites. *J. Chem. Ecol.* **28,** 2613–2625.

Hayes, R. A., Richardson, B. J., and Wyllie, S. G. (2003). To fix or not to fix: The role of 2-phenoxyethanol in rabbit, *Oryctolagus cuniculus*, chin gland secretion. *J. Chem. Ecol.* **29,** 1051–1064.

Hernández, M. R., Wenk, E. J., and Vittek, J. (1982). Autoradiographic localization of dexamethasone in the rabbit submandibular gland. *J. Dent. Res.* **61,** 821–823.

Hesterman, E. R., and Mykytowycz, M. (1968). Some observations on the odour of anal gland secretions from the rabbit, *Oryctolagus cuniculus* (L). *CSIRO Wildl. Res.* **13,** 71–81.

Hoffman, K. L., and González-Mariscal, G. (2006). Progesterone receptor activation signals behavioral transitions across the reproductive cycle of the female rabbit. *Horm. Behav.* **50,** 154–168.

Hoffman, K. L., and González-Mariscal, G. (2007). Relevante of ovarian signaling for the early behavioral transition from estrus to pregnancy in the female rabbit. *Horm. Behav.* **52,** 531–539.

Hoffman, K. L., Hernández Decasa, D. M., Beyer Ruíz, M. E., and González-Mariscal, G. (2010). Scent marking by the male domestic rabbit (*Oryctolagus cuniculus*) is stimulated by an object's novelty and its specific visual or tactile characteristics. *Behav. Brain Res.* **207,** 360–367.

Holst, D., von Hutzelmeyer, H., Kaetzke, P., Khaschei, M., Rôdel, H. G., and Schrutka, H. (2002). Social rank, fecundity and lifetime reproductive success in wild European rabbits (*Oryctolagus cuniculus*). *Behav. Ecol. Sociobiol.* **51,** 245–254.

Hudson, R., and Distel, H. (1982). The pattern of behavior of rabbit pups in the nest. *Behaviour* **85,** 260–275.

Hudson, R., and Distel, H. (1983). Nipple location by newborn rabbits: Behavioural evidence for pheromonal guidance. *Behaviour* **85,** 260–275.

Hudson, R., and Distel, H. (1984). Nipple-search pheromone in rabbits: Dependence on season and reproductive state. *J. Comp. Physiol. A* **155,** 13–17.

Hudson, R., and Distel, H. (1986). Pheromonal release of suckling in rabbits does not depend on the vomeronasal organ. *Physiol. Behav.* **37,** 123–129.

Hudson, R., and Distel, H. (1990). Sensitivity of female rabbits to changes in photoperiod as measured by pheromone emission. *J. Comp. Physiol. A* **167,** 225–230.

Hudson, R., and Vodermayer, T. (1992). Spontaneous and odor-induced chin marking in domestic female rabbits. *Anim. Behav.* **43,** 329–336.

Hudson, R., González-Mariscal, G., and Beyer, C. (1990). Chin-marking behavior, sexual receptivity, and pheromone emission in steroid-treated, ovariectomized rabbits. *Horm. Behav.* **24,** 1–13.

Hudson, R., Melo, A. I., and González-Mariscal, G. (1994). Effect of photoperiod and exogenous melatonin on correlates of estrus in the domestic rabbit. *J. Comp. Physiol.* **175,** 573–579.

Jilge, B. (1995). Ontogeny of the rabbit's circadian rhythms without an external zeitgeber. *Physiol. Behav.* **58,** 131–140.

Keil, W., von Stralendorff, F., and Hudson, R. (1990). A behavioral bioassay for analysis of rabbit nipple-search pheromone. *Physiol. Behav.* **47,** 525–529.

Kurosumi, K., Yamagishi, M., and Sekine, M. (1961). Mitochondrial deformation and apocrine secretory mechanism in the rabbit submandibular organ as revealed by electron microscopy. *Z. Zellforschung.* **55,** 297–312.

Lyne, A. G., Molyneux, G. S., Mykytowycz, R., and Parakkal, P. F. (1964). The development, structure, and function of the submandibular cutaneous (chin) glands in the rabbit. *Aust. J. Zool.* **12,** 340–348.

Martínez-Gómez, M., Lucio, R. A., Carro, M., Pacheco, P., and Hudson, R. (1997). Striated muscles and scent glands associated with the vaginal tract of the rabbit. *Anat. Rec.* **247,** 486–495.

McClintock, M. K. (1982). Group mating among Norway rats. II. The social dynamics of copulation: Competition, cooperation and mate choice. *Anim. Behav.* **30,** 410–425.

McDonald, P. G., Vidal, N., and Beyer, C. (1970). Sexual behavior in the ovariectomized rabbit after treatment with different amounts of gonadal hormones. *Horm. Behav.* **1,** 161–172.

Melo, A. I., Chirino, R., Jiménez, A., Cuamatzi, E., Beyer, C., and González-Mariscal, G. (2008). Effect of forebrain implants of testosterona or estradiol on scent-marking and sexual behavior in male and female rabbits. *Horm. Behav.* **54,** 676–683.

Monclús, R., Arroyo, M., Valencia, A., and De Miguel, F. J. (2009). Red foxes (*Vulpes vulpes*) use rabbit (*Oryctolagus cuniculus*) scent marks as territorial marking sites. *J. Ethol.* **27,** 153–156.

Moncomble, R. S., Coureaud, G., Quennedey, B., Langlois, D., Perrier, G., and Shaal, B. (2005). The mammary pheromone of the rabbit: From where does it come? *Anim. Behav.* **69,** 29–38.

Myers, K., and Poole, W. D. (1961). A study of the biology of the wild rabbit, *Oryctolagus cuniculus* (L) in confined population II. The effect of season and population increase on behaviour. *CSIRO Widl. Res.* **6,** 1–41.

Mykytowycz, R. (1962). Territorial function of chin gland secretion in the rabbit *Oryctolagus cuniculus* (L.). *Nature* **193,** 799.

Mykytowycz, R. (1965). Further observations on the territorial function and histology of the submandibular cutaneous (chin) glands in the rabbit, *Oryctolagus cuniculus* (L). *Anim. Behav.* **13,** 400–412.

Mykytowycz, R. (1968). Territorial marking by rabbits. *Sci. Am.* **218,** 116–126.

Mykytowycz, R. (1970). The role of skin glands in mammalian communication. *In* "Advances in Chemoreception," (J. B. Johnston, D. G. Moulton, and A. Turk. Eds.), Vol I: Communication by Chemical Signals, pp. 327-360. Appleton-Century-Crofts, New York.

Mykytowycz, R., and Dudzinski, M. L. (1966). A study of weight of odoriferous and other glands in relation to social status and degree of sexual activity in the wild rabbit, *Oryctolagus cuniculus* (L). *CSIRO Wildl. Res.* **11,** 31–47.

Mykytowycz, R., and Goodrich, B. S. (1974). Skin glands as organs of communication in mammals. *J. Invest. Dermatol.* **62,** 124–131.

Mykytowycz, R., and Ward, M. M. (1971). Some reactions of nestlings of the wild rabbit, *Oryctolagus cuniculus* (L.) when exposed to natural rabbit odors. *Forma Funct.* **4,** 137–148.

Mykytowycz, R., Hesterman, E. R., Gambale, S., and Dudzinski, M. L. (1976). A comparison of the effectiveness of the odors of rabbits, *Oryctolagus cuniculus*, in enhancing territorial confidence. *J. Chem. Ecol.* **2,** 13–24.

Ordinola, P., Martínez-Gómez, M., Manzo, J., and Hudson, R. (1997). Response of male domestic rabbits (*Oryctolagus cuniculus*) to inguinal gland secretion from intact and ovariectomized females. *J. Chem. Ecol.* **23,** 2079–2091.

Palka, Y. S., and Sawyer, C. H. (1966a). The effect of hypothalamic implants of ovarian steroids on oestrous behaviour in rabbits. *J. Physiol.* **185,** 251–269.

Palka, Y. S., and Sawyer, C. H. (1966b). Induction of estrous behavior in rabbit by hypothalamic implants of testosterone. *Am. J. Physiol.* **211,** 225–228.

Poindron, P., Lévy, F., and Keller, M. (2007). Maternal responsiveness and maternal selectivity in domestic sheep and goats: The two facets of maternal attachment. *Dev. Psychobiol.* **49,** 54–70.

Price, M. A., and Vandenbergh, J. G. (1992). Analysis of puberty-accelerating pheromones. *J. Exp. Zool.* **264,** 42–45.

Ramírez, V. D., and Beyer, C. (1988). The ovarian cycle of the rabbit: Its neuroendocrine control. *In* "The Physiology of Reproduction," (E. K. Knobil and J. D. Neils, Eds.), Vol. 2, pp. 1873–1892. Raven Press, New York.

Reece-Engel, C. (1988). Female choice of resident male rabbits *Oryctolagus cuniculus*. *Anim. Behav.* **36,** 1241–1242.

Reece-Engel, C. (1990). Scent marking, residency, and female choice in the European rabbit (*Oryctolagus cuniculus*). *In* "Chemical Signals in Vertebrates," (D. W. MacDonald, D. Müller-Schwarze, and S. E. Natynczuk, Eds.), Vol. 5, pp. 329–335. Oxford University Press.

Reiter, R. J. (1993). The melatonin rhythm: Both a clock and a calendar. *Experientia* **49,** 654–664.

Schaal, B., Coureaud, G., Langlois, D., Giniès, C., Sémon, E., and Perrier, G. (2003). Chemical and behavioural characterization of the rabbit mammary pheromone. *Nature* **424,** 68–72.

Schank, J. D., and McClintock, M. K. (1997). Ovulatory pheromone shortens ovarian cycles of female rats living in olfactory isolation. *Physiol. Behav.* **62,** 899–904.

Schley, P. (1976). Untersuchung zur künstlichen Aufzucht von Hauskaninchen Habilitation Thesis, Universität Giessen.

Soares, M. J., and Diamond, M. (1982). Pregnancy and chin marking in the rabbit, *Oryctolagus cuniculus*. *Anim. Behav.* **30,** 941–943.

Stoufflet, I., and Caillol, (1988). Relation between circulating sex steroid concentrations and sexual behavior during pregnancy and *post partum* in the domestic rabbit. *J. Reprod. Fert.* **82,** 209–218.

Wales, N. A. M., and Ebling, F. J. (1971). The control of the apocrine glands of the rabbit by steroid hormones. *J. Endocrinol.* **51,** 763–770.

CHAPTER SIXTEEN

Chemical Communication and Reproduction in the Gray Short-Tailed Opossum (*Monodelphis domestica*)

John D. Harder *and* Leslie M. Jackson

Contents

Abstract

The gray short-tailed opossum is one of the most widely studied of all marsupials and an important model for study of olfactory communication, particularly as it relates to pheromonal activation of reproduction. Males respond to differentially to female skin gland secretions and urine from anestrous females, while females respond only skin gland secretions, particularly that of the suprasternal gland. Divergent responses by male and female opossums to odors from these different

Department of Evolution, Ecology, and Organismal Biology, The Ohio State University, Columbus, Ohio

Vitamins and Hormones, Volume 83
ISSN 0083-6729, DOI: 10.1016/S0083-6729(10)83016-X

body sources are most likely related to sex-specific production and deposition of chemical signals in this species. Female opossums do not have an estrous cycle but are stimulated to estrus by male pheromone. Females nuzzle scent marks from male suprasternal gland secretions, and thereby facilitate delivery of a nonvolatile estrus-inducing pheromone to the chemosensory epithelium of vomeronasal organ. Neuroendocrine correlates of pheromonal induction of estrus include elevated plasma estradiol and upregulation of progesterone receptors in hypothalamic regions that control reproductive behavior.

I. Chemical Communication and Mammalian Reproduction

Mammals rely on their chemical senses to find food or investigate potential food, establish and maintain territories, and recognize individuals. Conspecific odor cues, or pheromones, are also involved in coordination of reproductive physiology and behavior. The term "pheromone" was first used as a descriptor of a chemical signal that acts as an innate releaser of insect behavior in a recipient of the same species (Karlson and Lüscher, 1959). For mammals, the definition of a pheromone was broadened to include a releaser pheromone that evokes an immediate behavioral response by the receiving individual, and a primer pheromone, that generates a long-term physiological or developmental change (Bronson, 1968; Wilson and Bosser, 1963). More recently, signaler pheromones have been distinguished from releaser pheromones as cues that provide immediate information, but do not necessarily elicit a behavioral response from the receiver (Johnston, 1983; Wysocki and Preti, 2004). A fourth category of pheromones, modulators, has been introduced as those pheromones that cause a change in the mood of an individual or affect the function of other sensory pathways (Jacob and McClintock, 2000). Pheromones in all four categories have been associated with many aspects of mammalian reproduction including sexual behavior, onset of puberty, partner preference, ovulation, conception, lactation, parental care, and social dominance hierarchies (Vandenbergh, 2006).

Much of our understanding of which reproductive functions are controlled by chemical cues and the neural circuitry connecting pheromone detection to reproductive response comes from more than 50 years of studies in rodent species, particularly mice. Primer pheromones in the urine of adult female mice delay the onset of puberty in juvenile females (Cowley and Wise, 1972; Drickamer, 1977), and suppress estrous cycles in group-housed adults (Whitten, 1959). By contrast, exposure of females to adult male urine accelerates the onset of puberty (Vandenbergh, 1969), induces and synchronizes estrous cycles in group-housed females (Whitten, 1956), and terminates a pregnancy conceived with another male (Bruce, 1960). More recent studies have expanded the list of possible sources of pheromones to include vaginal secretions (Kwan and Johnston, 1980), exudates from skin glands (Thiessen and Rice, 1976), and saliva (Smith and Block, 1991).

Two established neural pathways link chemical signals with reproductive function, the main olfactory system and the accessory olfactory system (Scalia and Winans, 1975). The main olfactory system includes chemoreceptors in the nasal epithelium and their projections to the main olfactory bulb and forebrain. The accessory olfactory system includes the sensory epithelium of the vomeronasal organ (VNO), which lies above the palate along the nasal septum, and the projections of the VNO to the accessory olfactory bulb, amygdala, and hypothalamus.

Experimental findings following ablation or disruption of one or the other of these olfactory systems demonstrate that both pathways participate in pheromone signaling, although it is widely accepted that the main olfactory system responds to volatile odors and the accessory olfactory system responds to the nonvolatile components of chemosignals. Pheromone effects on reproductive function via either one of the olfactory systems are now recognized in a variety of mammalian species including voles (Carter *et al.*, 1980), sheep (Knight and Lynch, 1980), goats (Walkden-Brown *et al.*, 1993), pigs (Dorries *et al.*, 1997), opossums (Fadem, 1987), and primates (Barrett *et al.*, 1990). In the vast majority of these studies, pheromones activate neuroendocrine responses that may either stimulate or inhibit ovarian function, and thereby impact female fertility. In only a few species studied to date, most notably the prairie vole (*Microtus orchrogaster*) and the gray short-tailed opossum (*Monodelphis domestica*; hereinafter referred to as the opossum), exposure to male pheromone is sufficient to activate an anestrous or quiescent ovary. This is unusual because ovarian function, as described below, is generally considered to be spontaneous and cyclical, although sometimes under the control of seasonal and other environmental factors. Because female opossums remain anestrous in the absence of male pheromones, they provide an opportunity for furthering our understanding of the cascade of neural and endocrine events that link chemical signals to changes in ovarian activity.

II. Reproductive Cycles and Seasonal Breeding in Female Mammals

In most female mammals, reproduction is characterized by regular ovarian cycles that include: (1) a follicular phase during which the female gametes mature in growing ovarian follicles, (2) the release of ova from the follicles at ovulation, and (3) a luteal phase in which the postovulatory follicular cells of the corpus luteum produce progestational hormones in anticipation of the ova being fertilized and subsequent implantation of embryos into the uterus. If conception does not occur, another follicular phase begins and the cycle is repeated. This cycle of follicular activity is accompanied by changes in the steroid hormones produced by the ovary. The follicular phase is associated with increasing concentrations of estradiol as follicles grow in size and the number of steroidogenic cells increases. Under these conditions, increasing concentrations of estradiol typically have a positive feedback effect on the secretion of hypothalamic gonadotropic releasing hormone (GnRH), which elicits a surge release of luteinizing hormone (LH) from the anterior pituitary gland. The LH surge stimulates ovulation, after which the remaining follicular cells luteinize and begin producing progesterone and, in some species, estradiol. The peak levels of estradiol at the time of ovulation also stimulate expression of estrus, that is, behavioral receptivity in the female. Thus, in most species, copulation coincides with the time of ovulation and increases the probability that conception will occur.

Energy balance is arguably the most critical factor regulating ovarian function. Without sufficient nutrition, the onset of puberty is delayed (Kennedy and Mitra, 1963) and adult females will have irregular cycles or cease cycling (Wade and Schneider, 1992). However, even with adequate food availability, relatively few mammalian species exhibit estrous cycles throughout the year. Their reproductive strategies have evolved under natural conditions in which food availability often varies on an annual basis. Natural selection has favored those strategies that anticipate seasonal variation in resources and optimize use of stored energy for courtship, gestation, and lactation, and maximize the probability that sufficient food will be available for offspring at the time of weaning (Bronson, 1985). Photoperiod is the predominant environmental cue controlling seasonal breeding in north temperate regions (Bronson, 1985), while annual patterns of precipitation, or wet and dry seasons, determine the availability of resources for reproduction in tropical areas (O'Connell, 1989; Perret and Atramentowicz, 1989).

The sheep is a well-studied example of a seasonal breeder in which reproductive activity is triggered annually by shortening day lengths in late summer or early autumn when females begin to have regular estrous cycles. As daylength increases in the spring, females cease cycling and generally remain anestrous until the onset of the next breeding season. Of interest to this review is the fact that photoperiodic suppression of ovarian activity in female sheep can be overridden by male odor cues. Estrus and ovulation will occur if anestrous ewes are exposed to odors in wool from a strange male (Knight and Lynch, 1980). A similar phenomenon has been demonstrated in goats (Walkden-Brown *et al.*, 1993), with the additional finding that pheromone exposure stimulates in increase in the multiunit activity of GnRH neurons, and an increase in the frequency of LH pulses (Murata *et al.*, 2009). These findings in the sheep and goat suggest that male odors are a dominant environmental signal regulating ovarian function, capable of overriding the inhibitory effects of photoperiod cues. However, female sheep and goats have spontaneous estrous cycles during permissive photoperiods, even in the absence of exposure to male odors.

Female opossums do not exhibit spontaneous ovarian cycles, but are reproductively active when exposed to male stimuli. This was first described by Fadem (1985). Subsequent studies demonstrated that unless directly exposed to males or their scent marks, adult females remain anestrous (Fadem, 1987), and juvenile females will not reach puberty (Harder and Jackson, 2003; Stonerook and Harder, 1992). In adult females, exposure to male odors results in ovarian activation and induction of estrus within 4–10 days of exposure. Activation of estrus by male odors in opossums differs from that observed in seasonally anestrous sheep in that the chemical signal is not, to our knowledge, overriding any other inhibitory environmental cue. Male odor cues are necessary and sufficient for induction of estrus in the opossum, a phenomenon that has been described in only one other species, the prairie vole (*Microtus ochrogaster*; Carter *et al.*, 1989; Richmond and Conaway, 1969). Thus, this unique aspect of female reproductive function exists in two very distantly related species, and is not simply related to the opossum being a marsupial or "nonplacental" mammal. The brief discussion of therian and metatherian mammal phylogeny and marsupial reproductive biology that follows is intended to clarify the differences in reproductive strategies between the two infraclasses, and place the unusual reproductive biology of the opossum in the context of phylogeny.

III. The Gray Short-Tailed Opossum: A Model for Pheromonal Control of Reproduction

Chemical communication plays a major role in the social behavior of mammals (Wyatt, 2003), including marsupials (Fadem, 1986; Hunsaker and Shupe, 1977). Best known in this regard among some 318 species of marsupials found worldwide is the gray short-tailed opossum. The opossum is also the most widely studied of all marsupials, and first to have its genome sequenced (Mikkelsen *et al.*, 2007). This small (60–150 g) opossum, native to the Caatinga region of southern Brazil (Streilein, 1982a), is typical of the 87 species in the neotropical family Didelphidae. The two infraclasses of therian mammals, Metatheria (marsupials), and Eutheria (all other viviparous mammals), diverged from a common ancestor 100 to 125 million years ago (Luo *et al.*, 2003; Marshall *et al.*, 1990), and the ancestral didelphid fauna of early cretaceous deposits in North America was similar in dental morphology to opossums of today. Thus, the reproductive patterns observed in extant members of Didelphidae may be viewed as primitive compared to those in more highly derived marsupials.

Didelphid marsupials are, with few exceptions, seasonally polyestrous with high ovulation rates. For example, about 60 ova are released per cycle in the Virginia opossum (*Didelphis virginiana*; Fleming and Harder, 1983). The brief gestation period does not interrupt the luteal phase of the estrous cycle (Harder and Fleming, 1981). The more highly derived kangaroos (Macropodidae) are monovular, exhibiting postpartum estrous and ovulation. Implantation of the newly conceived embryo is delayed as it enters diapause in response to stimuli associated with suckling of the neonate (Tyndale-Biscoe and Renfree, 1987). These differences aside, all marsupials share a common reproductive pattern, that is, a brief gestation period (11–30 days) and an extended period of lactation (2–12 months) that contrasts with the relatively long period of gestation and short lactation period in eutherian mammals.

"Placental mammal" is often used as a synonym for eutherian. This should be avoided, because metatherians are also placental mammals. The eutherian and metatherian placenta differs with regard to involvement of extraembryonic membranes (allantois vs. vitelline membrane), and the metatherian placenta does not invade the uterine epithelium. Nonetheless, the metatherian placenta is fully functional and efficient (Fig. 16.1). During the brief period of placentation (3–6 days), the embryo develops from a blastocyst (Harder *et al.*, 1993) to a fully formed embryo able to move on its own at birth, and find and attach to a teat where it is nourished for an extended period of body growth.

This brief review of metatherian and eutherian reproductive patterns is intended to provide an appreciation of the two infraclasses as representing

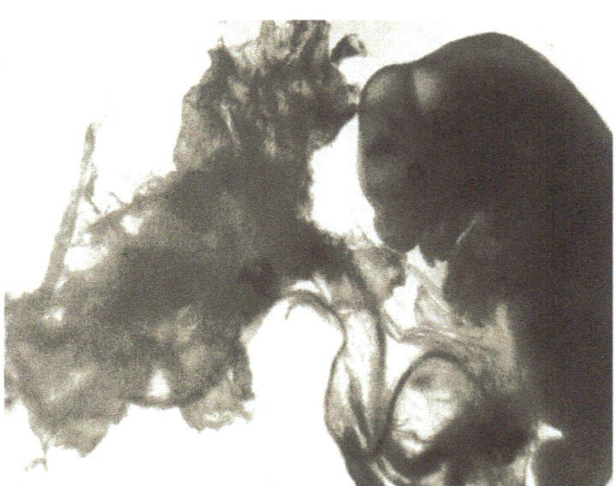

Figure 16.1 Photograph of a *Monodelphis domestica* embryo with the placenta attached taken 24 h before the expected time of parturition. Newborn opossums weigh approximately 100 mg and are 1 cm long. Photo by JDH.

alternative strategies for transfer of energy to young during gestation and lactation. The opossum merits attention as a representative metatherian, and as a model for study of olfactory inputs associated with reproductive activation. However, the unusual aspects of male pheromonal activation of reproduction seen in the opossum should not be considered typical or representative of metatherian reproduction. Although male-induced estrus and ovulation have been reported in the brush-tailed bettong (*Bettongia penicillata*; Hinds and Smith, 1992), this response appears to be rare among marsupials. Other studies of reproductive pheromones in marsupials have focused either on endocrine responses in males to female stimuli, as in *Macropus eugenii* (Catling and Sutherland, 1980; Inns, 1982) or synchronization of estrous cycles, as in woolly opossums (*Caluromys philander*; Perret and M'Barek, 1991).

IV. Olfactory Behavior; Sources and Reception of Chemical Signals

A. Olfactory behavior

Understanding olfactory communication in any species begins with knowledge of the body sources of odors and pheromones, the behaviors associated with their deposition, and some insight regarding the mechanisms used by the recipient for detection, reception, and transduction of chemical stimuli. Here, odor refers to any chemical released by one individual that is potentially detectable by another individual. As previously defined, a pheromone is an odor that elicits a predictable, stereotypic behavioral or physiological response, provides specific information, or modulates responses in the receiving individual. Mammalian odors and pheromones are secreted or released from diverse sources including skin glands, saliva, and urine. The chemical nature of odors and pheromones in scent marks is complex and not well characterized, but many of the behaviors associated with deposition of odors and another individual's response to those odors and pheromones are readily observed, and can be placed in the context of social communication. Streilein (1982a) first described sexually dimorphic scent marking behavior in the opossum, which involves use of the head, flank, and chest, particularly by males, in marking an object previously marked by other males (Fadem and Cole, 1985; Poran *et al.*, 1993a). Scent marking in males is an androgen-dependent behavior (Fadem *et al.*, 1989) that involves rubbing the head, chest, flank, and rump on hard surfaces, thereby depositing skin gland secretions from those parts of the body (Fadem and Cole, 1985). Female opossums scent mark less frequently than males and mark predominately with their head and flank, although rump dragging is a common proceptive behavior in estrous females, and males actively investigate the urine and feces of females (Streilein, 1982a).

Sniffing and nuzzling are behaviors involved with the reception of odors and pheromones. Sniffing, accompanied by a series of rapid upward jerks or vibrations of the nose, is associated with reception of volatile or airborne odors and is often a prelude to direct, nuzzling contact with a scent mark. Zuri and Halpern (2005) presented odors on cotton balls and observed that opossums first direct their snouts toward the balls, as if to access volatile cues, then touch the surface of the balls with their nose before grasping the ball and inserting their snouts deep inside. Perhaps the most prominent and stereotypic of all opossum olfactory behaviors is nuzzling, during which the opossum rapidly taps and rubs the moist surface of its nose and upper lip over a scent mark. Accompanied by an occasional licking, these actions apparently serve to dissolve components of the scent mark for delivery to the chemosensitive epithelium of the accessory olfactory organ, the VNO (Poran *et al.*, 1993b).

B. Diversity of chemosignals by body source

Much has been learned of the sources of pheromones through observation of behavioral responses to odors in scent marks collected manually from specific body regions. Zuri *et al.* (2003, 2005, 2007) used cotton balls, rubbed on skin glands or containing a drop of urine, as a standard substrate for presentation or odors from both sexes to males and females. Their findings confirm that different parts of the body produce different chemosignals (McClintock, 2002) and support previous evidence that these signals function in individual recognition (Holmes, 1992; Poran *et al.*, 1993a). Male opossums investigate odors from females more than those of males, and spend more time investigating odors from the flank skin of females than urine odors (Zuri *et al.*, 2007). Males also investigate the urine from anestrous females, but not urine from juveniles or estrous females, more than water controls (Zuri *et al.*, 2003). Because in most mammals males are attracted to urine from an estrous female, the lack of interest in or attraction to urine from estrous females is intriguing. Estrus is pheromonally induced in opossums, and so, males might enhance their chance of mating by locating an anestrous female and scent marking within her home range, particularly if estrous females are guarded or already bonded with another male.

Zuri *et al.* (2005) observed that female opossums investigated odors from male skin glands (suprasternal, flank, and submandibular) longer than those from female skin glands. Also, females were not attracted to urine from males or females; that is, investigation time of urine did not differ from water controls. Females investigated odors from the suprasternal gland of males longer than those from the flank gland of the same male (Zuri *et al.*, 2005). Most notably, females strongly investigate the odors of skin glands, particularly the suprasternal gland of males, but not urine of either males or females. These divergent responses by male and female opossums to odors from different body sources represent behavioral responses to signaler or releaser pheromones, and thus, they are most likely related to sex-specific production and deposition of chemical signals in this species.

In many mammals, urine is a primary source of chemosignal (Beauchamp, 1973; Drickamer, 1999). However, female opossums are an exception in this regard, as are golden hamsters (*Mesocricetus auratus*; Johnston and Bullock, 2001) and Belding's ground squirrels (*Spermophilus beldingi*; Mateo, 2006). Both hamsters and opossums live in arid environments that would favor persistence of oil-based scent marks and limited water loss due to excretion of urine for scent marking (Harder *et al.*, 2008; Poran *et al.*, 1993a; Zuri and Halpern, 2005).

C. Transduction of chemical signals

The VNO is a bilateral, tubular structure enclosed within a cartilaginous shell that lies dorsal to the anterior palate at the base of the nasal septum (Fig. 16.2). Chemical stimuli reach the VNO through the nasopalatine canal, which connects the nasal and oral cavities in carnivores and marsupials (Wysocki, 1979). An autonomically controlled vascular pump alters the pressure within the lumen of the VNO and, thereby aspirates airborne or nonvolatile mucus-borne chemical stimuli (Meredith *et al.*, 1980). Evidence for this in opossums comes from the study of Poran *et al.* (1993b) in which ^{3}H-proline, applied to male scent marks, was found in the VNO of females who had nuzzled the treated scent mark. At the cellular level, adding an extract of male suprasternal gland to homogenates of VNO sensory epithelium from adult females stimulated production of the second messenger IP_3 through activation of G-protein-coupled receptors (Wang *et al.*, 2007). Output from the sensory cells of the VNO pass through the vomeronasal nerve (VNN) to the accessory olfactory bulb. By contrast, the sensory epithelium of the main olfactory system, lining the nasal cavity, responds to small volatile molecules delivered during sniffing and inhalation, and nerves from this system project to the main olfactory bulb (Meredith, 1991).

The efferent projections from the accessory olfactory bulb terminate in several nuclei that have been associated with the release of hypothalamic GnRH and control of reproductive behavior (Halpern and Martinez-Marcos, 2003). The nuclei receiving accessory olfactory bulb input do not receive direct input from the main olfactory system (Meredith, 1991). Consequently, ablation of the peripheral chemoreceptors or transection of the nerves for one system (e.g., the VNO) leaves the other system intact such that the involvement of one pathway with a particular pheromonal signal can be evaluated.

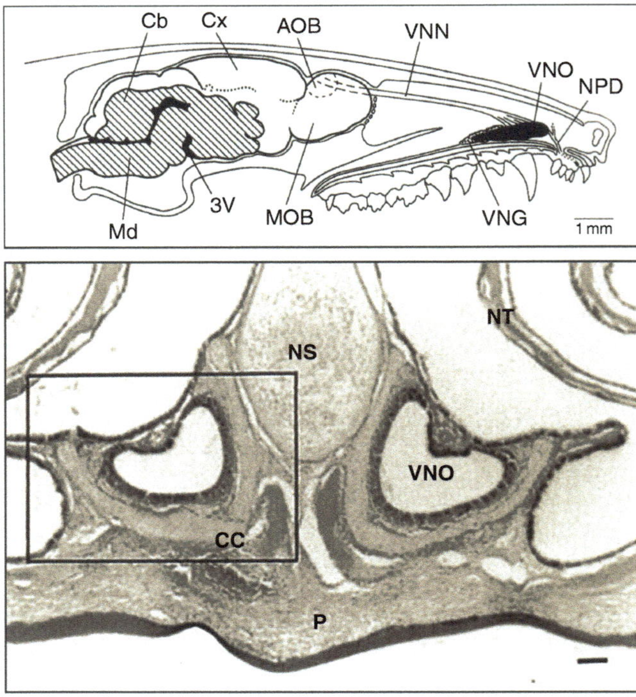

Figure 16.2 The vomeronasal organ of *Monodelphis domestica*. *Top*: Drawing of a parasagittal section through opossum skull illustrating the location of the nasopalatine duct (NPD), and the vomeronasal organ (VNO) above the rostral hard palate. The vomeronasal nerves (VNNs) perforate the cribiform plate of the ethmoid bone and terminate in the accessory olfactory bulb (AOB). 3V, third ventricle; Cb, cerebellum; Cx cerebral cortex; Md, medulla oblongata; MOB, main olfactory bulb. *Bottom*: Coronal section through the VNOs of a female after recovery from sham surgery in which the cartilaginous capsules (CC) encasing the VNOs were exposed by enlarging the incisive formina. NS, nasal septum; NT, nasal turbinates; P, palatal tissue. Drawing by Dave Dennis, photomicrograph by LMJ reprinted with permission from Jackson and Harder (1996).

D. Role of the accessory olfactory system in communication and reproduction

The VNO and accessory olfactory system of eutherian mammals is important for responses to odors of conspecifics and reproductive behavior as described in several recent reviews, including Brennan and Keverne (2003) and Halpern and Martinez-Marcos (2003). Experiments involving removal of the VNO or ablation of the accessory olfactory bulb have revealed sex and species differences in the involvement of the VNO in odor discrimination. For example, ablation of the VNO reduces the ability of male golden hamsters to discriminate between the vaginal odors of different females (Johnston, 1998; Steel and Keverne, 1985), and eliminates discrimination among females based on flank odors and feces (Johnston, 1998), but not when presented with urine (Johnston and Peng, 2000). By contrast, VNO ablation does not eliminate the ability of females to discriminate between flank gland or urine odors of individual males (Johnston and Peng, 2000).

The effects of ablation of the accessory olfactory system in opossums have been studied in several laboratories using different procedures. When considered together, the results of these studies provide a comprehensive understanding of the role of this chemosensory system in individual recognition and reproductive activation. Following a series of experiments that revealed differential responses of males and females to odors from skin glands and urine (Zuri *et al.*, 2003, 2005), Zuri and Halpern (2005) tested the role of the accessory olfactory system in odor discrimination by female opossums through observation of olfactory behavior before and after electrolytic ablation of the accessory olfactory bulb. Investigation of conspecific odors was diminished in females following this ablation, but in general, their ability to discriminate among odor sources was not compromised. One exception was the loss of the females' ability to discriminate between odors from the suprasternal gland and flank odors of the same males, which suggests that the accessory olfactory system may be important when the discrimination task is difficult, or when two odor sources differ in the secretion of nonvolatile components.

Adult female opossum remains anestrous, even when held in mixed-sex colonies, providing that they are isolated from direct contact with males or their scent marks (Fadem, 1987; Jackson and Harder, 2000), which suggests that the estrus-inducting pheromone is nonvolatile and is transduced in the VNO. Female prairie voles are similarly reliant on direct contact with males or their scent marks for induction of estrus, and blocking of reproductive activation by surgical removal of the VNO was first demonstrated in this species (Lepri and Wysocki, 1989; Wysocki *et al.*, 1991). Removal of the VNO also prevents pheromonal induction of estrus in opossums when females are exposed only to pheromones in male scent marks following surgery (Jackson and Harder, 1996). However, VNO ablation by cauterization fails to block reproductive activation when females are caged with males after surgery (Pelengaris *et al.*, 1992). These studies suggest that both the accessory and main olfactory systems may be involved in reproductive activation, and that ablation of both olfactory systems would block male-induced estrus and ovulation, as does olfactory bulbectomy in the musk shrew (*Suncus murinus*; Rissman and Li, 2000). It is likely, however, that under natural conditions of low density and an apparent solitary lifestyle (Streilein, 1982a), the VNO and the accessory olfactory system would be the primary route for reproductive activation. That is, females might well access the estrus-inducing pheromone by nuzzling male scent marks in the absence of direct contact with the male prior to onset of estrus and receptivity.

V. Male Estrus-Inducing Pheromone in Opossums

Early studies of estrus induction in opossums relied on a cage-switching technique to induce estrus (Fadem, 1987; Stonerook and Harder, 1992). Individual females were placed in cages previously occupied by males, which exposed the female to odors from urine and fecal deposits and scent marks left on the walls of the cage by the male. Male opossums have a prominent suprasternal gland and mark objects and surfaces in their environment by rubbing with their chest, as well as with several other parts of their body (Fadem and Cole, 1985; Poran *et al.*, 1993a). The suprasternal gland was first described by Fadem and Schwartz (1986) as a sexually dimorphic structure that is histologically similar to skin glands of small rodents that inhabit arid environments (Fig. 16.3). The gland is androgen dependent; it develops at puberty and will regress following castration (Fadem, 1986). When given a choice, adult, ovary-intact females show a preference for approaching and

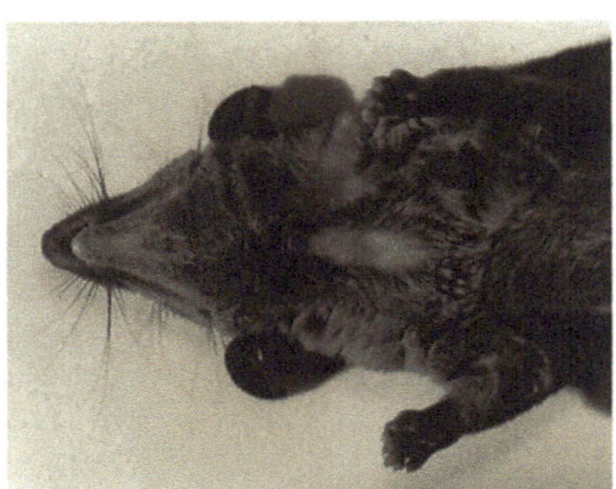

Figure 16.3 The suprasternal gland of male opossums (*Monodelphis domestica*). The gland is evident as a bare patch on the chest of an adult male. Histological examination of this gland revealed both sebaceous and apocrine glands in the underlying dermis (Fadem and Schwartz, 1986). Photograph by LMJ.

spending more time in the cage with an intact male than with a castrated male, which suggests that females are attracted to androgen-dependent odors (Fadem *et al.*, 2000). Interestingly, female response to male stimuli also appears to be steroid-dependent. Ovariectomized females did not show a preference for visiting intact males over castrates, but this preference was evident in ovariectomized females treated with estradiol implants. We have collected male urine, feces, and scent marks from both the flank and suprasternal gland and used them individually as stimuli for estrus induction (J.D. Harder and L.M. Jackson, unpublished data). To date, scent marks from the male suprasternal gland are the only potential source of pheromone to known to reliably induce estrus (Harder and Jackson, 1998).

The intense nuzzling behavior of female opossums directed toward scent marks from the male suprasternal gland (Jackson and Harder, 2000; Poran *et al.*, 1993a,b; Zuri *et al.*, 2005), strongly suggests that the estrus-inducing pheromone is nonvolatile. The concept of a nonvolatile pheromone is supported by the fact that females remain anestrous when they are individually caged in a colony that includes males housed in opaque cages on adjacent shelves. In this setting, females are exposed to ambient sounds and volatile odors, but are not exposed to nonvolatile, visual, or tactile cues. However, the different behavioral responses of females to secretions from the suprasternal and other male glands (Zuri *et al.*, 2005) suggest that females can detect a scent mark and selectively respond to it before making contact with it; that is, they are responding to a volatile signal.

The volatility of chemosignals in suprasternal gland secretions was recently examined by characterizing the behavioral and reproductive responses of female opossums with complete or restricted access to suprasternal gland scent marks (Harder *et al.*, 2008). Scent marks were collected by rubbing a glass vial across the suprasternal gland of an adult male, and anestrous females were presented with either the marked vial or a marked vial enclosed in a perforated shield that allowed for diffusion of volatile odors from the scent mark, but prevented the female from making contact with the scent mark. The investigatory behavior of the females directed toward marked vials was compared to behaviors directed toward clean, unshielded and shielded vials. The same procedure was followed when females were induced to estrus 5–10 days later. Both anestrous and estrous females detected volatile components in the male scent mark, as evidenced in higher nuzzling frequency on shielded, marked vials than on shielded, clean vials (Fig. 16.4). Nuzzling of unshielded, marked vials was higher in anestrous females than estrous females, suggesting a reduction in drive to access the estrous-inducing pheromone in females that had reached estrous (Harder *et al.*, 2008).

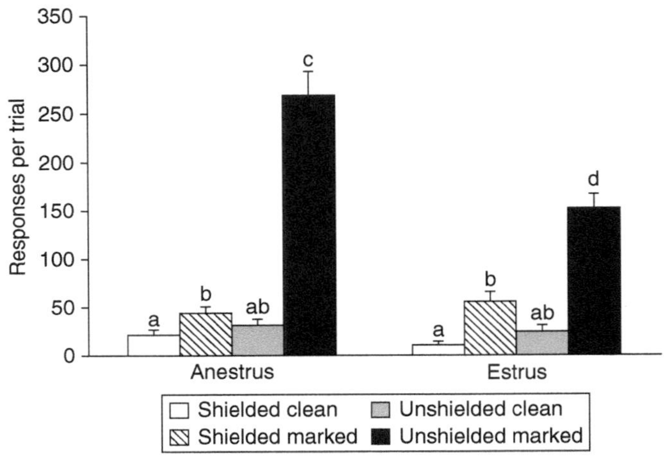

Figure 16.4 Mean (±SEM) nuzzling frequency during a 10-min test period on shielded and unshielded vials, with and without male scent marks by anestrous female opossums, and by the same females when in estrus. Different superscripts denote significant differences ($P < 0.05$) within and between reproductive states. Reprinted with permission from Harder *et al.* (2008).

The nonvolatile nature of the male estrus-inducing pheromone in secretions of the suprasternal gland was tested in females exposed for 14 days to a shielded, marked vial or to an unshielded, marked vial in a crossover design (Harder *et al.*, 2008). Estrus was induced in all 11 females exposed to unshielded vials and 10 of them copulated. Only 2 of the same 11 females, when exposed only to volatile odors from shielded marked vials, expressed estrus, and neither of them copulated. Taken together, these results clearly demonstrate that females respond behaviorally to both volatile and nonvolatile components in suprasternal gland secretion, but that the estrus-inducing pheromone in this secretion is nonvolatile. Thus, females are attracted to volatile components of the male scent mark, but contact with nonvolatile components is required for ovarian activation and expression of behavioral estrus.

VI. Endocrinology of Reproductive Activation

Activation of ovarian function by male pheromones is presumed to begin with stimulation of the GnRH neuronal system via signals from the main olfactory system or the accessory olfactory system, or both. An increase in GnRH secretion stimulates release of the gonadotropic hormones, LH and FSH, from the anterior pituitary gland, which ultimately stimulate follicular development and ovarian steroidogenesis. An increase in circulating concentrations of estradiol during pheromonal induction of estrus was first reported by Fadem (1989), and the effects of rising estradiol are evident in the thick smear of cornified epithelial cells in the cytology of the urogenital sinus (Baggott *et al.*, 1987; Fadem and Rayve, 1985), a 5% increase in body mass (Jackson and Harder, 2000), and hypertrophy of the uteri and lateral vaginal canals (Jackson and Harder, 1996; Stonerook and Harder, 1992) that are characteristic of induced estrus in adult opossums.

Estrogenic effects on reproductive tissues are also evident in females at the time of puberty, and like ovarian activation in the adult, puberty or first estrus is also dependent upon exposure to male pheromones. This was first determined in a study by Stonerook and Harder (1992) in which 90-day-old juvenile females housed in a mixed-sex colony were either indirectly exposed to ambient male chemical and auditory stimuli, or were directly exposed to male odors by regular cage-switching. Control females were maintained in a separate room and isolated from all male stimuli, and the onset of puberty was monitored using urogenital sinus cytology. All of the females directly exposed to male odors by cage-switching exhibited urogenital sinus estrus (UGSE) at a mean age of 126 days. Approximately 60% of the females indirectly exposed to ambient male odors exhibited estrus, but at a significantly later age of 162 days. None of the females that were isolated from all male stimuli expressed estrus before 180 days of age when the experiment ended. Uterine weights at first estrus were higher in direct exposure females than in indirect exposure females. Uteri collected from isolated females at 180 days of age were smaller than uteri from 105-day-old juvenile females from the same colony. Large, antral follicles were observed in ovaries from estrous females, but no corpora lutea were present, consistent with the fact that ovulation in the opossum is induced and requires the presence of a male (Baggott *et al.*, 1987; Harder *et al.*, 1993; Hinds *et al.*, 1992). Despite the 35–40 day difference in age at first estrus between direct and indirect exposure females, mean body mass at first estrus (60 g) was not different between the two groups, suggesting that sexual maturation is dependent on reaching a critical, threshold body mass, and that direct exposure of juvenile females to male scent marks results in acceleration of body growth.

The possibility that prepubertal exposure to male pheromone accelerates both somatic and sexual maturation was further examined in a later study (Harder and Jackson, 2003), in which females were exposed to male scent marks collected on glass vials beginning at 90 days of age. Unexposed, control females were exposed only to the ambient male stimuli of a mixed-sex colony. Urogenital sinus cytology and body mass were recorded daily for 60 days, and the reproductive tract and ovaries from randomly selected females in both groups were examined during necropsy at 90, 105, and 130 days; and at 150 days for the remaining unexposed females. Similar to the previous study, first estrus in exposed females occurred at a mean age of 127 days. In contrast to the results of Stonerook and Harder (1992), none of the unexposed females (held in a mixed-sex colony) reached puberty before the 150 days of age, and few of them attained the previously described critical body mass of 60 g. Exposed females had a significantly higher rate of growth (g/week) than unexposed females, and this difference preceded the onset of estrus in exposed females (Fig. 16.5). Male pheromones also stimulated follicular development such that antral follicle size was greater in ovaries from exposed females at 105 and 130 days, and the largest follicles (>500 μm) were observed only in ovaries from exposed females. Consistent with the pattern of follicular development in exposed females, mean uterine and lateral vaginal canal masses were higher in exposed females than in unexposed females. These findings further support the hypothesis that exposure to male pheromones stimulates body growth in juvenile females (Harder and Jackson, 2003). Furthermore, because follicular development was stimulated up to 3 weeks before first estrus, the results raise the possibility that accelerated somatic maturation is a consequence of pheromonal stimulation of the reproductive axis and increased production of ovarian estradiol and, perhaps, other growth factors. In this scenario, reproductive neuroendocrine function is stimulated by pheromone exposure, but full ovarian activation is inhibited until the female has reached a critical body size. The inhibitory factor could be one that inhibits GnRH

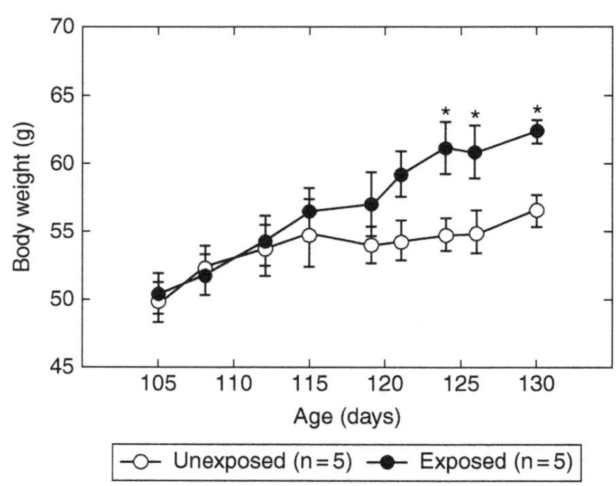

Figure 16.5 Growth curves for female opossums between 105 and 130 days of age. Asterisks indicate significant differences ($P < 0.05$) between mean body mass for females exposed to male pheromone beginning at 90 days of age, and unexposed females. Reprinted from Harder and Jackson (2003); http://www.RBEj.com/content/1/1/21.

neuronal function (or competes with the stimulatory pheromone signal), or it could be a permissive factor that is present in insufficient amounts until adult body size is reached.

Estrous female opossums appear to require direct exposure to males to induce ovulation because ovulation will not occur in response to continued exposure to male scent marks alone. However, copulation is not required because females who are mounted by a male, but separated before intromission occurs, will ovulate (Baggott *et al.*, 1987; Jackson, 2001). Further evidence that copulation is not the ovulatory stimulus is the existence of a preovulatory LH surge that occurs between 10 and 20 h after pairing but 10–12 h before copulation (Jackson *et al.*, 1999). The ovulatory signal could be other tactile or visual stimuli, or it could be a pheromone that is released by a male only when he is paired with an estrous female. Mating typically occurs only once, 2 days after pairing an estrous female with a male (Harder *et al.*, 1993), and ovulation occurs 18–30 h after copulation (Baggott *et al.*, 1987).

Peripheral concentrations of progesterone also begin to increase in estrous females approximately 10 h after pairing with a male (Harder *et al.*, 2005), and remain elevated throughout pairing and copulation. The increase in progesterone precedes ovulation by almost 48 h, and therefore, it is not luteal in origin. We speculate that the preovulatory progesterone in opossums is secreted by ovarian follicles, perhaps in response to the rising concentrations of LH. Concentrations of progesterone during the subsequent luteal phase are less than half of the maximum concentrations during the pericopulatory period (Jackson, 2001).

The precopulatory increase in progesterone is an important regulator of reproductive behavior. Estrous females who are paired with a male, but do not have an increase in plasma concentrations of progesterone, will not copulate (Harder *et al.*, 2005). Similarly, ovariectomized females that have been treated with both estradiol and progesterone are more sexually receptive than those treated with estradiol alone (Fadem *et al.*, 1996). In rodents, estradiol acts within the medial preoptic area (MPOA) and ventral medial hypothalamus (VMH) to increase progesterone receptors, and progesterone acting in these nuclei facilitates receptive behaviors and copulation (Pfaff *et al.*, 1994). A similar regulatory mechanism is found in opossums, except that the distribution and number of progesterone receptors are affected by exposure to male pheromone and contact with a male, rather than spontaneous, cyclical changes in ovarian hormones. Vitazka *et al.* (2009) examined progesterone receptor immunoreactivity in brains from four groups of female opossums: (1) naïve females never exposed to males or estrus-inducing pheromone, (2) anestrous females previously induced to estrus, (3) females in cytological estrus, and (4) estrous females who had copulated 1 h before brain tissue was collected. Naïve females had very little progesterone receptor expression in any of the nuclei examined. When compared to naïve females, previous or current exposure to males or their scent marks resulted in increased progesterone receptor expression in the MPOA and the anteroventral periventricular nucleus (AVPv), another hypothalamic nucleus involved with reproductive function (Gu and Simerly, 1994; Fig. 16.6). The persistence of progesterone receptor immunoreactivity in anestrous adults was apparently related to previous pheromone exposure or sexual experience. Pheromonal induction of estrus resulted in upregulation of progesterone receptors in the VMH when compared to experienced anestrus (EXPA) females, presumably as a consequence of increasing concentrations of plasma estradiol during reproductive activation.

Although anestrous female opossums are reliant on exposure to male pheromone for expression of estrus, female opossums spontaneously exhibit postlactational estrus (Jackson and Harder, 2000). Females that are individually caged in a mixed-sex colony will exhibit UGSE 7–10 days after removal of nursing young, either at the time of natural weaning of young at 8 weeks of age, or during midlactation (3–5 weeks postpartum). The

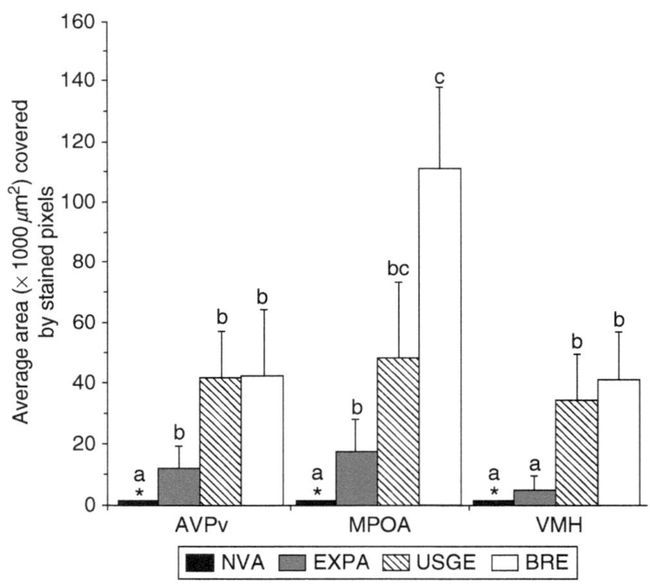

Figure 16.6 Average (±SEM) area covered by nuclear progesterone receptor immunoreactivity in three areas of the brain (AVPv, anteroventral periventricular nucleus; MPOA, medial preoptic area; VMH, ventromedial hypothalamus) in female opossums in four reproductive states. The reproductive states, represented by bars of different shading, are: naïve anestrus (NVA), experienced anestrus (EXPA), urogenital sinus estrus (UGSE), and behavioral receptive estrus (BRE). For bars representing data from one brain area, different letter superscripts represent significant differences between reproductive states ($P < 0.05$). *Averages of area covered in NVA females were too low to plot ($< 100\ \mu m^2$). Reprinted with permission from Vitazka *et al.* (2009).

interval between pup removal and estrus is similar to the interval between initial pheromone exposure and estrus in nonlactating females, and estradiol concentrations in postlactational and pheromone-induced estrous females are equivalent. The reproductive success (proportion giving birth and litter size) of females in postlactational estrus is equivalent to that of pheromone exposed females.

The discovery of postlactational estrus in a species that is otherwise dependent on male pheromone for reproductive activation is surprising. One explanation for this phenomenon is that postlactational females have a greater sensitivity to male odor cues and are, therefore, able to respond to volatile male odors that otherwise are ineffective at inducing estrus in anestrous adults. A second explanation is that the energy demands of nursing young peak in late lactation and drop sharply at weaning (Hsu *et al.*, 1999), leaving the postlactational female, on an *ad libitum* diet, in a positive energy balance with metabolic signals that could activate the GnRH neuronal system. Thirdly, lactation is recognized as nature's contraception because of the negative feedback action of prolactin on the secretion of GnRH. Cessation of lactation would release GnRH neurons from this inhibition, and this could potentially override the absence of stimulatory input from olfactory stimuli.

VII. Reproductive and Behavioral Ecology of Opossums

The opossum is typical of most small mammal models of olfactory communication. Little is known of the role of pheromones in natural populations of mammals, and even the basics of the ecology and natural history of some species have not been established. Studies of olfaction are typically based in laboratory settings with little opportunity or effort to corroborate the results in nature. A notable exception is represented in a series of studies by John Vandenbergh and colleagues with mice (*Mus musculus*) that revealed puberty-enhancing effects of male urine (Vandenbergh, 1969) and puberty-retarding effects of female urine (Drickamer, 1977). The results of these studies were extended to studies of feral mice in highway cloverleaf islands (Coppola and Vandenbergh, 1987), and large outdoor enclosures (Drickamer and Mikesic, 1990). Similarly, interpretation of the laboratory studies of chemosignals in prairie voles (Carter *et al.*, 1980) is facilitated with extensive knowledge of the natural history and ecology of this species (Getz and Carter, 1980; Getz *et al.*, 1987).

Since its introduction as a laboratory animal less than two decades ago (VandeBerg, 1983), the gray short-tailed opossum has become the most widely studied of all marsupials and first to have its genome sequenced

(Mikkelsen *et al.*, 2007). Unfortunately, relatively little is known of the ecology or natural history of this opossum, one of 15 species in the genus *Monodelphis*, which are distributed throughout much of tropical South America. *M. domestica* is best known in the Caatinga region of Brazil (8° S to 12° S), a semiarid area covered with scattered trees and shrubs. Here, it feeds on fruit, insects, and small vertebrates, and is most often captured around mesic rock outcroppings (Streilein, 1982b). *M. domestica* has also extended its range into cleared rainforest regions (Emmons, 1990). The breeding season of *M. domestica* in the Caatinga appears to be controlled by patterns of precipitation such that pregnancy rates are lowest in July through November, which are also the driest months (Bergallo and Cerqueira, 1994). A similar seasonality in reproduction was reported in a closely related species, *Monodelphis dimidiata*, a small insectivorous opossum that inhabits the grasslands of northern Argentina (Pine *et al.*, 1985).

Current understanding of olfactory communication and pheromonal activation of reproduction in opossums is sufficiently detailed and corroborated in several laboratories so as provide a basis for a reasonable proposal of how these aspects of opossum biology might operate under natural conditions. Young opossums are weaned at about 8 weeks of age, at which time their body mass is about half the threshold mass (60 g) for pheromonal induction of estrus (Harder and Jackson, 2003; Stonerook and Harder, 1992), and so, juvenile females probably remain in their natal area until they grow to about 50 g at 4 months of age. Young females, previously unexposed to males or their scent marks, are able to detect (Harder *et al.*, 2008) and perhaps evaluate, volatile components of the male scent mark. This might enable prepubertal females to avoid the nonvolatile estrus-inducing scent marks of closely related males, which would be particularly important if juvenile females do not disperse from their natal areas before the onset of puberty. Alternatively, the ability to discriminate among the quality of odor cues or scent marks may influence the direction and extent of dispersal in juvenile opossums.

Adult female opossums experience spontaneous, postlactational estrus (Jackson and Harder, 2000), and thus, following their first pregnancy, they are not dependent on male pheromone for induction of estrus. However, postlactational females might become anestrous, as in a seasonal drought, and require nuzzling access to male scent marks for pheromonal induction of estrus. Males appear to be more interested in the urine of anestrous than estrous females (Zuri *et al.*, 2003), and so, in the wild, males might be attracted to scent mark in the home ranges of anestrous females. Accordingly, the ability of females to detect volatile components of male scent marks and thereby locate them might be a factor in mate selection, because this would allow a female to evaluate the quality of a scent mark, particularly in regard to the relatedness of the source male. Subsequent nuzzling of the scent mark might not only induce estrus, but could also reinforce male identity cues and allow recognition of the same male several days later when the female is sexually receptive. Volatile components of gland secretions in Belding ground squirrels (*S. beldingi*) provide cues for individual recognition which appear to persist in the memory of recipients (Mateo, 2006). Nuzzling permits the release of molecules from dried, skin-based scent marks and thereby facilitates communication among individuals long after the signal has been released (Poran *et al.*, 1993a). Thus, reliance on skin gland secretions for scent marks in the gray short-tailed opossum might reflect a solitary lifestyle (Streilein, 1982a) and evolution of olfactory communication in a semiarid environment.

VIII. Summary and Conclusions

The gray short-tailed opossum merits attention as one of the most widely studied of all marsupials and as a model for study of olfactory communication, particularly as it relates to pheromonal activation of reproduction. Both males and females scent mark, but males utilize a greater diversity of body regions including the mandible, chest, flank, and rump. Divergent responses by male and female opossums to odors from these different body sources are likely related to sex-specific production and deposition of chemical signals in this species. Males respond differentially to female skin gland secretions and urine from anestrous females, while females respond only skin gland secretions, particularly from the suprasternal gland. Adult females do not have an estrous cycle and remain anestrous unless exposed to male pheromone. Similarly, juvenile females do not reach puberty when isolated from males or their scent marks. Female opossums nuzzle scent marks from male suprasternal gland secretion and access a nonvolatile estrus-inducing pheromone that is, as a result of this behavior, delivered to the chemosensory epithelium of vomeronasal organ. Neuroendocrine correlates of pheromonal induction of estrus include elevated plasma estradiol and upregulation of progesterone receptors in hypothalamic regions that control reproductive behavior and the release of GnRH. Pairing with a male stimulates a requisite rise in plasma progesterone that acts with elevated estradiol to stimulate the onset of sexual receptivity in the female.

The research discussed in this review has greatly enhanced our understanding of olfactory communication and the importance of pheromones for reproductive activation of female opossums. However, it is difficult to put this wealth of knowledge into an ecological context because so little is known about the life history and reproductive strategy of the opossum in its natural habitat. Many investigations of interactions between pheromones and mammalian reproduction arise from breeding attempts in laboratory colonies or agricultural populations. Animals in such populations may lack exposure to other sensory, nutritional, and social factors that influence reproduction under natural conditions, and thus, reproductive pheromones might appear to be more critical than they actually are in nature. Future studies of olfactory communication should focus on studies of population biology and the social behavior of opossums living in large outdoor enclosures, as well as ecological studies of this species in its natural habitat, the Caatinga of Brazil. Results of such studies would enable meaningful interpretation of the findings and conclusions from laboratory studies of olfactory communication and reproductive activation.

ACKNOWLEDGMENTS

Many of the studies from our laboratory that are cited in this review were supported by the National Science Foundation (IBN 9616588, 9723043, and 0527950) and The Ohio State University. We would also like to acknowledge the valuable contributions made by numerous undergraduate research assistants.

REFERENCES

Baggott, L. M., Davis-Butler, S., and Moore, H. D. M. (1987). Characterization of estrus and timed collection of oocytes in the gray short-tailed opossum (*Monodelphis domestica*). *J. Reprod. Fertil.* **79,** 109–114.

Barrett, J., Abbott, D. H., and George, L. M. (1990). Extension of reproductive suppression by pheromonal cues in subordinate female marmoset monkeys, *Callithrix jacchus*. *J. Reprod. Fertil.* **90,** 411–418.

Beauchamp, G. K. (1973). Attraction of male guinea pigs to conspecific urine. *Physiol. Behav.* **10,** 589–594.

Bergallo, H. G., and Cerqueira, R. (1994). Reproduction and growth of the opossum *Monodelphis domestica* (Mammalia: Didelphidae) in northeastern Brazil. *J. Zool.* **232,** 551–563.

Brennan, P. A., and Keverne, E. B. (2003). The vomeronasal organ. *In* "Handbook of Olfaction and Gestation," (R. L. Doty, Ed.), 2nd. edn., pp. 967–979. Marcel Dekker, New York.

Bronson, F. H. (1968). Pheromonal influences on mammalian reproduction. *In* "Perspectives in Reproduction and Sexual Behavior," (M. Diamond, Ed.), pp. 341–361. Indiana University Press, Bloomington.

Bronson, F. H. (1985). Mammalian reproduction: An ecological perspective. *Biol. Reprod.* **32,** 1–26.

Bruce, H. M. (1960). A block of pregnancy in the mouse caused by the proximity of strange males. *J. Reprod. Fertil.* **1,** 96–103.

Carter, C. S., Getz, L. L., Gavish, L., McDermott, J. L., and Arnold, P. (1980). Male-related pheromones and the activation of female reproduction in the prairie vole (*Microtus orchrogaster*). *Biol. Reprod.* **23,** 1038–1045.

Carter, C. S., Witt, D. M., Manock, S. R., Adams, K. A., Bahr, J. M., and Carlstead, K. (1989). Hormonal correlates of sexual behavior and ovulation in male-induced and postpartum estrus in female prairie voles. *Physiol. Behav.* **46,** 941–948.

Catling, P. C., and Sutherland, R. L. (1980). Effect of gonadectomy, season, and the presence of female tammar wallabies (*Macropus eugenii*) on concentrations of testosterone, luteinizing hormone, and follicle stimulating hormone in plasma of male tammar wallabies. *J. Endocrinol.* **86,** 25–33.

Coppola, D. M., and Vandenbergh, J. G. (1987). Induction of puberty-regulating chemosignals in wild mouse populations. *J. Mammal.* **68,** 86–91.

Cowley, J. J., and Wise, D. R. (1972). Some effects of mouse urine on neonatal growth and reproduction. *Anim. Behav.* **30,** 499–506.

Dorries, K. M., Adkins-Regan, E., and Halpern, B. P. (1997). Sensitivity and behavioral responses to the pheromone androstenone are not mediated by the vomeronasal organ in domestic pigs. *Brain Behav. Evol.* **49,** 53–62.

Drickamer, L. C. (1977). Delay of sexual maturation in female house mice by exposure to grouped females or urine from grouped females. *J. Reprod. Fertil.* **51,** 77–81.

Drickamer, L. C. (1999). Sexual attractants. *In* "Encyclopedia of Reproduction," (E. Knobil and J. D. Neill, Eds.), pp. 444–448. Academic Press, New York.

Drickamer, L. C., and Mikesic, D. G. (1990). Urinary chemosignals, reproduction, and population size for house mice (*Mus musculus*) living in field enclosures. *J. Chem. Ecol.* **16,** 2955–2968.

Emmons, L. H. (1990). Neotropical Rainforest Mammals, a Field Guide. The University of Chicago Press, Chicago. 281 pp.

Fadem, B. H. (1985). Evidence for the activation of female reproduction by males in a marsupial, the gray short-tailed opossum (*Monodelphis domestica*). *Biol. Reprod.* **33,** 112–116.

Fadem, B. H. (1986). Chemical communication in gray short-tailed opossums (*Monodelphis domestica*) with comparisons to other marsupials and with reference to monotremes. *In* "Chemical Signals in Vertebrates IV: Ecology, Evolution and Comparative Biology," (D. Duvall, D. Muller-Schwarze, and R. M. Silverstein, Eds.), pp. 587–607. Plenum Publishing Corp., New York.

Fadem, B. H. (1987). Activation of estrus by pheromones in a marsupial: Stimulus control and endocrine factors. *Biol. Reprod.* **36,** 328–332.

Fadem, B. H. (1989). The effects of pheromonal stimuli on estrus and peripheral plasma estradiol in female gray short-tailed opossums (*Monodelphis domestica*). *Biol. Reprod.* **41,** 213–217.

Fadem, B. H., and Cole, E. A. (1985). Scent marking in the gray short-tailed opossum (*Monodelphis domestica*). *Anim. Behav.* **33,** 730–738.

Fadem, B. H., and Rayve, R. S. (1985). Characteristics of the oestrus cycle and influence of social factors in grey short-tailed opossums (*Monodelphis domestica*). *J. Reprod. Fertil.* **73,** 337–342.

Fadem, B. H., and Schwartz, R. A. (1986). A sexually dimorphic suprasternal scent gland in gray short-tailed opossums (*Monodelphis domestica*). *J. Mammal.* **67,** 205–208.

Fadem, B. H., Erianne, G. S., and Karen, L. M. (1989). The hormonal control of scent marking and precopulatory behavior in male gray short-tailed opossums (*Monodelphis domestica*). *Horm. Behav.* **23,** 381–392.

Fadem, B. H., Taylor-Ali, L., and Erianne, D. C. (1996). The hormonal induction of mating behavior in female gray short-tailed opossums (*Monodelphis domestica*). *Horm. Behav.* **30,** 44–49.

Fadem, B. H., Dziadosz, D. R., Jackson, L. M., and Harder, J. D. (2000). Partner preference of intact and ovariectomized female gray short-tailed opossums (*Monodelphis domestica*). *Horm. Behav.* **38,** 187–192.

Fleming, M. W., and Harder, J. D. (1983). Luteal and follicular populations in the ovary of the opossum (*Didelphis virginiana*) after ovulation. *J. Reprod. Fertil.* **67,** 29–34.

Getz, L. L., and Carter, C. S. (1980). Social organization in *Microtus ochrogaster* populations. *Biologist* **62,** 56–69.

Getz, L. L., Hoffman, J. E., Klatt, B. J., Verner, L., Cole, F. R., and Lindroth, R. L. (1987). Fourteen years of population fluctuations of *Microtus ochrogaster* and *M. pennsylvanicus* in east central Illinois. *Can. J. Zool.* **65,** 1317–1325.

Gu, G., and Simerly, R. B. (1994). Hormonal regulation of opioid peptide neurons in the anteroventral periventricular nucleus. *Horm. Behav.* **28,** 503–511.

Halpern, M., and Martinez-Marcos, A. (2003). Structure and function of the vomeronasal system: An update. *Prog. Neurobiol.* **70,** 245–318.

Harder, J. D., and Fleming, M. W. (1981). Estradiol and progesterone profiles indicate a lack of endocrine recognition of pregnancy in the opossum. *Science* **212,** 1400–1402.

Harder, J. D., and Jackson, L. M. (1998). Pheromonal induction of estrus with secretions of the suprasternal gland in the gray short-tailed opossum. *Biol. Reprod.* **58**(Suppl. 1), 132–133.

Harder, J. D., and Jackson, L. M. (2003). Male pheromone stimulates ovarian follicular development and body growth in juvenile female opossums (*Monodelphis domestica*). *Reprod. Biol. Endocrinol.* **1,** 21–29.

Harder, J. D., Stonerook, M. J., and Pondy, J. (1993). Gestation and placentation in two New World opossums: *Didelphis virginiana* and *Monodelphis domestica*. *J. Exp. Zool.* **266,** 463–479.

Harder, J. D., Tadros, L. M., Rogier, R., Norfolk, J. R., and Fadem, B. H. (2005). Male-induced rise in progesterone precedes receptivity and ovulation in the gray short-tailed opossum (*Monodelphis domestica*). *Biol. Reprod.* **73**(Suppl 1), 225–226.

Harder, J. D., Jackson, L. M., and Koester, D. K. (2008). Behavioral and reproductive responses of female opossums to volatile and nonvolatile components of male suprasternal gland secretion. *Horm. Behav.* **54,** 741–747.

Hinds, L. A., and Smith, M. J. (1992). Evidence from plasma progesterone concentrations for male-induced ovulation in the brush-tailed bettong, *Bettongia penicillata*. *J. Reprod. Fertil.* **95,** 291–302.

Hinds, L. A., Reader, M., Wernberg-Moller, S., and Saunders, N. R. (1992). Hormonal evidence for induced ovulation in *Monodelphis domestica*. *J. Reprod. Fertil.* **95,** 303–312.

Holmes, D. J. (1992). Sternal odors as cues for social discrimination by female Virginia opossums, (*Didelphis virginiana*). *J. Mammal.* **73,** 286–291.

Hsu, M. J., Garton, D. W., and Harder, J. D. (1999). Energetics of offspring production: A comparison of a marsupial (*Monodelphis domestica*) and a eutherian (*Mesocricetus auratus*). *J. Comp. Physiol. B* **169,** 67–76.

Hunsaker, D., and Shupe, D. (1977). Behavior of new world marsupials. *In* "The Biology of Marsupials," (D. Shupe, Ed.), pp. 279–347. Academic Press, New York.

Inns, R. W. (1982). Seasonal changes in the accessory reproductive system and plasma testosterone levels of the male tammar wallaby, *Macropus eugenii*, in the wild. *J. Reprod. Fertil.* **66,** 675–680.

Jackson, L. M. (2001). Pheromonal Induction of Estrus and Ovulation in the Gray Short-tailed Opossum (*Monodelphis domestica*). Ph.D. thesis, The Ohio State University, Columbus.

Jackson, L. M., and Harder, J. D. (1996). Vomeronasal organ removal blocks pheromonal induction of estrus in gray short-tailed opossums (*Monodelphis domestica*). *Biol. Reprod.* **54,** 506–512.

Jackson, L. M., and Harder, J. D. (2000). Evidence for spontaneous postlactational estrus in gray short-tailed opossums (*Monodelphis domestica*). *Biol. Reprod.* **62,** 1823–1827.

Jackson, L. M., Danforth, D. R., and Harder, J. D. (1999). Luteinizing hormone and progesterone increase prior to copulation during induced ovulation in the gray short-tailed opossum (*Monodelphis domestica*). *Biol. Reprod.* (Suppl. 1)m 183.

Jacob, S., and McClintock, M. K. (2000). Psychological state and mood effects of steroidal chemosignals in women and men. *Horm. Behav.* **37,** 57–78.

Johnston, R. E. (1983). Chemical signals and reproductive behavior. *In* "Pheromones and Reproduction in Mammals," (J. G. Vandenbergh, Ed.), pp. 27–31. Academic Press, New York.

Johnston, R. E. (1998). Pheromones, the vomeronasal system, and communication. From hormonal responses to individual recognition. *Ann. NY Acad. Sci.* **855,** 333–348.

Johnston, R. E., and Bullock, T. A. (2001). Individual recognition by use of odours in golden hamsters: The nature of individual representation. *Anim. Behav.* **61,** 545–557.

Johnston, R. E., and Peng, M. (2000). The vomeronasal organ is involved in discrimination of individual odors by males but not by females in golden hamsters. *Physiol. Behav.* **70,** 537–549.

Karlson, P., and Lüscher, M. (1959). "Pheromones": A new term for a class of biologically active substances. *Nature* **183,** 55–56.

Kennedy, G. C., and Mitra, J. (1963). Body weight and food intake as initiating factors for puberty in the rat. *J. Physiol.* **166,** 408–418.

Knight, T. W., and Lynch, P. R. (1980). Source of ram pheromones that stimulate ovulation in the ewe. *Anim. Reprod. Sci.* **3,** 133–136.

Kwan, M., and Johnston, R. E. (1980). The role of vaginal secretion in hamster sexual behavior: Males' responses to normal and vaginectomized females and their odors. *J. Comp. Physiol. Psychol.* **94,** 905–913.

Lepri, J. J., and Wysocki, C. J. (1989). Removal of the vomeronasal organ disrupts the activation of reproduction in female voles. *Physiol. Behav.* **40,** 349–355.

Luo, Z.-X., Ji, Q., Wible, J. R., and Yuan, C.-X. (2003). An early Cretaceous tribosphenic mammal and metatherian evolution. *Science* **302,** 1934–1940.

Marshall, L. G., Case, J. A., and Woodburne, M. O. (1990). Phylogenetic relationships of the families of marsupials. *In* "Current Mammalogy," (H. H. Genoways, Ed.), pp. 433–481. Plenum Press, New York.

Mateo, J. M. (2006). The nature and representation of individual recognition odours in Belding's ground squirrels. *Anim. Behav.* **71,** 141–154.

McClintock, M. K. (2002). Pheromones, odors, and vasanas: The neuroendocrinology of social chemosignals in human and animals. *In* "Hormones, Brain, and Behavior," (D. W. Pfaff, A. P. Arnold, A. M. Etgen, S. E. Fahrbach, and R. T. Rubin, Eds.), Vol. 1, pp. 797–870. Academic Press, New York.

Meredith, M. (1991). Sensory processing in the main and accessory olfactory systems: Comparisons and contrasts. *J. Steroid Biochem.* **39,** 601–614.

Meredith, M., Marques, D. M., O'Connell, R. J., and Stern, F. L. (1980). Vomeronasal pump: Significance for male hamster sexual behavior. *Science* **207,** 1224–1226.

Mikkelsen, T. S., Wakefield, M. J., Aken, B., Amemiya, C. T., Chang, J. L., Duke, S., Gardber, M., Gentles, A. J., Goostadt, L., Heger, A., *et al.* (2007). Genome of the marsupial *Monodelphis domestica* reveals innovation in non-coding sequences. *Nature* **447,** 167–177.

Murata, K., Wakabayashi, Y., Kitago, M., Ohara, H., Watanabe, H., Tamogami, S., Warita, Y., Yamagishi, K., Ichikawa, M., Takeuchi, Y., Okamura, H., and Mori, Y. (2009). Modulation of gonadotrophin-releasing hormone pulse generator activity by the pheromone in small ruminants. *J. Neuroendocrinol.* **21,** 346–350.

O'Connell, M. A. (1989). Population dynamics of neotropical small mammals in seasonal habitats. *J. Mammal.* **70,** 532–548.

Pelengaris, S. A., Abbott, D. H., Barrett, J., and Moore, H. D. M. (1992). Induction of estrus and ovulation in female grey short-tailed opossums, *Monodelphis domestica*, involves the main olfactory epithelium. *In* "Chemical Signals in Vertebrates VI," (R. L. Doty and D. Müller-Schwarze, Eds.), pp. 253–257. Plenum Press, New York.

Perret, M., and Atramentowicz, M. (1989). Plasma concentrations of progesterone and testosterone in captive woolly opossums (*Caluromys philander*). *J. Reprod. Fertil.* **91,** 31–41.

Perret, M., and M'Barek, S. B. (1991). Male Influence on oestrous cycles in female woolly opossum (*Caluromys philander*). *J. Reprod. Fertil.* **91,** 557–566.

Pfaff, D. W., Schwartz-Giblin, S., McCarthy, M. M., and Kow, L. (1994). Cellular and molecular mechanisms of female reproductive behavior. *In* "Physiology of Reproduction," (E. Knobil and J. D. Neill, Eds.), 2nd. edn., pp. 107–220. Academic Press, New York.

Pine, R. H., Dalby, P. L., and Matson, J. O. (1985). Ecology, postnatal development, morphometrics, and taxonomic status of the short-tailed opossum, *Monodelphis dimidiata*, an apparently semelparous annual marsupial. *Ann. Carnegie Mus.* **54,** 195–231.

Poran, N. S., Tripoli, R., and Halpern, M. (1993a). Nuzzling in the gray short-tailed opossum II: Familiarity and individual recognition. *Physiol. Behav.* **53,** 969–973.

Poran, N. S., Vandoros, A., and Halpern, M. (1993b). Nuzzling in the gray short-tailed opossum I: Delivery of odors to vomeronasal organ. *Physiol. Behav.* **53,** 959–967.

Richmond, M. E., and Conaway, C. H. (1969). Induced ovulation and oestrus in *Microtus ochrogaster*. *J. Reprod. Fertil. Suppl.* **6,** 357–376.

Rissman, E. F., and Li, X. (2000). Olfactory bulbectomy blocks mating-induced ovulation in musk shrews (*Suncus murinus*). *Biol. Reprod.* **62,** 1052–1058.

Scalia, F., and Winans, S. S. (1975). The differential projections of the olfactory bulb and accessory bulb in mammals. *J. Comp. Neurol.* **161,** 31–56.

Smith, B. A., and Block, M. L. (1991). Male saliva cues and female social choice in Mongolian gerbils. *Physiol. Behav.* **2,** 379–384.

Steel, E., and Keverne, E. B. (1985). Effect of female odour on male hamsters mediated by the vomeronasal organ. *Physiol. Behav.* **35,** 195–200.

Stonerook, M. J., and Harder, J. D. (1992). Sexual maturation in female gray short-tailed opossums, *Monodelphis domestica*, is dependent upon male stimuli. *Biol. Reprod.* **46,** 290–294.

Streilein, K. E. (1982a). Behavior, ecology and distribution of South American marsupials. *In* "Mammalian Biology in South America," (M. A. Mores and H. H. Genoways, Eds.), Vol. 2, pp. 231–249. Pymatuning Laboratory of Ecology, Linesville, PA. Special Publication.

Streilein, K. E. (1982b). Ecology of small mammals in the semiarid Brazilian Caatinga I. Climate and faunal composition. *Ann. Carnegie Mus.* **51,** 79–107.

Thiessen, D., and Rice, M. (1976). Mammalian scent gland marking and social behavior. *Psychol. Bull.* **83,** 505–539.

Tyndale-Biscoe, H., and Renfree, M. B. (1987). Reproductive Physiology of Marsupials. Cambridge University Press, New York.

VandeBerg, J. L. (1983). The gray short-tailed opossum: A new laboratory animal. *ILAR News* **26,** 9–12.

Vandenbergh, J. G. (1969). Male odor accelerates female sexual maturation in mice. *Endocrinology* **84,** 658–660.

Vandenbergh, J. G. (2006). Pheromones and mammalian reproduction. *In* "Knobil and Neill's Physiology of Reproduction," (J. D. Neill, Ed.), 3rd edn., pp. 2041–2058. Academic Press, New York.

Vitazka, M. E., Càrdenas, H., Cruz, Y., Fadem, B. H., Norfolk, J. R., and Harder, J. D. (2009). Progesterone receptor in the forebrain of female gray short-tailed opossums: Effects of exposure to male stimuli. *Horm. Behav.* **55,** 190–196.

Wade, G. N., and Schneider, J. E. (1992). Metabolic fuels and reproduction in female mammals. *Neurosci. Biobehav. Rev.* **16,** 235–272.

Walkden-Brown, S. W., Restall, B. J., and Henniawati, (1993). The male effect in the Australian cashmere goat. 2. Role of olfactory cues from the male. *Anim. Reprod. Sci.* **32,** 55–67.
Wang, D., Chen, P., Wei, Q., and Halpern, M. (2007). Suprasternal gland secretion of male short-tailed opossum induces IP_3 generation in the vomeronasal organ. *Biochem. Biophys. Acta* **1770,** 725–732.
Whitten, W. K. (1956). Modification of the oestrous cycle of the mouse by external stimuli associated with the male. *J. Endocrinol.* **13,** 399–404.
Whitten, W. K. (1959). Occurrence of anoestrus in mice caged in groups. *J. Endocrinol.* **18,** 102–107.
Wilson, E. D., and Bosser, W. A. (1963). Chemical communication among animals. *Recent Prog. Horm. Res.* **19,** 673–710.
Wyatt, T. D. (2003). Pheromones and Animal Behavior, Communication by Smell and Taste. Cambridge University Press, Cambridge.
Wysocki, C. J. (1979). Neurobehavioral evidence for the involvement of the vomeronasal system in mammalian reproduction. *Neurosci. Biobehav. Rev.* **3,** 301–341.
Wysocki, C. J., and Preti, G. (2004). Facts, fallacies, fears, and frustrations with human pheromones. *Anat. Rec.* **281A,** 1201–1211.
Wysocki, C. J., Kruczek, M., Wysocki, L. M., and Lepri, J. J. (1991). Activation of reproduction in nulliparous and primiparous voles is blocked by vomeronasal organ removal. *Biol. Reprod.* **45,** 611–616.
Zuri, I., and Halpern, M. (2005). Modification of odor investigation and discrimination in female opossums *(Monodelphis domestica)* following the ablation of the accessory olfactory bulbs. *Behav. Neurosci.* **119,** 612–621.
Zuri, I., Su, W., and Halpern, M. (2003). Conspecific odor investigation by gray short-tailed opossums (*Monodelphis domestica*). *Physiol. Behav.* **80,** 225–232.
Zuri, I., Dombrowski, K., and Halpern, M. (2005). Skin and gland but not urine odours elicit conspicuous investigation by female grey short-tailed opossums, *Monodelphis domestica. Anim. Behav.* **69,** 635–642.
Zuri, I., Nguyen, D., Daniels, Y., and Halpern, M. (2007). Skin, gland, and urine odors elicit intense investigation by male gray short-tailed opossums, *Monodelphis domestica. Can. J. Zool.* **85,** 450–457.

CHAPTER SEVENTEEN

Pheromones in a Superorganism: From Gene to Social Regulation

C. Alaux, A. Maisonnasse, *and* Y. Le Conte

Contents

Abstract

Analogous to the importance of hormones in controlling organism homoeostasis, pheromones play a major role in the regulation of group homoeostasis at the social level. In social insects, pheromones coordinate the association of "unitary" organisms into a coherent social unit or so called "superorganism." For many years, honey bees have been a convincing model for studying pheromone regulation of social life. In addition, with the recent sequencing of its genome, a global view of pheromone communication is starting to emerge, and it is now possible to decipher this complex chemical language from the molecular to the social level. We review here the different pheromones regulating the main biological functions of the superorganism and detail their respective action on the genome, physiology and behavior of nestmates. Finally,

INRA, UMR 406 Abeilles et Environnement, Site Agroparc, Domaine Saint-Paul, Avignon, France

Vitamins and Hormones, Volume 83
ISSN 0083-6729, DOI: 10.1016/S0083-6729(10)83017-1

we suggest some future research that may improve our understanding of the remarkably rich syntax of pheromone communication at the social level.

I. Introduction

Social insect colonies have often been referred as "superorganisms" in analogy to the functional organization of complex higher organisms being composed of numerous cells (Wilson and Sober, 1989). Indeed, the colony organization of insect societies reveals numerous analogies to multicellular organisms. The first analogy is that both are associations of single units, cells, and individuals (organisms). Like cells, members of the colonies depend on the functioning of the higher unit and are unable to survive and develop outside this system. In the second analogy, the reproductive castes fulfill the role of the germ cells in organisms, and the sterile castes become analogous to the soma. Similar to somatic cells, sterile individuals follow organizational principles: the specialization into different functions and the coordination between the functional groups; this organization being governed by a well developed and sophisticated communication.

In organisms, the regulation of cell and organ activity is controlled by signals, like hormones, which elicit specific reactions in certain organs. Equivalent to the hormonal regulation in the individual organism, the colony is regulated chemically by pheromones (Fig. 17.1). Interactions between members of the society are mainly under the control of complex pheromone signaling, which spreads global information to further enable the colony homeostasis, provisioning, growth, defense, and reproduction but also mediate social conflicts (see Le Conte and Hefetz, 2008 for a review). Pheromones, defined also in the past as "ectohormones," are chemicals that are secreted externally and which produce dramatic and stereotyped changes in behavior and physiology of members of the same species (Karlson and Burtenandt, 1959). Pheromones are usually divided into two categories according to their effects: releaser pheromones induce an immediate behavioral response but primer pheromones alter behavioral repertoire through putative response threshold shifts (Wilson and Bossert, 1963). However, it has been shown recently that releaser pheromones can also modify response thresholds (Alaux and Robinson, 2007; Anderson *et al.*, 2007), which blurs the long-standing distinction between primer and releaser pheromone.

To function as coherent social units, social insects use a complex language based on specialized chemical signals that provide a remarkably rich syntax, which might be equivalent to the visual and auditory repertoire of higher vertebrates. The only social insect for which any primer pheromones have been identified is the honey bee (*Apis mellifera*), that has all the

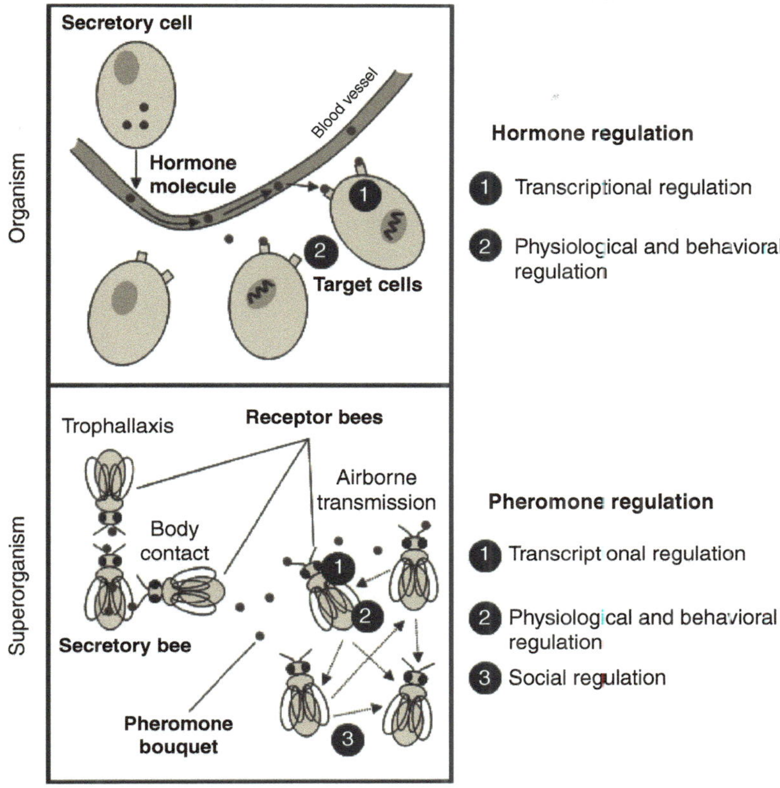

Figure 17.1 Analogy between organism hormones and superorganism pheromones. In organisms, hormones are synthesized by secretory cells and transported via the blood flow to target cells. Analogous communication scheme is observed at the social level with pheromones. The pheromone message is transported outside of the body and delivered through trophallaxis (transfer of food between group members), body contact or airborne transmission. Similarly to the hormone response, reception of the semiochemicals results generally in transcriptional responses, followed by changes in hormone levels and/or behavior. However, a higher level of regulation is observed in the superorganism with a modification of social interactions.

characteristics of a superorganism (Moritz and Fuchs, 1998). Honey bees live in societies that are characterized by a reproductive division of labor between the queen and workers, and a division of labor among workers for tasks related to colony growth and development. Far from being rigid, this social organization is highly flexible and mainly pheromone guided. Actually, around 50 chemical substances are known to be essential to the functioning of the society (Slessor *et al.*, 2005). With their unusually well characterized behaviors and pheromones (Le Conte and Hefetz, 2008; Slessor *et al.*, 2005) and their newly annotated genome sequence (Honey

Bee Genome Sequencing Consortium, 2006), honey bees are an emerging model for decoding the mechanism of pheromone language from molecular to social level. Here, we review, through a multilevel approach, this rapidly evolving field for honey bees that has been constantly fueled by the discovery of new pheromones and functions, and recently by the development of genomic tools. First, the main pheromones will be introduced by presenting their multiple effects on worker physiology and behavior. Then, we will detail the transcriptional changes occurring at the brain level upon pheromone perception and finally, we will explain how the pheromone language regulates social life.

II. Physiological and Behavioral Regulation

A. Reproduction

A hallmark of eusocial societies is the reproductive specialization, where the queen monopolizes reproduction and facultatively sterile workers contribute to the colony work force. In honey bees, despite workers being unable to mate, they have retained the capacity to develop ovaries and lay viable haploid eggs, which develop into males, since honey bees are haplodiploid (females are derived from fertilized eggs produced by the queen). However, only 0.01% of workers have fully developed ovaries and 1% of male eggs are derived from workers (Ratnieks, 1993). Worker reproduction is inhibited by the presence of the queen and/or brood (larvae), since a loss of one of them leads to the development of ovaries by workers. For example, in the absence of the queen, from 5% to 24% of workers possess developed ovaries (Page and Erickson, 1988). With several thousands of workers composing the colony, the queen cannot physically control this strong reproductive bias. Worker reproduction is rather inhibited through a primer pheromone mechanism, but also via worker policing (workers prevent each other from reproducing by removing worker-laid eggs, see Le Conte and Hefetz, 2008).

After some controversial research toward the identification of the queen pheromone, an active blend produced in the queen mandibular gland and composed of 5 molecules ((E)-9-oxodec-2-enoic acid (9-ODA), both enantiomers of 9-hydroxydec-2-enoic acid (9-HDA), methyl *p*-hydroxybenzoate (HOB) and 4-hydroxy-3-methoxyphenylethanol (HVA)) was identified (Slessor *et al.*, 1988). Later, Hoover *et al.* (2003) showed that this blend has a strong inhibitory effect on worker reproduction. Besides this queen mandibular pheromone (QMP), the brood produced by the queen also inhibits ovary development in workers by emitting two pheromones: the brood pheromone (BP), mainly composed of esters (Arnold *et al.*, 1994) and the highly volatile E-β-ocimene (Maisonnasse *et al.*, 2009). In reality, two esters from the BP have an effect on worker ovaries: ethyl palmitate and methyl linolenate (Mohammedi *et al.*, 1998). Interestingly, those inhibiting components produced by the brood were found to not be caste specific since the queen also produces the ethyl palmitate (Keeling and Slessor, 2005) and the E-β-ocimene (Gilley *et al.*, 2006). It is interesting to note that each of those compounds trigger a partial effect on ovary development (i.e., some workers still "escape" the reproductive control), which suggests synergistic effects between brood and queen pheromones on worker ovary inhibition.

In most insects, it has been documented that juvenile hormone (JH) controls ovary development by stimulating the production of vitellogenin (Vg, yolk protein precursor) in the fat body and its uptake by developing oocytes (Engelmann, 1983). In honey bees, QMP and BP inhibit JH biosynthesis by the corpora allata (Kaatz *et al.*, 1992; Le Conte *et al.*, 2001; Pankiw *et al.*, 1998), however, no direct effects of JH on ovary development have been found. Contrary to others insects, JH and Vg titers show an inverse pattern and behave antagonistically (Bloch *et al.*, 2002; Guidugli *et al.*, 2005), which explains the higher RNA levels of Vg induced by QMP (Fischer and Grozinger, 2008). Since Vg has multiple coordinating effects on social organization, it might regulate an alternative utilization of yolk protein other than oogenesis (Amdam *et al.*, 2003; see below).

B. Task allocation

A common feature of higher organisms and honey bee societies is the specialization of cells and workers, respectively, into various tasks. The many tasks associated to the maintenance of the hive are divided among the workers giving a division of labor. In honey bees, this task division can arise from genetic variability between workers (Oldroyd and Fewell, 2007; Robinson and Page, 1989). As a consequence, workers develop into specialists for certain tasks due to their low response threshold for this task. However, the main task division is age-related. During their life, workers undergo a behavioral maturation: they spend the first 2–3 weeks of their adult life working in the hive (feeding and taking care of the brood, building comb), and then the rest of their life outside of the hive (foraging for nectar and pollen to supply the colony growth). The nurse/forager ratio, crucial to the colony functioning, is not rigid, but highly plastic, depending on social environment and colony needs, which are communicated via pheromones.

The transition from nurse to forager is controlled by a colony-level network: the queen, brood, and foragers regulate the progression of young bees toward the typical tasks of older bees. QMP delays the onset of foraging (Pankiw *et al.*, 1998), but the action of BP is dose dependant. Below a certain threshold, BP stimulates behavioral maturation, but high doses (i.e., a large number of larvae) induce a delay (Le Conte *et al.*, 2001). Workers also inhibit the nestmate transition from nurse to forager via a pheromone, ethyl oleate (EO), which is mainly produced by foragers (Leoncini *et al.*, 2004). EO, which is also produced by the queen (Keeling and Slessor, 2005) and the brood (Le Conte *et al.*, 1989), stimulates the growth of hypopharyngeal gland used by nurses for the brood nourishment (Mohammedi *et al.*, 1996).

The hormonal mechanisms underlying honey bee behavioral maturation are well studied and reveal the major regulatory roles of JH and Vg (Bloch *et al.*, 2002; Guidugli *et al.*, 2005). The transition to a forager state is mediated by an increase in JH and a decrease of Vg titer (Page and Amdam, 2007). The higher level of Vg in nurses might be used for brood food production in the hypopharyngeal glands rather than for egg production in the ovaries (Amdam *et al.*, 2003). Pheromones are expected to regulate the division of labor through the modification of endocrine levels of JH and Vg. This was tested by different studies, which showed that QMP and high doses of BP decrease JH levels in workers during their behavioral maturation (Kaatz *et al.*, 1992; Le Conte *et al.*, 2001; Pankiw *et al.*, 1998). In addition, QMP and low doses of BP increases and decreases, respectively, Vg production (Fischer and Grozinger, 2008; Smedal *et al.*, 2009), which is consistent with their effect on the onset of foraging. Finally, it has been shown that QMP and BP modulate the sucrose response threshold of workers (Pankiw and Page, 2003). Since there is a robust association between worker sucrose responsiveness and foraging behavior (i.e., bees with low response threshold to sucrose mature faster into forager; Page *et al.*, 1998), the regulation of this behavioral module might directly affect behavioral maturation. The EO regulation on worker physiology is not yet known, but it is likely similar to the effects of QMP and BP due to their convergent effects.

C. Defense

Another important trait of honey bee biology is the shared defense of the colony upon disturbance by intruders or potential enemies. A rapid defense response is launched by guard bees when they detect a danger at the colony entrance. Alarm pheromones are immediately released by the guards to signal a threat to the colony members and coordinate the defensive response, which is characterized by either a dispersal of individuals or an attack against the potential danger. In this defensive context, guards play an analogous role to the T cells of the vertebrate immune system, which search out invaders in the body and release cytokines to mediate the immune response. In honey bees, two main alarm pheromones have been identified: the sting alarm pheromone, which is mainly composed of isopentyl acetate (IPA; Boch *et al.*, 1962) and 2-heptanone, produced in the mandibular glands (Shearer and Boch, 1965). If the role of IPA is well known in mediating defensive behavior, the role of 2-heptanone in colony defense is less clear. 2-Heptanone may act as a repellent scent-mark in the foraging context, because when applied by bees to flowers, subsequent floral visitors avoid these depleted flowers (Giurfa, 1993).

The primary role of IPA is to alert and recruit bees. However, defending bees need to localize the intruder, which would not be accurate if based on olfaction alone. Wager and Breed (2000) have shown that a second role of IPA is to release searching behavior and enhance response to moving targets. A third role of IPA in mediating defense response has been identified by rating sting extension in bees subjected to electrical shocks. Prior exposure to small doses of IPA increased the sting extension reflex to the electrical shocks, but higher doses resulted in decreased responsiveness (Nunez *et al.*, 1998). This reduction was antagonized by application of naloxone, a specific antagonist of opioids, indicating that large doses of IPA activated an endogenous opioid system leading to stress-induced analgesia (Nunez *et al.*, 1998). The opioid system is believed to inhibit pain to trigger alternative behavioral responses (Dyakonova, 2001). Therefore, Nunez *et al.* (1998) suggested that the activation of opioid analgesia by IPA decreases the probability of withdrawal when facing an enemy thus increasing its defensive efficiency.

Besides inducing a quick hard-wired defensive response, IPA also affects longer latency behavioral responsiveness. The colony responsiveness to IPA increases after subsequent exposures, meaning that a brief exposure to IPA without association to reward can modify the behavioral response threshold (Alaux and Robinson, 2007). It is possible that a shift in responsiveness to IPA enables the colony to respond more rapidly and vigorously to intruders that have been encountered previously. Such a phenomenon is analogous to the immunological memory of mammals, which is a fundamental feature of an adaptive immune system. In that context, previously aroused guards resemble memory T cells, by mounting a faster and stronger immune response toward foreign invaders that were encountered during a prior infection.

D. Longevity

In honey bees, adult lifespan can be influenced by the social environment via pheromones. QMP-treated bees live longer, when starved, compared to control bees (Fischer and Grozinger, 2008), but bees exposed to low doses of BP have a reduced lifespan (Smedal *et al.*, 2009). Despite QMP and BP having antagonistic effects on bee longevity, they share the same mechanism. Both affect Vg levels and nutrient storage capacity, which are known to increase worker survival (e.g., Vg protects bees from oxidative stress; Corona *et al.*, 2007; Seehuus *et al.*, 2006). QMP increased and low doses of BP decreased both Vg levels and nutrient storage (Fischer and Grozinger, 2008; Smedal *et al.*, 2009). Since, Vg levels and nutrient storage are higher in nurses compared to foragers (Fluri *et al.*, 1982; Toth and Robinson, 2005), their regulation by pheromones are consistent with QMP and BP effects on worker division of labor. In that context, one would expect that high doses of BP, which delay the onset of foraging (Le Conte *et al.*, 2001), increase bee lifespan.

E. Learning

The olfactory system of honey bees undergoes significant maturation during early adult life, a process that is influenced by environmental stimuli (Gascuel and Masson, 1987), but also by the presence of the queen (Morgan *et al.*, 1998). While the role of QMP in regulating olfactory maturation is not known, a recent series of studies have shown that QMP can affect olfactory learning and memory. Vergoz *et al.* (2007b) first showed that exposure to QMP significantly blocks aversive learning in young bees. QMP attracts young workers to the queen and entices them to feed her, but also to lick and antennate her body, which allow a distribution of her QMP bouquet throughout the colony (Slessor *et al.*, 1988). Vergoz *et al.* (2007b) explained that the effects of QMP on aversive learning would increase the likelihood of workers attending the queen by preventing them from forming an aversion to her pheromones. This effect was mediated by a single component of QMP (HVA), which has a similar structure to a dopamine molecule and affects dopamine signaling in the brain of young bees (Beggs *et al.*, 2007). Finally, Beggs and Mercer (2009) found that HVA actually interacts with dopamine receptors in the bee brain, and thus targets directly the dopamine pathways, which play an essential role in aversive learning (Vergoz *et al.*, 2007a).

III. Gene Regulation

Before eliciting a response, pheromone signals are processed in the brain. Identification of neural pathways and olfactory sensory maps in the honey bee brain has given new clues about pheromone processing and representation (see Sandoz *et al.*, 2007 for a review). A complementary approach is to determine how pheromones are molecularly transduced in the brain. Indeed, molecular signaling pathways connect pheromone signals to the regulation of neural functions and, ultimately to behavioral and physiological responses. Since its genome has been sequenced (Honey Bee Genome Sequencing Consortium, 2006), it has been possible to analyze the pheromone-regulated transcription. And thanks to genomic approaches using microarrays, a global view of gene regulation by pheromone signaling is beginning to emerge. In this section, we will review how pheromones are orchestrating gene expression changes in the honey bee brain.

A. Long-term regulation

In order to better understand how pheromones affect neuronal responsiveness and behavioral state, studies started to trace the molecular changes that occur throughout the brain in response to pheromone perception. Tracking the long-term changes in brain gene expression is needed to reflect the long-term changes in physiology and behavior induced by primer pheromones. QMP influences behavior by affecting neural and endocrine systems that specify responsiveness to specific social and environmental stimuli (Beggs *et al.*, 2007; Morgan *et al.*, 1998; Pankiw *et al.*, 1998). Using cDNA microarray analysis, Grozinger *et al.* (2003) showed that QMP affects the expression levels of hundreds of genes in the brain of adult honey bees. A previous study reported widespread differences in gene expression between nurses and foragers, with some genes being more highly expressed in nurse brain compared to forager brain (nurse genes), and inversely other genes being more highly expressed in forager brain compared to nurse brain (forager genes; Whitfield *et al.*, 2003). Comparing QMP-regulated genes to behavioral genes, Grozinger *et al.* (2003) found that QMP tends to activate genes in the brain that are upregulated in nurses but repress genes that are upregulated in foragers. Similarly, BP, when administered in high doses, leads to a delay in the onset of honey bee foraging (Le Conte *et al.*, 2001) and modifies the expression of genes in the honey bee brain (Alaux *et al.*, 2009a). BP tended to upregulate nurse genes but down-regulate forager genes in the brain of young bees. Those findings were consistent with results for QMP and supported the idea that the effects of pheromones on behavior are due to effects on brain gene expression.

The effects of pheromones on behavioral genes are not hard-wired and independent of age but are modulated by maturational processes as shown by age-dependent effects of BP on the "molecular signature" of the brain (Alaux *et al.*, 2009a). On one hand, BP tended to repress forager genes in young honey bees, but, on the other hand, forager genes were stimulated in older honey bees. These differences might be related to the dose-dependent effects of BP on behavioral maturation (Le Conte *et al.*, 2001). Perhaps, bees become less sensitive to BP with age and this leads to the differences in brain gene expression detected here; age-related changes in responsiveness to pheromones are well known (Grozinger and Robinson, 2007; Pham-Delegue *et al.*, 1993; Robinson, 1987a). The conclusion that pheromones modulate behavior by regulating the expression level of behavioral genes was further confirmed by the upregulation of the gene *malvolio* in old bees (Alaux *et al.*, 2009a). *Malvolio* encodes a manganese transmembrane transporter and is upregulated in the forager brain compared with the nurse brain (Ben-Shahar *et al.*, 2004). In addition, manganese treatment causes an increase in sucrose responsiveness (Ben-Shahar *et al.*, 2004), which is associated with an earlier age at onset of foraging and a tendency to forage for pollen rather than nectar (Page *et al.*, 1998). The effects of *malvolio* are consistent with the dual effects of BP on the onset of foraging and the tendency to specialize on pollen foraging (Pankiw, 2004a,b).

QMP and BP are two different chemical blends with pleiotropic effects but which have in common the effect of delaying the transition from nurse to foraging behavior and inhibiting worker ovary development. It is not clear why such redundancy exists in chemical communication, but this is a common theme in insect societies (Slessor *et al.*, 2005). Perhaps, such redundancy leads to finer levels of control or increased resiliency in the event of a communication failure. Pheromones with overlapping functions could have evolved to converge on the same molecular targets in the brain, or they could engage parallel pathways. The very low number of genes regulated by both QMP and BP suggest that they both elicit effects on different sets of genes in the brain (Alaux *et al.*, 2009a). Cautious conclusion should be drawn from this comparison, because the two pheromones were analyzed with different microarray platforms (cDNA mircroarrays generated from brain expressed sequenced tags for QMP and oligonucleotide microarrays generated from the whole genome for BP). However, because they likely use different peripheral receptors, they are expected to affect different neural and molecular pathways. The weak overlap of brain gene expression could also be explained by the different behavioral and physiological processes regulated by QMP and BP. Indeed, BP also increases larval feeding (Le Conte *et al.*, 1995; Mohammedi *et al.*, 1996) and QMP stimulates "retinue" behavior (Slessor *et al.*, 1988).

Another main effect of QMP is the inhibition of worker ovary development (Hoover *et al.*, 2003). One prediction from the previously observed effect of QMP on behavioral genes is that QMP-regulated genes are associated with ovary development. However, by analyzing the differences in brain gene expression between reproductive and sterile workers, Grozinger *et al.* (2007) did not find a significant bias for genes upregulated in reproductive workers to be downregulated by QMP. This does not preclude the idea that pheromones regulate the behavior and physiology of workers by regulating behaviorally and physiologically relevant genes. Because the main effect observed here is at the level of ovaries, monitoring, in those tissues, the expression patterns of genes regulated by QMP might provide a better characterization of the pheromonal effect on worker reproduction.

B. Short-term regulation

It is well established that short social interactions elicit strong genomic responses in the brain, suggesting that perception of social signal may modify the brain neurogenomic state to allow individuals to respond adaptively to subsequent social interactions (Clayton, 2000; Robinson *et al.*, 2008). Similar responses have been observed in honey bees stimulated by the stinging alarm pheromone. A brief exposure of workers to IPA causes, within 30 min, an increase in mRNA expression of the transcription factor (TF), *c-Jun*, in the antennal lobes (main olfactory center in the brain; Alaux and Robinson, 2007). This response is associated with an increase in colony responsiveness to subsequent exposure to alarm pheromone (Alaux and Robinson, 2007). Thus, honey bees have the capacity to mount a rapid genomic response to pheromone stimulation coupled with neural and behavioral plasticity. In addition, Alaux *et al.* (2009b) analyzed the transcriptional cascade activated by *c-Jun* in response to alarm pheromone and found that a 1 min exposure affects brain expression of hundreds of genes 1 h later. Even a quick behavioral response to a brief stimulus is likely to be associated with many changes in gene expression, thereby changing the experience of the organisms to the given stimulus.

Some genes involved in biogenic amine signaling (*Dopa decarboxylase* and *Tyramine receptor*) were upregulated by alarm pheromone in the honey bee brain (Alaux *et al.*, 2009b). This signaling pathway is implicated in the regulation of aggression in invertebrates (Dierick and Greenspan, 2007; Hunt *et al.*, 2007). In addition, the expression level of the gene encoding the corticotropin-releasing hormone-binding protein, a key protein involved in animals' "fight-or-flight" stress–response (Huising and Flik, 2005), was modified by this short exposure to alarm pheromone. This rapid genome-wide response to alarm pheromone showed a significant overlap with genes that are differentially expressed between the extremely aggressive Africanized honey bee (AHB) and the more docile European honey bees (EHB; Alaux *et al.*, 2009b). The detection of alarm pheromone activates genes that are highly expressed in unexposed AHB and represses genes highly expressed in EHB suggesting that alarm pheromone causes an AHB-like gene expression profile.

Using a gene ontology analysis, Alaux *et al.* (2009b) showed that functions involved in visual perception and the response to stimuli were significantly overrepresented in the gene set upregulated by alarm pheromone. This is consistent with the fact that aggressive behavior is visually guided and that alarm pheromone, besides recruiting nestmates, also increases flight activity and enhances the response to moving targets (Wager and Breed, 2000). It would be important to extend this type of genome-wide analysis to other releaser pheromones (like attraction and sex pheromones) to determine if the rapid induction of a genomic response in the brain, coupled with an increase in arousal, is a general response to pheromones.

C. Pheromone-regulated transcription factors

The high proportion of TFs regulated by QMP and BP (Alaux *et al.*, 2009a; Grozinger *et al.*, 2003) suggests that they might be key mediators of pheromone signaling responses. TFs function as transcriptional activators or repressors by binding to sequence-specific enhancer or promoter regions of DNA adjacent to the genes that they regulate. Putative TF-binding sites can be identified via bioinformatic methods and can provide additional information about the mechanisms of pheromone-regulated transcription. Alaux *et al.* (2009a) showed that the promoter regions of genes regulated by BP are enriched for putative TF-binding *cis*-regulatory motifs. An increase or a decrease in the behavioral response to the same pheromone is well known in invertebrates (see Anton *et al.*, 2007 for a review). This plasticity of pheromone response is usually influenced by endocrine factors like JH (Anton and Gadenne, 1999; Grozinger and Robinson, 2007; Robinson, 1987b). However, as discussed above, BP induces "opposite" effects on brain gene expression depending on the age of individuals. The mechanisms underlying such changes remain to be elucidated, but the age specificity of the DNA motif-gene set associations provides some first insights about the mechanisms (Alaux *et al.*, 2009a). Among those, the *cis*-regulatory DNA motif *Adf1* was enriched in gene sets regulated by BP in young bees as compared to old bees and has been shown to be associated with genes regulated by JH (Sinha *et al.*, 2006), which increases pheromone sensitivity (Anton and Gadenne, 1999). This motif could represent a key factor in the age-dependant sensitivity to BP discussed previously.

The *cis*-regulatory DNA motifs associated with QMP-regulated genes have not yet been identified, so it is not known whether they are shared by both pheromones. However, some studies have begun to provide new insights into the relationships between QMP and TF regulation in the inhibition of honey bee behavioral maturation. For example, Grozinger *et al.* (2003) found the honey bee ortholog of *Drosophila melanogaster Krüppel-homolog 1* (*Kr-h1*) to be strongly and chronically downregulated over several days by QMP. The regulation of this zinc finger TF by QMP is influenced by the endocrine status of the honey bee (Grozinger and Robinson, 2007) and a previous study indicated that it is more highly expressed in foragers compared to nurses (Whitfield *et al.*, 2003). *Kr-h1* may play a role in orchestrating ecdysone-regulated transcriptional pathways and neuronal morphogenesis (Shi *et al.*, 2007).

All of these connections suggest a functional linkage between pheromone, behavior, and molecular regulation. Due to known similarities in pheromone signaling across organisms, it is reasonable to assume that studies of model organisms, such as the honey bee, will have general significance. Also future genomic studies will undoubtedly continue to increase our knowledge of pheromone-regulated gene expression. For example, combining the standard chromatin immunoprecipitation assay with microarrays or high-throughput sequencing, will enable researchers to localize the binding sites of TFs in the genome and to establish a genomic landscape of pheromone-regulated TFs, similar to what has been done in hormone research (Cheung and Kraus, 2010).

IV. Social Regulation

Collective decision-making requires an informational flow that is effective in reaching the majority of the workers. Contrary to volatile substances, which do not require close proximity between members of the society to be effective at the group level, nonvolatile substances need a continuous transport analogous to the transport of hormones by the blood in vertebrates. Workers can actively transport pheromones through trophallaxis and body contact. This quick and constant circulation of pheromones provides flow of information important to the maintenance of colony organization and functionality (e.g., reproduction and growth).

A. Reproduction

Honey bee colonies follow a yearly cycle starting with a "somatic" growth stage, which is characterized by an increase in worker number, and followed by colony reproduction (i.e., production of drones and queens). Reproduction in honey bee colonies occurs at two levels: individual and colonial, both being regulated by the same pheromone, QMP. This primary superorganismic pheromone inhibits the development of ovaries in all members of the colony as discussed above, but also prevents the construction of new queen cells and, thus, the rearing of new queens (Winston *et al.*, 1990). QMP is rapidly moved among members by messenger bees that have body contact with the queen and extensively lick her (Naumann *et al.*, 1991). These messenger bees contribute to the dispersal of QMP and thus the maintenance of colony stability. However, instability occurs when the colony population grows and the QMP distribution becomes less efficient (Naumann *et al.*, 1993). Because of this congestion the QMP is diluted and fails to be transmitted. Workers behave as if they were queenless and begin to build new queen cells and larvae, the precursors of colony reproduction by swarming (Winston *et al.*, 1991).

The reproductive capability of workers is normally inhibited by primer pheromones (QMP and BP), which target ovary development. This suppression is essential to the colony stability and functionality given that reproductive workers do not work as hard as normal worker bees (Dampney *et al.*, 2004). The importance of pheromonal control in maintaining colony reproductive harmony is better appreciated in the cases in which it breaks down. A rare behavioral syndrome in EHB populations (*A. mellifera*) illustrates this breakdown. In some colonies, called "anarchistic" colonies, a large proportion of workers activate their ovaries and lay eggs, affecting colony functionality, despite the inhibitory presence of the queen and BP (Oldroyd *et al.*, 1999). The pheromonal control could be inefficient, however these "anarchistic" colonies are headed by queens who have normal QMP production (Hoover *et al.*, 2005a), suggesting that workers are less sensitive to the QMP or that its transmission or reception is less effective (Hoover *et al.*, 2005b). Also, anarchistic workers seem to have a higher threshold to brood signal compared to wild-type bees (Oldroyd *et al.*, 2001). In some extreme cases, the failure of the pheromonal control can lead to a destructive state of the colony, as is the case for the uncontrolled replication of *Apis mellifera capensis* workers (Cape honey bee) in *Apis mellifera scutellata* host colonies. *A. m. capensis* workers can parasitize *A. m. scutellata* colonies and reproduce via thelytokous parthenogenesis, by producing clones of themselves (Oldroyd, 2002). In a few weeks, replication of *A. m. capensis* workers leads to an increase in number of parasitic workers within the host colony but also to reduced foraging activity and food supplies caused by an underrepresentation of *A. m. capensis* in the foraging force, which can lead to the death of the colony (Martin *et al.*, 2002). The ability of *A. m. capensis* parasitic workers to activate their ovaries inside the host society suggests that they are not inhibited by the pheromones that usually repress oogenesis. Parasitic workers are actually able to produce queen-like pheromones (Simon *et al.*, 2001). Therefore *A. m. capensis* workers look like pseudoqueens, with regards to their reproductive capacities and pheromone bouquet, which suggests that they are not inhibited by the queen (i.e. own) pheromones. The breakdown of reproductive order in the superorganism is analogous to the spread of cancer in vertebrates with the uncontrolled replication of malignant cell and consequently has been assimilated to a social cancer (Oldroyd, 2002). Like cancerous cells, which escape from the immune system, parasitic workers have the potential to bypass the pheromonal control of the colony.

B. Colony growth

During the "somatic" growth of the colony, each worker needs to obtain information about the colony requirements and to respond accordingly. The sensitivity and the ability of the society to reallocate tasks in response to changing conditions is a key component of colony development (Robinson, 1992). In that context, the role of pheromones is analogous to the biochemicals that coordinate the functions of distinct cell subpopulation during the development of multicelullar organisms.

After having selected a nest site, the honey bee swarm needs to build up a new comb for brood rearing and storing food. At that time, the colony needs to produce a worker force for the development of the colony, instead of reproductive individuals. Similar to growth hormone in vertebrates, Ledoux *et al.* (2001) found that QMP actually stimulates the secretion of wax and the production of worker-size cells. Therefore, QMP regulates both the development of the nest and task allocation. This centralized control is operated by a single queen, who produces a baseline amount of pheromone. However, colony needs change with colony size and time of the year. Workers need to acquire this information, but whether the queen can modulate her pheromone output according to the colony requirement is not known.

The dynamic regulation of task allocation is decentralized, governed not by a single colony leader but rather by regular interactions between colony members (self-organization). For example, to optimize colony and brood development, an effective ratio of nurse to forager is needed. The colony response to an increased need for brood rearing (large amount of brood) should involve a lengthening of the nursing phase. On the other hand, a reduced amount of brood suggests that more food is needed for the colony to increase the rate of brood production. These colony requirements are communicated through BP production: high doses lengthen the nursing phase whereas low doses accelerate the transition from nurse to forager phase (Le Conte *et al.*, 2001). In addition to its primer effects, BP can also induce a quick increase in pollen foraging within a few hours (Pankiw, 2007; Pankiw and Page, 2001). This decentralized control is mediated as well by interactions between adult workers. This was demonstrated by experimental manipulations of old or young bees population (Huang and Robinson, 1992). Later it has been found that chemical extracts of nurses have stimulating effects on the foraging behavior of young bees (Pankiw, 2004b), but the pheromone produced by foragers (EO) inhibits the behavioral maturation of young bees (Leoncini *et al.*, 2004). Altogether these results suggest a feedback mechanism between nurses and foragers, particularly adapted to regulate the size of the colony foraging force. For example, an abrupt loss of foragers due to predation or bad weather might be communicated through a decreased amount of EO and thus followed by a quick behavioral maturation of nurse bees. In summary, in the organism and superorganism, cells and honey bee workers, respectively coordinate their action through similar general mechanisms involving centralized control, self-organization and feedback loops with hormones and pheromones being the key coordinators.

V. Conclusions and Future Directions

Great progress has been made toward deciphering the chemical language. It is now known that pheromones in honey bees modulate individual interaction through their action on behavioral genes and individual physiology. However, by including the importance of synergy, dose and context, pheromone communication in honey bees appears to be remarkably complex (Slessor *et al.*, 2005; Fig. 17.2). Pheromones have been well studied

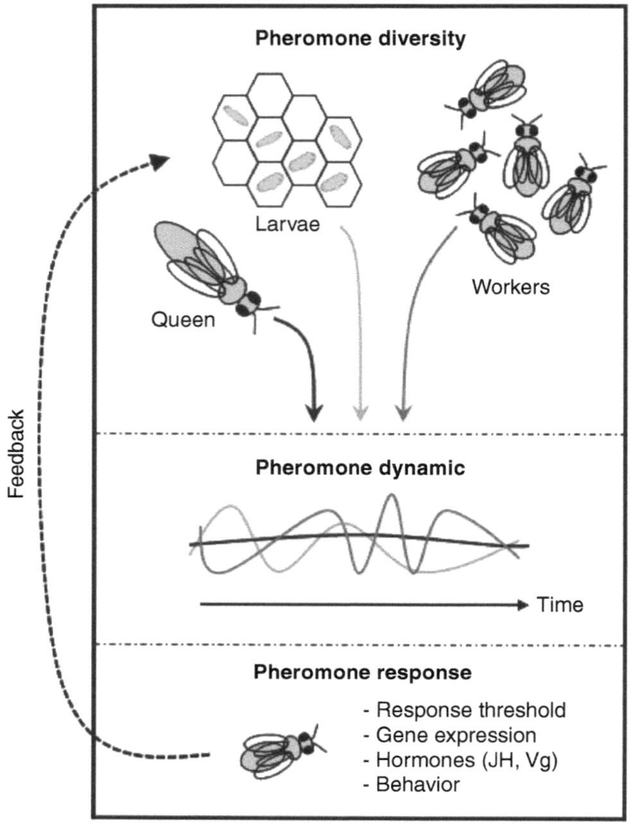

Figure 17.2 Complexity of pheromone language in honey bees. Pheromone language is remarkably complex since it is based on different levels of variation providing different nuances. First, there is a great diversity of pheromones produced by the different castes. Second, pheromone production is not rigid but dynamic and depends on the number of individuals, which follow temporal variation. Even if the single queen of the colony produces a baseline amount of QMP, its transmission is affected by the numbers of individual in the colony. Finally, variations might occur upon reception with different individuals having different response thresholds depending on their age (Pham-Delegue *et al.*, 1993) and genetic background (Kocher *et al.*, 2010; Pankiw *et al.*, 1994). This results in different genomic, physiological, and behavioral responses, which will affect in return pheromone production.

independently, but they may interact to further regulate the social life. For example, different chemicals like QMP and BP may not interact to inhibit ovary development (Hoover *et al.*, 2005b) but may have a synergistic effect on development of the hypopharyngeal glands (Peters *et al.*, 2010).

Individuals need to constantly integrate chemical information originating from their nestmates and answer in the correct way. Therefore, research integrating more than one pheromone promises to give a better representation of pheromone communication in this superorganism.

Pheromone signaling involves the secretion of chemical blends and their detection and processing by receivers. Although recent electrophysiological and molecular approaches have provided new insights into the mechanisms of pheromone integration and processing in the bee brain, less is known about pheromone biosynthesis and receptors. In that context, encouraging progress has been made thanks to the first identification of genes regulating QMP biosynthesis (Malka *et al.*, 2009) and the 9-ODA receptor, the main compound of QMP (Wanner *et al.*, 2007). Analysis of the honey bee genome sequence highlighted a remarkable expansion of the odorant receptor (Or) family (170 Ors) relative to solitary insects (62 and 79 Ors for *Drosophila melanogaster* and *Anopheles gambiae*, respectively; Robertson and Wanner, 2006). This high diversity in Ors perhaps allows the bees to recognize diverse floral odors and pheromone blends. Future studies on the biosynthetic processes that regulate pheromone production and the identification of pheromone receptors will improve our knowledge of chemical communication and open new avenues of investigation.

Finally, another promising area of research is to determine how chemical communication is affected by infectious disease of the colony. Since colonies are typically composed of thousands of bees with frequent interactions, living in groups increases risk of pathogens transmission, with each individual being a potential host. Experimental evidence in insects has shown that parasites cannot only evade immune responses but also exploit the endocrine system of the host to favor their growth and reproduction (Hurd, 2009). In honey bees, studies revealed that the cuticular hydrocarbon profile involved in social recognition can be modified by the activation of the immune system (Richard *et al.*, 2008) and parasitization by the ectoparasitic mite *Varroa destructor* (Salvy *et al.*, 2001). However, it is not know whether, analogous to the modification of hormone signaling in the organism, pathogen infection would affect pheromone signaling in the colony. Disruption of pheromone communication could occur in two ways: either a pathogen could exploit the pheromone system of the colony to its own advantage or during an infection the maintenance of this system would be too costly for the colony. Either way, a progressive modification of pheromone production and/or detection at the individual level could lead to the colony collapse. We believe that such findings would provide new insights into how pheromone signaling is integrated and operates a dynamic regulation of the different units of the superorganism.

ACKNOWLEDGMENTS

We thank C. M. McDonnell and C. M. Grozinger for comments that improved the manuscript. C. Alaux and A. Maisonnasse were supported by an INRA young researcher position (INRA SPE department) and a HFSP grant (RGP0042/2007-C101), respectively.

REFERENCES

Alaux, C., and Robinson, G. E. (2007). Alarm pheromone induces immediate-early gene expression and slow behavioral response in honey bees. *J. Chem. Ecol.* **33,** 1346–1350.

Alaux, C., Le Conte, Y., Adams, H. A., Rodriguez-Zas, S., Grozinger, C. M., Sinha, S., and Robinson, G. E. (2009a). Regulation of brain gene expression in honey bees by brood pheromone. *Genes Brain Behav.* **8,** 309–319.

Alaux, C., Sinha, S., Hasadsri, L., Hunt, G. J., Guzman-Novoa, E., DeGrandi-Hoffman, G., Uribe-Rubio, J. L., Southey, B. R., Rodriguez-Zas, S., and Robinson, G. E. (2009b). Honey bee aggression supports a link between gene regulation and behavioral evolution. *Proc. Natl. Acad. Sci. USA* **106,** 15400–15405.

Amdam, G. V., Norberg, K., Hagen, A., and Omholt, S. W. (2003). Social exploitation of vitellogenin. *Proc. Natl. Acad. Sci. USA* **100,** 1799–1802.

Anderson, P., Hansson, B. S., Nilsson, U., Han, Q., Sjoholm, M., Skals, N., and Anton, S. (2007). Increased behavioral and neuronal sensitivity to sex pheromone after brief odor experience in a moth. *Chem. Senses* **32,** 483–491.

Anton, S., and Gadenne, C. (1999). Effect of juvenile hormone on the central nervous processing of sex pheromone in an insect. *Proc. Natl. Acad. Sci. USA* **96,** 5764–5767.

Anton, S., Dufour, M. C., and Gadenne, C. (2007). Plasticity of olfactory-guided behaviour and its neurobiological basis: Lessons from moths and locusts. *Entomol. Exp. Appl.* **123,** 1–11.

Arnold, G., Le Conte, Y., Trouiller, J., Hervet, H., Chappe, B., and Masson, C. (1994). Inhibition of worker honeybee ovaries development by a mixture of fatty acid esters from larvae. *C. R. Acad. Sci. Paris, Ser. III* **317,** 511–515.

Beggs, K. T., and Mercer, A. R. (2009). Dopamine receptor activation by honey bee queen pheromone. *Curr. Biol.* **19,** 1206–1209.

Beggs, K. T., Glendining, K. A., Marechal, N. M., Vergoz, V., Nakamura, I., Slessor, K. N., and Mercer, A. R. (2007). Queen pheromone modulates brain dopamine function in worker honey bees. *Proc. Natl. Acad. Sci. USA* **104,** 2460–2464.

Ben-Shahar, Y., Dudek, N. L., and Robinson, G. E. (2004). Phenotypic deconstruction reveals involvement of manganese transporter *malvolio* in honey bee division of labor. *J. Exp. Biol.* **207,** 3281–3288.

Bloch, G., Wheeler, D. L., and Robinson, G. E. (2002). Endocrine influences on the organization of insect societies. *In* "Hormones, Brain, and Behavior," (D. W. Pfaff, A. P. Arnold, A. M. Etgen, S. E. Fahrbach, and R. T. Rubin, Eds.), Vol. 3, pp. 195–236. Academic Press, New York.

Boch, R., Shearer, D. A., and Stone, B. C. (1962). Identification of iso-pentyl acetate as an active component in the sting pheromone of the honey bee. *Nature* **195,** 1018–1020.

Cheung, E., and Kraus, W. L. (2010). Genomic analyses of hormone signaling and gene regulation. *Ann. Rev. Physiol.* **72,** 5.1–5.28.

Clayton, D. F. (2000). The genomic action potential. *Neurobiol. Learn. Mem.* **74,** 185–216.

Corona, M., Velarde, R. A., Remolina, S., Moran-Lauter, A., Wang, Y., Hughes, K. A., and Robinson, G. E. (2007). Vitellogenin, juvenile hormone, insulin signaling, and queen honey bee longevity. *Proc. Natl. Acad. Sci. USA* **104,** 7128–7133.

Dampney, J. R., Barron, A. B., and Oldroyd, B. P. (2004). Measuring the cost of worker reproduction in honeybees: Work tempo in an "anarchic" line. *Apidologie* **35**, 83–88.
Dierick, H. A., and Greenspan, R. J. (2007). Serotonin and neuropeptide F have opposite modulatory effects on fly aggression. *Nat. Genet.* **39**, 678–682.
Dyakonova, V. E. (2001). Role of opioid peptides in behavior of invertebrates. *J. Evol. Biochem. Physiol.* **37**, 335–347.
Engelmann, F. (1983). Vitellogenesis controlled by juvenile hormone. *In* "Endocrinology of Insects," (R. G. H. Downer and H. Laufer, Eds.), pp. 259–270. Alan R. Liss, New York.
Fischer, P., and Grozinger, C. M. (2008). Pheromonal regulation of starvation resistance in honey bee workers (*Apis mellifera*). *Naturwissenschaften* **95**, 723–729.
Fluri, P., Luscher, M., Wille, H., and Gerig, L. (1982). Changes in the weight of the pharyngeal gland and haemolymph titres of juvenile hormone, protein and vitellogenin in worker honey bees. *J. Insect Physiol.* **28**, 61–68.
Gascuel, J., and Masson, C. (1987). Influence of olfactory deprivation on synapse frequency in developing antennal lobe of the honeybee *Apis mellifera*. *Neurosci. Res. Commun.* **1**, 173–180.
Gilley, D. C., DeGrandi-Hoffman, G., and Hooper, J. E. (2006). Volatile compounds emitted by live European honey bee (*Apis mellifera* L.) queens. *J. Insect Physiol.* **52**, 520–527.
Giurfa, M. (1993). The repellent scent-mark of the honeybee *Apis mellifera ligustica* and its role as communication cue during foraging. *Insect. Soc.* **40**, 59–67.
Grozinger, C. M., and Robinson, G. E. (2007). Endocrine modulation of a pheromone-responsive gene in the honey bee brain. *J. Comp. Physiol. A* **193**, 461–470.
Grozinger, C. M., Sharabash, N. M., Whitfield, C. W., and Robinson, G. E. (2003). Pheromone-mediated gene expression in the honey bee brain. *Proc. Natl. Acad. Sci. USA* **100**, 14519–14525.
Grozinger, C. M., Fan, Y., Hoover, S. E., and Winston, M. L. (2007). Genome-wide analysis reveals differences in brain gene expression patterns associated with caste and reproductive status in honey bees (*Apis mellifera*). *Mol. Ecol.* **16**, 4837–4848.
Guidugli, K. R., Piulachs, M. D., Belles, X., Lourenco, A. P., and Simoes, Z. L. P. (2005). Vitellogenin regulates hormonal dynamics in the worker caste of a eusocial insect. *FEBS Lett.* **579**, 4961–4965.
Honey Bee Genome Sequencing Consortium, (2006). Insights into social insects from the genome of the honeybee *Apis mellifera*. *Nature* **443**, 931–949.
Hoover, S. E. R., Keeling, C. I., Winston, M. L., and Slessor, K. N. (2003). The effect of queen pheromones on worker honey bee ovary development. *Naturwissenschaften* **90**, 477–480.
Hoover, S. E. R., Oldroyd, B. P., Wossler, T. C., and Winston, M. L. (2005a). Anarchistic queen honey bees have normal queen mandibular pheromones. *Insect. Soc.* **52**, 6–10.
Hoover, S. E. R., Winston, M. L., and Oldroyd, B. P. (2005b). Retinue attraction and ovary activation: Responses of wild type and anarchistic honey bees (*Apis mellifera*) to queen and brood pheromones. *Behav. Ecol. Sociobiol.* **59**, 278–284.
Huang, Z. Y., and Robinson, G. E. (1992). Honeybee colony integration: Worker–worker interactions mediate hormonally regulated plasticity in division of labor. *Proc. Natl. Acad. Sci. USA* **89**, 11726–11729.
Huising, M. O., and Flik, G. (2005). The remarkable conservation of corticotropin-releasing hormone (CRH)-binding protein in the honeybee (*Apis mellifera*) dates the CRH system to a common ancestor of insects and vertebrates. *Endocrinology* **146**, 2165–2170.
Hunt, G. J., Amdam, G. V., Schlipalius, D., Emore, C., Sardesai, N., Williams, C. E., Rueppell, O., Guzman-Novoa, E., Arechavaleta-Velasco, M., Chandra, S., Fondrk, M. K., Beye, M., *et al.* (2007). Behavioral genomics of honeybee foraging and nest defense. *Naturwissenschaften* **94**, 247–267.

Hurd, H. (2009). Evolutionary drivers of parasite-induced changes in insect life-history traits from theory to underlying mechanisms. *Adv. Parasitol.* **68,** 85–110.

Kaatz, H. H., Hildebrandt, H., and Engels, W. (1992). Primer effect of queen pheromone on juvenile hormone biosynthesis in adult worker honey bees. *J. Comp. Physiol. B* **162,** 588–592.

Karlson, P., and Burtenandt, A. (1959). Pheromones (ectohormones) in insects. *Ann. Rev. Entomol.* **4,** 39–58.

Keeling, C. I., and Slessor, K. N. (2005). A scientific note on the aliphatic esters in queen honey bees. *Apidologie* **36,** 559–560.

Kocher, S. D., Ayroles, J. F., Stone, E. A., and Grozinger, C. M. (2010). Individual variation in pheromone response correlates with reproductive traits and brain gene expression in worker honey bees. *PLoS ONE* **5**(2), e9116.

Le Conte, Y., and Hefetz, A. (2008). Primer pheromones in social Hymenoptera. *Ann. Rev. Entomol.* **53,** 523–542.

Le Conte, Y., Arnold, G., Trouiller, J., Masson, C., Chappe, B., and Ourisson, G. (1989). Attraction of the parasitic mite *Varroa* to the drone larvae of honey bees by simple aliphatic esters. *Science* **245,** 638–639.

Le Conte, Y., Sreng, L., and Poitout, S. H. (1995). Brood pheromone can modulate the feeding behavior of *Apis mellifera* workers (Hymenoptera: Apidae). *J. Econ. Entomol.* **88,** 798–804.

Le Conte, Y., Mohammedi, A., and Robinson, G. E. (2001). Primer effects of a brood pheromone on honeybee behavioural development. *Proc. R. Soc. B* **268,** 163–168.

Ledoux, M. N., Winston, M. L., Higo, H., Keeling, C. I., Slessor, K. N., and LeConte, Y. (2001). Queen and pheromonal factors influencing comb construction by simulated honey bee (*Apis mellifera* L.) swarms. *Insect. Soc.* **48,** 14–20.

Leoncini, I., Le Conte, Y., Costagliola, G., Plettner, E., Toth, A. L., Wang, M. W., Huang, Z., Becard, J. M., Crauser, D., Slessor, K. N., and Robinson, G. E. (2004). Regulation of behavioral maturation by a primer pheromone produced by adult worker honey bees. *Proc. Natl. Acad. Sci. USA* **101,** 17559–17564.

Maisonnasse, A., Lenoir, J. C., Costagliola, G., Beslay, D., Choteau, F., Crauser, D., Becard, J. M., Plettner, E., and Le Conte, Y. (2009). A scientific note on E-β-ocimene, a new volatile primer pheromone that inhibits worker ovary development in honey bees. *Apidologie* **40,** 562–564.

Malka, O., Karunker, I., Yeheskel, A., Morin, S., and Hefetz, A. (2009). The gene road to royalty—differential expression of hydroxylating genes in the mandibular glands of the honeybee. *FEBS J.* **276,** 5481–5490.

Martin, S. J., Beekman, M., Wossler, T. C., and Ratnieks, F. L. W. (2002). Parasitic Cape honeybee workers, *Apis mellifera capensis*, evade policing. *Nature* **415,** 163–165.

Mohammedi, A., Crauser, D., Paris, A., and Le Conte, Y. (1996). Effect of a brood pheromone on honeybee hypopharyngeal glands. *C. R. Acad. Sci. Paris, Ser. III* **319,** 769–772.

Mohammedi, A., Paris, A., Crauser, D., and Le Conte, Y. (1998). Effect of aliphatic esters on ovary development of queenless bees (*Apis mellifera* L.). *Naturwissenschaften* **85,** 455–458.

Morgan, S. M., Butz Huryn, V. M., Downes, S. R., and Mercer, A. R. (1998). The effects of queenlessness on the maturation of the honey bee olfactory system. *Behav. Brain Res.* **91,** 115–126.

Moritz, R. F. A., and Fuchs, S. (1998). Organization of honeybee colonies: Characteristics and consequences of a superorganism concept. *Apidologie* **29,** 7–21.

Naumann, K., Winston, M. L., Slessor, K. N., Prestwich, G. D., and Webster, F. X. (1991). Production and transmission of honey bee queen (*Apis mellifera* L.) mandibular gland pheromone. *Behav. Ecol. Sociobiol.* **29,** 321–332.

Naumann, K., Winston, M. L., and Slessor, K. N. (1993). Movement of honey bee (*Apis mellifera* L.) queen mandibular gland pheromone in populous and unpopulous colonies. *J. Insect Behav.* **6,** 211–223.

Nunez, J., Almeida, L., Balderrama, N., and Giurfa, M. (1998). Alarm pheromone induces stress analgesia via an opioid system in the honeybee. *Physiol. Behav.* **63,** 75–80.

Oldroyd, B. P. (2002). The Cape honeybee: An example of a social cancer. *Trends Ecol. Evol.* **17,** 249–251.

Oldroyd, B. P., and Fewell, J. H. (2007). Genetic diversity promotes homeostasis in insect colonies. *Trends Ecol. Evol.* **22,** 408–413.

Oldroyd, B. P., Halling, L., and Rinderer, T. E. (1999). Development and behaviour of anarchistic honeybees. *Proc. R. Soc. B* **266,** 1875–1878.

Oldroyd, B. P., Wossler, T. C., and Ratnieks, F. R. (2001). Regulation of ovary activation in worker honey-bees (*Apis mellifera*): Larval signal production and adult response thresholds differ between anarchistic and wild-type bees. *Behav. Ecol. Sociobiol.* **50,** 366–370.

Page, R. E. Jr., and Amdam, G. V. (2007). The making of a social insect: Developmental architectures of social design. *Bioessays* **29,** 334–343.

Page, R. E., and Erickson, E. H. (1988). Reproduction by worker honey bees (*Apis mellifera* L.). *Behav. Ecol. Sociobiol.* **23,** 117–126.

Page, R. E. Jr., Erber, J., and Fondrk, M. K. (1998). The effect of genotype on response thresholds to sucrose and foraging behavior of honey bees (*Apis mellifera* L.). *J. Comp. Physiol. A* **182,** 489–500.

Pankiw, T. (2004a). Brood pheromone regulates foraging activity of honey bees (Hymenoptera: Apidae). *J. Econ. Entomol.* **97,** 748–751.

Pankiw, T. (2004b). Worker honey bee pheromone regulation of foraging ontogeny. *Naturwissenschaften* **91,** 178–181.

Pankiw, T. (2007). Brood pheromone modulation of pollen forager turnaround time in the honey bee (*Apis mellifera* L.). *J. Insect Behav.* **20,** 173–180.

Pankiw, T., and Page, R. E. Jr. (2001). Brood pheromone modulates honeybee (*Apis mellifera* L.) sucrose response thresholds. *Behav. Ecol. Sociobiol.* **49,** 206–213.

Pankiw, T., and Page, R. E. Jr. (2003). Effect of pheromones, hormones, and handling on sucrose response thresholds of honey bees (*Apis mellifera* L.). *J. Comp. Physiol. A* **189,** 675–684.

Pankiw, T., Winston, M. L., and Slessor, K. N. (1994). Variation in worker response to honey bee (*Apis mellifera* L) queen mandibular pheromone (Hymenoptera Apidae). *J. Insect Behav.* **7,** 1–15.

Pankiw, T., Huang, Z.-Y., Winston, M. L., and Robinson, G. E. (1998). Queen mandibular gland pheromone influences worker honey bee (*Apis mellifera* L.) foraging ontogeny and juvenile hormone titers. *J. Insect Physiol.* **44,** 685–692.

Peters, L., Zhu-Salzman, K., and Pankiw, T. (2010). Effect of primer pheromones and pollen diet on the food producing glands of worker honey bees (*Apis mellifera* L.). *J. Insect Physiol.* **56,** 132–137.

Pham-Delegue, M. H., Trouiller, J., Caillaud, C. M., Roger, B., and Masson, C. (1993). Effect of queen pheromone on worker bees of different ages: Behavioural and electrophysiological responses. *Apidologie* **24,** 267–281.

Ratnieks, F. L. W. (1993). Egg-laying, egg-removal, and ovary development by workers in queenright honey-bee colonies. *Behav. Ecol. Sociobiol.* **32,** 191–198.

Richard, F.-J., Aubert, A., and Grozinger, C. M. (2008). Modulation of social interactions by immune stimulation in honey bee, *Apis mellifera*, workers. *BMC Biol.* **6,** 50.

Robertson, H. M., and Wanner, K. W. (2006). The chemoreceptor superfamily in the honey bee, Apis mellifera: Expansion of the odorant, but not gustatory, receptor family. *Genome Res.* **16,** 1395–1403.

Robinson, G. E. (1987a). Modulation of alarm pheromone perception in the honey bee: Evidence for division of labor based on hormonal regulated response thresholds. *J. Comp. Physiol. A* **160,** 613–619.
Robinson, G. E. (1987b). Regulation of honey bee age polyethism by juvenile hormone. *Behav. Ecol. Sociobiol.* **20,** 329–338.
Robinson, G. E. (1992). Regulation of division of labor in insect societies. *Ann. Rev. Entomol.* **37,** 637–665.
Robinson, G. E., and Page, R. E. (1989). Genetic basis for division of labor in an insect society. *In* "The Genetics of Social Evolution," (M. D. Breed and R. E. Page, Eds.), pp. 61–81. West View Press, Boulder.
Robinson, G. E., Fernald, R. D., and Clayton, D. F. (2008). Genes and social behavior. *Science* **322,** 896–900.
Salvy, M., Martin, C., Bagneres, A. G., Provost, E., Roux, M., Le Conte, Y., and Clement, J. L. (2001). Modifications of the cuticular hydrocarbon profile of *Apis mellifera* worker bees in the presence of the ectoparasitic mite *Varroa jacobsoni* in brood cells. *Parasitology* **122,** 145–159.
Sandoz, J. C., Deisig, N., de Brito Sanchez, M. G., and Giurfa, M. (2007). Understanding the logics of pheromone processing in the honeybee brain: From labeled-lines to across-fiber patterns. *Front. Behav. Neurosci.* **1,** 5.
Seehuus, S. C., Norberg, K., Gimsa, U., Krekling, T., and Amdam, G. V. (2006). Reproductive protein protects functionally sterile honey bee workers from oxidative stress. *Proc. Natl. Acad. Sci. USA* **103,** 962–967.
Shearer, D. A., and Boch, R. (1965). 2-Heptanone in the mandibular gland secretion of the honey bee. *Nature* **206,** 530.
Shi, L., Lin, S., Grinberg, Y., Beck, Y., Grozinger, C. M., Robinson, G. E., and Lee, T. (2007). Roles of *Drosophila Kruppel-homolog 1* in neuronal morphogenesis. *Dev. Neurobiol.* **67,** 1614–1626.
Simon, U. E., Moritz, R. F. A., and Crewe, R. M. (2001). The ontogenetic pattern of mandibular gland components in queenless worker bees (*Apis mellifera capensis*). *J. Insect Physiol.* **47,** 735–738.
Sinha, S., Ling, X., Whitfield, C. W., Zhai, C. X., and Robinson, G. E. (2006). Genome scan for *cis*-regulatory DNA motifs associated with social behavior in honey bees. *Proc. Natl. Acad. Sci. USA* **103,** 16352–16357.
Slessor, K. N., Kaminski, L.-A., King, G. G. S., Borden, J. H., and Winston, M. L. (1988). Semiochemical basis of the retinue response to queen honey bees. *Nature* **332,** 354–356.
Slessor, K. N., Winston, M. L., and Le Conte, Y. (2005). Pheromone communication in the honeybee (*Apis mellifera* L.). *J. Chem. Ecol.* **31,** 2731–2745.
Smedal, B., Brynem, M., Kreibich, C. D., and Amdam, G. V. (2009). Brood pheromone suppresses physiology of extreme longevity in honey bees (*Apis mellifera*). *J. Exp. Biol.* **212,** 3795–3801.
Toth, A. L., and Robinson, G. E. (2005). Worker nutrition and division of labour in honeybees. *Anim. Behav.* **69,** 427–435.
Vergoz, V., Roussel, E., Sandoz, J.-C., and Giurfa, M. (2007a). Aversive learning in honeybees revealed by the olfactory conditioning of the sting extension reflex. *PLoS ONE* **2,** e288.
Vergoz, V., Schreurs, H. A., and Mercer, A. R. (2007b). Queen pheromone blocks aversive learning in young worker bees. *Science* **317,** 384–386.
Wager, B. R., and Breed, M. (2000). Does honey bee sting alarm pheromone give orientation information to defensive bees? *Ann. Entomol. Soc. Am.* **93,** 329–1332.
Wanner, K. W., Nichols, A. S., Walden, K. K., Brockmann, A., Luetje, C. W., and Robertson, H. M. (2007). A honey bee odorant receptor for the queen substance 9-oxo-2-decenoic acid. *Proc. Natl. Acad. Sci. USA* **104,** 14383–14388.

Whitfield, C. W., Cziko, A. M., and Robinson, G. E. (2003). Gene expression profiles in the brain predict behavior in individual honey bees. *Science* **302,** 296–299.
Wilson, E. O., and Bossert, W. H. (1963). Chemical communication among animals. *Recent Prog. Horm. Res.* **19,** 673–716.
Wilson, D. S., and Sober, E. (1989). Reviving the superorganism. *J. Theor. Biol.* **136,** 337–356.
Winston, M. L., Higo, H. A., and Slessor, K. N. (1990). Effect of various dosages of queen mandibular gland pheromone on the inhibition of queen rearing in the honey bee (Hymenoptera: Apidae). *Entomol. Soc. Am.* **83,** 234–238.
Winston, M. L., Higo, H. A., Colley, S., Pankiw, T., and Slessor, K. N. (1991). The role of queen mandibular pheromone and colony congestion in honey bee (*Apis mellifera* L.) reproductive swarming (Hymenoptera: Apidae). *J. Insect Behav.* **4,** 649–660.

CHAPTER EIGHTEEN

Unraveling the Pheromone Biosynthesis Activating Neuropeptide (PBAN) Signal Transduction Cascade that Regulates Sex Pheromone Production in Moths

Shogo Matsumoto, Atsushi Ohnishi, Jae Min Lee, *and* J. Joe Hull[1]

Contents

Molecular Entomology Laboratory, RIKEN Advanced Science Institute, Wako, Saitama, Japan

[1] Current address: USDA-ARS Arid Land Agricultural Research Center, 21881 N Cardon Lane, Maricopa, Arizona, USA

Vitamins and Hormones, Volume 83

ISSN 0083-6729, DOI: 10.1016/S0083-6729(10)83018-3

Abstract

Studies over the past three decades have demonstrated that female moths usually produce sex pheromones as multicomponent blends in which the ratios of the individual components are precisely controlled, making it possible to generate species-specific pheromone blends. Most moth pheromone components are *de novo* synthesized from acetyl-CoA in the pheromone gland (PG) through modifications of fatty acid biosynthetic pathways. Pheromone biosynthesis activating neuropeptide (PBAN), a neurohormone produced by a cephalic organ (subesophageal ganglion) stimulates sex pheromone biosynthesis in the PG via an influx of extracellular Ca^{2+}. In recent years, we have expanded our knowledge of the precise mechanisms underlying silkmoth (*Bombyx mori*) sex pheromone production by characterizing a number of key molecules. In this review, we want to highlight our efforts in elucidating these mechanisms in *B. mori* and to understand how they relate more broadly to lepidopteran sex pheromone production in general.

I. Introduction

While significant progress has been made over the years in elucidating the chemical structures of the species-specific multicomponent blends of sex pheromones that adult female moths use to attract conspecific males (Ando *et al.*, 2004), the molecular mechanisms underlying sex pheromone production in pheromone gland (PG) cells have remained poorly understood. To address this, we focused our efforts on using diverse methodological approaches to elucidate the intricate molecular events occurring within silkmoth (*Bombyx mori*) PG cells during pheromonogenesis (the period just prior to and including pheromone production) and to determine at the molecular level how the external signal of pheromone biosynthesis activating neuropeptide (PBAN) is transmitted into the biological response of pheromone production and release. Our research endeavors have lead to the successful identification and characterization of several key molecules essential to silkworm sex pheromone biosynthesis (Matsumoto *et al.*, 2007). In addition to broadening our understanding of the cellular events occurring in lepidopteran sex pheromone biosynthesis, we feel that our identification of many of these components and their associated pathways also provides insights into a number of topics relevant to modern cellular biology including mechanisms of lipid uptake, lipogenesis, hormone-regulated lipolysis, membrane trafficking associated with lipid transport/release, intracellular calcium signaling, etc. By characterizing these unsolved mechanisms in PG cells, we seek to provide a basic, novel understanding of the fundamental aspects of lipid and cellular biology, knowledge that can then be applied to elucidate similar mechanisms in organisms of different phyla.

II. Physiological Background

A. Pheromone gland

Because moth PGs are functionally differentiated organs that originate in the intersegmental membrane between the eighth and ninth abdominal segments, they are fundamentally uniform in their location and histological composition regardless of species (Percy-Cunningham and MacDonald, 1987). In *B. mori*, the PG is distinguishable as a pair of eversible, ventrolateral sacs (*sacculi laterals*, Fig. 18.1A; Fónagy *et al.*, 2001). Sex pheromone-producing cells in the PG are homogeneous single-layered epidermal cells consisting of about 9000 cells that are in direct contact with the overlying cuticular surface (Fig. 18.1B); these cells can be microscopically discerned by the presence of cytoplasmic lipid droplets (LDs; Fónagy *et al.*, 2000, 2001).

In the PG cells of *B. mori*, numerous cellular events culminating in the production of sex pheromone (i.e., *E,Z*-10,12-hexadecadien-1-ol, commonly known as bombykol) take place in concert before and after eclosion. This process, referred to as "pheromonogenesis" has a preadult eclosion phase that involves robust accumulation of cytoplasmic LDs and upregulation of numerous PG-specific genes, and a postadult eclosion phase that is characterized by: (1) PBAN-stimulated influx of extracellular Ca^{2+}, and (2) lipolysis of cytoplasmic LDs followed by conversion of the stored precursors to bombykol (see below) (Matsumoto *et al.*, 2007).

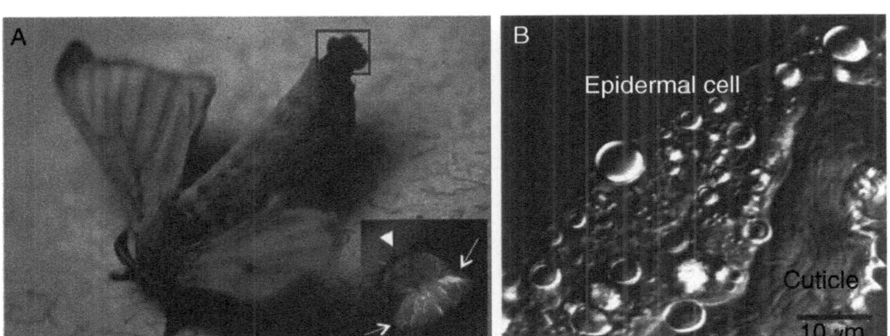

Figure 18.1 *B. mori* pheromone gland (PG). (A) Image of a female *B. mori* moth exhibiting stereotypical calling behavior with an extruded PG. Inset—image of a dissected PG (arrows) and ovipositor (arrowhead). (B) High magnification image of one of the pheromone-producing cells that comprise the PG. The large reflective lipid droplets that are distinguishing characteristics of PG cells can be clearly seen. (From Fónagy *et al.*, 2000.)

B. Hormonal regulation of moth sex pheromone production

Because mating is often limited to a specific phase of the photoperiod, the biochemical processes that comprise sex pheromone biosynthesis must be precisely regulated. In most moth species, these processes are regulated by PBAN, a neuropeptide consisting of 33–34 amino acids with the core C-terminal pentapeptide, FSPRLamide. Initially purified and sequenced from the corn earworm, *Helicoverpa zea* (Raina *et al.*, 1989), and the silkmoth, *B. mori* (Kitamura *et al.*, 1989), PBAN has since been identified in numerous other lepidopteran species (Rafaeli and Jurenka, 2003). In most species, PBAN acts directly on the PG following adult emergence to stimulate sex pheromone production by activating various steps in lepidopteran sex pheromone biosynthetic pathways (Rafaeli, 2009).

To date, sex pheromones from more than 530 moth species have been chemically identified (Ando *et al.*, 2004). Most moth species utilize Type I pheromone components, which consist of relatively simple straight-chain C_{10}-C_{18} aliphatic compounds that usually contain several double bonds and an oxygenated functional group of a primary alcohol, aldehyde, or acetate ester (Jurenka, 2003). A small subset of moths use Type II components (unsaturated hydrocarbons or hydrocarbon epoxides) as sex pheromones (Millar, 2000). A general scheme for the biosynthetic pathway of Type I pheromone components has become apparent in which the components are synthesized *de novo* in the PG cells from acetyl-CoA using modified fatty acid biosynthetic pathways (Bjostad *et al.*, 1987; Jurenka, 2003). The long-chain fatty acid (LCFA) intermediates, palmitic and stearic acids, are converted stepwise to the final pheromone components through a combination of desaturation and chain-shortening reactions, followed by reductive modifications of the carbonyl carbon via fatty alcohol precursors. Various combinations of limited chain-shortening and regio- and stereospecific desaturation steps significantly contribute to the production of a large number of species-specific pheromone components in moths (Martinez *et al.*, 1990; Roelofs *et al.*, 2002). In these sex pheromone biosynthetic pathways, PBAN regulates, in a species-dependent manner, either the initial or the terminal steps of the pathways. In *Argyrotaenia velutinana* (Tang *et al.*, 1989), *H. zea* (Jurenka *et al.*, 1991a), *Mamestra brassicae* (Jacquin *et al.*, 1994), *Cadra cautella* and *Spodoptera exigua* (Jurenka, 1997), PBAN regulates a step (or steps) in fatty acid biosynthesis, most likely acetyl-CoA carboxylase as shown in *Helicoverpa armigera* (Tsfadia *et al.*, 2008). In *Thaumetopoea pityocampa* (Arsequell *et al.*, 1990), *Spodoptera littoralis* (Fabrias *et al.*, 1994; Martinez *et al.*, 1990), *B. mori* (Ozawa *et al.*, 1993), and *Manduca sexta* (Fang *et al.*, 1995), the pheromonotropic control point is the terminal step of fatty-acyl reduction. It was later demonstrated in *B. mori* that PBAN also regulates lipolysis of the cytoplasmic LDs to liberate stored sex pheromone precursor fatty acids (see below) in addition to regulation of the terminal

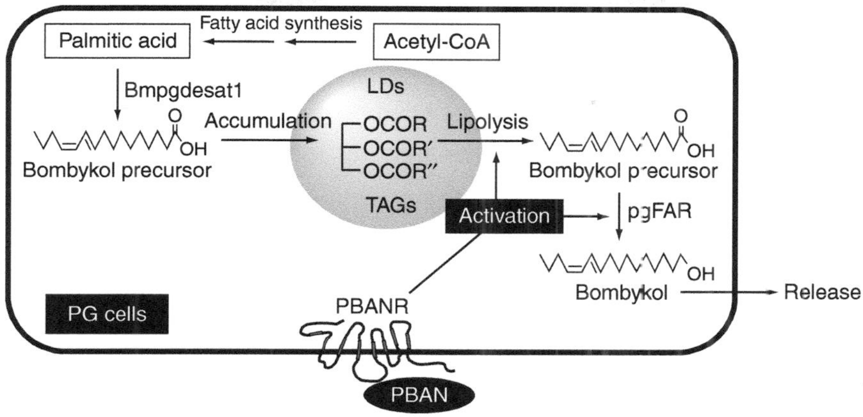

Figure 18.2 General scheme of bombykol biosynthesis. Prior to eclosion, the bombykol precursor ((*E*,*Z*)-10,12-hexadecadienoic acid) is generated from fatty acid synthesis-derived palmitic acid and stored as a triacylglycerol (TAG) within the PG cytoplasmic lipid droplets (LDs). Following eclosion, PBANR activation triggers release of the stored bombykol precursor and its subsequent reduction to bombykol.

reductase (Fig. 18.2; Matsumoto *et al.*, 2007). Similar two-step regulation by PBAN was also reported in *Heliothis virescens*, in which PBAN controls steps near the beginning and end of the pheromone biosynthetic process (Eltahlawy *et al.*, 2007).

C. Requirement of extracellular Ca^{2+}

Regardless of species, extracellular Ca^{2+} is required to turn the PBAN signal into the biological response of sex pheromone production, as demonstrated by the loss of pheromonotropic activity in isolated PG assays performed in the absence of extracellular Ca^{2+} in *H. zea*, *H. armigera*, *H. virescens*, *A. velutinana*, and *Ostrinia nubilalis* (Rafaeli, 2002). Furthermore, the pheromonotropic effects of PBAN have been mimicked by ionomycin in *B. mori* and *H. armigera* and by the ionophore A23187 in *B. mori*, *Spodoptera litura*, *O. nubilalis*, *A. velutinana*, and *H. virescens* (Rafaeli, 2002). In addition, the inorganic Ca^{2+} channel blocker, La^{3+}, inhibited sex pheromone production in *B. mori*, *H. zea*, and *A. velutinana* (Rafaeli, 2002). These findings suggested that the PBAN stimulus triggers an influx of extracellular Ca^{2+} into PG cells. Recently, this crucial event was directly demonstrated in isolated *B. mori* PGs using fluorescent Ca^{2+} imaging techniques (see below) (Hull *et al.*, 2007b).

Early pharmacological studies designed to characterize the PBAN-activated Ca^{2+} channel in *H. zea* and *H. virescens* suggested the involvement of a receptor-activated Ca^{2+} channel (RACC; Jurenka, 1996; Jurenka *et al.*, 1991b); however, the mechanism of activation and the molecular nature of the PBAN-activated Ca^{2+} channel remained to be resolved (see below).

D. Role of cyclic nucleotides as second messengers

While extracellular Ca^{2+} has been shown to be an absolute requirement for pheromonotropic activity in every moth species studied to date, accumulating evidence suggests that the intracellular signal transduction cascade triggered by the PBAN stimulus is species-dependent. This is particularly evident when comparing *B. mori* and the heliothine species (*H. zea* and *H. armigera*), the two lepidopteran models in which PBAN pheromonotropic activity has been most extensively studied. In heliothine species, the cyclic nucleotide second messenger, cyclic adenosine-3′,5′-monophosphate (cAMP), is a crucial component in PBAN signaling (Rafaeli, 2002; Rafaeli and Jurenka, 2003), whereas in *B. mori* cAMP is not involved (Hull *et al.*, 2007a). In *B. mori*, PBAN stimulation results in activation of the terminal fatty-acyl reduction step, which generates the final fatty alcohol product (bombykol) from the bombykol precursor fatty acid (Ozawa *et al.*, 1993). In heliothine moths, however, PBAN regulates a step (most likely acetyl-CoA carboxylase) in fatty acid biosynthesis (Jurenka *et al.*, 1991a; Rafaeli *et al.*, 1990; Tsfadia *et al.*, 2008). The involvement of cAMP in PBAN signaling has also been suggested in *A. velutinana*, in which PBAN likewise regulates a step in fatty acid biosynthesis (Jurenka *et al.*, 1994; Tang *et al.*, 1989). Conversely, in *S. litura*, another species in which PBAN regulates the fatty-acyl reductase (FAR), cAMP analogs and the adenylate cyclase activator forskolin had no effect on pheromone production (Matsumoto *et al.*, 1995). These findings further support the trend that PBAN regulation is linked to and differentiated by adenylate cyclase activity as those species in which fatty acid biosynthesis is modified by PBAN are dependent on cAMP production whereas those species, such as *B. mori*, that rely on PBAN activation of the terminal reductase are not (Hull *et al.*, 2007a; Matsumoto, 1997; Rafaeli, 2009).

III. Molecular Background: Essential Components of *B. mori* Sex Pheromone Production

To identify the functional proteins involved in *B. mori* pheromonogenesis, we generated a PG expressed-sequence tag (EST) database by constructing a normalized PG cDNA library prepared from newly emerged female moths of the inbred p50 strain (Yoshiga *et al.*, 2000). Expression analyses of EST clones using various tissues and PGs isolated during different developmental stages revealed that a dozen genes were specifically expressed in the PG and upregulated the day prior to adult eclosion. In addition, using the public *B. mori* EST databases SilkBase and CYBERGATE (http://morus.ab.a.u-tokyo.ac.jp/cgi-bin/index.cgi; http://150.26.71.213/cgi-bin/main_MX), we screened *in silico* for PG-specific genes. Of the approximate 11,000 independent clones in SilkBase, we found 312 expressed in the PG. Expression analyses followed by RNA interference (RNAi) screening of these clones has resulted in identification of a number of intriguing PG-specific and PG-selective genes.

A. Bombykol biosynthesis enzymes

1. Fatty-acyl desaturase (Bmpgdesat1)

In bombykol biosynthesis, palmitate is converted stepwise to bombykol through two desaturation steps followed by fatty-acyl reduction (Ando *et al.*, 1988). Bombykol biosynthesis (Fig. 18.2) is a rather simple process that differs from those of most other Type I pheromone biosynthetic pathways in that it does not require chain-shortening or further modification of the terminal hydroxyl group. The first desaturation step appears to be a general step presumably catalyzed by a *Z*11 desaturase frequently seen in the pheromone biosynthetic pathways of numerous moth species (Roelofs *et al.*, 2002). In contrast, the second desaturation step is less common in that it generates a conjugated diene system through 1,4-elimination of two hydrogen atoms at the allylic positions of the double bond in the *Z*11-monoene C_{16} intermediate. Similar 1,4-desaturation reactions involving monoene acyl precursors have only been observed in a handful of sex pheromone biosynthetic pathways. In experiments designed to clone the acyl-CoA desaturase genes responsible for bombykol biosynthesis, we found that a single desaturase, initially referred to as Desat1 but since renamed for clarification purposes Bmpgdesat1, produced both the *Z*11 monoene and the Δ10, 12 dienes, indicating that this enzyme is a unique bifunctional desaturase that has diverged from other lepidopteran Δ11 desaturases (Moto *et al.*, 2004; Ohnishi *et al.*, 2006). Following our publication, desaturases similarly exhibiting dual- or tri-catalytic activity have been identified in *S. littoralis* (Serra *et al.*, 2006), *M. sexta* (Matousková *et al.*, 2007), and *T. pityocampa* (Serra *et al.*, 2007), suggesting that these multifunctional Δ11 desaturases may represent a subfamily of lepidopteran desaturases.

2. PG-specific fatty-acyl reductases (pgFAR)

In the biosynthesis of Type I pheromones, the key enzyme required for the production of oxygenated functional groups is a FAR that converts fatty-acyl pheromone precursors to the corresponding alcohols (Fig. 18.2). Depending on the moth species, these alcohols can be acetylated or oxidized to the corresponding aldehydes. Despite the significant role, pgFAR has in generating the diverse species-specific oxygenated constituents of moth sex pheromones, this enzyme had eluded molecular identification and characterization. Surprisingly, this type of long-chain FAR had also not been characterized in either vertebrates or other invertebrates. Consequently, the quality of our *B. mori* PG EST database proved to be crucial in our efforts. In support of earlier biochemical characterizations (Ozawa and Matsumoto, 1996), we found that *B. mori* pgFAR contained the consensus N-terminal NAD(P)H binding motif observed in other reductases, and exhibited a strong substrate specificity for the bombykol precursor fatty acid, (*E,Z*)-10,12-hexadecadienoic acid (Moto *et al.*, 2003). This was a surprising finding because reduction of pheromone precursor fatty acids to their corresponding alcohols is a common step in the biosynthesis of oxygenated sex pheromone components regardless of the moth species. Although the published pgFAR genes currently in the literature are limited to those of *B. mori* and *Ostrinia scapulalis* (Anthony *et al.*, 2009), our finding implies that pgFARs from different moth species constitute a family of pgFARs with varying substrate specificities.

B. Molecules associated with LD dynamics

1. Constituents of the LDs

As explained below, characterization of the cytoplasmic LDs within the PG cells significantly advanced our understanding of the molecular mechanisms underlying sex pheromone production in *B. mori* (Matsumoto *et al.*, 2002). Prior to eclosion, bombykol-producing cells are characterized by an abundance of LDs within the cytoplasm. Staining these LDs with the fluorescent lipid marker, Nile Red facilitated our ability to monitor their progression throughout pheromonogenesis (Fig. 18.3); these LDs begin to form 1-2 d prior to eclosion, and they accumulate rapidly on the day of eclosion. After eclosion, the density of the LDs decreases over the course of the day in accordance with female calling behavior, the period when female moths are actively releasing bombykol. The LDs then reaccumulate during the night when the females are inactive (Fónagy *et al.*, 2000, 2001).

Posteclosion decrease in the LD density can be prevented by decapitation (inhibition of PBAN release) and restimulated with a pheromonotropic stimulus (PBAN injection after decapitation; Fig. 18.3), an indication that the LDs function to store bombykol precursors that are then released upon PBAN stimulation (Fónagy *et al.*, 2000). We confirmed this hypothesis by analyzing the chemical composition of the LD contents. HPLC separation of the LD contents and mass-spectrometric structure analyses confirmed that they are various triacylglycerols (TAGs) with the bombykol precursor, Δ10, 12-hexadecadienoate, predominantly sequestered as a major component at the *sn*-1 and/or *sn*-3 position of the glycerides (Matsumoto *et al.*,

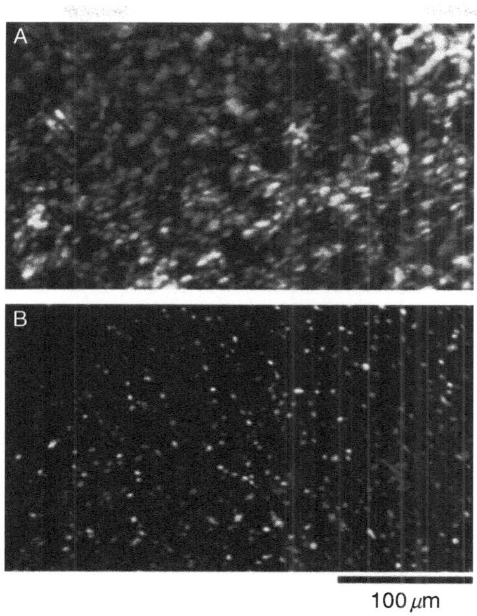

Figure 18.3 *B. mori* PG cytoplasmic lipid droplets function as bombykol precursor repositories. Images are of PG cells dissected from 1-day-old decapitated females injected with phosphate buffered saline ± PBAN. PG cells have been stained with Nile Red (a fluorescent lipid marker). (A) PBS alone. (B) PBS + 5 pmol Bom-PBAN. (From Ohnishi *et al.*, 2006.) (See Color Insert.)

2002). These results indicate that the LDs do indeed play a role in storing the bombykol precursor in the form of TAGs and in releasing it for bombykol biosynthesis in response to PBAN stimulus. As mentioned above, PBAN had previously been shown to stimulate fatty-acyl reduction in *B. mori* (Ozawa *et al.*, 1993). With the publication of our LD findings, we demonstrated that PBAN stimulates bombykol production by coincidently activating the two steps essential for bombykol biosynthesis, lipolysis of the LD TAGs (release of stored Δ10, 12-hexadecadienoate) and fatty-acyl reduction (conversion to bombykol; Fig. 18.2).

2. Fatty acid transport protein (BmFATP)

A gene encoding the *B. mori* FATP homolog (BmFATP) was found to be predominantly expressed in the PG where it undergoes remarkable upregulation 1 d prior to adult emergence. This expression profile is highly reminiscent of other gene products involved in the bombykol biosynthetic pathway and suggested that BmFATP might also be involved. In support of this hypothesis, *in vivo* RNAi knockdown of the BmFATP gene significantly suppressed bombykol production (Ohnishi *et al.*, 2009).

FATPs belong to an evolutionarily conserved family of membrane-bound proteins that facilitate the uptake of extracellular LCFAs and/or very LCFAs across the plasma membrane (Lewis *et al.*, 2001; Schaffer and Lodish, 1994; Stahl, 2004) and catalyze the ATP-dependent esterification of these fatty acids to their corresponding acyl-CoA derivatives (Hall *et al.*, 2003; Hirsch *et al.*, 1998).

For the cytoplasmic LDs in the PG, fatty acyls sequestered in the TAGs are restricted to five long-chain fatty acyls: two unsaturated C_{16} fatty acyls (Δ11-hexadecenoate and Δ10, 12-hexadecadienoate) and three conventional C_{18} fatty acyls (oleate, linoleate, and linolenate) with the bombykol precursor, Δ10, 12-hexadecadienoate, as the major component (Matsumoto *et al.*, 2002). While the bombykol biosynthesis precursors, Δ11-hexadecenoate and Δ10, 12-hexadecadienoate, are synthesized *de novo* in PG cells (Arima *et al.*, 1991), the essential fatty acids (linoleic and linolenic acids) derived from dietary fatty acids (Stanley-Samuelson *et al.*, 1988) must be taken up across the plasma membrane. Because RNAi-mediated knockdown of BmFATP *in vivo* significantly suppressed LD accumulation by preventing TAG synthesis, it is clear that BmFATP plays an essential role in preeclosion LD accumulation (Ohnishi *et al.*, 2009). Furthermore, in conjunction with the findings that BmFATP stimulates the uptake of extracellular LCFAs and that BmFATP knockdown reduces cellular long-chain acyl-CoA synthetase activity (Ohnishi *et al.*, 2009), these results suggest that BmFATP plays a role in stimulating the TAG synthesis required for LD accumulation via a process similar to the so-called vectorial acylation that couples the uptake of extracellular fatty acids with activation to CoA thioesters (Obermeyer *et al.*, 2007).

3. Acyl-CoA binding proteins (pgACBP and mgACBP)

Two distinct ACBPs are expressed specifically (pgACBP) or selectively (mgACBP) in the *B. mori* PG and undergo upregulation 1 d prior to adult emergence. mgACBP is also highly expressed in the midgut during the larval feeding stages (Matsumoto *et al.*, 2001). ACBP is a well-conserved 10-kDa *N*-acetylated polypeptide that is expressed in a wide variety of species ranging from yeast to mammals (Faergeman and Knudsen, 1997). Because ACBPs are known to specifically bind straight-chain (C_{14}–C_{22}) fatty acyl-CoA esters with high affinity, and to protect them from hydrolysis (Kragelund *et al.*, 1993; Mogensen *et al.*, 1987; Rasmussen *et al.*, 1993, 1994), it was speculated that they might function as carriers or cellular deposits of the acyl-CoAs utilized in pheromone biosynthesis. The use of dsRNAs to knock down the expression of pgACBP and mgACBP demonstrated that this was indeed the case, since loss of either pgACBP or mgACBP function prevented TAG accumulation within the cytoplasmic LDs, and consequently the availability of the bombykol precursors (Ohnishi *et al.*, 2006). In *M. sexta*, ACBP expression is highest during periods of active feeding and lipid transport from the midgut (Snyder and Antwerpen, 1997). The high abundance of mgACBP transcripts in the midgut of larval *B. mori* suggests that the role of mgACBPs in pheromone biosynthesis is secondary to a dietary role, which would indicate that mgACBP likely donates conventional C_{18} fatty acyl-CoAs derived from dietary lipids whereas pgACBP specifically donates *de novo* synthesized pheromone precursor fatty acyl-CoAs. As mentioned above, because BmFATP facilitates both the uptake of extracellular C_{18} fatty acids and their conversion to corresponding C_{18} fatty acyl-CoAs via vectorial acylation, our results further imply essential but distinct roles for BmFATP, pgACBP, and mgACBP in the formation of the cytoplasmic LDs that are essential for storing and releasing the bombykol precursor fatty acid during pheromonogenesis (Ohnishi *et al.*, 2009).

It is interesting to note that while searching for factors regulating transcription of PG-specific genes, we found that *β*-D-glucosyl-*O*-L-tyrosine, a humoral factor that appears in the pupal hemolymph 1 d prior to eclosion, regulates pgACBP transcription (Ohnishi *et al.*, 2005). Surprisingly, while *β*-D-glucosyl-*O*-L-tyrosine titers rise dramatically prior to eclosion and reach the maximum level on the day preceding eclosion, this factor had no effect on the transcription of other PG-specific genes, such as pgFAR and Bmpgdesat1.

IV. Essential Components and Mechanisms of the *B. mori* PBAN Signal Transduction Cascade

A. PBAN receptor (PBANR)

It has been known since the mid-80s that sex pheromone production in moths is triggered by PBAN. However, because early attempts using traditional biochemical methods proved inconclusive, molecular identification and characterization of the cell surface PBANR would have to wait for the advent of modern bioinformatics. Identification of mammalian neuromedin U receptor-like sequences following annotation of the *Drosophila* genome significantly aided the discovery process. The presence of these gene sequences was noteworthy as the biologically essential C-terminal pentapeptide motifs present in PBAN (FSPRLamide) and mammalian neuromedin U (FRPRNamide) are highly conserved. Furthermore, one of the *Drosophila* neuromedin U receptor homologs could be activated by PBAN (Park *et al.*, 2002), indicating that the PBAN and neuromedin U receptors are also conserved. Consequently, using a homology-based molecular approach, full-length clones encoding the PBANR were independently amplified from the PGs of *H. zea* and *B. mori* (Choi *et al.*, 2003;

Hull *et al.*, 2004). While both genes encode G protein-coupled receptors (GPCR) with significant sequence similarity (76%), the two receptors are differentiated by the presence of a 67 amino acid C-terminal extension in *B. mori* PBANR. PBANR homologs have also been identified in *Plutella xylostella* (accession # AAY34744.1), *S. littoralis* (accession # ABD52277.1; Zheng *et al.*, 2007), *H. armigera*; (accession #AAW47417.1; Rafaeli *et al.*, 2007), and *S. exigua* (accession # ABY62317.2). Surprisingly, multiple PBANR isoforms were identified in both *M. sexta* (accession #s FJ240221.1–FJ240224) and *H. virescens* (accession #s ABU93812.1, ABU93813.1, ABV58013.1; Kim *et al.*, 2008). Interestingly, the *H. virescens* PBANR-C isoform, which contains a C-terminus that is more similar to *B. mori* than *H. zea*, was preferentially amplified from PGs (Kim *et al.*, 2008).

Northern blot analysis of *B. mori* PBANR showed that it is predominantly expressed in the PG and that it undergoes significant upregulation one day prior to adult emergence. Transient expression assays further showed that *B. mori* PBANR triggers an influx of extracellular Ca^{2+} in response to PBAN binding. *B. mori* PBANR cell surface localization was confirmed by fluorescent confocal imaging of cells transiently expressing a fluorescent chimera of the receptor tagged at the C terminus with a green fluorescent protein variant (EGFP). This construct specifically bound Rhodamine Red labeled-PBAN (RR-PBAN) as evidenced by the loss of RR-PBAN associated fluorescence in the presence of unlabeled PBAN but not in the presence of an unrelated peptide (Hull *et al.*, 2004). Further characterization of the *B. mori* PBANR-EGFP construct in conjunction with RR-PBAN indicated that *B. mori* PBANR undergoes ligand-induced internalization (Fig. 18.4). Removal of the 67 amino acid C terminal extension prevented internalization, suggesting that the *B. mori* and *H. zea* PBANRs exhibit different internalization kinetics and thus have distinctive regulatory mechanisms associated with receptor desensitization (Hull *et al.*, 2005).

B. PBAN-mediated activation of store-operated channels

As mentioned above, moth sex pheromone biosynthetic pathways are dependent on the presence of extracellular Ca^{2+}, suggesting that PBAN triggers the opening of cell surface ion channels and the concomitant influx of Ca^{2+}. This crucial event was recently demonstrated using isolated *B. mori* PGs loaded with a cell permeable fluorescent probe for Ca^{2+} (Fura PE-3AM; Hull *et al.*, 2007b). In the presence of external Ca^{2+}, a sharp increase in fluorescence was observed following PBAN stimulation (Fig. 18.5A). No increase in fluorescence was seen in the absence of external Ca^{2+} (Fig. 18.5B) and fluorescence intensity decreased with repeated PBAN stimulation (Fig. 18.5C), suggesting partial desensitization of either the channel or the receptor as observed in the heterologous expression assays (see above).

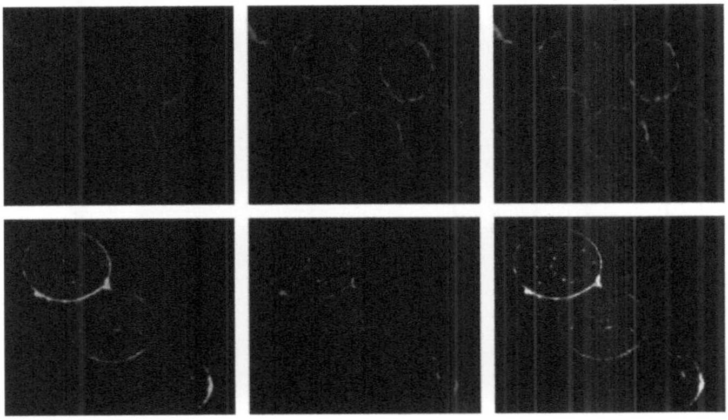

Figure 18.4 PBAN-induced internalization of transiently expressed PBANR. Fluorescent confocal images of Sf9 cells transiently expressing *B. mori* PBANR-EGFP. Cells were incubated in the presence of 50 nM RR-PBAN for 60 min at 4 °C. RR-PBAN was removed and the cells were incubated for 30 min at 27 °C and then fixed. EGFP fluorescence (green) was obtained using an argon laser (488-nm), while Rhodamine Red fluorescence (red) was obtained using a krypton/argon laser (568-nm). Figures were merged using Photoshop 6.0. Yellow color indicates colocalization of PBANR-EGFP and RR-PBAN. Note the presence of numerous intracellular fluorescent puncta following 30 min incubation at 27 °C. (From Hull *et al.*, 2004.) (See Color Insert.)

Because numerous biological processes are mediated by fluctuations in Ca^{2+} levels, entry into the cell is tightly regulated (Berridge *et al.*, 2000). The two most pervasive Ca^{2+}-permeable cation channels are voltage-operated channels (VOCs; Lacinova, 2005) and RACCs (Berridge *et al.*, 2000), which can be subdivided into two subgroups: diacylglycerol (DAG)-dependent channels and store-operated channels (SOCs). DAG-dependent channels open in response to phospholipase C (PLC)-generated DAG or one of its downstream metabolites, such as arachidonic acid (Hardie, 2007; Shuttleworth *et al.*, 2004). SOCs open in response to IP_3-mediated depletion of endoplasmic reticulum (ER) Ca^{2+} stores (Parekh and Putney, 2005). SOCs can also be pharmacologically activated by thapsigargin (Tg). The pharmacological profile of the PBAN-activated channel in *B. mori* PGs was consistent with the involvement of SOCs: bombykol production is blocked by classical SOC inhibitors, activators of DAG-dependent channels are ineffective, and the pheromonotropic effects of PBAN can be mimicked by Tg (Hull *et al.*, 2007b).

Since SOCs are ultimately dependent on the soluble IP_3-generated downstream of PLC activation (Putney *et al.*, 2001; Venkatachalam *et al.*,

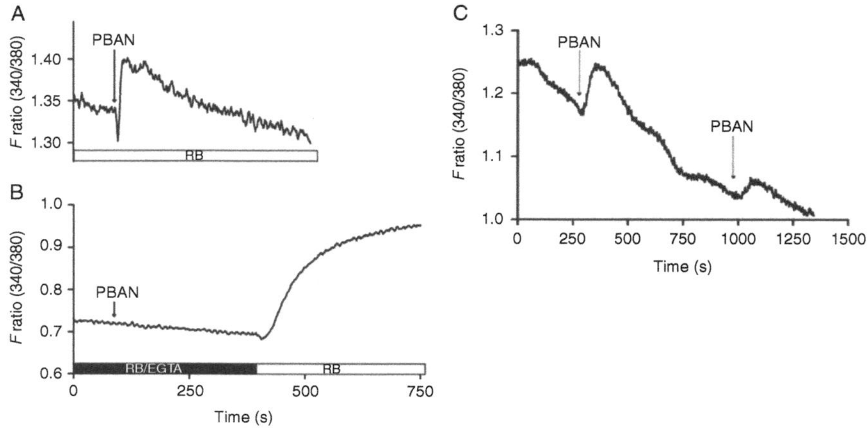

Figure 18.5 Effect of PBAN on Ca^{2+} influx in Fura3PE-AM loaded *B. mori* PG cells. (A) Representative fluorescence intensity tracing of the Ca^{2+}-associated response in PG cells following stimulation with 120 nM PBAN. (B) Representative fluorescence intensity tracing of the Ca^{2+}-associated response in PG cells initially stimulated with 120 nM PBAN in Ca^{2+}-deficient buffer and then transferred to Ca^{2+}-replete buffer. (C) Representative fluorescence intensity tracing of the Ca^{2+}-associated response in PG cells following repeated stimulation using increasing concentrations of PBAN (first arrow: 500 nM PBAN; second arrow: 700 nM PBAN). (From Hull *et al.*, 2007b.)

2002), the effect of PBAN on total inositol phosphate levels in B. *mori* PGs was examined. In the presence of $LiCl_2$, an inhibitor of inositol monophosphatase, there is a significant increase in the levels of PG total inositol phosphates following PBAN stimulation (Hull *et al.*, 2010). Furthermore, the pharmacological profile of PLC inhibitors on bombykol production is consistent with PBAN-mediated PLC activation. To establish the molecular identity of the heterotrimeric G protein activated downstream of PBAN binding, homology-based PCR methods were used to clone PG-expressed Gα subunits, which included two Gαs, one Gαq and one Gαo. Other signal transduction gene products were also cloned, including multiple G protein β and γ subunits, two isoforms of PLCβ, PLCγ, and a portion of the IP_3 receptor activated by the soluble IP_3 released upon PLC activation. *In vivo* RNAi-mediated knockdown studies revealed that the *B. mori* PBAN signal is transmitted via a canonical pathway utilizing Gq-mediated PLC activation, and that BmGq1, BmPLCβ1, BmIP_3R, and BmPLCγ are necessary components (Hull *et al.*, 2010). The determination that BmPLCγ plays a role in transmitting the PBAN stimulus was unexpected, although not without precedent. We anticipate that further studies into BmPLCγ function will help define its precise role in the PBAN signal transduction cascade.

C. BmSTIM1 and BmOrai1B

Stromal interaction molecule 1 (STIM1) and Orai1 have recently been shown to be essential for some SOC Ca^{2+} entry mechanisms (Hewavitharana *et al.*, 2007; Wu *et al.*, 2007). STIM1 is an ER membrane protein that communicates the state of ER Ca^{2+} stores to the cell surface SOCs. A conformational change in STIM1 in response to diminished luminal Ca^{2+} levels promotes its translocation from or within the ER to regions of the plasma membrane (Stathopulos *et al.*, 2008). Orai (or Ca^{2+}release-activated Ca^{2+} channel modulator 1, CRACM1) is a four transmembrane domain protein organized as a dimer in the plasma membrane under resting conditions. Interaction with the C-terminus of STIM1 induces tetramerization of the Orai dimers and the subsequent influx of extracellular Ca^{2+} (Penna *et al.*, 2008). Because the pharmacological profile of the channel opened in response to PBAN binding was consistent with SOC activation, the potential role of STIM1 and Orai1 in bombykol production was investigated. Using the available EST and genomic databases, we cloned *B. mori* homologs of both proteins. BmSTIM1 is a 577 amino acid protein characterized by an intraluminal EF-hand Ca^{2+} binding domain, a single transmembrane domain, and a highly conserved C-terminal domain containing a cluster of basic amino acids (residues 380–385) shown to be necessary for Orai1 interaction (Hull *et al.*, 2009). Two variants of Orai1 (BmOrai1A and BmOrai1B), which are differentiated by the presence of a 37 amino acid N-terminal extension in BmOrai1A, have been identified in *B. mori*; however, only the BmOrai1B variant is actively expressed in the PG. Functional expression of BmSTIM1 and BmOrai1B in cultured insect cells and *in vivo* dsRNA-mediated RNAi knockdown effects showed that both proteins are integral components of the PBAN signaling cascade (Hull *et al.*, 2009).

V. Model for PBAN Signaling in *B. mori*

Based on these data, we have generated the following model to describe the molecular mechanisms underlying bombykol production (Fig. 18.6). Before eclosion, the bombykol precursor is synthesized *de novo* from acetyl-CoA through fatty acid biosynthesis. At this time, however, the bombykol precursor is not converted to bombykol, but is rather stored as TAGs in PG cytoplasmic LDs. After eclosion, PBAN is released into the hemolymph where it interacts with PBANR on the cell surface of PG cells. This binding triggers an influx of Ca^{2+} via a canonical signal transduction cascade that culminates in the activation of BmSTIM1 and BmOrai1. The concomitant rise in intracellular Ca^{2+} accelerates both lipolysis and fatty-acyl reduction

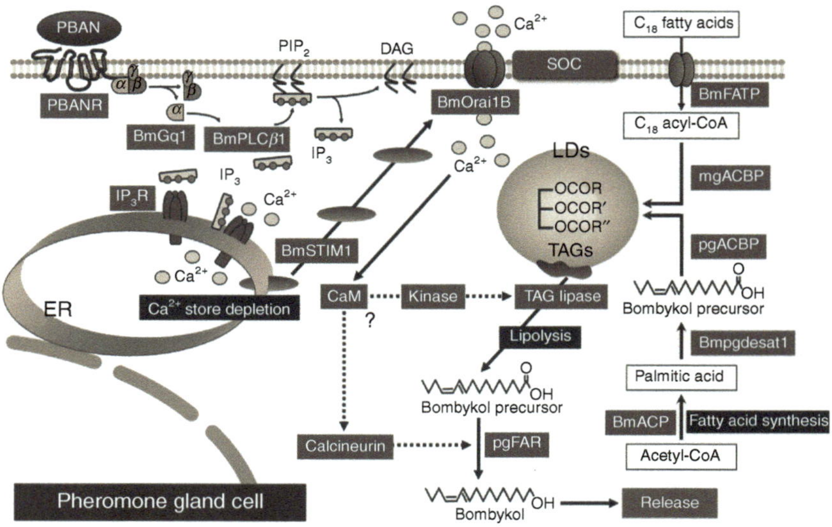

Figure 18.6 Proposed model of the molecular events underlying *B. mori* pheromonogenesis. (See Color Insert.)

through a calmodulin/calcineurin-mediated phosphorylation/dephosphorylation cascade culminating in bombykol production. The precise mechanisms underlying the phosphorylation/dephosphorylation cascade, however, have yet to be determined.

VI. Conclusions

In our endeavor to understand the molecular mechanisms underlying sex pheromone production in the silkmoth *B. mori*, we have taken advantage of the available *B. mori* genomic information to facilitate characterization of PG-specific and PG-selective genes (*Bmpgdesat1*, *pgFAR*, *PBANR*, *BmFATP*, *pgACBP*, and *mgACBP*). We have also demonstrated the specific roles of these genes in bombykol biosynthesis *in vivo* using an RNAi-mediated approach (Ohnishi *et al.*, 2006). In conclusion, effective use of the loss-of-function approach that we established for *B. mori* not only provided unambiguous evidence regarding the *in vivo* functional relevance of these genes, but also demonstrated the potential for this method to dissect the molecular interactions that constitute biosynthetic pathways. Our next challenge is to determine the mechanism (i.e., the phosphorylation/dephosphorylation cascade) by which the external PBAN signal activates the dual activities of lipolysis of the cytoplasmic TAGs and fatty-acyl reduction.

To begin to address this, we have made more extensive use of RNAi screening to facilitate cloning of a PG-specific lipase gene that is most likely responsible for TAG lipolysis. In addition, we have found that numerous PG proteins are phosphorylated in response to PBAN stimulation (Ohnishi, unpublished observation).

ACKNOWLEDGMENTS

We wish to thank Shinji Atsusawa and Masaaki Kurihara of the Molecular Entomology Laboratory at the RIKEN Advanced Science Institute for their technical support. This work was supported by the Lipid Dynamics Research Project of RIKEN, the Targeted Proteins Research Program (TPRP) of the Ministry of Education, Culture, Sports, Science, and Technology of Japan, and Grants-in-Aid for Scientific Research (B) 20380040 from the Japan Society for the Promotion of Science.

REFERENCES

Ando, T., Hase, R., Arima, R., and Uchiyama, M. (1988). Biosynthetic pathway of bombykol, the sex pheromone of the female silkworm moth. *Agric. Biol. Chem.* **52,** 473–478.

Ando, T., Inomata, S., and Yamamoto, M. (2004). Lepidopeteran sex pheromones. *Top. Curr. Chem.* **239,** 51–96.

Anthony, B., Fujii, T., Moto, K., Matsumoto, S., Fukuzawa, M., Tatsuki, S., and Ishikawa, Y. (2009). Pheromone-gland-specific fatty-acyl reductase in the adzuki bean borer, *Ostrinia scapulalis* (Lepidoptera: Crambidae). *Insect Biochem. Mol. Biol.* **39,** 90–95.

Arima, R., Takahara, K., Kadoshima, T., Numazaki, F., Ando, T., Uchiyama, M., Nagasawa, H., Kitamura, A., and Suzuki, A. (1991). Hormonal regulation of pheromone biosynthesis in the silkworm moth, *Bombyx mori* (Lepidoptera: Bombycidae). *Appl. Entomol. Zool.* **26,** 137–147.

Arsequell, G., Fabrias, G., and Camps, F. (1990). Sex pheromone biosynthesis in the processionary moth *Thaumetopoea pityocampa* by delta-13 desaturation. *Arch. Insect Biochem. Physiol.* **14,** 47–56.

Berridge, M. J., Lipp, P., and Bootman, M. D. (2000). The versatility and universality of calcium signaling. *Nat. Rev. Mol. Cell Biol.* **1,** 11–21.

Bjostad, L. B., Wolf, W. A., and Roelofs, W. L. (1987). Pheromone biosynthesis in lepidopterans: Desaturation and chain shortening. *In* "Pheromone Biochemistry," (G. D. Prestwich and G. J. Blomquist, Eds.), pp. 77–120. Academic Press, Orlando.

Choi, M. Y., Fuerst, E. J., Rafaeli, A., and Jurenka, R. (2003). Identification of a G protein-coupled receptor for pheromone biosynthesis activating neuropeptide from pheromone glands of the moth *Helicoverpa zea. Proc. Natl. Acad. Sci. USA* **100,** 9721–9726.

Eltahlawy, H., Buckner, J. S., and Foster, S. P. (2007). Evidence for two-step regulation of pheromone biosynthesis by the pheromone biosynthesis-activating neuropeptide in the moth *Heliothis virescens. Arch. Insect Biochem. Physiol.* **64,** 120–130.

Fabrias, G., Marco, M. P., and Camps, F. (1994). Effect of the pheromone biosynthesis activating neuropeptide on sex pheromone biosynthesis in *Spodoptera littoralis* isolated glands. *Arch. Insect Biochem. Physiol.* **27,** 77–87.

Faergeman, N. J., and Knudsen, J. (1997). Role of long-chain fatty acyl-CoA esters in the regulation of metabolism and in cell signalling. *Biochem. J.* **323,** 1–12.

Fang, N., Teal, P. E. A., and Tumlinson, J. H. (1995). PBAN regulation of pheromone biosynthesis in female tobacco hornworm moths, *Manduca sexta* (L). *Arch. Insect Biochem. Physiol.* **29,** 35–44.

Fónagy, A., Yokoyama, N., Okano, K., Tatsuki, S., Maeda, S., and Matsumoto, S. (2000). Pheromone-producing cells in the silkmoth, *Bombyx mori*: Identification and their morphological changes in response to pheromonotropic stimuli. *J. Insect Physiol.* **46,** 735–744.

Fónagy, A., Yokoyama, N., and Matsumoto, S. (2001). Physiological status and change of cytoplasmic lipid droplets in the pheromone-producing cells of the silkmoth, *Bombyx mori* (Lepidoptera, Bombicidae). *Arthropod Struct. Dev.* **30,** 113–123.

Hall, A. M., Smith, A. J., and Bernlohr, D. A. (2003). Characterization of the Acyl-CoA synthetase activity of purified murine fatty acid transport protein 1. *J. Biol. Chem.* **278,** 43008–43013.

Hardie, R. C. (2007). TRP channels and lipids: From *Drosophila* to mammalian physiology. *J. Physiol.* **578,** 9–24.

Hewavitharana, T., Deng, X., Soboloff, J., and Gill, D. L. (2007). Role of STIM and Orai proteins in the store-operated calcium signaling pathway. *Cell Calcium* **42,** 173–182.

Hirsch, D., Stahl, A., and Lodish, H. F. (1998). A family of fatty acid transporters conserved from mycobacterium to man. *Proc. Natl. Acad. Sci. USA* **95,** 8625–8629.

Hull, J. J., Ohnishi, A., Moto, K., Kawasaki, Y., Kurata, R., Suzuki, M. G., and Matsumoto, S. (2004). Cloning and characterization of the pheromone biosynthesis activating neuropeptide receptor from the silkmoth, *Bombyx mori*: Significance of the carboxyl terminus in receptor internalization. *J. Biol. Chem.* **279,** 51500–51507.

Hull, J. J., Ohnishi, A., and Matsumoto, S. (2005). Regulatory mechanisms underlying pheromone biosynthesis activating neuropeptide (PBAN) induced internalization of the *Bombyx mori* PBAN receptor. *Biochem. Biophys. Res. Commun.* **334,** 69–78.

Hull, J. J., Kajigaya, R., Imai, K., and Matsumoto, S. (2007a). The *Bombyx mori* sex pheromone biosynthetic pathway is not mediated by cAMP. *J. Insect Physiol.* **53,** 782–793.

Hull, J. J., Kajigaya, R., Imai, K., and Matsumoto, S. (2007b). Sex pheromone production in the silkworm, *Bombyx mori*, is mediated by store-operated Ca^{2+} channels. *Biosci. Biotech. Biochem.* **71,** 1993–2001.

Hull, J. J., Lee, J. M., Kajigaya, R., and Matsumoto, S. (2009). *Bombyx mori* homologs of STIM1 and Orai1 are essential components of the signal transduction cascade that regulates sex pheromone production. *J. Biol. Chem.* **284,** 31200–31213.

Hull, J. J., Lee, J. M., and Matsumoto, S. (2010). Gqα-linked PLCβ1 and PLCγ are essential components of the pheromone biosynthesis activating neuropeptide (PBAN) signal transduction cascade. *Insect Mol. Biol.* **19**, 553–566.

Jacquin, E., Jurenka, R. A., Ljungberg, H., Nagnan, P., Lofstedt, C., Descoins, C., and Roelofs, W. L. (1994). Control of sex pheromone biosynthesis in the moth *Mamestra brassicae* by the pheromone biosynthesis activating neuropeptide. *Insect Biochem. Mol. Biol.* **24,** 203–211.

Jurenka, R. A. (1996). Signal transduction in the stimulation of sex pheromone biosynthesis in moths. *Arch. Insect Biochem. Physiol.* **33,** 245–258.

Jurenka, R. A. (1997). Biosynthetic pathway for producing the sex pheromone component (Z,E)-9,12-tetradecadienyl acetate in moths involves a delta 12 desaturase. *Cell. Mol. Life Sci.* **53,** 501–505.

Jurenka, R. A. (2003). Biochemistry of female moth sex pheromones. *In* "Insect Pheromone Biochemistry and Molecular Biology," (G. J. Blomquist and R. G. Vogt, Eds.), pp. 53–80. Elsevier Academic Press, Oxford.

Jurenka, R. A., Jacquin, E., and Roelofs, W. L. (1991a). Control of the pheromone biosynthetic pathway in *Helicoverpa zea* by the pheromone biosynthesis activating neuropeptide (PBAN). *Arch. Insect Biochem. Physiol.* **17,** 81–91.

Jurenka, R. A., Jacquin, E., and Roelofs, W. L. (1991b). Stimulation of pheromone biosynthesis in the moth *Helicoverpa zea*: Action of a brain hormone on pheromone glands involves Ca^{2+} and cAMP as second messengers. *Proc. Natl. Acad. Sci. USA* **88,** 8621–8625.

Jurenka, R. A., Fabrias, G., DeVoe, L., and Roelofs, W. L. (1994). Action of PBAN and related peptides on pheromone biosynthesis in isolated pheromone glands of the red-banded leafroller moth, *Argyrotaenia velutinana. Comp. Biochem. Physiol.* **108C,** 153–160.

Kim, Y. J., Nachman, R. J., Aimanova, K., Gill, S., and Adams, M. E. (2008). The pheromone biosynthesis activating neuropeptide (PBAN) receptor of *Heliothis virescens*: Identification, functional expression, and structure-activity relationships of ligand analogs. *Peptides* **29,** 268–275.

Kitamura, A., Nagasawa, H., Kataoka, H., Inoue, T., Matsumoto, S., Ando, T., and Suzuki, A. (1989). Amino acid sequence of pheromone biosynthesis activating neuropeptide (PBAN) of the silkworm, *Bombyx mori. Biochem. Biophys. Res. Commun.* **163,** 520–526.

Kragelund, B. B., Andersen, K. V., Madsen, J. C., Knudsen, J., and Poulsen, F. M. (1993). Three-dimensional structure of the complex between acyl-coenzyme A binding protein and palmitoyl-coenzyme A. *J. Mol. Biol.* **230,** 1260–1277.

Lacinova, L. (2005). Voltage-dependent calcium channels. *Gen. Physiol. Biophys.* **24,** 1–78.

Lewis, S. E., Listenberger, L. L., Ory, D. S., and Schaffer, J. E. (2001). Membrane topology of the murine fatty acid transport protein 1. *J. Biol. Chem.* **276,** 37042–37050.

Martinez, T., Fabrias, G., and Camps, F. (1990). Sex pheromone biosynthetic pathway in *Spodoptera littoralis* and its activation by a neurohormone. *J. Biol. Chem.* **265,** 1381–1387.

Matousková, P., Pichová, I., and Svatos, A. (2007). Functional characterization of a desaturase from the tobacco hornworm moth (*Manduca sexta*) with bifunctional Z11- and 10,12-desaturase activity. *Insect Biochem. Mol. Biol.* **37,** 601–610.

Matsumoto, S. (1997). Intracellular signal transduction of pheromone biosynthesis activating neuropeptide (PBAN) in lepidopteran insects. *Recent Res. Dev. Agric. Biol. Chem.* **1,** 33–49.

Matsumoto, S., Ozawa, R., Uchiumi, K., Kurihara, M., and Mitsui, T. (1995). Intracellular signal transduction of PBAN action in the common cutworm, *Spodoptera litura*: Effect of pharmacological agents on sex pheromone production in vitro. *Insect Biochem. Mol. Biol.* **25,** 1055–1059.

Matsumoto, S., Yoshiga, T., Yokoyama, N., Iwanaga, M., Koshiba, S., Kigawa, T., Hirota, H., Yokoyama, S., Okano, K., Shimada, T., and Tatsuki, S. (2001). Characterization of acyl-CoA-binding protein (ACBP) in the pheromone gland of the silkworm, *Bombyx mori. Insect Biochem. Mol. Biol.* **31,** 603–609.

Matsumoto, S., Fónagy, A., Yamamoto, M., Wang, F., Yokoyama, N., Esumi, Y., and Suzuki, Y. (2002). Chemical characterization of cytoplasmic lipid droplets in the pheromone-producing cells of the silkmoth, *Bombyx mori. Insect Biochem. Mol. Biol.* **32,** 1447–1455.

Matsumoto, S., Hull, J. J., Ohnishi, A., Moto, K., and Fónagy, A. (2007). Molecular mechanisms underlying sex pheromone production in the silkmoth, *Bombyx mori*: Characterization of the molecular components involved in bombykol biosynthesis. *J. Insect Physiol.* **53,** 752–759.

Millar, J. G. (2000). Polyene hydrocarbons and epoxides: A second major class of lepidopteran sex attractant pheromones. *Ann. Rev. Entomol.* **45,** 575–604.

Mogensen, I. B., Schulenberg, H., Hansen, H. O., Spener, F., and Knudsen, J. (1987). A novel acyl-CoA-binding protein from bovine liver. Effect on fatty acid synthesis. *Biochem. J.* **241,** 189–192.

Moto, K., Yoshiga, T., Yamamato, M., Takahashi, S., Okano, K., Ando, T., Nakata, T., and Matsumoto, S. (2003). Pheromone gland-specific fatty-acyl reductase of the silkmoth, *Bombyx mori. Proc. Natl. Acad. Sci. USA* **100,** 9156–9161.

Moto, K., Suzuki, M. G., Hull, J. J., Kurata, R., Takahashi, S., Yamamato, M., Okano, K., Imai, K., Ando, T., and Matsumoto, S. (2004). Involvement of a bifunctional fatty-acyl desaturase in the biosynthesis of the silkmoth, *Bombyx mori*, sex pheromone. *Proc. Natl. Acad. Sci. USA* **101,** 8631–8636.

Obermeyer, T., Fraisl, P., DiRusso, C. C., and Black, P. N. (2007). Topology of the yeast fatty acid transport protein Fat1p: Mechanistic implications for functional domains on the cytosolic surface of the plasma membrane. *J. Lipid Res.* **48,** 2354–2364.

Ohnishi, A., Koshino, H., Takahashi, S., Esumi, Y., and Matsumoto, S. (2005). Isolation and characterization of a humoral factor that stimulates transcription of the acyl-CoA binding protein in the pheromone gland of the silkmoth, *Bombyx mori*. *J. Biol. Chem.* **280,** 4111–4116.

Ohnishi, A., Hull, J. J., and Matsumoto, S. (2006). Targeted disruption of genes in the *Bombyx mori* sex pheromone biosynthetic pathway. *Proc. Natl. Acad. Sci. USA* **103,** 4398–4403.

Ohnishi, A., Hashimoto, K., Imai, K., and Matsumoto, S. (2009). Functional characterization of the *Bombyx mori* fatty acid transport protein (BmFATP) within the silkmoth pheromone gland. *J. Biol. Chem.* **284,** 5128–5136.

Ozawa, R., and Matsumoto, S. (1996). Intracellular signal transduction of PBAN action in the silkworm, *Bombyx mori*: Involvement of acyl CoA reductase. *Insect Biochem. Mol. Biol.* **26,** 259–265.

Ozawa, R., Ando, T., Nagasawa, H., Kataoka, H., and Suzuki, A. (1993). Reduction of the acyl group: The critical step in bombykol biosynthesis that is regulated *in vitro* by the neuropeptide hormone in the pheromone gland of *Bombyx mori*. *Biosci. Biotech. Biochem.* **57,** 2144–2147.

Parekh, A. B., and Putney, Jr., J. W. (2005). Store-operated calcium channels. *Physiol. Rev.* **85,** 757–810.

Park, Y., Kim, Y. J., and Adams, M. E. (2002). Identification of G protein-coupled receptors for *Drosophila* PRXamide peptides, CCAP, corazonin, and AKH supports a theory of ligand–receptor coevolution. *Proc. Natl. Acad. Sci. USA* **99,** 11423–11428.

Penna, A., Demuro, A., Yeromin, A. V., Zhang, S. L., Safrina, O., Parker, I., and Cahalan, M. D. (2008). The CRAC channel consists of a tetramer formed by Stim-induced dimerization of Orai dimers. *Nature* **456,** 116–120.

Percy-Cunningham, J. E., and MacDonald, J. A. (1987). Biology and ultrastructure of sex pheromone-producing glands. *In* "Pheromone Biochemistry," (G. D. Prestwich and G. J. Blomquist, Eds.), pp. 27–75. Academic Press, Orlando.

Putney, Jr., J. W., Broad, L. M., Braun, F. J., Lievremont, J. P., and Bird, G. S. (2001). Mechanisms of capacitative calcium entry. *J. Cell Sci.* **114,** 2223–2229.

Rafaeli, A. (2002). Neuroendocrine control of pheromone biosynthesis in moths. *Int. Rev. Cytol.* **213,** 49–91.

Rafaeli, A. (2009). Pheromone biosynthesis activating neuropeptide (PBAN): Regulatory role and mode of action. *Gen. Comp. Endocrinol.* **162,** 69–78.

Rafaeli, A., and Jurenka, R. A. (2003). PBAN regulation of pheromone biosynthesis in female moths. *In* "Insect Pheromone Biochemistry and Molecular Biology," (G. J. Blomquist and R. G. Vogt, Eds.), pp. 107–136. Elsevier Academic Press, Oxford.

Rafaeli, A., Soroker, V., Kamensky, B., and Raina, A. K. (1990). Action of pheromone biosynthesis activating neuropeptide on *in vitro* pheromone glands of *Heliothis armigera* females. *J. Insect Physiol.* **36,** 641–646.

Rafaeli, A., Bober, R., Becker, L., Choi, M. Y., Fuerst, E. J., and Jurenka, R. (2007). Spatial distribution and differential expression of the PBAN receptor in tissues of adult *Helicoverpa* spp. (Lepidoptera: Noctuidae). *Insect Mol. Biol.* **16,** 287–293.

Raina, A., Jaffe, K., Kempe, T. G., Keim, P., Blacher, R. W., Fales, H. M., Riley, C. T., Klun, J. A., Ridgway, R. L., and Hayes, D. K. (1989). Identification of a neuropeptide hormone that regulates sex pheromone production in female moths. *Science* **244,** 796–798.

Rasmussen, J. T., Rosendal, J., and Knudsen, J. (1993). Interaction of acyl-CoA binding protein (ACBP) on processes for which acyl-CoA is a substrate, product or inhibitor. *Biochem. J.* **292,** 907–913.

Rasmussen, J. T., Faergeman, N. J., Kristiansen, K., and Knudsen, J. (1994). Acyl-CoA-binding protein (ACBP) can mediate intermembrane acyl-CoA transport and donate acyl-CoA for β-oxidation and glycerolipid synthesis. *Biochem. J.* **299,** 165–170.

Roelofs, W. L., Liu, W., Hao, G., Jiao, H., Rooney, A. P., and Linn, Jr., C. E. (2002). Evolution of moth sex pheromones via ancestral genes. *Proc. Natl. Acad. Sci. USA* **99,** 13621–13626.

Schaffer, J. E., and Lodish, H. F. (1994). Expression cloning and characterization of a novel adipocyte long chain fatty acid transport protein. *Cell* **79,** 427–436.

Serra, M., Pina, B., Bujons, J. L., Camps, F., and Fabrias, G. (2006). Biosynthesis of 10,12-dienoic fatty acids by a bifunctional Delta11 desaturase in *Spodoptera littoralis. Insect Biochem. Mol. Biol.* **36,** 634–641.

Serra, M., Pina, B., Abad, J. L., Camps, F., and Fabrias, G. (2007). A multifunctional desaturase involved in the biosynthesis of the processionary moth sex pheromone. *Proc. Natl. Acad. Sci. USA* **104,** 16444–16449.

Shuttleworth, T. J., Thompson, J. L., and Mignen, O. (2004). ARC channels: A novel pathway for receptor-activated calcium entry. *Physiology (Bethesda)* **19,** 355–361.

Snyder, M. J., and Antwerpen, R. V. (1997). Cellular distribution, levels, and function of the diazepam-binding inhibitor/acyl-CoA-binding protein in last instar *Manduca sexta* midgut. *Cell Tissue Res.* **288,** 177–184.

Stahl, A. (2004). A current review of fatty acid transport proteins (SLC27). *Pflugers Arch.* **447,** 722–727.

Stanley-Samuelson, D. W., Jurenka, R. A., Cripps, C., Blomquist, G. J., and deRenobales, M. (1988). Fatty acids in insects: Composition, metabolism and biological significance. *Arch. Insect Biochem. Physiol.* **9,** 1–33.

Stathopulos, P. B., Zheng, L., Li, G. Y., Plevin, M. J., and Ikura, M. (2008). Structural and mechanistic insights into STIM1-mediated initiation of store-operated calcium entry. *Cell* **135,** 110–122.

Tang, J. D., Charlton, R. E., Jurenka, R. A., Wolf, W. A., Phelan, P. L., Sreng, L., and Roelofs, W. L. (1989). Regulation of pheromone biosynthesis by a brain hormone in two moth species. *Proc. Natl. Acad. Sci. USA* **86,** 1806–1810.

Tsfadia, O., Azrielli, A., Falach, L., Zada, A., Roelofs, E., and Rafaeli, A. (2008). Pheromone biosynthetic pathways: PBAN-regulated rate-limiting steps and differential expression of desaturase genes in moth species. *Insect Biochem. Mol. Biol.* **38,** 552–567.

Venkatachalam, K., van Rossum, D. B., Patterson, R. L., Ma, H. T., and Gill, D. L. (2002). The cellular and molecular basis of store-operated calcium entry. *Nat. Cell Biol.* **4,** E263–E272.

Wu, M. M., Luik, R. M., and Lewis, R. S. (2007). Some assembly required: Constructing the elementary units of store-operated Ca^{2+} entry. *Cell Calcium* **42,** 163–172.

Yoshiga, T., Okano, K., Mita, K., Shimada, T., and Matsumoto, S. (2000). cDNA cloning of acyl-CoA desaturase homologs in the silkworm, *Bombyx mori. Gene* **246,** 339–345.

Zheng, L., Lytle, C., Njauw, C. N., Altstein, M., and Masrtins-Green, M. (2007). Cloning and characterization of the pheromone biosynthesis activating neuropeptide receptor gene in *Spodoptera littoralis* larvae. *Gene* **393,** 20–30.

CHAPTER NINETEEN

Pheromones in Social Wasps

Bruschini Claudia,* Cervo Rita,* *and* Turillazzi Stefano*,†

Contents

Abstract

Social wasps need an efficient communication system to coordinate their members in the numerous activities of the colony. In this regard, the chemical channel is the most utilized by social wasps to transfer information in intraspecific (pheromones) and interspecific (allomones) communication. In this chapter, we reviewed the main chemical substances which mediate recognition between colony members and coordinate nest defense, alarm and recruitment. Due to their central role in the colonial life, the majority of pheromones have

* Dipartimento di Biologia Evoluzionistica, Università degli Studi di Firenze, Firenze, Italy
† Centro Interdipartimentale di Spettrometria di Massa (C.I.S.M.), Università degli Studi di Firenze, Firenze, Italy

Vitamins and Hormones, Volume 83
ISSN 0083-6729, DOI: 10.1016/S0083-6729(10)83019-5

been identified and their functions have been deeply investigated in many species. On the contrary, sex pheromones which are the most studied in insects, have been quite neglected in social wasps.

I. Introduction

Social wasps are Aculeate Hymenoptera belonging to the family Vespidae. The term social, or more properly eusocial, refers to the life style of species which live in colonies defined by three fundamental traits: (i) overlapping of at least two adult generations, (ii) cooperative brood care and, overall, (iii) extreme reproductive division of labor into fertile reproductive castes—queens—and sterile non-reproductive castes—workers (Michener, 1969).

Social wasps share these traits with ants, bees, and the group of social cockroaches called Termites (Inward *et al.*, 2007). While all termites and ants are eusocial, bees and wasps show a wide range of social organization, from solitary to highly eusocial. For this reason, bees and wasps are considered key groups for the study of social evolution and, in particular, "Vespidae is the only insect family in which diverse genera and species span a full spectrum of levels of social organization" (Hunt, 2007).

A. Social wasps' systematic

According to Carpenter (1982) the family Vespidae is divided in six subfamilies (Fig. 19.1A) showing different lifestyle and biology. Euparagiinae and Masarinae include only solitary species. On the other hand, the Eumeninae, the largest subfamily with more than one thousand species, presents a range of parental behaviors that is particularly important for the study of the origin of eusociality.

The Stenogastrinae wasps are eusocial but due to the low levels of social organization, they represent a key group for the evolution of social behavior (Hunt, 2007; Turillazzi, 1989, 1991). These wasps live in tropical forests of South East Asia and New Guinea where they build their nests without peduncles on trees, on rootlets hanging from earth trenches or on the walls of caves perfectly camouflaged with leaves, sticks, or mud pieces. Their colonies are very small with maximally a dozen individuals (Turillazzi, 1991). The subfamily comprises seven genera (Carpenter and Starr, 2000) with more than 70 described species (Turillazzi, unpublished).

The eusocial subfamily Polistinae is the most diversified group of social wasps, both in terms of number of species, morphological and behavioral diversity (Carpenter, 1991). Polistine social wasps are cosmopolitan, although concentrated primarily in the tropics, especially in the New World. They are divided in four tribes (Polistini, Myschocittarini, Ropalidiini, Epiponini),

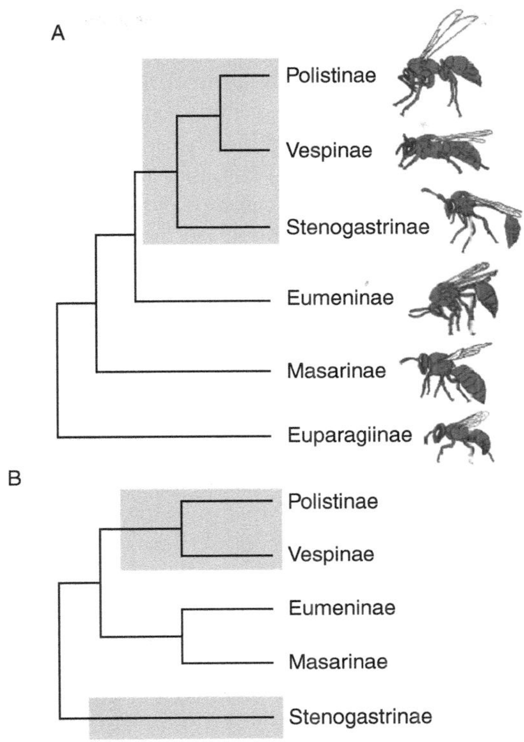

Figure 19.1 Phylogenetic trees representing the Vespidae subfamilies: A) the phylogenetic tree based on morphological and behavioral characters (Carpenter, 1982; Pickett and Carpenter, 2010); B) a more recent phylogenetic tree based only on molecular data (Schmitz and Moritz, 2000) (from Hines *et al.*, 2007, *Proc. Natl. Acad. Sci.*, Copyright (2007), National Academy of Sciences, U.S.A.).

comprising 28 genera and more than 800 species (Carpenter, 1991) with a variable population size ranging from a few individuals to more than one million (in the colonies of the South American species *Agelaia vicina*). According to the colony foundation strategy they are divided in: "independent-founding" species, when the nest is founded by solitary fertilized females (which can be joined by other fertilized females), and "swarm-founding" species, when a new nest is founded by a swarm composed by one (or more) fertilized females, together with a group of workers or sterile females (Jeanne, 1991). *Polistes* is the only genus of the tribe Polistini and it comprises exclusively independent-founding species. This genus represents a key model for the study of social evolution because it shows only slight caste differentiation. Moreover, the wide geographical distribution, the limited size of their colonies and the nest without envelope suspended by a pedicel, make the genus *Polistes* a suitable model for scientific researches (Starks and Turillazzi, 2006; Turillazzi and West-Eberhard, 1996). All the species belonging to the genus *Mischocyttarus*, the only representative of the South American tribe Mischocyttarini, are independent-founding species (Gadagkar, 1991). The tribe Ropalidiini, instead, shows both modes of colony founding: the genus *Parapolybia* (Asian distribution) includes only independent-founding species as well as the African genus *Belonogaster*. The genus *Polybioides* has both African and Asian species all of which are swarm-founding. The genus *Ropalidia* is distributed both in Africa and in the South Asian and Australian tropics and includes both independent- and swarm-founding species (Gadagkar, 1991). The last tribe, the South American Epiponini, includes 24 swarm-founding genera (Jeanne, 1991).

The subfamily Vespinae (yellowjackets and hornets) presents only highly eusocial species and this implies morphological differentiation between queens and workers. They are mainly distributed in the temperate areas of the Old and New World where they build large nests with envelopes which protect a pile of cell combs where up to thousands individuals live. The subfamily includes four genera: *Provespa*, *Vespa*, *Dolichovespula* and *Vespula* (Greene, 1991; Matsuura, 1991; Spradbery, 1973).

Many morphological, developmental, and behavioral differences shown by Stenogatrinae wasps with respect to the other two eusocial subfamilies (resumed in Hunt, 2007; Turillazzi, 1991), together with biomolecular evidences (Hines *et al.*, 2007; Schmitz and Moritz, 2000), may suggest that the similarities in the social biology among the three subfamilies can be due to evolutionary convergences. In this case, that the evolution of social behavior in these wasps could be an independent evolutionary pathway to eusociality in the family Vespidae (see Hunt, 2007; but see Pickett and Carpenter, 2010; Fig. 19.1B).

B. Social communication

The large number of individuals of an insect colony, requires an efficient communication system that involves the transfer of information among colony members and allows the coordination of both the common activities and the different tasks of its inhabitants. Among several communication channels used by social insects the visual channel is the cheapest and often the less flexible, as it requires the visibility of the signaler to the receivers, an enlightened environment as well as efficient receptors. On the other hand, an acoustic signal can be perceived even if the emitter is not visible but, usually, the energy required to maintain this kind of signal for a long time is extremely high. For these reasons, the chemical channel has been selected for intracolonial communication in almost all social insects, including wasps. For example, in ants and termites, which usually nest underground, or in wasps and bees with enveloped combs, visual signals are useless to transfer information with respect to chemical ones. Even if the structure and the nest-building material of social bees and wasps favor the transmission of vibratory signals, chemical communication is the most convenient way to rapidly and efficiently share the information inside the colony. Social insects are defined as "chemical factories" owing to the great number of exocrine glands which can be found in their bodies (Billen and Morgan, 1998). These glands are known to be the source of chemical substances with both intraspecific and interspecific communicative functions (pheromones and allomones, respectively). Analogously to the other social insects, in social wasps numerous exocrine glands have been described, but only few of them were reported as the source of compounds with proven or probable pheromonal function (Fig. 19.2, Table 19.1); they can be mainly found in the head and gastrum but some additional glands have been discovered in other body parts as legs and antennae (see Billen and Morgan, 1998; Downing, 1991; Jeanne, 1996; Landolt and Akre, 1979).

Since social wasps are model organisms for the study of the evolution of social behavior, due to the different levels of social organization, they could be also key species for the study of the evolution of communication (West-Eberhard, 1996). Analytical techniques, sensible enough to study the limited quantities of chemical substances used by these insects, permit the deciphering of the complex world of colony odors (Wyatt, 2003).

II. Nestmate Recognition Pheromones

Wasp colonies, analogously to colonies of other social insects, are closed systems where the access to non-group members is denied by colony inhabitants (Howard and Blomquist, 2005). The maintenance of colony integrity is a fundamental feature of social groups as it prevents alien individuals from entering the colony and exploiting the social life advantages and resources usually devoted to relatives. In this context, the ability to recognize relatives (kin recognition) or, at least, colony members (nestmate recognition) is fundamental for social life since it prevents dispensing altruistic behaviors to non-relative individuals.

Although, some recent studies (Cervo *et al.*, 2008a; Tibbetts, 2002, 2004; Tibbetts and Curtis, 2007; Tibbetts and Dale, 2004) have explored the possibility that, at least in some species of *Polistes*, visual signals can play a role in the recognition of colony members, there are robust evidences that nestmate-recognition ability in social wasps, as well as in other social insects, is mediated by chemical signals (reviewed by Dani, 2006; Gamboa, 1996, 2004; Lenoir *et al.*, 1999; Lorenzi, 2006; Singer *et al.*, 1998).

The wasp body surface is covered by a thin layer of wax substances (mainly cuticular hydrocarbons, CHCs) that play a crucial role to reduce

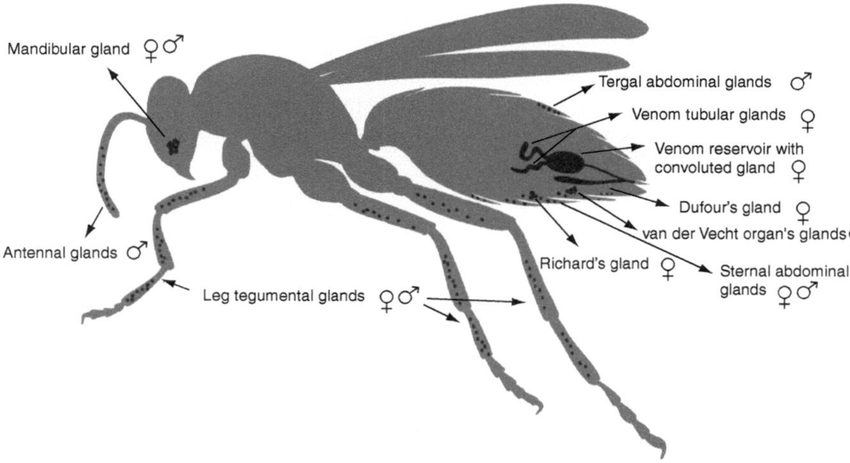

Figure 19.2 Schematic drawing of locations of exocrine glands on the body of a generic social wasp for which a pheromonal function in males and females has been reported; locations and scales are approximate only.

both internal water loss and the entrance of pathogens and parasites (Blomquist and Dillwith, 1985). However, this epicuticular blend of waxes plays a communicative role as well as it functions as a source of information for other individuals of the same or different species (Howard, 1993).

This epicuticular layer of lipids is synthesized by cells associated with the epidermis (Nelson and Blomquist, 1995). However, it has been demonstrated that the Dufour's gland also contains a mixture of lipids similar to the mixture of the epicuticular blend (Cervo *et al.*, 2002a; Dani *et al.*, 1996a; Ruther *et al.*, 1998; Turillazzi *et al.*, 2008). Although, these results have suggested that the Dufour's gland could be involved in the production of these pheromones in social wasps (Dani *et al.*, 1996a; Ruther *et al.*, 1998), studies to confirm the contribution of this gland to the production of the epicuticular layer are necessary. Moreover, the same CHCs found on the cuticle and in the Dufour's gland are also the main compounds of the abdominal sternal glands (Dani *et al.*, 2003).

A. Species level

Chemical analyses, based mainly on Gas Chromatography coupled to Mass Spectrometry (GC–MS), have deciphered the chemical nature of the epicuticular substances and their relative amounts for many species of social wasps; in six species of Stenogastrinae (Beani *et al.*, 2002; Cervo *et al.*, 2002a; Turillazzi *et al.*, 2004, 2008; Zanetti *et al.*, 2001), 11 species of Vespinae (Brown *et al.*, 1991; Butts and Espelie, 1995; Butts *et al.*, 1991;

Table. 19.1 Presence/absence of the principal compounds or classes of compounds with proven or probable pheromonal function in the three social subfamilies of Vespidae [Stenogastrinae, Polistinae, Vespinae]

Pheromone	Subfamily			Source	Main compound(s)
Nestmate recognition	S		+	Epidermis and Dufour's gland	Hydrocarbons
	P	IF	+		
		SF	+		
	V		+		
Queen	S		–		
	P	IF	–		
		SF	–		
	V		+	Head glands	δ-*n*-Hexadecalactone
Alarm	S		–	Venom apparatus	
	P	IF	+		Acetates, amides, spiroacetals
		SF	+		Amide, spiroacetals
	V		+		Amide, alcohol, hydrocarbons
Trail	S		–		
	P	IF	–		
		SF	+	Richards's gland and Dufour's gland	Aldehydes, ketones, aromatics, alcohol
	V		–		
Sex attractant (♀)	S		+		
	P	IF	+	Venom apparatus	
		SF	–		
	V		+	Various glands	
Substrate marking (♂)	S		+	Abdominal glands	
	P	IF	+	Antennal, abdominal mandibular and leg glands	
		SF	+	Abdominal glands	
	V		+	Antennal glands	

The ascertained and/or hypothetical source of these compounds are also reported.
S, Stenogastrinae; P, Polistinae; V, Vespinae
IF, indipendent-founding; SW, swarm-founding
+, presence; –, absence.

Dani *et al.*, 2004; Martin *et al.*, 2008; Ruther *et al.*, 1998) and among Polistinae, 12 species of *Polistes* (11 reviewed by Dani, 2006 and *Polistes satan*, Tannure-Nascimento *et al.*, 2007) as well as two species of swarming Polistinae (*Parachartergus atzecus*, Espelie and Hermann, 1988; *Ropalidia opifex*, Dapporto *et al.*, 2006). Recently, Dani (2006) reviewed the general characteristics of this complex epicuticular mixture to highlight the differences among species. These compounds are mainly hydrocarbons (*n*-alkanes, *n*-alkenes, methyl branched alkanes) with a chain length ranging from 20 to 40 carbon atoms and, at a minor extent, also esters, alcohols, fatty acids and long chained amides. Methyl-alkanes are the compounds numerically and quantitatively more represented in the epicuticular mixture of *Polistes* species, but this is not the case for Stenogastrinae and Vespinae (Dani, 2006). CHCs are relatively non-volatile molecules that can be detected only by direct contact or at very short range (Brandstaetter *et al.*, 2008; Brockmann *et al.*, 2003).

From the above mentioned studies, it emerges that the epicuticular lipids blend is qualitatively and/or quantitatively different among the species of wasps. CHCs could be involved in species isolation and could be particularly important for sympatric speciation, as reported for the fruit fly (*Drosophila melanogaster*) and its sibling species (Cobb and Ferveur, 1996), but investigations of this aspect of recognition are still lacking for social wasps.

B. Population level

An epicuticular profile variation has been found also at the population level in *Polistes dominulus* where it has been shown that wasps of neighboring localities possess more similar CHCs profiles than wasps of more distant ones (Dapporto *et al.*, 2004a,b,c). At the end of the overwintering period, *P. dominulus* gynes belonging to different populations are able to recognize individuals of their original population. Laboratory evidences indicated that they prefer to associate with gynes coming from the same locality, suggesting a possible mechanism to avoid association with non-relatives (Cervo *et al.*, 2002b; Dapporto *et al.*, 2004b). However, Dapporto and colleagues (2004b) demonstrated that such recognition ability disappears when gynes from different populations overwintered in mixed laboratory clusters; the overwintering experience (in homo- or in mixed-population groups) is crucial for co-foundresses choice at the beginning of the Spring (Dapporto *et al.*, 2004b). Wasps of mixed hibernation clusters possess a similar cuticular blend with respect to wasps of the same localities hibernated in homo-population clusters (Dapporto *et al.*, 2004b). Philopatry—that is, the spring tendency of foundresses to return to their natal nests—is a common strategy among *Polistes* wasps (see Reeve, 1991) that probably facilitates the association among previously nestmates (generally full sisters) and "refreshes" the natal colony hydrocarbon blend, even if it was homogenized in mixed hibernation clusters during winter (Sumana *et al.*, 2005). In fact, Sumana *et al.* (2005) showed that the nests maintain their own CHCs blend throughout the winter, from autumn to the following spring, facilitating the association among previous nestmates to found a new colony.

C. Colony level

However, the most relevant CHCs variation for nestmate recognition context is among different colonies of the same population (see Gamboa, 1996, 2004). Although a colonial CHCs signature is a common assumption for the nestmate recognition process, such CHCs colonial variation within a species is often indirectly inferred instead of being revealed by chemical analyses. Evidences showing colonial hydrocarbon blends are usually obtained from behavioral assays by recording differential reactions toward nestmate and non-nestmate conspecific female lures. These studies have been carried out on the three subfamilies of social wasps (Cervo *et al.*, 1996, 2002a; Dani *et al.*, 1996b; Dapporto *et al.*, 2006; Kudo *et al.*, 2007; Lorenzi *et al.*, 1997; Ruther *et al.*, 1998; Sledge *et al.*, 2001a). However, when discriminant analyses were performed to demonstrate the colonial nature of CHCs blends, each individual was correctly assigned to its own nest as expected (Butts and Espelie, 1995; Butts *et al.*, 1993; Cervo *et al.*, 2002a; Cotoneschi *et al.*, 2007; Dapporto *et al.*, 2006; Espelie *et al.*, 1994; Layton *et al.*, 1994; Singer *et al.*, 1992; Sledge *et al.*, 2001a; Sumana *et al.*, 2005; Tannure-Nascimento *et al.*, 2007; Zanetti *et al.*, 2001). These studies showing a quantitative variation of compounds blend among wasp colonies indicate but do not prove that CHCs are involved in the nestmate recognition process. Bioassays performed with CHCs removed from single individuals (by washing the wasps in non-polar solvents) and then reapplied on dead individuals (Cervo *et al.*, 2002a; Dani *et al.*, 1996b; Lorenzi *et al.*, 1997; Ruther *et al.*, 1998; Sledge *et al.*, 2001a) have definitely assigned to the CHC components the role of nestmate recognition cues.

Even if our current general knowledge of the different components of the CHCs blend in different social wasps and their variation at different levels (species, populations, intercolonies, intracolony) is fairly advanced, more research is necessary to understand the communicative meaning of this complex mixture. In the 1990s, the analysis of the results obtained by correlational studies on *Polistes* wasps (Bonavita-Cougourdan *et al.*, 1991; Espelie *et al.*, 1994; Gamboa *et al.*, 1996) suggested that branched hydrocarbons could be more important than linear hydrocarbons for nestmate recognition. More recently, some researchers (Dani *et al.*, 2001; Lorenzi *et al.*, 2004a; Ruther *et al.*, 2002) have tested which compound or set of compounds were responsible for nestmate recognition by experimentally adding single compounds (naturally present in the original chemical profile) to the cuticular mixture of live wasps and then recording nestmates reactions. The aggressive response toward nestmates with signature manipulated by branched compounds augmentation (Dani *et al.*,

2001) supports the idea that, at least in *P. dominulus*, this class of compounds rather than the linear CHCs represents the recognition cues. This result is confirmed by similar experiments carried out on other social insect species (Dani *et al.*, 2005; Lucas *et al.*, 2005) but in contrast (see Dani, 2006) with the results of different bioassays performed on the same species, *P. dominulus* (Lorenzi *et al.*, 2004a) and on the European hornet (Ruther *et al.*, 2002).

Although several studies (see Gamboa, 2004 for a review) provided evidences that the recognition odor has both heritable and environmental (from food and/or nesting material) components, it is not easy to understand the relative importance of one component over the other one (Gamboa, 2004).

According to the optimal acceptance threshold model developed by Reeve (1989), nestmate acceptance or rejection is context-dependent; the efficiency of nestmate recognition could be affected by several factors as colony size, queen number, experience and/or proximity with the intruder's colony. A weak recognition ability is expected in large colonies of multiple-queens (polygyny) swarming species where the genetic variation is higher compared to that of single queen colonies, yet bioassays carried out on several species have produced different results. Field experiments on *R. opifex*, a swarming species with relative small colonies and queens number, showed a well-functioning nestmate recognition system (Dapporto *et al.*, 2006). Despite the queens number of *Polybia paulista* colonies is the highest among polygynous species, also this species shows a good nestmate discrimination ability and allows only colony members to enter the society (Kudo *et al.*, 2007). However, Gastreich *et al.* (1990) did not find any evidence for nestmate-alien conspecific discrimination in the polygynous species *Parachartergus colobopterus*. The factor linked to the colony proximity effect on nestmate recognition ability has been investigated in two stenogastrine wasp species belonging to the genus *Liostenogaster* (*Liostenogaster flavolineata* and *Liostenogaster vechti*) that build large clusters of nests, often very close to each other (Cervo *et al.*, 1996), and in four species of *Polistes* (Gamboa *et al.*, 1991; Lorenzi and Caprio, 2000; Pfenning, 1990) that found their nests in aggregations. The former studies show that a wasp is able to discriminate between the CHCs' blend of its own colony (either of a nestmate or of the nest) from that of neighboring colonies. However, the individuals of those stenogastrine species living in clusters, perform a high percentage of erroneous acceptances when compared with non-clustering congeneric species (Cervo *et al.*, 2002a). Probably, as predicted by Reeve's model (1989), the acceptance threshold could be altered when continuous alien rejection becomes costly. Moreover, females of *Polistes exclamans* (Pfenning, 1990) and *Polistes fuscatus* (Gamboa *et al.*, 1991) were more tolerant toward conspecifics belonging to nearby colonies than toward those belonging to more distant colonies (more than 10 km); according to Gamboa (2004), this differential tolerance may be due to the share of both genetic and environmental components of recognition odor.

All these studies suggest that nestmate recognition is a very efficient system in all the species of social wasps where it has been studied (with the only exception of *P. colobopterus*); in fact, such ability is a feature of the small societies of the most primitively subfamily of social wasps, the Stenogastrinae, as well as of the large and complex societies of highly eusocial wasps, the Vespinae.

D. The mechanism of recognition

Although the nestmate discrimination capacity has been investigated in numerous species belonging to the three Vespidae subfamilies, the mechanism underlining the nestmate recognition process has been researched intensively only in *Polistes* wasps (see Gamboa, 1996, 2004; Singer *et al.*, 1998). However, it is probable that the same mechanism works also for the other social wasp species. The classic studies on the ontogeny of *Polistes* nestmate recognition showed that, at emergence, each wasp learns the colonial CHCs blend by the paper of its own natal nest. This blend is used as a template to compare the chemical phenotypes of the individuals encountered by each wasp throughout its life (reviewed by Gamboa, 1996, 2004; Singer *et al.*, 1998). This comparison allows each wasp to discriminate between nestmates (when the template and the chemical phenotype pattern match) and non-nestmates (when the two patterns do not match). The nest material signature mirrors the signature of the colony inhabitants (Cotoneschi *et al.*, 2007; Espelie and Hermann, 1990; Espelie *et al.*, 1990; Lorenzi, 1992; Singer *et al.*, 1992), and the nest's odor is the central element of the reference template (Gamboa *et al.*, 1986). Recognition cues learning process based on the nest material occurs immediately after the emergence and it is updated throughout the adult life according to colony odor changes (Gamboa, 1996, 2004).

Females of *Polistes* wasps, both foundresses and workers, are reported to stroke the comb with the ventral part of their gasters. Stroking behavior has been described for the first time in queens of *Polistes gallicus* forced to accept an alien conspecific comb (Cervo and Turillazzi, 1989). Afterward, it was reported for queens of other species artificially driven in a similar situation (Lorenzi and Cervo, 1992; Van Hooser *et al.*, 2002) or for intraspecific (Cervo and Lorenzi, 1996), interspecific facultative social parasites (Cervo *et al.*, 2004), and obligate social parasites (Turillazzi *et al.*, 1990; Zacchi *et al.*, 1996). Although abdominal stroking behavior is also exhibited by foundresses on their own combs, with a differential frequency (Dani *et al.*, 1992) according to their rank in the dominance hierarchy (Pardi, 1948), it is performed more vigorously and frequently by female social parasites on alien intra- or interspecific nests (see Cervo, 2006; Cervo and Dani, 1996). It was suggested by the latter authors that paper wasp females performed the stroking behavior to apply their own odor (CHCs) to the comb in order to guarantee their acceptance by the new emerged workers.

Although numerous evidences suggest that the mechanism of recognition is common within the genus *Polistes*, it has been studied only in three American species (*Polistes fuscatus*, *Polistes metricus*, *Polistes carolina*; Pfenning *et al.*, 1983a,b; Shellmann and Gamboa, 1982) out of the 206 species belonging to the genus (Carpenter, 1996). Analogous studies performed on other *Polistes* species living in different habitats and under different ecological pressures (e.g., social parasitism) would be necessary to confirm the general applicability of the *Polistes* recognition model. However, an additional study performed on the independent-founding species *Ropalidia marginata* (Venkataraman *et al.*, 1988) showed a similar mechanism of recognition.

Although the "recognition template" model is easily applicable to species with paper nests, as this material is a very good absorbent substrate, it could work less efficiently for wasp species with mud nests as some stenogastrine wasps. In fact, a different mechanism for colony template acquisition has been proposed and discussed for *L. flavolineata* (Cervo *et al.*, 2002a). Since its nest is built with mud, and this material carries only a little quantity of CHCs, the abdominal substance secreted by the Dufour's gland-rich of the same compounds of the wasp cuticle (Cervo *et al.*, 2002a; Keegans *et al.*, 1993), and deposited on the eggs and on small larvae-seems a more suitable substrate for CHCs template acquisition (Cervo *et al.*, 2002a). Unfortunately, too few bioassays on this topic have been performed on Stenogastrinae wasps (Cervo *et al.*, 2002a; Turillazzi *et al.*, 2008) to designate this secretion as an alternative source of recognition template.

E. Males and brood CHCs

The cuticular mixture composition reported so far for each species is referred to adult females as these individuals are the main subjects of sociobiological studies. The CHCs composition of males, rather neglected members of wasp colony life (Beani, 1996), has been studied only in a few species (Espelie and Hermann, 1990; Layton *et al.*, 1994; Spiewok *et al.*, 2006). However, more intensive investigations on male chemical profiles would be needed to understand the possible involvement of CHCs in mating strategies and mate selection in social wasps. Ryan and Gamboa (1986) investigated the male-recognition process in a mating context in *Polistes fuscatus* showing that males discriminate between nestmates and alien individuals (both females and males) and prefer to copulate with unrelated females.

Slightly more information is available for CHCs profile of the immature brood although very few studies have been carried out on the capacity of females to discriminate their own brood from the alien one. In general, the CHCs blend of the immature brood (larvae and eggs) resembles the cuticular chemical mixture of the females of the same species (as reported by Espelie and Hermann, 1990 for *Polistes annularis*). Recently, additional details on chemical signatures of immature stages have been reported.

Cuticular signature of *P. dominulus* eggs resembles the chemical profile of the egg-layer female (Dapporto *et al.*, 2007a) providing profitable recognition cues to perform differential oophagy (Dapporto *et al.*, 2010) reported among co-foudresses of this species (Dapporto *et al.*, 2007a; Gervet, 1964; Liebig *et al.*, 2005; Lorenzi and Filippone, 2000; Pardi, 1946). The cuticle of larvae possesses its own specific CHCs profile that differs from the one of the adults (Brown *et al.*, 1991 for *Vespula germanica*; Cotoneschi *et al.*, 2007 for *P. dominulus*); moreover, larvae of *P. dominulus* possess a characteristic colony-specific signature that allow the adults to discriminate among larvae odor according to the colony of origin, as behavioral assays have shown (Cotoneschi *et al.*, 2007). These results have also been confirmed for *P. fuscatus*, where workers in a binary test show more aggressive reactions toward alien larvae than against their own larvae (Panek and Gamboa, 2000). Chemical analyses and bioassays on larvae of *P. dominulus* have also shown that the larvae could be discriminated on the basis of their gender, but such differences do not seem to be used by the adult wasps to the advantage of one of the two sexes (Cotoneschi *et al.*, 2009). Other studies (Panek and Gamboa, 2000; Strassmann *et al.*, 2000) did not provide behavioral evidences that queens of two American *Polistes* species are able to discriminate among larvae on the basis of relatedness. However, Dani *et al.* (2004) reported that both *P. dominulus* and *Vespa crabro* adult females of different patrilines can be statistically discriminated on the basis of their CHCs profiles providing evidence for a potential cue in kin recognition.

Differently from the immature brood (eggs and larvae) carrying a specific chemical signature, responsible for their recognition both within colony and between colonies, the newly emerged individuals of *Polistes* wasps are "chemically insignificant" (*sensu* Lenoir *et al.*, 2001). This feature allows them to be accepted, up to 24 h after eclosion, in different colonies without aggression by colony members (Lorenzi *et al.*, 2004a). Between the first and third day from their emergence, the young wasps acquire more complex chemical signatures (Panek *et al.*, 2001) with a substantial increase of branched CHCs (Lorenzi *et al.*, 2004a). Behavioral tests (Lorenzi *et al.*, 2004a) demonstrated that young females adsorb chemicals from the surrounding environment at a major extent than older females; this capacity probably allows new emerged individuals to acquire a colonial signature. Similar acceptance of newly emerged individuals in unrelated colonies has been reported for females of *R. marginata* (Arathi *et al.*, 1997) and for males of *P. paulista* (Kudo and Zucchi, 2006).

F. Nestmate recognition breakdown

The most impressive proof of the CHCs importance in the nestmate recognition process is provided by the deep changes in chemical cuticular signatures observed in the wasp social parasites (recently reviewed by

Lorenzi, 2006). Obligate social parasites are rare species present both in the Vespinae (four species) and in the Polistinae (three species) but unknown in the Stenogastrinae (Cervo, 2006; Cervo and Dani, 1996). The females of the obligate social parasite species are unable to found a nest and lack the worker force; these reduced colonial capacities make them obligatorily dependent on the worker force of another species to rear their own brood (Wilson, 1971). To succeed in host colony exploitation, an obligate social parasite must become a member of the host colony, chemically overcoming the host nestmate recognition system. The chemical strategies adopted by the obligate social parasites to fool the host females about their real identity have been deeply investigated in *Polistes* wasps opening fascinating scenarios. Before usurpation, parasite females possess a hydrocarbon signature both simpler and different from that of the females of the host species, but after usurpation their chemical signatures match those of the host species (Bagnères *et al.*, 1996; Lorenzi *et al.*, 2004b; Turillazzi *et al.*, 2000). Additional studies carried out on *Polistes sulcifer*, obligate social parasite of *P. dominulus*, demonstrated a finely tuned match with the host. After usurpation, the parasite female shows the specific signature of the host colony she has usurped promoting, in this way, her acceptance into the host nest as a colony member (Sledge *et al.*, 2001a); moreover, the parasite female shows the characteristic CHCs signature of the dominant female that she has displaced (Dapporto *et al.*, 2004d). In addition, before the host nest usurpation, the parasite cuticles are poorer in hydrocarbons quantity compared to individuals of the host species (Lorenzi and Bagnères, 2002; Lorenzi *et al.*, 2004b). According to the "insignificant hypothesis" proposed by Lenoir *et al.* (2001) for parasitic ants, the lower CHCs quantity on the parasite may limit or eliminate the aggressive reaction of the hosts as this quantity is under the CHCs perception threshold. Even if a quantitative threshold for chemical recognition is the necessary general assumption for this hypothesis, its existence has been only recently demonstrated in *P. dominulus* (Cini *et al.*, 2009). Alternatively, a poor CHCs quantity profile of the pre-usurpation parasites could furnish a "blank chemical status" of the cuticle to better adsorb or/and acquire a new signature (Lorenzi *et al.*, 2004b). While the chemical strategies adopted by the parasite usurpers to elude the host recognition system are now understood, the mechanisms allowing the immature parasitic brood to be accepted by the host have only recently been addressed in social insects. A cuticular mixture with a low proportion of branched compounds seems to be the chemical strategy that makes the social parasite immature brood tolerated within the host colony; this kind of signature, not meaningful for the host, has been found on the cuticle of *P. sulcifer* larvae (Cervo *et al.*, 2008b) as well as on eggs of the social parasite *Vespa dybowskii* (Martin *et al.*, 2008).

III. Queen Pheromones and Fertility/Rank Pheromones

In most social Hymenoptera as ants, bees, and wasps, the individuals are highly specialized both behaviorally and morphologically. Queens produce eggs and workers perform all the activities needed for colony development, exhibiting either a reversible or irreversible reduction of ovarian activity and generally renouncing direct reproduction in the presence of their queen (Hölldobler and Wilson, 1990; Jeanne, 1991; West-Eberhard, 1996; Wilson, 1971).

In the Vespinae, where the castes are strikingly morphologically distinguishable, there are evidences of a pheromonal control on workers physiology and behavior by the queen (Fletcher and Ross, 1985), and, if the queen is experimentally removed, the workers are able to produce male-destined eggs (Bourke, 1988). The workers of *Vespa*, *Vespula*, and *Dolichovespula* cease foraging and performing nest tasks when the queen is absent or experimentally removed, but resume their works once the queen is replaced on its own nest (Matsuura and Yamane, 1990). In *Vespa orientalis* the queen pheromone, *δ-n*-hexadecalactone, has been identified and isolated from the head of the queen (Ikan *et al.*, 1969; Ishay *et al.*, 1965). The pheromone induces workers, once they have approached and licked the queen and formed a circle around her, to perform nest activities, although suppression of workers' ovarian development has not been demonstrated (Spradbery, 1991). In *Vespula atropilosa* and *Vespula pensylvanica* (Landolt *et al.*, 1977) workers in queen-less colonies exhibit reduced foraging, brood care, and nest activities as well as increased ovarian development. The transmission of the pheromone in these species occurs either by thropallaxis or by contact with the substrate (Greene, 1991). The queen in *V. pensylvanica* and *Vespula vulgaris* probably deposits a pheromone on the comb that inhibits worker ovarian development, even if no pheromonal-mediated behavioral response to queens has been demonstrated (Akre and Reed, 1983).

Circumstantial evidence of queen pheromones exist even among the swarm-founding Polistinae (*Polybia*, *Protopolybia*, and *Agelaia*, Landolt *et al.*, 1998) and recently in the independent-founding *R. marginata* (Sumana *et al.*, 2008). Queens of *Metapolybia aztecoides* are recognized by their nestmates on the basis of a substance secreted by the head; however, queen recognition does not necessarily imply queen control (West-Eberhard, 1977).

Nonetheless, despite great evidences of a strong queen influence over workers' physiology and behavior, queen's control over workers is thought to be affected through dominance–subordinance interactions in many social wasps (Keller and Nonacs, 1993; West-Eberhard, 1969). Conflicts among individuals over reproduction are widespread especially in those species which lack morphological differences between queen and workers (Strassmann *et al.*, 2004). In these species, colony sizes are characteristically small, and reproductive division of labor is regulated by behavioral interactions among individuals that have (for the most part) equivalent reproductive potentials. Physical contests between foundresses at the early stages of the nesting cycle are common in several polistine species (Gamboa and Dropkin, 1979; Gamboa and Stump, 1996; Pardi, 1942, 1946; Premnath *et al.*, 1996; Röseler, 1991; Tindo and Dejean, 2000) leading to reproductive hierarchies where the rank is correlated with reproductive success (Pardi, 1948; Peeters, 1993) and ovarian activity (Dietemann *et al.*, 2003; Monnin *et al.*, 1998; Sledge *et al.*, 2001b).

Polistes wasps are one of the most studied organisms in terms of the evolution of social behavior (Starks and Turillazzi, 2006) and CHCs have been shown to function as tokens of dominance and reproductive status. In fact, differences between the hydrocarbon mixtures of queens and workers have been reported (*P. dominulus*, Bonavita-Cougourdan *et al.*, 1991; *P. metricus*, Layton *et al.*, 1994; *Polistes fuscatus*, Espelie *et al.*, 1994; *Polistes biglumis bimaculatus*, Lorenzi *et al.*, 1994; *P. satan*, Tannure-Nascimento *et al.*, 2008). Moreover, in *P. gallicus* queens are distinguished from workers by the hydrocarbon mixtures of the van der Vecht organ secretion (Dapporto *et al.*, 2007b), but the chemical signatures of workers are not dependent on their social situation (queenless/queenright colonies) and on their fertility status. Indeed, the profile of orphaned workers with developed ovaries does maintain the worker specificity showed in queenright colonies (Dapporto *et al.*, 2007b). A completely different situation occurs in the sympatric, congeneric *P. dominulus*, where it has been demonstrated that worker blends are clearly dependent on social context (Dapporto *et al.*, 2007a), since orphaned workers rapidly change their CHCs profiles to resemble that of their lost dominant and subordinate foundresses (Dapporto *et al.*, 2005). In fact, *P. dominulus* workers developing ovaries in orphaned nests showed cuticular profiles similar to those of dominant foundresses thus suggesting an influence of both social context and fertility on CHCs, while the rest of the workers retained undeveloped ovaries but changed as well their cuticular profiles matching those of subordinate foundresses suggesting a strong influence of social context, even in the absence of any change in their fertility. Overall, this study suggested that in *P. dominulus* CHCs are not determined at a preimaginal stage (Dapporto *et al.*, 2005). Moreover, in *P. dominulus*, that presents solitary or associative colony foundation, CHCs have also been shown to differ among foundresses depending on their reproductive rank (Dapporto *et al.*, 2004c; Sledge *et al.*, 2001b). Actually differences between co-foundresses are not distinguishable at the beginning of the nesting season before ranks are established (Sledge *et al.*, 2001b) but, as soon as workers emerge, alpha-females are easily chemically distinguished from their subordinate foundresses and new workers. Workers and subordinates are characterized by increased relative percentages of *n*-alkanes and monomethyl alkanes, whereas the alpha-female is characterized by higher fractions of alkenes and dimethyl alkanes (Sledge *et al.*, 2001b). A relationship between CHCs profiles and the size of the corpora allata, the source of juvenile hormone that modulates ovarian development and sexual maturation has also been found (Sledge *et al.*, 2001b, 2004). Furthermore, in this species despite low relatedness in foundresses associations (Queller *et al.*, 2000), the alpha-females lay almost all the eggs destined to hatch (Pardi, 1942) and consequently indirect fitness appears too low to compensate for helper costs (Queller *et al.*, 2000). Recent studies have also reported that the cuticle and egg surface of a female of *P. dominulus* show similar hydrocarbon profiles (Dapporto *et al.*, 2007a) resulting in dominant and subordinate laid eggs with distinctive chemical blends. Downing and Jeanne (1983) suggested that the Dufour's gland is the source of the cues used by dominant females of *Polistes fuscatus* to recognize their own eggs from those laid by other females. This chemical cue could be a marker for egg recognition also in *P. dominulus* (Dapporto *et al.*, 2007a). The dominant individual probably performs a dominance behavior toward subordinates to test their cuticular signatures and to assess the eggs' profiles in order to efficiently police them (Dapporto *et al.*, 2010a). In *Polistes* paper wasps, the simple presence of the dominant female (and thus of her pheromones) is not sufficient to suppress worker and subordinate reproduction (Dapporto *et al.*, 2007a; Liebig *et al.*, 2005), and dominance, rather than fertility, determines chemical signatures in *Polistes* wasps because fully fertile subordinate wasps do not change their profile to match that of the dominant females (Dapporto *et al.*, 2007a,b, 2010a). Another recent and opposite study on *P. dominulus* (Izzo *et al.*, 2010) states instead, that fertility rather than dominance drives the chemical signatures of the different females of the colony. This contradictory conclusion on the same species, could be linked to the operational definition of the concept of dominance in different stages of *Polistes* annual cycle as clarified by Dapporto and coworkers (2010b).

On the contrary, Stenogastrinae colonies often have more than one potential egg-layer and, in a few species, but differently from the above Polistinae wasps, dominance hierarchies, when present, are relatively mild and not linear (Turillazzi, 1991). Despite this, the cuticular lipid profile of fertile individuals differs in the levels of one or more compounds from that of non-fertile individuals in four Stenogastrinae species (Turillazzi *et al.*, 2004). Moreover, in all four species, the concentration of one or more compounds was correlated with the degree of ovarian development.

IV. Sex Pheromones

Sex pheromones are chemical substances capable of eliciting behaviors related to mate-finding, mate-selection, and copulation. In social wasps they can be divided in: (1) sex attractant and recognition pheromones produced by females to attract males and stimulate copulatory behavior and (2) territorial marking pheromones produced by males (Ayasse *et al.*, 2001; Jeanne, 1996; Landolt *et al.*, 1998; Shorey, 1977; Wilson, 1971). Even if the use of male-attracting pheromones is common in social Hymenoptera (reviewed by Ayasse *et al.*, 2001; Keeling *et al.*, 2004), and although there is evidence for sex pheromones in some species of the Vespidae, not a single one has been identified yet (Spiewok *et al.*, 2006).

A. Female sex pheromones

Ono *et al.* (1985) observed several males of *Vespa mandarinia* flying to the entrance of an underground nest and hypothesized that they were attracted by pheromones emanating from the nest. Pheromonal communication of sexual receptivity by females has also been shown in several other vespine and stenogastrine wasps, where males form clusters, trying to mate with single females (for Vespinae: *Dolichovespula sylvestris*, Sanderman, 1938; *Vespa crabro*, Batra, 1980; *V. atropilosa*, MacDonald *et al.*, 1974; for Stenogastrinae: Turillazzi, 1991; Turillazzi and Pardi, 1982) or with males that had been in contact with receptive females (*V. germanica*, Thomas, 1960; *Vespula maculifrons*, Ross, 1983). Ono and Sasaki (1987) were able to elicit mating attempts by males in six *Vespa* species even on freeze-dried dead males which had been previously treated with the extracts of virgin queens. Only queens but not workers induced copulatory responses in the six *Vespa* species even if they were not species specific (Ono and Sasaki, 1987); in fact interspecific cross-activities of the pheromones were found for all pair-wise combinations between five of the six sympatric species, *Vespa analis*, *Vespa mandarinia*, *Vespa tropica*, *Vespa simillima xanthoptera*, and *V. crabro*. The first demonstration of male attraction by female-produced sex pheromones was reported for the southern yellowjacket, *Vespula squamosa* (Reed and Landolt, 1990a). Males flew upwind in a flight tunnel in response both to caged queens and hexane extract of unmated queens, with the greatest response to the extract of the thorax, suggesting that the possible sources of pheromones were pro/mesothoracic glands, and/or, at minor extent, the venom and Dufour's glands in the abdomen (Reed and Landolt, 1990a). Also males of *P. exclamans* exhibit upwind flights in response to conspecific females, female odor, or solvent extract of females even if all body parts seem to stimulate attraction, indicating a possible spread of the pheromone over the body by grooming (Reed and Landolt, 1990b).

The venom components of *Polistes fuscatus*, *P. exclamans* (Post and Jeanne, 1983a, 1984), and *Belonogaster petiolata* (Keeping *et al.*, 1986) have a male-attracting effect and induce a copulatory behavior. The females seem to spread the venom secretion over the surface of their body by grooming (Post and Jeanne, 1984). The active component of the venom of the two *Polistes* species, which seems to be part of its volatile fraction, has not been identified but its effect is not species-specific: males of *P. fuscatus* respond to the venom of *P. exclamans* and *V. maculifrons* even if at a lesser extent (Post and Jeanne, 1984). In contrast, Bruschini *et al.* (2006b) reported that the venom volatile profiles are both qualitatively and quantitatively different among females of European *Polistes* species, even if bioassays testing the male attractant function have not been performed. Nevertheless, sting extrusion during the copulatory sequence in *Polistes* suggests a possible active role of the venom as a sex-attractant (Romani *et al.*, 2005).

Females of *Polistes fuscatus* regardless of age, caste, and whether or not they have been mated, are attractive to males and stimulate reproductive behavior (Post and Jeanne, 1985). This result suggests that males have not evolved the ability to discriminate between gynes and workers. A recent work on *V. crabro* showed that drones were attracted to both live caged gynes and to dead workers treated with gyne extracts, indicating the presence of a female-produced sex attractant (Spiewok *et al.*, 2006). Extracts from gynes, workers, and drones contained exclusively cuticular lipids, and the profile from gynes was much more diverse than that of workers and drones; the most striking differences related to the alkenes, monomethyl- and dimethylalkanes suggested a potential role as attracting and copulation-releasing semiochemicals in *V. crabro* (Spiewok *et al.*, 2006).

Post and Jeanne (1984) reported that *Polistes* males respond to a "contact pheromone", probably CHCs present on female's body, that apparently communicates species identity and that could be of primary importance in maintaining reproductive isolation. A similar close-range or contact pheromone that may be involved in the recognition of conspecifics was found in *Mischocyttarus flavitarsis* (Litte, 1979), *V. crabro* (Batra, 1980), and *V. maculifrons* females (Post, 1980). It has been suggested that both sexes (e.g. *P. exclamans*; Reed and Landolt, 1990b) carry individual pheromonal signatures that function in sex attraction.

B. Male sex pheromones

There are several behavioral evidences for the existence of male marking pheromones in male territorial contexts, even if the chemical evidence for the related pheromones is not yet provided.

Males of several species of *Polistes* (see Beani, 1996), at the end of the colonial cycle, occupy small territories, often contiguous to each others, that they continuously patrol and defend both from neighboring territorial males and from intruders. Each time a male lands on such territories it rotates almost half circle around while rubbing its gastral sterna on the substratum and then it performs a complete grooming of the posterior legs and abdomen. This rubbing behavior, described for the first time for males of *Polistes nimphus* (Turillazzi and Cervo, 1982), has been reported for males of several other species of *Polistes* (Beani and Turillazzi, 1988, 1990a,b; Polak, 1993; Post and Jeanne, 1983b;

Reed and Landolt, 1991; Wenzel, 1987). Male rubbing behavior has been reported also in two species of *Mischocyttarus* (Litte, 1979, 1981), in some Stenogastrinae species (Turillazzi and Francescato, 1990) and in *Polybia* (West-Eberhard, 1982). Rubbing, as well as prolonged grooming at perches (Beani and Calloni, 1991a), seems associated with the release of pheromones (Beani *et al.*, 1992; Reed and Landolt, 1990b; Turillazzi and Cervo, 1982; Wenzel, 1987) probably secreted by abdominal and leg glands (Beani and Calloni, 1991a,b; Turillazzi, 1979; Turillazzi and Calloni, 1983). A different marking behavior has been reported for *Polistes* males that also rub perch sites with their mandibles, which contain enlarged mandibular glands (Reed and Landolt, 1991; Wenzel, 1987). Furthermore, a more volatile pheromone is probably released by *Polistes jadwigae* males in their territories as they bend their abdomens exposing the sternal glands (Kasuya, 1981). Recently, sex--dimorphic secretory cells have been described in the antennomeres of *P. dominulus* and *V. crabro*; the occurrence of "antennal courtship" movements, species-specific and prolonged, suggests the release of contact or low-volatile sex pheromones that have not been identified yet (Romani *et al.*, 2005).

Similarly, males of some Stenogastrinae stretch their abdomen during their patrolling flights, exposing a band of tegumental glands along the anterior margin of the third tergite (Turillazzi and Calloni, 1983; Turillazzi and Francescato, 1990). Although the activity of the males of one of these species occurs mainly in flight, they also perform two scent-marking behaviors of the substrate: one involves the extrusion of the mouthparts, while the other involves the rubbing of the abdomen tip on the leaf borders leaving small dark spots (Beani and Landi, 2000; Beani *et al.*, 2002). Chemical analysis of these spots revealed the presence of CHCs mixture similar to the cuticle and hindgut content suggesting a possible role of these marking spots in species and sex recognition (Beani *et al.*, 2002).

However, further studies are needed to shed light on the chemical nature of male secretions and their role in mating behavior.

V. Alarm Pheromones

In social insects, the defense of the colony is critical for all colony members (Hermann and Blum, 1981; Schmidt, 1990). For this reason, a strong selection for rapid communication to recruit nestmates against predators or intruders led to the evolution of alarm pheromones (Wyatt, 2003). Alarm pheromones of social insects are, after sex pheromones, the most commonly produced class of chemical signals and they have evolved independently within all major taxa (Blum, 1985).

Alarm behavior has been defined as "any response to a disturbance of the colony that increases the likelihood that colony members will take defensive actions" (Landolt *et al.*, 1998). Alarm pheromones are responsible to arouse colony members' awareness of a potential threat to the colony, to direct the wasps toward the target in an aggressive manner and finally to attack it. Alarm pheromones are challenging to be defined as it is often difficult, during bioassays, to dissociate these stimuli from others - and thus alarm response is often confused with strict defense, recruitment or attraction (Blum, 1985). Actually, an alarm pheromone consists of several components where only one or few could be the active compounds responsible of eliciting alarm behavior, while the others could either work synergistically with those or serve to other functions (Billen and Morgan, 1998).

In social wasps, alarm pheromones are highly volatile compounds primarily secreted by the exocrine glands associated with the sting apparatus (Akre, 1982; Ali and Morgan, 1990; Billen and Morgan, 1998; Downing, 1991; Landolt and Akre, 1979) to induce stereotyped reactions (Starr, 1990) among insects that function to recruit workers and to accelerate movements and attack toward intruders (Ali and Morgan, 1990).

Maschwitz (1964a,b) was the first to demonstrate in the yellowjackets *V. vulgaris* and *V. germanica* an alarm response to crushed entire bodies and body parts of wasps, and the venom was identified as the source of the alarm stimulus (Maschwitz, 1964a,b; Moritz and Bürgin, 1987). Pheromone-mediated alarm has since then been observed in several other vespines: the oriental European hornet *V. orientalis* (Ishay *et al.*, 1965), *Dolichovespula saxonica* (Maschwitz, 1984), the southern yellowjacket *V. squamosa* (Landolt and Heath, 1987), the eastern yellowjacket *V. maculifrons* (Landolt *et al.*, 1995), the European hornet *V. crabro* (Veith *et al.*, 1984), *Provespa anomala* Saussure (Maschwitz and Hanel, 1988), and the giant-hornet *V. mandarinia* (Ono *et al.*, 2003). The evidence of alarm pheromones, eliciting defensive behaviors in many species belonging to the 4 genera, suggests that they could be universal in the subfamily Vespinae (Landolt *et al.*, 1998), even if old studies did not find alarm pheromones in *Vespula atropilosa* and *V. pensylvanica* (Akre, 1982; Hermann and Blum, 1981). Chemical investigation on the nature of the volatile components of the venom has been carried out in *V. orientalis* (Saslavasky *et al.*, 1973), *V. vulgaris* (Aldiss, 1983), *V. crabro* (Veith *et al.*, 1984), *V. squamosa* (Heath and Landolt, 1988), *V. maculifrons* (Landolt *et al.*, 1995), and *V. mandarinia* (Ono *et al.*, 2003), all species for which the presence of alarm pheromones in the venom has been demonstrated through bioassays (see above paragraph). A series of alkanes with chain length ranging from C10 to C34 have been reported in the venom of *V. orientalis* and bioassays have shown that those varying from C11 to C14 show a weak alarm-eliciting effect (Saslavasky *et al.*, 1973). The amide, *N*-(3-methylbutyl)acetamide has been isolated and identified in the venom of *V. vulgaris* (Aldiss, 1983), *V. squamosa* (Heath and Landolt, 1988) and *V. maculifrons* (Landolt *et al.*, 1995). Only in the last two species, bioassays have shown that the amide elicits alarm behavior (Heath and Landolt, 1988; Landolt *et al.*, 1995), even if at unnaturally high doses, suggesting that other volatiles from the sting apparatus may also act in synergy as alarm pheromones (Landolt *et al.*, 1995). Moreover, Aldiss (1983) demonstrated that crushed heads of *V. vulgaris* applied to cotton dental rolls attracted conspecific workers and elicited attacks when tested on certain colonies in the reproductive phase. Observations of *V. squamosa* wasps attacking corks placed close to the nest entrance showed that these wasps bite and chew the target in addition to stinging it, still corroborating the hypothesis of a second alarm pheromone originating from the head (Landolt *et al.*, 1999). Furthermore, Reed and Landolt (2000) demonstrated that the alarm pheromone is atipically long lasting on a target attacked by *V. squamosa* wasps. Moreover, the alarm pheromone can be deposited either from the sting or the mandibles to mark an attacking vertebrate predator so that the predator is quickly detected and attacked again upon its return to a wasp colony. However, the head extracts of *V. germanica* workers did not elicit any alarm response either at the nest entrance or under foraging conditions, even when testing different doses (D'Adamo *et al.*, 2004). The authors concluded that *V. germanica* head extract works as an attractant and no evidence exists to date to indicate alarm activity, in agreement with previous studies on ants and bees (Billen and Morgan, 1998). Veith *et al.* (1984) have found methylbutanols and their corresponding acetic esters in the venom sac of the hornet *V. crabro* and that one of the identified alcohols, 2-methyl-3-buten-2-ol elicits alarm among the hornets during behavioral experiments. A quantitative analysis about the effectiveness of these alarm pheromone components has been conducted measuring the heat production rates of the hornets by means of direct calorimetry (MacLean and Schmolz, 2004). This kind of test can be appropriate to quantify specific parameters of an alarm response when a substance has already been proven to be alarm-inducing (Schmolz *et al.*, 1999). Hornets exhibited a strong response to all alarm pheromone components, mainly 2-methyl-3-butane-2-ol in agreement with the previous study. They also reacted intensively to the main alarm pheromone component of the honey bee, isopentylacetate, but less intensively to the alarm pheromone component of yellowjackets, *N*-(3-methylbutyl)acetamide. Recently, Ono *et al.* (2003) have shown with field bioassays that 2-pentanol is the most active component among the venom volatiles in *V. mandarinia*, with 3-methyl-1-butanol and 3-methylbutyl-1-methylbutanoate acting in synergy with it.

Among the swarm-founding Polistinae there are some species, such as *Protopolybia fuscatus* and *Polybia emaciata*, which do not attack an intruder but retreat to their nests without showing any alarm or recruitment response (Landolt *et al.*, 1998). Instead, venom structures (sac/sting apparatus) of *Polybia occidentalis* induce alarm with recruitment of a large number of wasps to the outer surface of the envelope (Jeanne, 1981a). Outside the nest, the venom odor reduces the threshold for attack behavior but attack itself seems to be released only if associated with an appropriate (dark and moving) visual cue. Neither the single chemical nor the visual cue is sufficient to elicit the full sequence of alarm recruitment ending with the attack (Jeanne, 1981a). An alarm response elicited by the venom glands was also found in *Polybia rejecta* (Overal *et al.*, 1981), *Ropalidia romandi* (Kojima, 1994), *P. paulista* (Manzolli-Palma *et al.*, 1998), and *Polybioides raphigastra* (Sledge *et al.*, 1999). The venom content of this latter species showed a complex mixture of mainly saturated and unsaturated linear hydrocarbons with chain length varying from C11 to C18, saturated 2-alcohols, and the spiroacetal 2,8-dimethyl-1,7-dioxaspiro[5.5]undecane (Sledge *et al.*, 1999). The same spiroacetal, along with *N*-(3-methylbutyl)acetamide and several other compounds, was found in the venom content of *Polybia sericea* and *P. occidentalis*, and field bioassays carried out with *P. occidentalis* clearly showed the alarm-eliciting effect of that spiroacetal (Dani *et al.*, 2000). Fortunato *et al.* (2004) reported the repertoires of alarm response behavior of five swarming *Ropalidia* species. *R. opifex* and three species of the *R. flavopitcta* group possessed alarm pheromones in the venom (in accordance with results on *R. romandi*, Kojima, 1994), while *Ropalidia sumatrae* did not show any chemically mediated alarm as the alarm behavior response in this species seems to be coordinated only by visual stimuli (Fortunato *et al.*, 2004). Interestingly, the venom volatiles content of the five species did not differ markedly, suggesting that alarm compounds have no semiochemical effect as alarm recruitment in *R. sumatrae* (Fortunato *et al.*, 2004). An alarm pheromone seems also to be missing in *P. colobopterus,* a species that builds cryptic nests. An external disturbance to the nest induces some workers to produce a rustling sound by vibrating their gasters on the nest envelope, that functions as an alarm signal. Additional workers come out of the nest, and while standing on it, spray a sticky mist of venom toward the intruder (Jeanne and Keeping, 1995). If the disturbance continues, the workers fly away abandoning the colony rather than attempting to sting the intruder (Strassmann *et al.*, 1990). The venom of *P. colobopterus* has evolved in a sticky spray probably replacing its function as alarm pheromone. Similarly, venom spraying has been reported also for *V. germanica* and *V. vulgaris* (Maschwitz, 1964b), *Dolichovespula arenaria* (Greene *et al.*, 1976) and *V. orientalis* (Saslavasky *et al.*, 1973), but neither the context nor the stimuli eliciting this behavior have been described for these species.

For independent-founding Polistinae, Landolt *et al.* (1998) hypothesized that species building nests without envelopes less likely possess an alarm communication system based on pheromones. Bioassays did not show pheromonal mediation of alarm in *B. petiolata* (Keeping, 1995) and *Mischocyttarus immarginatus* (London and Jeanne, 1996). *M. immarginatus* did not respond with alarm behavior to its venom nor to the venom of *P. occidentalis* that builds nests in close proximity; whereas the latter species responds with alarm behavior to its own venom (Jeanne, 1981a) and to the venom of *M. immarginatus*, although with less intensity.

Early works failed to find any evidence of alarm pheromones in *P. gallicus* [=*P. dominulus*], *Polistes nimpha* [=*P. nimphus*] (Freisling, 1943) and in *P. dubia* [=*P. biglumis*] (Maschwitz, 1964a). However, the venom of *Polistes canadensis* (Jeanne, 1982a), *P. exclamans*, and *Polistes fuscatus* (Post *et al.*, 1984a) was found to elicit an alarm response. The odor of the venom was able to reduce the threshold for attack and works as an attractant but only if associated with an appropriate, black and moving, visual stimulus. Recently, the same results were obtained with the venom of workers of *P. nimphus*, *P. dominulus*, and *P. gallicus* (Bruschini, 2005; Bruschini *et al.*, 2006a, 2008a). The venom extracts presented to the colony induced a very aggressive behavior in the wasps as the number of stings on a target was significantly higher than after presentation of a control (Bruschini *et al.*, 2006a). Chemical analyses of the venom volatile fraction of four European *Polistes* species (*P. dominulus*, *P. gallicus*, *P. nimphus* and the social parasite *P. sulcifer*) and of the South Asian *P. olivaceus* showed a complex mixture of compounds and, within each single species, both qualitative and quantitative differences were observed (Bruschini *et al.*, 2006b,c). This means that venom volatiles could be used as good systematic characters to discriminate among aculeate-related species (Bruschini *et al.*, 2007). The most common volatile compounds found in the venom were spiroacetals, amides, and acetates and propanoates of aliphatic secondary alcohols. In particular, 2,8-dimethyl-1,7-dioxaspiro[5.5]undecane has already been reported in the venom of several other wasps (Dani *et al.*, 1998, 2000; Sledge *et al.*, 1999) and it was shown to elicit alarm communication in *P. occidentalis* (Dani *et al.*, 2000), while *N*-(3-methylbutyl)acetamide is the alarm pheromone in *V. squamosa* and *V. maculifrons* (Heath and Landolt, 1988; Landolt *et al.*, 1995). At present however, it is not clear if a single compound of the venom, maybe the amide or the spiroacetal, or a combination of compounds acting synergistically are responsible for the alarm reaction in *Polistes* species. Venom volatiles are also caste-specific in *P. dominulus* (Bruschini *et al.*, 2008b) and field bioassays conducted on the same species indicated that the presence of worker venom extract near the colony stimulates a greater number of workers to perform the entire alarm sequence ending in attack and stinging. Foundress venom seemed to be less effective in alarming the colony (Bruschini *et al.*, 2008b), suggesting that venom volatiles of foundresses may have additional functions possibly linked to conspecific interactions (i.e., sex pheromones).

The colonies of wasps belonging to the Stenogastrinae family are composed by only a few individuals (see Turillazzi, 1996). These wasps possess an effective sting and an apparently functional venom apparatus (Turillazzi, 1989), but they normally show little aggression toward predators (Turillazzi, 1991). Moreover, their stings cause much less pain than those of other social wasps at least from a human point of view (Turillazzi, 1990). If these wasps are disturbed on the nests, they drop passively from it, except when the disturbance is caused by conspecifics or ants (Turillazzi, 1991). The volatile compounds present in the venom reservoir of seven species of Stenogastrinae belonging to three genera *Eustenogaster*, *Liostenogaster*, and *Parischnogaster* were analyzed by Dani *et al.* (1998). They were mainly a mixture of linear alkanes and alkenes, with a chain length ranging from C11 to C17, in all the species. Behavioral experiments failed to demonstrate any pheromonal function of the venom (Landi *et al.*, 1998).

From this overview, the alarm pheromones appear to be heterogeneously distributed among social wasps raising questions on how many times they have evolved and if, in some more ancestral groups or species (i.e., Stenogastrinae), they have never evolved or have been lost. At present, there is no evidence that the signaling wasps are able to actively release alarm pheromones and emission might only occur after the object of disturbance has been stung. Only circumstantial evidences in *P. occidentalis* show that the alarm response spreads from an alarmed worker to all the others on the nest in less than 1.5 s (Jeanne, unpublished). Moreover, venom spraying has been reported for *Vespula*, *Dolichovespula*, and *Vespa* (Greene *et al.*, 1976; Maschwitz, 1964b; Saslavasky *et al.*, 1973), but all the observations were conducted on wasps that were aroused or attempting to sting some surfaces so that these behaviors could be only abortive sting attempts.

VI. Trail and Substrate Marking Pheromones

The production of substances to trail or mark a substrate is widespread in animals; however, it is among social insects that we can find some of the most impressive examples of this kind of communication. In social insects, trail pheromones are produced in many species and they play a central role both for the colonial cycle and/or for colony survival (Wyatt, 2003). These substances allow recruiting colony members to a new nest site, to a food source, or to other places where a great number of individuals are necessary to exploit resources (see Wilson, 1971). For this reason, the use of recruitment communication represents probably one of the principal factors determining the ecological dominance of social insects in many habitats (Wyatt, 2003). A wide range of trail pheromones are reported and chemically identified for ants and termites that live on the ground (see Vander Meer *et al.*, 1998; Wyatt, 2003); however, among social bees and social wasps, trail pheromones are less widespread probably because they spend their life mainly in an airborne environment.

Among social wasps, there are numerous behavioral evidences indicating that swarm-founding species use chemical substances to trail the swarm from the old nest to a new nesting site (see Jeanne, 1991, 1996). Descriptions of workers stop-overing along the route on prominent objects, where they drag the ventral part of their gaster, have been reported for several species that perform swarm emigration (reviewed by Jeanne, 1991, 1996; Landolt *et al.*, 1998; Smith *et al.*, 2002), suggesting the releasing of trail pheromones along the flight path. Even if founding the nests by swarms has been reported also for the vespine genus *Protovespa* (Matsuura, 1991), this nest foundation mode is probably regularly used by all the 24 genera of the New World tribe Epiponini and in some species of the Old World tribe Ropalidiini (Jeanne, 1991, 1996; Smith *et al.*, 2002). Jeanne (1981b) was the first to perform a field bioassay during the emigration of *P. sericea* swarms by experimentally inducing workers to follow an artificial route trailing with the secretion of the fifth gastral sternite glands (Richards' glands in the epiponine wasps). In this species, these glands produce a secretion that accumulates on the anterior margin of the fifth sternite where it becomes visible (a brownish wax) and presents a characteristic leather odor (Jeanne, 1981b). The chemical analysis of the secretion of this gland showed a complex mixture of volatile substances where the major compounds were alkyl and aromatic aldehydes, fatty acids, 3-phenylpropanoic acid, ketones, a macrolactone, a pyranone compound and nerolidol (Clarke *et al.*, 1999). A similar experiment demonstrated the existence of a trail pheromone in *Polybiodies tabidus*, an African ropalidine swarming species (Francescato *et al.*, 1993). The authors suggested the Dufour's gland as the possible source of this trail substance as this species lacks sternal glands. Moreover, the chemical analysis of the Dufour's gland secretion of *P. tabidus* showed a mixture of compounds much simpler than those found in the Richard's gland secretion of *P. sericea* (Dani *et al.*, 1997). The compounds were also less volatile, mainly high molecular weight hydrocarbons and a few esters, while the major compound was shown to be 1-hexadecanol (Dani *et al.*, 1997). However, bioassays to investigate the role of the Dufour's gland secretion during the swarming behavior of *P. tabidus* have not been carried out yet. Behavioral observations performed during swarming of *Apoica*, a nocturnal genus sister group to all the other epiponine genera (Carpenter, 1991), suggested a different communication mode of emigration (Howard *et al.*, 2002; Hunt *et al.*, 1995; Jeanne *et al.*, 1983). During swarm emigration, *Apoica pallens* does not perform the gaster-dragging behavior on the substrate along the way between the new and the old-nesting sites as other swarm-founding species do; once at the new site individuals of *A. pallens* seem to release chemicals into the air medium by holding the gaster in a calling-display to recruit the swarm (Howard *et al.*, 2002).

A different context in which chemicals help to orient the wasps is related to the localization of the nest entrance in independent-founding species with comb surrounded by an envelope. After the first report of this nest-entrance marking behavior in *V. vulgaris* (Butler *et al.*, 1969), recent studies (Jandt *et al.*, 2005; Steinmetz and Schmolz, 2003; Steinmetz *et al.*, 2002) on four species of Vespinae wasps have provided evidences that both ground-nesting (*V. vulgaris*, *V. crabro*, *V. germanica*) and aerial-nesting species

(*D. saxonica*) use chemical substances to find the nest entrance. Nest-entrance marking behavior could be particularly useful to returning foragers when the nest entrance is hidden by vegetation, but it can also be commonly used to easily find the colony in the last phase of the approaching flight to the nest. Chemical analyses carried out around the nest-entrance of *V. vulgaris* have shown the same mixture of hydrocarbons found on the workers cuticle (Steinmetz *et al.*, 2003). Although the hydrocarbons could be deposited by the wasps through the exocrine glands (Steinmetz *et al.*, 2003), the hydrocarbons accumulation at the nest entrance is probably the indirect effect induced by workers stroking their abdomens while entering/exiting the nest (Jandt *et al.*, 2005; Steinmetz *et al.*, 2003). About 200 individuals passing through the entrance are needed to evoke a similar response in *V. germanica* workers (Jandt *et al.*, 2005). This experimental evidence supports the idea that the nest-entrance trail of *V. germanica* is an accidental cue due to passing wasps (Jandt *et al.*, 2005), otherwise the response should have been elicited by very few passing individuals, if it was a signal evolved for communicative purposes.

As this trail marking seems to be accidentally deposited by the individuals while entering/exiting the colony, it should have a colonial signature. However, bioassays on *V. vulgaris* showed that the response elicited by the odors of different colonies is similar when workers belonging to different nests were tested (Steinmetz *et al.*, 2003). According to Gamboa (2004), the lack of colonial specificity in the response could be due to a more permissive acceptance thresholds in the context of chemical trails.

Differently from other social insects species, where trail pheromones are used to locate food sources, they seem not widespread in social wasps (see Jeanne, 1996). The giant-hornet *V. mandarinia japonica* is the only hornet species known to have evolved *en masse* predation of other social bees and wasps (Ono *et al.*, 1995). A single *Vespa* scout releases a foraging-site marking pheromone from the van der Vecht organ's glands, rubbing the basal tuft of the terminal gastral sternite around the entrance of the nest of a honeybee colony. This is used by the other hornet nestmates to congregate and attack the marked site *en masse* (Ono *et al.*, 1995).

VII. Defense Allomones

Social wasp colonies, being a great source of nourishing material in the form of defenseless immature brood, are attractive targets for several invertebrate and vertebrate predators (Jeanne, 1982b).

Ants are important natural enemies of eusocial wasps and represent a major selective force on wasp social and defensive behavior (Chadab, 1979; Jeanne, 1975, 1979; Kojima, 1993; Post and Jeanne, 1981) especially in the tropics where ants have generated a high diversity among the vespid subfamily Polistinae (O'Donnell and Jeanne, 1990).

The five independent-founding genera of the Polistinae wasps make nests consisting of an exposed comb, which, in most species, is suspended from the substrate by a single, narrow petiole (Wenzel, 1991). The colonies are initiated by one or more queens without the aid of workers, thus leaving the nests often unattended, making chemical defenses very important at all times. Gaster rubbing, which is a movement of the female abdomen against the nest petiole from one side to the other several times, was first described by Jeanne (1970) for *Mischocyttarus drewseni*. This repeated movement allows the females to apply an ant-repellent allomone secreted from the van der Vecht organ's glands, located on the sixth sternite of the gaster (Downing, 1991; Jeanne, 1996; Vecht, 1968). The ant defense function of the rubbing behavior has been shown in the remaining four independent-founding polistine genera *Polistes*, *Ropalidia*, *Parapolybia*, and *Belonogaster* (European *Polistes*, Turillazzi and Ugolini, 1979; *Polistes fuscatus*, Post and Jeanne, 1981; *Ropalidia fasciata*, Kojima, 1983; *Parapolybia indica*, Kojima, 1992; *B. petiolata*, Keeping, 1990). Two active ant repellent components have been found in the secretion of *Polistes fuscatus* (Post *et al.*, 1984b) and field bioassays showed that methylpalmitate and its methyl ester homolog, methylmyristate, have an ant repellent activity against ants (Post *et al.*, 1984b). The repellent effect of the two substances has also been tested on four ant species tending aphids. All four ant species were repelled, but at different degrees of repellency depending on the social mode of foraging: ant species lacking plasticity in their foraging strategy and relying on trail odors were repelled much more extensively than ants using a variety of cues for locating food (Henderson and Jeanne, 1989). Observations on pre-emergence, single-foundress colonies of Japanese paper wasps (*Polistes chinensis antennalis*) revealed that there is also a latitudinal gradient in the intensity of application of an ant-repellent substance to the nest petiole. Thus the lower the latitude, the more frequently a foundress rubbed an ant repellent substance onto the nest petiole probably as an evolution in the tropical regions of the world of a defensive mechanism against ant predation on wasp brood (Kojima, 1993). Furthermore, Post and Jeanne (1981) observed that in simulated ant attacks on wasps of the species *Polistes fuscatus*, small colonies were more likely to use chemical defenses than large ones where, instead, the active defense played a relatively more important role. Even *Mischocyttarus cerberus* wasps used both behavioral and chemical strategies for nest defense depending on the colony stage, suggesting that both the number of wasps and of immature brood on the nest are important factors in the kind and in the intensity of the defense behavior against ant attacks (Togni and Giannotti, 2007, 2008).

Chemical and behavioral evidences showed that among the long-chain carboxylic acids identified in fifth and sixth sternal gland secretion of *P. dominulus* and its obligate social parasite *P. sulcifer*, the unsaturated fatty acids were repellent against three ant species, while the saturated ones were not (Dani *et al.*, 1995, 1996c). Recently, performing chemical analysis with a different sampling technique, these authors found the same carboxylic acid to be present in a variety of tissues other than the glands (Dani *et al.*, 2003) and new bioassays have shown that long-chain methyl esters, alkanes, and alkenes have a similar repellent effect as fatty acids on the ant *Monomorium pharaonis* suggesting that any aliphatic long-chain compounds liquid at room temperature may also play a significant role in the defense of the nest against ants (Dani *et al.*, 2003).

In contrast to independent-founders, swarm-founding Polistinae species never leave new nest sites unattended so they should not require the ant repellent secretion of van der Vecht organ's gland. In fact, in every swarm-founding lineage where the sixth sternal gland has been studied, either the gland or the ant-repellent function of its secretion has been lost. Only three out of the 24 swarm-founding genera possess van der Vecht organ's gland. In two of these genera (*Agelaia* and *Apoica*), van der Vecht organ's gland secretion does not repel ants (London and Jeanne, 2000), while the third genus (the vespine *Provespa*) has not been tested. Moreover, most of the swarm-founding Polistinae build nests that are broadly attached to the substrate and covered with an envelope, so it could be argued that nest envelope protects against ants (Jeanne, 1975) allowing the evolutionary loss of an ant-repellent secretion. However, all Vespinae wasps (yellowjackets and hornets, the sister clade to the Polistinae) build enclosed nests (Wenzel, 1991, 1993) and all of them retained the van der Vecht organ's gland, even if in the majority of the species its ant repellent ability has not been tested (Matsuura and Yamane, 1990). Moreover, only Martin (1992) reported the production of an ant-repellent by the sixth and seventh sternal glands in *Vespa affinis* and *V. tropica* (L.). The two epiponine swarm-founding genera without nest envelopes (*Apoica* and most *Agelaia*) are the only ones that retained the van der Vecht organ's gland, but the gland's ant-repellency has been lost (London and Jeanne, 2000). Although nest envelopes are undoubtedly important in colony defense (Jeanne, 1975), these data suggest that their presence or absence is less informative than the mode of colony founding (independent vs. swarm-founding) for explaining patterns of loss of van der Vecht organ's gland and/or ant-repellent function (Smith *et al.*, 2001). Chemical defense against ants in the Epiponini species was lost with the evolution of swarm founding rather than with the appearance of the nest envelope. Moreover, London and Jeanne (2000) reported that *Agelaia multipicta*, *P. sericea*, and *Polistes myersi* actively defend their nests against ants even if only *P. myersi* produces an ant repellent. This implies that the difference between independent founding and swarm-founding wasps is that the first ones use both chemical and active defense to protect their brood from ants whereas the latter appear to rely completely on active defense having lost the chemical defense.

Stenogastrine wasps, lacking the van der Vecht organ's gland, produce an ant blocking secretion from a different exocrine gland, the Dufour's gland (Turillazzi, 1985; Turillazzi and Pardi, 1981). The ant guards of several stenogastrine species are barriers composed of a mixture of alkanes, alkenes, and methyl branched alkanes with only small amounts of fatty acids (Sledge *et al.*, 2000) and their function seems to be a physical rather than a chemical one.

Wasps, mainly belonging to the genus *Vespa*, are among the major predators of other social wasps and honeybees, especially in the South-East Asia (Matsuura and Yamane, 1990; Ono *et al.*, 1995). An interesting study showed that the yellow-hornet *V. simillima xanthoptera* is able to detect the foraging-site marking pheromone secreted from the giant-hornet *V. mandarinia* van der Vecht glands in order to coordinate an intra- and intercolonial defensive response (Ono, 2006). 1-Methylbutyl-3-methylbutanoate has been identified as the major component of the giant-hornet marking secretion (Ono *et al.*, 2003), and it elicits a strong defensive reaction of *V. simillima* wasps identical to the response when it detects the foraging-site marking pheromone.

In temperate regions, in addition to ant predation, birds of various genera and species can prey on single wasps or on the small colonies of *Polistes* (Strassmann, 1981; Turillazzi, 1984), while other vertebrates, such as badgers, skunks, and bears can dare to attack great colonies of yellowjackets (Starr, 1985). In *P. dominulus*, the mandibular glandular secretion contained mainly a series of aliphatic acids from C2 to C18 and small amounts of aldehydes and alcohols (Fortunato *et al.*, 2001). Laboratory bioassays did not show an alarm function of the mandibular gland secretion. The authors suggest that this secretion could be a warning signal released on the nest by disturbed wasps, particularly at night, against vertebrate nocturnal predators (Fortunato *et al.*, 2001).

VIII. Future Directions

Although increasing progress on the chemical communication systems of social wasps has been achieved and numerous pheromones were identified as highlighted in this chapter, still many aspects of the chemical communication world of these social insects have not been yet deeply investigated. Several behavioral patterns and wasp postures observed in well-defined life contexts suggest the probable emission of substances with communicative values. On the other hand, the existence of exocrine glands in specific body parts supports their possible implication in pheromone production. Future attention should be paid to these behavioral and physiological aspects which could lead to the discovery of new chemical substances involved in social wasp interactions.

Moreover, the recent finding of a complex blend of polar substances present, together with the hydrocarbons, on the cuticle of *Polistes* wasps (Turillazzi *et al.*, 2006a) opens the possibility that CHCs are not the only compounds with a recognition pheromone role. In fact, this blend of polar substances of a molecular weight (MW) between 900 and 3000 Da, presumably proteinaceous in most part, has been found to be different among species (Baracchi *et al.*, 2009; Turillazzi *et al.*, 2007) and among wasp castes—foundresses and workers (Dapporto *et al.*, 2008). This variability roughly resembles the complex variation of CHCs mixture found at different organizational levels in social wasps. Moreover, it has been demonstrated that wasps are able to perceive these substances (Turillazzi *et al.*, 2006b) that can be used by future *Polistes* foundresses as chemical cues to find suitable hibernation sites to overwinter (Turillazzi *et al.*, 2006b).

At the same time, the volatile compounds of the venom were shown both to be variable at different organizational levels in *Polistes* wasps (species, colonies, castes) and to be perceived by the wasps (Bruschini, 2005; Bruschini *et al.*, 2006a,b, 2007, 2008a,b). Future research to discover whether these venom volatiles can be emitted "voluntarily" by the wasps, even without stinging, could open new perspectives on chemical communication aspects of social wasps.

ACKNOWLEDGMENTS

The current knowledge of the social wasps pheromones has been largely improved by the work of Dr. Francesca R. Dani and Dr. Leonardo Dapporto that we greatly thank for their critical reading and precious suggestions. The collaboration with the staff of the Mass Spectrometry Center (C.I.S.M.) of Florence, in particular Prof. Gloriano Moneti and Dr. Giuseppe Pieraccini, has been fundamental for the study of the chemical communication in social wasps. We also greatly thank Dr. Davide Baracchi, Dr. Federico Cappa, Dr. Alessandro Cini, and Prof. Laura Beani for reading and commenting the manuscript, and Dr. Gerald Litwack for the english revision.

REFERENCES

Akre, R. D. (1982). Social wasps. *In* "Social Insects," (H. R. Herman, Ed.), Vol. 4, pp. 1–105. Academic Press, New York.

Akre, R. D., and Reed, H. C. (1983). Evidence for a queen pheromone in *Vespula*. *Can. Entomol.* **115,** 371–377.

Aldiss, J. B. J. F. (1983). Chemical Communication in British Social Wasps (Hymenoptera: Vespidae) Ph.D. Dissertation, University of Southampton, United Kingdom. (pp. 252).

Ali, M. F., and Morgan, E. D. (1990). Chemical communication in insect communities: A guide to insect pheromones with special emphasis to social insects. *Biol. Rev.* **65,** 227–247.

Arathi, H. S., Shakarad, M., and Gadagkar, R. (1997). Factors affecting the acceptance of alien conspecifics on nests of the primitively eusocial wasp, *Ropalidia marginata* (Hymenoptera: Vespidae). *J. Insect Behav.* **10,** 343–353.

Ayasse, M., Paxton, R. J., and Tengö, J. (2001). Mating behaviour and chemical communication in the order Hymenoptera. *Annu. Rev. Entomol.* **46,** 31–78.

Bagnères, A., Lorenzi, M. C., Clément, J. L., Dusticier, G., and Turillazzi, S. (1996). Chemical usurpation of a nest by paper wasp parasites. *Science* **272,** 889–892.

Baracchi, D., Dapporto, L., Teseo, S., Hashim, R., and Turillazzi, S. (2010). Medium molecular weight polar substances of the cuticle as tools in the study of the taxonomy, systematics and chemical ecology of tropical hover wasps (Hymenoptera: Stenogastrinae). *J. Zool. Syst. Evol. Res.* **48,** 109–114.

Batra, S. W. T. (1980). Sexual behaviour and pheromones of the European hornet, *Vespa crabro* germana (Hymenoptera: Vespidae). *J. Kansas Entomol. Soc.* **53,** 461–469.

Beani, L. (1996). Lek-like courtship in paper-wasps: "A prolonged, delicate, and troublesome affair". *In* "Natural History and Evolution of Paper Wasps," (S. Turillazzi and M. J. West-Eberhard, Eds.), pp. 113–125. Oxford University Press, Oxford.

Beani, L., and Calloni, C. (1991a). Leg tegumental glands and male rubbing behaviour at leks in *Polistes dominulus* (Hymenoptera: Vespidae). *J. Insect Behav.* **4,** 449–462.

Beani, L., and Calloni, C. (1991b). Male rubbing behavior and the hypothesis of pheromonal release in polistinae wasps (Hymenoptera: Vespidae). *Ethol. Ecol. Evol.* **1,** 51–54. (Special Issue).

Beani, L., and Landi, M. (2000). Aerial leks and marking behaviour in *Parischnogaster mellyi* males (Hymenoptera Stenogastrinae). *Insect Soc. Life* **3,** 3–10.

Beani, L., and Turillazzi, S. (1988). Alternative mating tactics in males of *Polistes dominulus* (Hymenoptera: Vespidae). *Behav. Ecol. Sociobiol.* **22,** 257–264.

Beani, L., and Turillazzi, S. (1990a). Overlap at landmarks by lek-territorial and swarming males of two sympatric polistine wasps. (Hymenoptera: Vespidae). *Ethol. Ecol. Evol.* **2,** 419–431.

Beani, L., and Turillazzi, S. (1990b). Male swarms at landmarks and scramble competition polygyny in *Polistes gallicus* (Hymenoptera: Vespidae). *J. Insect Behav.* **3,** 545–556.

Beani, L., Cervo, R., Lorenzi, M. C., and Turillazzi, S. (1992). Landmark-based mating systems in four *Polistes* Species (Hymenoptera: Vespidae). *J. Kansas Entomol. Soc.* **65,** 211–217.

Beani, L., Sledge, M. F., Maiani, S., Boscaro, F., Landi, M., Fortunato, A., and Turillazzi, S. (2002). Behavioral and chemical analyses of scent-marking in the lek system of a hover-wasp (Vespidae, Stenogastrinae). *Insect Soc.* **49,** 275–281.

Billen, J., and Morgan, E. D. (1998). Pheromone communication in social insects: Sources and secretions. *In* "Pheromone Communication in Social Insects," (R. K. Vander Meer, M. D. Breed, K. E. Espelie, and M. L. Winston, Eds.), pp. 3–33. Westview Press, Boulder.

Blomquist, J. G., and Dillwith, J. W. (1985). Cuticular lipids. *In* "Comprehensive Insect Physiology, Biochemistry and Pharmacology," (G. A. Kerkut and L. I. Gilbert, Eds.), Vol. 3, pp. 117–154. Pergamon Press, Oxford.

Blum, M. S. (1985). Alarm pheromones. *In* "Comprehensive Insect Physiology, Biochemistry and Pharmacology," (G. A. Kerkut and L. I. Gilbert, Eds.), Vol. 9, pp. 193–224. Pergamon Press, Oxford.

Bonavita-Cougourdan, A., Theraulaz, G., Bagnères, A. G., Roux, M., Pratte, M., Provost, E., and Clément, J. L. (1991). Cuticular hydrocarbons, social organization and ovarian development in a polistine wasp: *Polistes dominulus* Christ. *Comp. Biochem. Physiol.* **100B,** 667–680.

Bourke, A. F. G. (1988). Worker reproduction in the higher eusocial Hymenoptera. *Q. Rev. Biol.* **63,** 291–311.

Brandstaetter, A. S., Endler, A., and Kleineidam, C. J. (2008). Nestmate recognition in ants is possible without tactile interaction. *Naturwissenschaften* **95,** 601–608.

Brockmann, A., Groh, C., and Fröhlich, B. (2003). Wax perception in honeybees: Contact is not necessary. *Naturwissenschaften* **90,** 424–427.

Brown, W. V., Spradbery, J. P., and Lacey, M. J. (1991). Changes in the cuticular hydrocarbon composition during development of the social wasp, *Vespula germanica* (F.) (Hymenoptera, Vespidae). *Comp. Biochem. Physiol.* **99B,** 553–562.

Bruschini, C. (2005). Difesa della colonia e feromoni di allarme in vespe europee del genere *Polistes* (Hymenoptera, Vespidae). PhD Thesis, University of Florence, Italy.

Bruschini, C., Cervo, R., and Turillazzi, S. (2006a). Evidence of alarm pheromones in the venom of *Polistes dominulus* workers (Hymenoptera: Vespidae). *Physiol. Entomol.* **31,** 286–293.

Bruschini, C., Dani, F. R., Pieraccini, G., Guarna, F., and Turillazzi, S. (2006b). Volatiles from the venom of five species of paper wasps (*Polistes dominulus, P. gallicus, P. nimphus, P. sulcifer* and *P. olivaceus*). *Toxicon* **47,** 812–825.

Bruschini, C., Dani, F. R., Pieraccini, G., Guarna, F., and Turillazzi, S. (2006c). Erratum to "Volatiles from the venom of five species of paper wasps (*Polistes dominulus, P. gallicus, P. nimphus, P. sulcifer* and *P. olivaceus*)". *Toxicon* **48,** 473–475.

Bruschini, C., Cervo, R., and Turillazzi, S. (2007). Can venom volatiles be a taxonomic tool for *Polistes wasps* (Hymenoptera, Vespidae)? *J. Zool. Syst. Evol. Res.* **45,** 202–205

Bruschini, C., Cervo, R., and Turillazzi, S. (2008a). Nesting habit and alarm pheromones in *Polistes gallicus* (Hymenoptera, Vespidae). *J. Insect Behav.* **21,** 123–129.

Bruschini, C., Cervo, R., Protti, I., and Turillazzi, S. (2008b). Caste differences in venom volatiles and their effect on alarm behaviour in the paper wasp *Polistes dominulus* (Christ). *J. Exp. Biol.* **211,** 2442–2449.

Butler, C. G., Fletcher, D. J. C., and Watler, D. (1969). Nest-entrance marking with pheromones by the honeybee *Apis mellifera* L., and by a wasp, *Vespula vulgaris* L. *Anim. Behav.* **17,** 142–147.

Butts, D. P., and Espelie, K. E. (1995). Role of nest-paper hydrocarbons in nestmate recognition of *Dolichovespula maculata* (L.) workers (Hymenoptera, Vespidae). *Ethology* **100,** 39–49.

Butts, D. P., Espelie, K. E., and Hermann, H. R. (1991). Cuticular hydrocarbons of four species of social wasps in the subfamily Vespinae: *Vespa crabro* (L.), *Dolichovespula maculata* (L.), *Vespula squamosa* (Drury), and *Vespula maculifrons* (Buysson). *Comp. Biochem. Physiol.* **99B,** 87–91.

Butts, D. P., Camann, M. A., and Espelie, K. E. (1993). Discriminant analysis of cuticular hydrocarbons of the baldfaced hornet, *Dolichovespula maculata* (Hymenoptera: Vespidae). *Sociobiology* **21,** 193–201.

Carpenter, J. M. (1982). The phylogenetic relationships and natural classification of the Vespoidae (Hymenoptera). *Syst. Entomol.* **7,** 11–38.

Carpenter, J. M. (1991). Phylogenetic relationships and the origin of social behavior in the Vespidae. *In* "The Social Biology of Wasps," (K. G. Ross and R. W. Matthews, Eds.), pp. 7–32. Comstock Publication Associates, Ithaca, NY.

Carpenter, J. M. (1996). Phylogeny and biogeography. *In* "Natural History and Evolution of Paper Wasps," (S. Turillazzi and M. J. West-Eberhard, Eds.), pp. 18–57. Oxford University Press, Oxford.

Carpenter, J. M., and Starr, C. K. (2000). A new genus of hover wasps from Southeast Asia (Hymenoptera: Vespidae; Stenogastrinae). *Am. Mus. Novit.* **3291,** 1–12.

Cervo, R. (2006). An overview on *Polistes* parasites and their hosts. *Ann. Zool. Fenn.* **43,** 531–549.

Cervo, R., and Dani, F. R. (1996). Social parasitism and its evolution in *Polistes*. *In* "Natural History and Evolution of Paper Wasps," (S. Turillazzi and M. J. West-Eberhard, Eds.), pp. 98–112. Oxford University Press, Oxford.

Cervo, R., and Lorenzi, M. C. (1996). Behaviour in usurpers and late joiners of *Polistes biglumis bimaculatus* (Hymenoptera, Vespidae). *Insect. Soc.* **41,** 1–11.

Cervo, R., and Turillazzi, S. (1989). Nest exchange experiments in *Polistes gallicus* (L.). *Ethol. Ecol. Evol.* **1,** 185–193.

Cervo, R., Dani, F. R., and Turillazzi, S. (1996). Nestmate recognition in three species of stenogastrinae wasps (Hymenoptera, Vespidae). *Behav. Ecol. Sociobiol.* **39,** 311–316.

Cervo, R., Dani, F. R., Zanetti, P., Massolo, A., and Turillazzi, S. (2002a). Chemical nestmate recognition in a stenogastrine wasp, *Liostenogaster flavolineata* (Hymenoptera: Vespidae). *Ethol. Ecol. Evol.* **14,** 351–363.

Cervo, R., Stagi, M., and Turillazzi, S. (2002b). From overwintering group disgregation to nets foundation in *Polistes dominulus* (Hymenoptera, Vespidae): Laboratory observations. *Insect Soc. Life* **4,** 141–144.

Cervo, R., Stemmer, C., Castle, W., Queller, D., and Strassmann, J. (2004). Social parasitism of *P. dominulus* by *P. nimphus* (Hymenoptera, Vepidae). *Insect. Soc.* **51,** 1–8.

Cervo, R., Dapporto, L., Beani, L., Strassmann, J. E., and Turillazzi, S. (2008a). On status badges and quality signals in the paper wasp *Polistes dominulus*: Body size, facial colour patterns and hierarchical rank. *Proc. R. Soc. B* **275,** 1189–1196.

Cervo, R., Dani, F. R., Cotoneschi, C., Scala, C., Lotti, I., Strassmann, J. E., Queller, D. C., and Turillazzi, S. (2008b). Why are larvae of the social parasite wasp *Polistes sulcifer* not removed from the host nest? *Behav. Ecol. Sociobiol.* **62,** 1319–1331.

Chadab, R. (1979). Army-Ant Predation on Social Wasps. PhD dissertation, University of Connecticut, Storrs, CT.

Cini, A., Gioli, L., and Cervo, R. (2009). A quantitative threshold for nestmate recognition in a paper social wasp. *Biol. Lett.* **5,** 459–461.

Clarke, S. R., Dani, F. R., Jones, G. R., Morgan, E. D., and Turillazzi, S. (1999). Chemical analysis of the swarming trail pheromone of the social wasp *Polybia sericea* (Hymenoptera: Vespidae). *J. Insect Physiol.* **45,** 877–883.

Cobb, M., and Ferveur, J. F. (1996). Evolution and genetic-control of mate recognition and stimulation in *Drosophila. Behav. Process.* **35,** 35–54.

Cotoneschi, C., Dani, F. R., Cervo, R., Sledge, M. F., and Turillazzi, S. (2007). *Polistes dominulus* (Hymenoptera: Vespidae) larvae have their own chemical signatures. *J. Insect Physiol.* **53,** 954–963.

Cotoneschi, C., Dani, F. R., Cervo, R., Scala, C., Strassmann, J. E., Queller, D. C., and Turillazzi, S. (2009). *Polistes dominulus* (Hymenoptera, Vespidae) larvae show different cuticular patterns according to their sex: Workers seem not use this chemical information. *Chem. Senses* **34,** 195–202.

D'Adamo, P., Lozada, M., and Corley, J. C. (2004). An attraction pheromone from heads of worker *Vespula germanica* Wasps. *J. Insect Behav.* **17,** 809–821.

Dani, F. R. (2006). Cuticular lipids as semiochemicals in paper wasps and other social insects. *Ann. Zool. Fenn.* **43,** 500–514.

Dani, F. R., Cervo, R., and Turillazzi, S. (1992). Abdomen stroking behaviour and its possible functions in *Polistes dominulus* (Christ) (Hymenoptera, Vespidae). *Behav. Process.* **28,** 51–58.

Dani, F. R., Morgan, E. D., and Turillazzi, S. (1995). Chemical analysis of sternal gland secretion of paper wasp *Polistes dominulus* (Christ) and its social parasite *Polistes sulcifer* (Zimmermann) (Hymenoptera: Vespidae). *J. Chem. Ecol.* **21,** 1709–1718.

Dani, F. R., Morgan, E. D., and Turillazzi, S. (1996a). Dufour gland secretion of *Polistes* wasp: Chemical composition and possible involvement in nestmate recognition (Hymenoptera. Vespidae). *J. Insect Physiol.* **6,** 541–548.

Dani, F. R., Fratini, S., and Turillazzi, S. (1996b). Behavioural evidence for the involvement of Dufour's gland secretion in nestmate recognition in the social wasp *Polistes dominulus* (Hymenoptera: Vespidae). *Behav. Ecol. Sociobiol.* **38,** 311–319.

Dani, F. R., Cannoni, S., Turillazzi, S., and Morgan, E. D. (1996c). Ant repellent effect of the sternal gland secretion of *Polistes dominulus* (Christ) and *P. sulcifer* (Zimmermann) (Hymenoptera: Vespidae). *J. Chem. Ecol.* **22,** 37–48.

Dani, F. R., Morgan, E. D., Jones, G. R., Francescato, E., Turillazzi, S., and Dejean, A. (1997). Search for a trail pheromone in a social swarming wasp of the old world (*Polybioides tabidus* Hymenoptera: Vespidae). Proceedings of the C.N.R.S. Jacques Monod Conference: Chemical Communication in Vertebrates and Invertebrates, p. 41. La Londe-les-Maures, France.

Dani, F. R., Morgan, E. D., Jones, G. R., Turillazzi, S., Cervo, R., and Francke, W. (1998). Species-specific volatile substances in the venom sac of hover wasps. *J. Chem. Ecol.* **24,** 1091–1104.

Dani, F. R., Jeanne, R. L., Clarke, S. R., Jones, G. R., Morgan, E. D., Francke, W., and Turillazzi, S. (2000). Chemical characterization of the alarm pheromone in the venom of *Polybia occidentalis* and of volatiles form the venom of *P. sericea*. *Physiol. Entomol.* **25,** 363–369.

Dani, F. R., Jones, G. R., Destri, S., Spencer, S. H., and Turillazzi, S. (2001). Deciphering the recognition signature within the cuticular chemical profile of paper wasps. *Anim. Behav.* **62,** 165–171.

Dani, F. R., Jones, G. R., Morgan, E. D., and Turillazzi, S. (2003). Reevaluation of the chemical secretion of the sternal glands of *Polistes* social wasps (Hymenoptera Vespidae). *Ethol. Ecol. Evol.* **15,** 73–82.

Dani, F. R., Foster, K. R., Zacchi, F., Seppa, P., Massolo, A., Carelli, A., Arevalo, E., Queller, D. C., Strassmann, J. E., and Turillazzi, S. (2004). Can cuticular lipids provide sufficient information for within-colony nepotism in wasps? *Proc. R. Soc. Lond. B* **271,** 745–753.

Dani, F. R., Jones, G. R., Corsi, S., Beard, R., Pradella, D., and Turillazzi, S. (2005). Nestmate recognition cues in the honey bee: Differential importance of cuticular alkanes and alkenes. *Chem. Senses* **30,** 477–489.

Dapporto, L., Palagi, E., and Turillazzi, S. (2004a). Cuticular hydrocarbons of *Polistes dominulus* as a biogeographic tool: A study of populations from Tuscan Archipelago and surrounding areas. *J. Chem. Ecol.* **30,** 2139–2151.

Dapporto, L., Pansolli, C., and Turillazzi, S. (2004b). Hibernation clustering and its consequences for associative nest foundation in *Polistes dominulus* (Hymenoptera, Vespidae). *Behav. Ecol. Sociobiol.* **56,** 315–321.

Dapporto, L., Theodora, P., Spacchini, C., Pieraccini, G., and Turillazzi, S. (2004c). Rank and epicuticular hydrocarbons in different populations of the paper wasp *Polistes dominulus* (Christ) (Hymenoptera, Vespidae). *Insect. Soc.* **51,** 279–285.

Dapporto, L., Cervo, R., Sledge, M. F., and Turillazzi, S. (2004d). Rank integration in dominance hierarchies of host colonies by the paper wasp social parasite *Polistes sulcifer* (Hymenoptera, Vespidae). *J. Insect Physiol.* **50,** 217–223.

Dapporto, L., Sledge, F. W., and Turillazzi, S. (2005). Dynamics of cuticular chemical profiles of *Polistes dominulus* workers in orphaned nests (Hymenoptera, Vespidae). *J. Insect Physiol.* **51,** 969–973.

Dapporto, L., Fondelli, L., and Turillazzi, S. (2006). Nestmate recognition and identification of cuticular hydrocarbons composition in the swarm founding paper wasp *Ropalidia opifex*. *Biochem. Syst. Ecol.* **34,** 617–625.

Dapporto, L., Dani, F. R., and Turillazzi, S. (2007a). Social dominance molds cuticular and egg chemical blends in a paper wasp. *Curr. Biol.* **17,** R504–R505.

Dapporto, L., Santini, A., Dani, F. R., and Turillazzi, S. (2007b). Workers of a *Polistes* paper wasp detect the presence of their queen by chemical cues. *Chem. Senses* **32,** 795–802.

Dapporto, L., Lambardi, D., and Turillazzi, S. (2008). Not only cuticular lipids: First evidence of differences between foundresses and their daughters in polar substances in the paper wasp *Polistes dominulus*. *J. Insect Physiol.* **54,** 89–95.

Dapporto, L., Bruschini, C., Cervo, R., Petrocelli, I., and Turillazzi, S. (2010a). To eat or not to eat? Hydrocarbon rank signatures explain differential oophagy and dominance in a paper wasp. *J. Exp. Biol.* **213,** 453–458.

Dapporto, L., Bruschini, C., Cervo, R., Dani, F. R., Jackson, D. E., Petrocelli, I., and Turillazzi, S. (2010b). Timing matters when assessing dominance and chemical signatures in the paper wasp *Polistes dominulus*. *Behav. Ecol. Sociobiol.* **64,** 1363–1365.

Dietemann, V., Peeters, C., Liebig, J., Thivet, V., and Hölldobler, B. (2003). Cuticular hydrocarbons mediate discrimination of reproductives and nonreproductives in the ant *Myrmecia gulosa*. *Proc. Natl. Acad. Sci. USA* **100,** 10341–10346.

Downing, H. A. (1991). The function and evolution of exocrine glands. *In* "The Social Biology of Wasps," (K. G. Ross and R. W. Matthews, Eds.), pp. 540–569. Comstock Publication Associates, Ithaca, NY.
Downing, H. A., and Jeanne, R. L. (1983). Correlation of season and dominance status with activity of exocrine glands in *Polistes fuscatus* (Hymenoptera: Vespidae). *J. Kansas Entomol. Soc.* **56,** 387–397.
Espelie, K. E., and Hermann, H. R. (1988). Congruent cuticular hydrocarbons: Biochemical convergence of a social wasp, an ant and a host plant. *Biochem. Syst. Ecol.* **16,** 5050–5508.
Espelie, K. E., and Hermann, H. R. (1990). Surface lipid of the social wasp *Polistes annularis* (L.) and its nest and nest pedicel. *J. Chem. Ecol.* **16,** 1841–1852.
Espelie, K. E., Wenzel, J. W., and Chang, G. (1990). Surface lipids of social wasp *Polistes metricus* say and its nest and pedicel and their relation to nestmate recognition. *J. Chem. Ecol.* **16,** 2229–2241.
Espelie, K. E., Gamboa, G. J., Grudzien, T. A., and Bura, E. A. (1994). Cuticular hydrocarbons of the paper wasp, *Polistes fuscatus*: A search for recognition pheromones. *J. Chem. Ecol.* **20,** 1677–1687.
Fletcher, D. J. C., and Ross, K. G. (1985). Regulation of reproduction in eusocial Hymenoptera. *Ann. Rev. Entomol.* **30,** 319–343.
Fortunato, A., Maile, R., Turillazzi, S., Morgan, E. D., Moneti, G., Jones, G. R., and Pieraccini, G. (2001). Defensive role of secretion of ectal mandibular glands of the wasp *Polistes dominulus*. *J. Chem. Ecol.* **27,** 569–579.
Fortunato, A., Dani, F. R., Sledge, M. F., Fondelli, L., and Turillazzi, S. (2004). Alarm communication in *Ropalidia* social wasps. *Insect. Soc.* **51,** 299–305.
Francescato, E., Turillazzi, S., and Dejean, A. (1993). Swarming behaviour in *Polybioides tabida* (Hymenoptera Vespidae). *Act. Colloq. Insect. S.* **8,** 121–126.
Freisling, J. (1943). Zur psychologie der feldwespe. *Z. Tierpsychol.* **5,** 438–463.
Gadagkar, R. (1991). *Belonogaster. Mischocyttarus. Parapolybia*, and independent founding *Ropalidia*. *In* "The Social Biology of Wasps," (K. G. Ross and R. W. Matthews, Eds.), pp. 149–190. Comstock Publication Associates, Ithaca, NY.
Gamboa, G. J. (1996). Kin recognition n social wasps. *In* "Natural History and Evolution of Paper Wasps," (S. Turillazzi and M. J. West-Eberhard, Eds.), pp. 161–177. Oxford University Press, Oxford.
Gamboa, G. J. (2004). Kin recognition in eusocial wasps. *Ann. Zool. Fenn.* **41,** 789–808.
Gamboa, G. J., and Dropkin, J. A. (1979). Comparison of behaviors in early versus late foundress associations of the paper wasp *Polistes metricus* (Hymenoptera: Vespidae). *Can. Entomol.* **111,** 919–926.
Gamboa, G. J., and Stump, K. A. (1996). The timing of conflict and cooperation among cofoundresses of the social wasp *Polistes fuscatus* (Hymenoptera: Vespidae). *Can. J. Zoolog.* **74,** 70–74.
Gamboa, G. J., Reeve, H. K., Ferguson, I. D., and Wacker, T. L. (1986). Nestmate recognition in social wasps. The origin and acquisition of recognition odours. *Anim. Behav.* **34,** 685–695.
Gamboa, G. J., Foster, R. L., Scope, J. A., and Bitterman, A. M. (1991). Effects of stage of colony cycle, context, and intercolony distance on conspecific tolerance by paper wasp (*Polistes fuscatus*). *Behav. Ecol. Sociobiol.* **29,** 87–94.
Gamboa, G. J., Grudzier, T. A., Espelie, K. A., and Bura, E. A. (1996). Kin recognition in social wasps: Combining behavioural and chemical evidence. *Anim. Behav.* **51,** 625–629.
Gastreich, K. R., Queller, D. C., Hughes, C. R., and Strassmann, J. E. (1990). Kin discrimination in the tropical swarm-founding wasp, *Parachartergus colobopterus*. *Anim. Behav.* **40,** 598–601.
Gervet, J. (1964). le comportement d'oophagie différentielle chez *Polistes gallicus* L. (Hymen. Vesp.). *Insect. Soc.* **11,** 343–382.

Greene, A. (1991). *Dolichovespula* and *Vespula*. *In* "The Social Biology of Wasps," (K. G. Ross and R. W. Matthews, Eds.), pp. 263–305. Comstock Publication Associates, Ithaca, NY.

Greene, A., Akre, R. D., and Landolt, P. J. (1976). The aerial yellowjacket, *Dolichovespula arenaria* (Fab.): Nesting biology, reproductive production, and behavior (Hymenoptera: Vespidae). *Melanderia* **26,** 1–34.

Heath, R. R., and Landolt, P. J. (1988). The isolation, identification and synthesis of the alarm pheromone of *Vespula squamosa* (Drury) (Hymenoptera: Vespidae) and associated behavior. *Experientia* **44,** 82–83.

Henderson, G., and Jeanne, R. L. (1989). Response of aphid-tending ants to a repellent produced by wasps (Hymenoptera: Formicidae, Vespidae) *Ann. Entomol. Soc. Am.* **82,** 516–519.

Hermann, H. R., and Blum, M. S. (1981). Defensive mechanisms in the social Hymenoptera. *In* "Social Insects," (H. R. Hermann, Ed.), pp. 77–197. Academic Press, New York.

Hines, H. M., Hunt, J. H., O'Connor, T. K., Gillespie, J. J., and Cameron, S. A. (2007). Multigene phylogeny reveals eusociality evolved twice in vespid wasps. *Proc. Natl. Acad. Sci. USA* **104,** 3295–3299.

Hölldobler, B., and Wilson, E. O. (1990). The Ants Springer, Berlin, Heidelberg, New York. pp. XIV+732.

Howard, R. W. (1993). Cuticular hydrocarbons and chemical communication. *In* "Insect Lipids," (D. W. Stanley-Samuelson and D. R. Nelson, Eds.), pp. 177–226. University of Nebraska Press, Lincon.

Howard, R. W., and Blomquist, G. J. (2005). Ecological, behavioral, and biochemical aspects of insect hydrocarbons. *Annu. Rev. Entomol.* **50,** 371–393.

Howard, K. J., Smith, A. R., O'Donnell, S., and Jeanne, R. L. (2002). Novel method of swarm emigration by the epiponine wasp, *Apoica pallens* (Hymenoptera Vespidae). *Ethol. Ecol. Evol.* **14,** 365–371.

Hunt, J. H. (2007). The Evolution of Social Wasps. Oxford University Press, New York. pp. IX+259.

Hunt, J. H., Jeanne, R. L., and Keeping, M. G. (1995). Observations on *Apoica pallens*. A nocturnal Neotropical social wasp (Hymenoptera: Vespidae, Polistinae, Epiponini). *Insect. Soc.* **42,** 223–236.

Ikan, R., Gottlieb, R., Bergmann, E. D., and Ishay, J. (1969). The pheromone of the queen of the Oriental hornet, *Vespa orientalis*. *J. Insect Physiol.* **15,** 1709–1712.

Inward, D., Beccaloni, G., and Eggleton, P. (2007). Death of an order: A comprehensive molecular phylogenetic study confirms that termites are eusocial cockroaches. *Biol. Lett.* **3,** 331–335.

Ishay, I., Ikan, R., and Bergmann, E. D. (1965). The presence of pheromones in the Oriental hornet, *Vespa orientalis* F. *J. Insect Physiol.* **11,** 1307–1309.

Izzo, A., Wells, M., Huang, Z., and Tibbetts, E. (2010). Cuticular hydrocarbons correlate with fertility, not dominance, in a paper wasp, *Polistes dominulus*. *Behav. Ecol. Sociobiol.* **64,** 857–864.

Jandt, J. M., Curry, C., Hemauer, S., and Jeanne, R. J. (2005). The accumulation of a chemical cue: Nets-entrance trail in the German yellowjacket, *Vespula germanica*. *Naturwissenschaften* **92,** 242–245.

Jeanne, R. L. (1970). Chemical defense of brood by a social wasp. *Science* **168,** 1465–1466.

Jeanne, R. L. (1975). The adaptiveness of social wasp nest architecture. *Q. Rev. Biol.* **50,** 267–287.

Jeanne, R. L. (1979). A latitudinal gradient in rates of ant predation. *Ecology* **60,** 1211–1224.

Jeanne, R. L. (1981a). Alarm recruitment, attack behaviour, and the role of the alarm pheromone in *Polybia occidentalis* (Hymenoptera: Vespidae). *Behav. Ecol. Sociobiol.* **9,** 143–148.

Jeanne, R. L. (1981b). Chemical communication during swarm emigration in the social wasp *Polybia sericea* (Olivier). *Anim. Behav.* **29,** 102–113.

Jeanne, R. L. (1982a). Evidence for an alarm substance in *Polistes canadensis*. *Experientia* **38,** 329–330.

Jeanne, R. L. (1982b). Predation, defense and colony size and cycle in the social wasps. *In* "The Biology of Social Insects," (M. C. Breed, C. D. Michener, and H. E. Evans, Eds.), pp. 280–284. Westview Press, Boulder, CO.

Jeanne, R. L. (1991). The swarm-founding Polistinae. *In* "The Social Biology of Wasps," (K. G. Ross and R. W. Matthews, Eds.), pp. 191–231. Comstock Publication Associates, Ithaca, NY.

Jeanne, R. L. (1996). The evolution of exocrine gland function in wasps. *In* "Natural History and Evolution of Paper Wasps," (S. Turillazzi and M. J. West-Eberhard, Eds.), pp. 144–159. Oxford University Press, Oxford.

Jeanne, R. L., and Keeping, M. G. (1995). Venom spraying in *Parachartergus colobopterus*: A novel defensive behavior in a social wasp (Hymenoptera: Vespidae). *J. Insect Behav.* **8,** 433–442.

Jeanne, R. L., Downing, G. A., and Post, D. C. (1983). Morphology and function of sternal glands in polistine wasps (Hymenoptera: Vespidae). *Zoomorphology* **103,** 149–164.

Kasuya, E. (1981). Male mating territory in a Japanese paper wasp, *Polistes jadwigae* Dalla Torre (Hymenoptera: Vespidae). *Kontyu* **49,** 607–614.

Keegans, S. J., Morgan, E. D., Turillazzi, S., Jackson, B. D., and Billen, J. (1993). The Dufour gland and the secretion placed on eggs of two species of social wasps, *Liostenogaster flavolineata* and *Parischnogaster jacobsoni* (Vespidae: Stenogastrinae). *J. Chem. Ecol.* **19,** 279–290.

Keeling, C. I., Plettner, E., and Slessor, K. N. (2004). Hymenopteran semiochemicals. *Top. Curr. Chem.* **239,** 133–177.

Keeping, M. G. (1990). Rubbing behavior and morphology of van der Vecht's gland in *Belonogaster petiolata* (Hymenoptera: Vespidae). *J. Insect Behav.* **3,** 85–104.

Keeping, M. G. (1995). Absence of chemical alarm in a primatively eusocial wasp (*Belonogaster petiolata*, Hymeoptera: Vespidae). *Insect. Soc.* **42,** 317–320.

Keeping, M. G., Lipschitz, D., and Crewe, R. M. (1986). Chemical mate recognition and release of male sexual behavior in a polybiine wasp, *Belanogaster petiolata* (DeGeer) (Hymenoptera: Vespidae). *J. Chem. Ecol.* **12,** 773–779.

Keller, L., and Nonacs, P. (1993). The role of queen pheromones in social insects: Queen control or queen signal? *J. Chem. Ecol.* **12,** 773–779.

Kojima, J. (1983). Defense of the pre-emergence colony against ants by means of a chemical barrier in *Ropalidia fasciata* (Hymenoptera: Vespidae). *Jpn. J. Ecol.* **33,** 213–223.

Kojima, J. (1992). The ant repellent function of the rubbing substance in an Old World polistine, *Parapolybia indica* (Hymenoptera: Vespidae). *Ethol. Ecol. Evol.* **4,** 183–185.

Kojima, J. (1993). A latitudinal gradient in intensity of applying ant-repellent substance to the nest petiole in paper wasp (Hymeoptera: Vespidae). *Insect. Soc.* **40,** 403–421.

Kojima, J. (1994). Evidence for an alarm pheromone in the old world, swarm-founding paper wasp, *Ropalidia romandi* (Le Guillou) (Hymenoptera: Vespidae). *J. Aust. Entomol. Soc.* **33,** 45–47.

Kudo, K., and Zucchi, R. (2006). Effect of a foreign male's age on acceptance into a conspecific colony in a Neotropical wasp. *Entomol. Sci.* **9,** 355–357.

Kudo, K., Tsuchida, K., Mateus, S., and Zucchi, R. (2007). Nestmate recognition in a neotropical polygynous wasp. *Insect. Soc.* **54,** 29–33.

Landi, M., Coster-Longman, C., and Turillazzi, S. (1998). Alarm response in a laboratory population of *Parischnogaster mellyi* (Stenogastrinae). *Insect Soc. Life* **2,** 59–63.

Landolt, P. J., and Akre, R. D. (1979). Occurrence and location of exocrine glands in some social vespidae (Hymenoptera). *Ann. Entomol. Soc. Am.* **72,** 141–148.

Landolt, P. J., and Heath, R. R. (1987). Alarm pheromone behavior of *Vespula squamosa* (Hymenoptera: Vespidae). *Fla. Entomol.* **70,** 222–225.

Landolt, P. J., Akre, R. D., and Greene, A. (1977). Effects of colony division on *Vespula atropilosa* (Sladen) (Hymenoptera: Vespidae). *J. Kansas Entomol. Soc.* **50,** 135–147.

Landolt, P. J., Heath, R. R., Reed, H. C., and Manning, K. (1995). Pheromonal mediation of alarm in the eastern yellowjacket (Hymenoptera: Vespidae). *Fla. Entomol.* **78,** 101–108.

Landolt, P. J., Jeanne, R. L., and Reed, H. C. (1998). Chemical communication in social wasps. *In* "Pheromone Communication in Social Insects. Ants, Wasps, Bees and Termites," (R. K. Vander Meer, M. D. Breed, M. L. Winston, and K. E. Espelie, Eds.), pp. 216–235. Westview Press, Boulder, CO.

Landolt, P. J., Reed, H. C., and Heath, R. R. (1999). An alarm pheromone from heads of worker *Vespula squamosa* (Hymenoptera: Vespidae). *Fla. Entomol.* **82,** 356–359.

Layton, J. M., Camann, M. A., and Espelie, K. E. (1994). Cuticular lipid profiles of queens, workers, and males of social wasp *Polistes metricus* Say are colony-specific. *J. Chem. Ecol.* **20,** 2307–2321.

Lenoir, A., Fresneau, D., Errard, C., and Hefetz, A. (1999). Individual and colonial identity in ants: The emergence of the social representation concept. *In* "Information Processing in Social Insects," (C. Detrain, J. L. Deneubourg, and J. M. Pasteels, Eds.), pp. 219–237. Birkhauser Verlag, Basel, Switzerland.

Lenoir, A., D'Ettorre, P., and Errard, C. (2001). Chemical ecology and social parasitism in ants. *Annu. Rev. Entomol.* **46,** 573–599.

Liebig, J., Monnin, T., and Turillazzi, S. (2005). Direct assessment of queen and lack of worker suppression in a paper wasp. *Proc. R. Soc. Lond. B* **272,** 1339–1344.

Litte, M. (1979). *Mischocyttarus flavitarsis* in Arizona: Social and nesting biology of a pollistine wasp. *Z. Tierpsychol.* **50,** 282–312.

Litte, M. (1981). Social biology of the polistine wasp *Mischocyttarus labiatus*: Survival in a Columbian rain forest. *Contrib. Zool.* **327,** 1–27.

London, K. B., and Jeanne, R. L. (1996). Alarm in a wasp–wasp nesting association: Do members signal cross-specifically? *Insect Soc.* **43,** 211–215.

London, K. B., and Jeanne, R. L. (2000). The interaction between mode of colony founding, nest architecture and ant defense in polistine wasps. *Ethol. Ecol. Evol.* **12,** 13–25.

Lorenzi, M. C. (1992). Epicuticular hydrocarbons of *Polistes biglumis bimaculatus* (Hymenoptera, Vespidae): Preliminary results. *Ethol. Ecol. Evol.* **3,** 61–63, (Special Issue).

Lorenzi, M. C. (2006). The results of an arms race: Mechanical strategies of *Polistes* social parasites. *Ann. Zool. Fenn.* **43,** 550–563.

Lorenzi, M. C., and Bagnères, A. G. (2002). Concealing identity and mimicking hosts: A dual chemical strategy for a single social parasite? (*Polistes atrimandibularis*, Hymenoptera: Vespidae). *Parasitology* **125,** 507–512.

Lorenzi, M. C., and Caprio, P. (2000). Nest recognition in neighboring colonies: A comparison of two European species of *Polistes* wasps (*P. dominulus* and *P. nimphus*, Hymenoptera, Vespidae). *J. Ethol.* **18,** 65–68.

Lorenzi, M. C., and Cervo, R. (1992). Behaviour of *Polistes biglumis bimaculatus* (Hymenoptera, Vespidae) foundresses on alien conspecific nests. *In* "Biology and Evolution of Social Insects," (J. Billen, Ed.), pp. 273–279. Leuven University Press, Belgium.

Lorenzi, M. C., and Filippone, F. (2000). Opportunistic discrimination of alien eggs by social wasps (*Polistes biglumis*, Hymenoptera: Vespidae): A defense against social parasitism? *Behav. Ecol. Sociobiol.* **48,** 402–406.

Lorenzi, M. C., Bagnères, A. G., Clement, J. L., and Turillazzi, S. (1994). Mechanisms of colony recognition: Features of the epicuticular hydrocarbons of *Polistes biglumis bimaculatus* (Hymenoptera Vespidae). *Ethol. Ecol. Evol.* **6,** 428–429.

Lorenzi, M. C., Bagnères, A. G., Clèment, J. L., and Turillazzi, S. (1997). *Polistes biglumis bimaculatus* epicuticular hydrocarbons and nestmate recognition (Hymenoptera, Vespidae). *Insect. Soc.* **44,** 123–128.
Lorenzi, M. C., Sledge, M. F., Laiolo, P., Sturlini, E., and Turillazzi, S. (2004a). Cuticular hydrocarbon dynamics in young adult *Polistes dominulus* (Hymenoptera: Vespidae) and the role of linear hydrocarbons in nestmate recognition systems. *J. Insect Physiol.* **50,** 935–941.
Lorenzi, M. C., Cervo, R., Zacchi, F., Turillazzi, S., and Bagnères, A. G. (2004b). Dynamics of chemical mimicry in the social parasite wasp *Polistes semenowi* (Hymenoptera: Vespidae). *Parasitology* **129,** 643–651.
Lucas, C., Pho, D. B., Jallon, J. M., and Fresneau, D. (2005). Role of cuticular hydrocarbons in the chemical recognition between ant species in the *Pachicondila villosa* species complex. *J. Insect Physiol.* **51,** 1148–1157.
MacDonald, J. F., Akre, R. D., and Hill, W. B. (1974). Comparative biology and behavior of *Vespula atropilosa* and *V. pensylvanica* (Hymenoptera: Vespidae). *Melanderia* **181,** 1–66.
MacLean, C., and Schmolz, E. (2004). Calorimetric investigations on the action of alarm pheromones in the hornet *Vespa crabro. Thermochim. Acta* **414,** 71–77.
Manzolli-Palma, M. F., Gobbi, N., and Palma, M. S. (1998). Alarm pheromones and the influence of pupal odor on the aggressiveness of *Polybia paulista* (Ihering) (Hymenoptera: Vespidae). *J. Venom. Anim. Toxins* **4,** 61–69.
Martin, S. J. (1992). Colony defence against ants in *Vespa. Insect. Soc.* **39,** 99–112.
Martin, S. J., Takahashi, J., Ono, M., and Drijfhout, F. P. (2008). Is the social parasite *Vespa dybowskii* using chemical transparency to get her eggs accepted? *J. Insect Physiol.* **54,** 700–707.
Maschwitz, U. (1964a). Alarm substances and alarm behavior in social Hymenoptera. *Nature* **204,** 324–327.
Maschwitz, U. (1964b). Gefahrenalarmstoffe and Gefahrenalarmierung bei sozialen Hymenopteren. *Z. Vergl. Physiol.* **47,** 596–655.
Maschwitz, U. (1984). Alarm behavior in the long cheeked wasp *Dolichovespula saxonica* (Hymenoptera: Vespidae). *Dtsch. Entomol. Z.* **31,** 33–34.
Maschwitz, U. W., and Hanel, H. (1988). Biology of the southeast Asian nocturnal wasp, *Provespa anomala* (Hymenoptera: Vespidae). *Entomol. Gen.* **14,** 47–52.
Matsuura, M. (1991). *Vespa* and *Provespa*. *In* "The Social Biology of Wasps," (K. G. Ross and R. W. Matthews, Eds.), pp. 232–262. Comstock Publication Associates, Ithaca, NY.
Matsuura, M., and Yamane, S. (1990). Biology of the Vespine Wasps Sprinter-Verlag, Berlin, Heidelberg. pp. 323.
Michener, C. D. (1969). Comparative Social Behavior of Bees. *Annu. Rev. Entomol.* **14,** 299–342.
Monnin, T., Malosse, C., and Peeters, C. (1998). Solid Phase MicroExtraction and cuticular hydrocarbon differences related to reproductive activity in the queenless ant *Dinoponera quadriceps. J. Chem. Ecol.* **24,** 473–490.
Moritz, F. A., and Bürgin, H. (1987). Group response to alarm pheromones in social wasps and honeybee. *Ethology* **76,** 15–26.
Nelson, D. R., and Blomquist, G. J. (1995). Insect waxes. *In* "Waxes: Chemistry, Molecular Biology and Functions," (R. J. Hamilton and W. W. Christie, Eds.), pp. 1–90. The Oily Press, England.
O'Donnell, S., and Jeanne, R. L. (1990). Notes on an army ant (*Eciton burchelli* Westwood) raid on a social wasp nest (*Agelaia vespocapa* Richards) in Costa Rica. *J. Trop. Ecol.* **6,** 507–509.
Ono, M. (2006). Defensive strategy of yellow-hornet against predation by giant hornet. Proc. XV Inter. Cong. Int. Union Study Soc. Insects, 233 .
Ono, M., and Sasaki, M. (1987). Sex pheromones and there cross–activities in six Japanese sympatric species of the genus *Vespa. Insect. Soc.* **34,** 252–260.

Ono, M., Sasaki, M., and Okada, I. (1985). Mating behavior of the giant hornet, *Vespa mandarinia* Smith and its pheromonal regulation. Proc. XXX Int. Apic. Congr., Nagoya, Japan. pp. 255–259.
Ono, M., Igarashi, T., Ohno, E., and Sasaki, M. (1995). Unusual thermal defence by a honeybee against mass attack by hornets. *Nature* **377,** 334–336.
Ono, M., Terabe, H., Hori, H., and Sasaki, M. (2003). Components of giant hornet alarm pheromone. *Nature* **424,** 637–638.
Overal, W. L., Simões, D., and Gobbi, N. (1981). Colony defense and sting autotomy in *Polybia rejecta* (F) (Hymenoptera: Vespidae). *Rev. Bras. Entomol.* **25,** 41–47.
Panek, L. M., and Gamboa, G. J. (2000). Queens of the paper wasp *Polistes fuscatus* (Hymenoptera: Vespidae) discriminate among larvae on the basis of relatedness. *Ethology* **106,** 159–170.
Panek, L. M., Gamboa, G. J., and Espelie, K. E. (2001). The effect of a wasp's age on its cuticular hydrocarbon and its tolerance by nestmate and non-nestmate conspecics (*Polistes fuscatus,* Hymenoptera: Vespidae). *Ethology* **107,** 55–63.
Pardi, L. (1942). Ricerche sui Polistini. V. La poliginia iniziale in *Polistes gallicus* (L.). *Boll. Ist. Entomol. Univ. Bologna* **14,** 1–106.
Pardi, L. (1946). Ricerche sui Polistini VII. La "dominazione" ed il ciclo ovarico annuale di *Polistes gallicus* (L.). *Boll. Ist. Entomol. Univ. Bologna* **15,** 25–84.
Pardi, L. (1948). Dominance order in *Polistes* wasps. *Physiol. Zool.* **21,** 1–13.
Peeters, C. (1993). Monogyny and polygyny in ponerine ants with or without queens. *In* "Queen Number and Sociality in Insects," (L. Keller, Ed.). pp. 234–261. Oxford University Press, Oxford.
Pfenning, D. W. (1990). Nestmate and nest discrimination among workers from neighbouring colonies of social wasps *Polistes exclamans. Can. J. Zool.* **68,** 268–271.
Pfenning, D. W., Reeve, H. K., and Shellmann, J. S. (1983a). Learned component of nestmate discrimination in workers of a social wasp, *Polistes fuscatus* (Hymenoptera, Vespidae). *Anim. Behav.* **31,** 412–416.
Pfenning, D. W., Gamboa, G. J., Reeve, H. K., Shellmann, J. S., Reeve, J. S., and Ferguson, I. D. (1983b). The mechanism of nestmate discrimination in social wasps (Hymenoptera: Vespidae). *Behav. Ecol. Sociobiol.* **13,** 299–305.
Pickett, K. M., and Carpenter, J. M. (2000). Simultaneous analysis and the origin of eusociality in the Vespidae (Insecta: Hymenoptera). *Arthro. System. & Phylog.* **61,** 3–33.
Polak, M. (1993). Landmark territoriality in the neotropical paper wasps *Polistes canadensis* (L.) and *P.* carnifex (F.) (Hymenoptera: Vespidae). *Ethology* **95,** 278–290.
Post, D. C. (1980). Observations on male behaviour of the eastern yellowjacket, *Vespula maculifrons* (Hymenoptera: Vespidae). *Entomol. News* **91,** 113–116.
Post, D. C., and Jeanne, R. L. (1981). Colony defense against ants by *Polistes fuscatus* (Hymenoptera: Vespidae) in Wisconsin. *J. Kansas Entomol. Soc.* **54,** 599–625.
Post, D. C., and Jeanne, R. L. (1983a). Venom: Source of a sex pheromone in the social wasp *Polistes fuscatus* (Hymenoptera: Vespidae). *J. Chem. Ecol.* **9,** 259–266.
Post, D. C., and Jeanne, R. L. (1983b). Male reproductive behavior of the social wasp *Polistes fuscatus* (Hymenoptera: Vespidae). *Z. Tierpsychol.* **62,** 157–171.
Post, D. C., and Jeanne, R. L. (1984). Venom as interspecific sex pheromone and species recognition by a cuticular pheromone in paper wasps (*Polistes,* Hymenoptera: Vespidae). *Physiol. Entomol.* **9,** 65–75.
Post, D. C., and Jeanne, R. L. (1985). Sex pheromone in *Polistes fuscatus* (Hymenoptera: Vespidae). Effect of age, caste, and mating. *Insect. Soc.* **32,** 70–77.
Post, C. D., Downing, H. A., and Jeanne, R. L. (1984a). Alarm response to venom by social wasp *Polistes exclamans* and *P. fuscatus* (Hymenoptera: Vespidae). *Chem. Ecol.* **10,** 1425–1433.

Post, D. C., Mohamed, M. A., Coppel, H. C., and Jeanne, R. L. (1984b). Identification of ant repellent allomone produced by social wasp *Polistes fuscatus* (Hymenoptera: Vespidae). *J. Chem. Ecol.* **10,** 1799–1807.

Premnath, S., Sinha, A., and Gadagkar, R. (1996). Dominance relationship in the establishment of reproductive division of labour in a primitively eusocial wasp (*Ropalidia marginata*). *Behav. Ecol. Sociobiol.* **39,** 125–132.

Queller, D. C., Zacchi, F., Cervo, R., Turillazzi, S., Henshaw, M. T., Santorelli, L. A., and Strassmann, J. E. (2000). Unrelated helpers in a social insect. *Nature* **405,** 784–787.

Reed, H. C., and Landolt, P. J. (1990a). Queens of the southern yellowjacket, *Vespula squamosa*, produce sex attractant (Hymenoptera: Vespidae). *Fla. Entomol.* **73,** 687–689.

Reed, H. C., and Landolt, P. J. (1990b). Sex attraction in a paper wasp, *Polistes exclamans* Viereck (Hymenoptera: Vespidae), in a wind tunnel. *J. Chem. Ecol.* **16,** 1277–1287.

Reed, H. C., and Landolt, P. J. (1991). Swarming of paper wasps (Hymenoptera: Vespidae) sexuals at towers in Florida. *Ann. Entomol. Soc. Am.* **84,** 628–635.

Reed, H. C., and Landolt, P. J. (2000). Application of alarm pheromone to targets by southern yellowjackets (Hymenoptera: Vespidae). *Fla. Entomol.* **83,** 193–196.

Reeve, H. K. (1989). The evolution of conspecific acceptance thresholds. *Am. Nat.* **133,** 407–435.

Reeve, H. K. (1991). Polistes. *In* "The Social Biology of Wasps," (K. G. Ross and R. W. Matthews, Eds.), pp. 99–148. Comstock Publication Associates, Ithaca, NY.

Romani, R., Beani, L., Isidoro, N., Fortunato, A., Riolo, P., Bin, F., and Turillazzi, S. (2005). A new role for antennation in paper wasps (Hymenoptera: Vespidae): Antennal courtship and sex dimorphic glands in antennomeres. *Insect. Soc.* **52,** 96–102.

Röseler, P.-F. (1991). Reproductive competition during colony establishment. *In* "The Social Biology of Wasps," (K. G. Ross and R. W. Matthews, Eds.), pp. 309–335. Comstock Publication Associates, Ithaca, NY.

Ross, K. G. (1983). Laboratory studies of the mating biology of the eastern yellowjacket, *Vespula maculifrons* (Hymenoptera: Vespidae). *J. Kansas Entomol. Soc.* **56,** 523–527.

Ruther, J., Sieben, S., and Schricker, B. (1998). Role of cuticular lipids in nestmate recognition of the European hornet *Vespa crabro* L. (Hymenoptera, Vespidae). *Insect. Soc.* **45,** 169–179.

Ruther, J., Sieben, S., and Schricker, B. (2002). Nestmate recognition in social wasps: Manipulation of hydrocarbon profiles induces aggression in the European hornet. *Naturwissenschaften* **89,** 111–114.

Ryan, R., and Gamboa, G. J. (1986). Nestmate recognition between males and gynes of the social wasp *Polistes fuscatus* (Hymenoptera: Vespidae). *Ann. Entomol. Soc. Am.* **79,** 572–575.

Sanderman, R. G. (1938). The swarming of the males of *Vespula sylvestris* (scop.) around a queen. *Proc. R. Entomol. Soc. A* **13,** 87–88.

Saslavasky, H., Ishay, J., and Iran, R. (1973). Alarm substances as toxicants of oriental hornet, *Vespa orientalis*. *Life Sci.* **12,** 135–144.

Schmidt, J. O. (1990). Hymenopteran venoms: Striving toward the ultimate defense against vertebrates. *In* "Insect Defenses," (L. D. Evans and J. O. Schmidt, Eds.), pp. 387–419. State University of New York Press, Albany.

Schmitz, J., and Moritz, R. F. A. (2000). Molecular evolution in social wasps. *In* "Hymenoptera: Evolution, Biodiversity and Biological Control," (A. D. Austin and M. Dowton, Eds.), pp. 84–89. CSIRO Publishing, Australia.

Schmolz, B., Scholz, T., and Lamprecht, I. (1999). Alarm pheromones in social insects. *Nachr. Chem. Tech. Lab.* **4,** 1095–1098.

Shellmann, J. S., and Gamboa, G. J. (1982). Nestmate discrimination in social wasps: The role of exposure to nest and nestmates (*Polistes fuscatus*, Hymenoptera, Vespidae). *Anim. Behav.* **33,** 331–332.

Shorey, H. H. (1977). Interactions of insects with their chemical environments. *In* "Chemical Control and Insect Behavior, Theory and Application," (H. H. Ahorey and J. J. McKelvey, Eds.), pp. 1–5. Wiley-Interscience, New York.

Singer, T. L., Camann, M. A., and Espelie, K. E. (1992). Discriminant analysis of cuticular hydrocarbons of social wasp *Polistes exclamans* Viereck and surface hydrocarbons of its nest paper and pedicel. *J. Chem. Ecol.* **18,** 785–797.

Singer, T. L., Espelie, K. E., and Gamboa, G. J. (1998). Nest and nestmate discrimination in independent-founding paper wasps. *In* "Pheromone Communication in Social Insects," (R. K. Vander Meer, M. D. Breed, M. D. Wiston, and K. E. Espelie, Eds.), pp. 104–125. Westview Press, Boulder, CO.

Sledge, M. F., Dani, F. R., Fortunato, A., Maschwitz, U., Clarke, S. R., Francescato, E., Hashim, R., Morgan, E. D., Jones, G. R., and Turillazzi, S. (1999). Venom induces alarm behaviour in the social wasp *Polybioides raphigastra* (Hymenoptera: Vespidae): An investigation of alarm behaviour, venom volatiles and sting autotomy. *Physiol. Entomol.* **24,** 234–239.

Sledge, M. F., Fortunato, A., Turillazzi, S., Francescano, E., Hashim, R., Moneti, G., and Jones, G. R. (2000). Use of Dufour's gland secretion in nest defence and brood nutrition by hover wasps (Hymenoptera, Stenogastrinae). *J. Insect Physiol.* **46,** 753–761.

Sledge, M. F., Dani, F. R., Cervo, R., Dapporto, L., and Turillazzi, S. (2001a). Recognition of social parasites as nestmates: Adoption of colony-specific host cuticular odours by the paper wasp parasite *Polistes sulcifer. Proc. R. Soc. Lond. B* **268,** 2253–2260.

Sledge, M. F., Boscaro, F., and Turillazzi, S. (2001b). Cuticular hydrocarbons and reproductive status in the social wasp *Polistes dominulus. Behav. Ecol. Sociobiol.* **49,** 401–409.

Sledge, M. F., Trinca, I., Massolo, A., Boscaro, F., and Turillazzi, S. (2004). Variation in cuticular hydrocarbon signatures, hormonal correlates and establishment of reproductive dominance in a polistine wasp. *J. Insect Physiol.* **50,** 73–83.

Smith, A. R., O'Donnell, S., and Jeanne, R. L. (2001). Correlated evolution of colony defence and social structure: A comparative analysis in eusocial wasps (Hymenoptera: Vespidae). *Evol. Ecol. Res.* **3,** 331–344.

Smith, A. R., O'Donnell, S., and Jeanne, R. L. (2002). Evolution of swarm communication in eusocial wasps (Hymenoptera: Vespidae). *J. Insect Behav.* **15,** 751–764.

Spiewok, S., Schmolz, E., and Ruther, J. (2006). Mating system of the European hornet *Vespa crabro*: Male seeking strategies and evidence for the involvement of a sex pheromone. *J. Chem. Ecol.* **32,** 2777–2788.

Spradbery, J. P. (1973). Wasps. An Account of the Biology and Natural History of Solitary and Social Wasps. University of Washington Press, Seattle. pp. xv+408.

Spradbery, J. P. (1991). Evolution of queen number and queen control. *In* "The Social Biology of Wasps," (K. G. Ross and R. W. Matthews, Eds.), pp. 336–388. Comstock Publication Associates, Ithaca, NY.

Starks, P.T. and Turillazzi, S. (Eds.). (2006). *Polistes* Wasps: The Emergence of a Model Genus *Ann. Zool. Fenn.*Vol. 43, p. 624.

Starr, C. K. (1985). Enabling mechanism in the origin of sociality in the Hymenoptera: The sting's the thing. *Ann. Entomol. Soc. Am.* **78,** 171–173.

Starr, C. K. (1990). Holding the fort: Colony defence in some primitively social wasps. *In* "Insect Defense, Adaptive Mechanisms and Strategies of Prey and Predators," (D. L. Evans and J. O. Schmidt, Eds.), pp. 421–463. State University of New York Press, Stony Brook.

Steinmetz, I., and Schmolz, E. (2003). Use of terrestrial chemical trails for nest orientation in an open nesting wasp, *Dolichovespula saxonica* F. *Insect. Soc.* **50,** 292–294.

Steinmetz, I., Sieben, S., and Schmolz, E. (2002). Chemical trails used for orientation in nest cavities by two vespine wasps, *Vespa crabro* and *Vespula vulgaris. Insect. Soc.* **49,** 354–356.

Steinmetz, I., Schmolz, E., and Ruther, J. (2003). Cuticular lipids as trail pheromone in a social wasp. *Proc. R. Soc. Lond. B* **270,** 385–391.

Strassmann, J. E. (1981). Parasitoids, predators and group size in the paper wasp, *Polistes exlamans*. *Ecology* **62,** 1225–1233.
Strassmann, J. E., Hughes, C. R., and Queller, D. C. (1990). Colony defense in the social wasp, *Parachartergus colobopterus*. *Biotropica* **22,** 324–327.
Strassmann, J. E., Seppä, P., and Queller, D. C. (2000). Absence in within-colony kin discrimination: Foundresses of the social wasp, *Polistes carolina*, do not prefer their own larvae. *Naturwissenschaften* **87,** 266–269.
Strassmann, J. E., Fortunato, A., Cervo, R., Turillazzi, S., Damon, J. M., and Queller, D. C. (2004). The cost of queen loss in the social wasp *Polistes dominulus* (Hymenoptera: Vespidae). *J. Kansas Entomol. Soc.* **74,** 343–355.
Sumana, A., Liebert, A. E., Berry, A. S., Switz, G. T., Orians, C. M., and Starks, P. T. (2005). Nest hydrocarbons as cues for phylopatry in a paper wasp. *Ethology* **111,** 469–477.
Sumana, A., Deshpande, S. A., Bhadra, A., and Gadagkar, R. (2008). Workers of the primitively eusocial wasp *Ropalidia marginata* do not perceive their queen across a wire mesh partition. *J. Ethol.* **26,** 207–212.
Tannure-Nascimento, I. C., Nascimento, F. S., Turatti, I. C., Lopes, N. P., Trigo, J. R., and Zucchi, R. (2007). Colony membership is reflected by variations in cuticular hydrocarbon profile in a Neotropical paper wasp, *Polistes satan* (Hymenoptera, Vespidae). *Genet. Mol. Res.* **6,** 390–395.
Tannure-Nascimento, I. J., Nascimento, F. S., and Zucchi, R. (2008). The look of royalty: Visual and odour signals of reproductive status in a paper wasp. *Proc. R. Soc. Lond. B* **275,** 2555–2561.
Thomas, C. R. (1960). The European wasp (*Vespula germanica* Fab.) in New Zealand. *NZ Dept. Sci. Ind. Res. Inf. Ser.* **27,** 1–74.
Tibbetts, E. A. (2002). Visual signals of individual identity in the wasp *Polistes fuscatus*. *Proc. R. Soc. Lond. B* **269,** 1423–1428.
Tibbetts, E. A. (2004). Complex social behaviour can select for variability in visual features: A case study in *Polistes* wasps. *Proc. R. Soc. Lond. B* **271,** 1955–1960.
Tibbetts, E. A., and Curtis, T. R. (2007). Rearing conditions influence quality signals but not individual identity signals in *Polistes* wasps. *Behav. Ecol.* **18,** 602–607.
Tibbetts, E. A., and Dale, J. (2004). A socially enforced signal of quality in a paper wasp. *Nature* **432,** 218–222.
Tindo, M., and Dejean, A. (2000). Dominance hierarchy in colonies of *Belonogaster juncea juncea* (Vespidae, Polistinae). *Insect. Soc.* **47,** 158–163.
Togni, O. C., and Giannotti, E. (2007). Nest defense behavior against the attack of ants in colonies of pre-emergent *Mischocyttarus Cerberus* (Hymenoptera, Vespidae). *Sociobiology* **50,** 1–20.
Togni, O. C., and Giannotti, E. (2008). Nest defense behavior against ant attacks in post-emergent colonies of wasp *Mischocyttarus Cerberus* (Hymenoptera, Vespidae). *Acta Ethol.* **11,** 43–54.
Turillazzi, S. (1979). Tegumental glands in the abdomen of some European *Polistes* (Hymenoptera, Vespidae). *Monit. Zool. Ital.* **13,** 67–70.
Turillazzi, S. (1984). Defensive mechanisms in *Polistes* wasps. *In* "Defensive Mechanisms in Social Insects," (H. R. Herman, Ed.), pp. 33–58. New York Academic Press, New York.
Turillazzi, S. (1985). Function and characteristics of the abdominal substance secreted by wasps of the genus *Parischnogaster* (Hymenoptera Stenogastrinae). *Monit. Zool. Ital.* **19,** 91–99.
Turillazzi, S. (1989). The origin and evolution of social life in the Stenogastrinae (Hymenoptera: Vespidae). *J. Insect Behav.* **2,** 649–661.
Turillazzi, S. (1990). Social biology of *Liostenogaster vechti* Turillazzi 1988 (Hymenoptera Stenogastrinae). *Trop. Zool* **3,** 68–87.
Turillazzi, S. (1991). The Stenogastrinae. *In* "The Social Biology of Wasps," (K. G. Ross and R. W. Matthews, Eds.), pp. 74–98. Cornell University Press, Ithaca, NY.

Turillazzi, S. (1996). *Polistes* in perspective: Comparative social biology in *Belonogaster* and Stenogastrinae. *In* "Natural History and Evolution of Paper Wasps," (S. Turillazzi and M. J. West-Eberhard, Eds.), pp. 235–247. Oxford University Press, Oxford.
Turillazzi, S., and Calloni, C. (1983). Tegumental glands in the third gastral tergites of male *Parischnogaster nigricans serrei* (Du Buysson) and *P. Mellyi* (Saussure) (Hymenoptera Stenogastrinae). *Insect. Soc.* **30,** 455–460.
Turillazzi, S., and Cervo, R. (1982). Territorial behaviour in males of *P. nimpha* (Christ) (Hymenoptera, Vespidae). *Z. Tierpsychol.* **58,** 174–180.
Turillazzi, S., and Francescato, E. (1990). Patrolling behaviour and related secretory structures in the males of some stenogastrine wasps (Hymenoptera, Vespidae). *Insect. Soc.* **37,** 146–157.
Turillazzi, S., and Pardi, L. (1981). Ant guards on nests of *Parischnogaster nigricans serrei* (Buysson) (Stenogastrinae). *Monit. Zool. Ital. (N.S.)* **15,** 1–17.
Turillazzi, S., and Pardi, L. (1982). Social behavior of *Parischnogaster nigricans serrei* (Hymenoptera: Vespoidea) in Java. *Ann. Entomol. Soc. Am.* **75,** 657–664.
Turillazzi, S., and Ugolini, A. (1979). Rubbing behaviour in some European *Polistes* (Hymenoptera: Vespidae). *Monit. Zool. Ital. (N.S.)* **16,** 75–88.
Turillazzi, S. and West-Eberhard, M.J. (Eds.), (1996). Natural History and Evolution of Paper Wasps. Oxford University Press, Oxford. p. XIV+400.
Turillazzi, S., Cervo, R., and Cavallari, I. (1990). Invasion of the nest of *Polistes dominulus* by the social parasite *Sulcopolistes sulcifer* (Hymenoptera, Vespidae). *Ethology* **84,** 47–59.
Turillazzi, S., Sledge, M. F., Dani, F. R., Cervo, R., Massolo, A., and Fondelli, L. (2000). Social hackers: Integration in the host chemical recognition system by a paper wasp social parasite. *Naturwissenschaften* **87,** 172–176.
Turillazzi, S., Sledge, M. F., Dapporto, L., Landi, M., Fanelli, D., Fondelli, L., Zanetti, P., and Dani, F. R. (2004). Epicuticular lipids and fertility in primitively social wasps (Hymenoptera Stenogastrinae). *Physiol. Entomol.* **29,** 464–471.
Turillazzi, S., Mastrobuoni, G., Dani, F. R., Moneti, G., Pieraccini, G., La Marca, G., Bartolucci, G., Perito, B., Lambardi, D., Cavallini, V., and Dapporto, L. (2006a). Dominulin A and B: Two new antibacterial peptides identified on the cuticle and in the venom of the social paper wasp Polistes dominulus using MALDI-TOF, MALDI-TOF/TOF, and ESI-Ion Trap. *J. Am. Soc. Mass Spectr.* **17,** 376–383.
Turillazzi, S., Dapporto, L., Pansolli, C., Boulay, R., Dani, F. R., Moneti, G., and Pieraccini, G. (2006b). Habitually used hibernation sites of paper wasps are marked with venom and cuticular peptides. *Curr. Biol.* **16,** R530–R553.
Turillazzi, S., Bruschini, C., Lambardi, D., Francese, S., Spadolini, I., and Mastrobuoni, G. (2007). Comparison of the medium molecular weight venom fractions from five species of common social wasps by MALDI-TOF spectra profiling. *J. Mass Spectrom.* **42,** 199–205.
Turillazzi, S., Fanelli, D., Theodora, P., Lambardi, D., Ortolani, I., Hashim, R., and Baracchi, D. (2008). Determinant of immature brood and nest recognition in a stenogastrine wasp (Hymenoptera Vespidae). *Ethol. Ecol. Evol.* **20,** 17–33.
Van Hooser, C. A., Gamboa, G. J., and Fishwild, T. G. (2002). The function of abdominal stroking in the paper wasp, *Polistes fuscatus* (Hymenoptera Vespidae). *Ethol. Ecol. Evol.* **14,** 141–148.
Vander Meer, R.K., Breed, M.D., Winston, M.L., and Espelie, K.E. (Eds.), (1998). Pheromone Communication in Social Insects. Ants, Wasps, Bees and Termites. Westview Press, Boulder, CO. p. xi+368.
van der Vecht, J. (1968). The terminal gastral sternite of female and worker social wasps (Hymenoptera, Vespidae). *P. K. Ned. Akad. C Biol.* **71,** 411–422.
Veith, H. J., Koeniger, N., and Maschwitz, U. (1984). 2-Methyl-3-buten-2-ol a major component of the alarm pheromone of the hornet *Vespa crabro*. *Naturwissenschaften* **71,** 328–329.

Venkataraman, A. B., Swarnalatha, V. B., Nair, P., Vinutha, C., and Gadagkar, R. (1988). The mechanism of nestmate discrimination in the tropical social wasp *Ropalidia marginata* and its implications for the evolution of sociality. *Behav. Ecol. Sociobiol.* **23,** 271–279.

Wenzel, J. W. (1987). Male reproductive behaviour and mandibular glands in *Polistes major* (Hymenoptera: Vespidae). *Insect. Soc.* **34,** 44–57.

Wenzel, J. W. (1991). Evolution of nest architecture. *In* "The Social Biology of Wasps," (K. G. Ross and R. W. Matthews, Eds.), pp. 480–519. Cornell University Press, Ithaca, NY.

Wenzel, J. W. (1993). Application of the biogenetic law to behavioral ontogeny: A test using nest architecture in paper wasps. *J. Evol. Biol.* **6,** 229–247.

West-Eberhard, M. J. (1969). The Social Biology of Polistine Wasps. Miscellaneous Publications Museum of Zoology, University of Michigan. pp. 101.

West-Eberhard, M. J. (1977). The establishment of reproductive dominance in social wasp colonies. Proc. 8th Inter. Cong. Int. Union Study Soc. Insects pp. 223–227.

West-Eberhard, M. J. (1982). The nature and evolution of swarming in tropical social wasps (Vespidae, Polistine, Polybiini). *In* "Social Insects in the Tropics," (P. Jaisson, Ed.), Vol. 1, pp. 97–128. Université de Paris-Nord, Paris.

West-Eberhard, M. J. (1996). Wasp societies as microcosms for the study of development and evolution. *In* "Natural History and Evolution of Paper-Wasps," (S. Turillazzi and M. J. West-Eberhard, Eds.), pp. 290–317. Oxford University Press, Oxford.

Wilson, E. O. (1971). The Insect Societies. Harvard University Press, Cambridge, MA. pp. 548.

Wyatt, T. D. (2003). Pheromones and animal behaviour. Communication by Smell and Taste Cambridge University Press, Cambridge. pp. 391.

Zacchi, F., Cervo, R., and Turillazzi, S. (1996). How *Polistes semenowi*, obligate social parasite, invades the nests of its host, *Polistes dominulus* (Hymenoptera, Vespidae). *Insect Soc. Life* **1,** 125–130.

Zanetti, P., Dani, F. R., Destri, S., Fanelli, D., Massolo, A., Moneti, G., Pieraccini, G., and Turillazzi, S. (2001). Nestmate recognition in *Parischnogaster striatula* (Hymenoptera, Stenogastrinae), visual and olfactory recognition cues. *J. Insect Physiol.* **47,** 1013–1020.

CHAPTER TWENTY

New Pheromones and Insect Control Strategies

Gadi V. P. Reddy* *and* Angel Guerrero†

Contents

Abstract

A survey of the new environmentally safe strategies used for insect control is presented. The survey includes mating disruption, pheromone antagonists as chemical communication inhibitors, pheromones and plant-based volatiles, attractant-and-kill, and push–pull strategies. Important successes have been obtained, particularly in mating disruption with significant reduction in pesticide use in low to moderate pest infestations. One important factor of concern is the high cost of semiochemicals and formulations containing them in comparison to the conventional insecticide treatments, and a combined effort by scientists, producers, and farmers should be made to reduce the cost of application of these semiochemicals. © 2010 Elsevier Inc.

* Western Pacific Tropical Research Center, College of Natural and Applied Sciences, University of Guam, Mangilao, Guam, USA

† Department of Biological Chemistry and Molecular Modeling, Institute of Advanced Chemistry of Catalonia (CSIC), Barcelona, Spain

Vitamins and Hormones, Volume 83
ISSN 0083-6729, DOI: 10.1016/S0083-6729(10)83020-1

I. Introduction

Pheromones are chemicals produced by insects to induce a certain behavioral response on conspecific individuals. These compounds have many different effects and are named according to the elicited response, for example, sex pheromones, aggregation pheromones, alarm pheromones, etc. Some pheromones function as attractants, allowing individuals to detect and locate mates, whereas others induce trail-following, oviposition or aggregation in other congeners. Pheromones have become important tools for monitoring and controlling agricultural pest populations, and as such, a large compendium of over 1600 pheromones and sex attractants has been published in the past four decades (Witzgall *et al.*, 2004). Structurally, pheromones are mostly long chain unsaturated esters (mainly acetates), alcohols, and aldehydes, and species specificity is governed by the identity of the different components of the pheromone blend and by their relative proportions in the mixture.

Insect control by pheromones alone has precincts but they can be used in integrated control in conjunction with other practices (Howse *et al.*, 1998). The importance of pheromone-based strategies is emphasized by the continuously increasing problems associated with the use of conventional pesticides. Although insecticides have been traditionally precluded in integrated pest management (IPM) programs, the new concept of IPM, which includes set action thresholds, monitoring and identification of pests, prevention and control, allows also the use of minimum applications of low-risk pesticides. However and without doubt, pheromones play a dominant role in all stages of IPM programs.

In the past four decades, there has been a substantial volume of literature on insect pheromones and new opportunities have arisen to exploit the use of semiochemicals in managing insect pest problems (Reddy and Guerrero, 2004). In this review, we present a number of examples which emphasize the new concepts and ways insect pheromones have been used in new insect control strategies. The review, which covers the work done in the past 10 years, deals with the prospects and constraints of the current insect control strategies and outlines the need of developing novel approaches in IPM programs.

II. Mating Disruption in Insect Control Programs

Mating disruption has been the most successful approach for pest control over the past few decades. The release of large amounts of pheromone into a crop to prevent or delay mating has been remarkably efficient in a variety of cases, so that it is now an accepted control option for a number of lepidopteran pests of fruits, vegetables, and forests (Gut *et al.*, 2004) (Table 20.1). Important successes of mating disruption include control of the codling moth *Cydia pomonella* in pome fruit, the oriental fruit moth *Grapholita molesta* in stone fruit peaches and nectarines, the tomato pinworm *Keiferia lycopersicella* in vegetables, the pink bollworm *Pectinophora gossypiella* in cotton, and the omnivorous leafroller *Platynota stultana* in vineyards (Il'ichev *et al.*, 2006; Welter *et al.*, 2005)

There has been a strong debate about the mechanisms underlying mating disruption, which fall into two main categories either through "false trails" or by sensory overload. There is general agreement, however, in that the proposed mechanisms by which mating disruption works are not mutually exclusive, and that several mechanisms may be present for a specific pest under different conditions and different species respond differently to prolonged exposures to pheromone (Howse *et al.*, 1998).

The effectiveness of mating disruption is strongly related to population density. In many cases, high-density insect populations are more difficult to control than less dense infestations. For example, Borchert and Walgenbach (2000) found that mating disruption was not effective in orchards with high-density populations of the tufted apple bud moth *Platynota idaeusalis*. Also, Vickers *et al.* (1998) reported that neither mating disruption alone nor when supplemented with insecticides gave commercially acceptable levels (<0.2% damage at harvest) of control of the codling moth *Cydia pomonella* in other than low-density populations. In this case, the surface treated to control this moth by mating disruption in the Northwest United States increased from 1000 ha in 1991 to ~45,000 ha in 2000 (Brunner *et al.*, 2002). Other successful mating disruption experiments in low-density infestations have been reported to control the gypsy moth *Lymantria dispar* (Onufrieva *et al.*, 2008; Sharov *et al.*, 2002), and the chestnut tortrix *Cydia splendana* (Antonaroli, 2000) (Table 20.1).

In open landscapes, such as parks, residential areas, commercial sites, etc. with a much lower density of trees than in a forest, mating disruption has resulted in an effective treatment for the eradication of isolated, low-density gypsy moth populations when males and females were initially deployed at least 1 m apart on separate trees (Onufrieva *et al.*, 2008). However, mating disruption was not as effective when the infestation was concentrated on a small number of trees and males and females were close to each other in space and time (Onufrieva *et al.*, 2008).

An important issue in mating disruption experiments is to measure the efficacy of the formulations. Capture of zero (complete shutdown) or very few moths in pheromone-baited traps within the crop is the most common parameter used to indicate successful disruption of the pest. However, it is not uncommon to record low catches in traps and still detect a substantial number of mated females (Atanasov *et al.*, 2002). One of the successful

Table 20.1 Recent examples of pheromone mediated mating disruption as promising strategy shown in Lepidopteran insects

Scientific name	Common name	Family	Host plants	References
Adoxophyes honmai	Smaller tea tortrix moth	Tortricidae	Tea	Mochizuki *et al.* (2002)
Adoxophyes orana	Summer fruit tortrix moth	Tortricidae	Orchard	Navrozidis *et al.* (2005)
Adoxophyes orana fasciata	Summer fruit tortrix moth	Tortricidae	Orchard	Okazaki *et al.* (2001)
Anarsia lineatella	Peach twig borer	Tortricidae	Orchard	Trematerra *et al.* (2000)
Argyrotaenia velutinana	Redbanded leafroller	Tortricidae	Orchard	Stelinski *et al.* (2004)
Ascotis selenaria cretacea	Japanese giant looper	Geometridae	Garden	Ohtani *et al.* (2001)
Bonagota cranaodes	Brazilian apple leafroller	Tortricidae	Apple	Coracini *et al.* (2001)
Cameraria ohridella	Horse chestnut leafminer	Gracillariidae	Horse chestnut	Grodner *et al.* (2008) and Siekmann *et al.* (2009)
Chilo suppressalis	Rice stripped stem borer	Pyralidae	Rice	Sheng *et al.* (2000), Yang *et al.* (2001), and Alfaro *et al.* (2009)
Choristoneura rosaceana	Obliquebanded leafroller	Tortricidae	Apple	Trimble and Appleby (2004)
Cryptophlebia illepida	Koa seedworm	Tortricidae	Koa	Jones and Aihara-Sasaki (2001)
Cryptoblabes gnidiella	Honeydew moth	Pyralidae	Vineyards	Gordon *et al.* (2003)
Cydia fagiglandana	Beech moth	Tortricidae	Chestnut	Antonaroli (2000)
Cydia nigricana	Pea moth	Tortricidae	Pea	Witzgall *et al.* (1996, 2008)
Cydia pomonella	Codling moth	Tortricidae	Fruits/orchards	Femenia-Ferreri *et al.* (2007) and Welter and Cave (2007)
Cydia splendana	Chestnut tortrix	Tortricidae	Chestnut	Antonaroli (2000)
Cydia strobilella	Spruce cone moth	Tortricidae	Orchard	Trudel *et al.* (2006)
Cydia trasias	Chinese tortrix	Tortricidae	Pagoda tree	Zhang *et al.* (2003)
Dioryctria amatella	Southern pine coneworm	Pyralidae	Orchard	Debarr *et al.* (2000)
Ectomyelois ceratoniae	Carob moth	Pyralidae	Orchard	Vetter *et al.* (2006)
Endopiza viteana	Grape berry moth	Tortricidae	Grape	Trimble *et al.* (2003)

Ephestia cautella	Almond moth	Pyralidae	Stored products	Shani and Clearwater (2001) and Ryne *et al.* (2006)
Ephestia kuehniella	Mediterranean flour moth	Pyralidae	Stored products	Sieminska *et al.* (2009) and Camilla *et al.* (2007)
Epiphyas postvittana	Light brown apple moth	Tortricidae	Orchards	Il'ichev (2006) and Mo *et al.* (2006)
Eucosma sonomana	Western pine shoot borer	Tortricidae	Pine	Gillette *et al.* (2006)
Eupoecilia ambiguella	Vine moth	Tortricidae	Grape	Ciglar *et al.* (2002)
Euproctis pseudoconspersa	Tea tussock moth	Tea	Tea	Wang *et al.* (2005)
Euzophera pinguis	Olive pyralid moth	Pyralidae	Olive	Ortiz *et al.* (2007)
Grapholita molesta (previously known as *Cydia molesta*)	Oriental fruit moth	Tortricidae	Peaches and nectarines	Kovanci *et al.* (2004), Il'ichev *et al.* (2006), and Welter *et al.* (2005)
Helicoverpa armigera	American bollworm	Noctuidae	Cotton and vegetables	Toyoshima *et al.* (2001) and Kehat and Dunkelblum (1990)
Ichneumonoptera chrysophanes	Clearwing borer	Sesiidae	Persimmon	Vickers (2002)
Keiferia lycopersicella	Tomato pinworm	Gelechiidae	Vegetables	Welter *et al.* (2005)
Leucoptera coffeella	Coffee leaf miner	Lyonetiidae	Coffee	Ambrogi *et al.* (2006)
Lobesia botrana	European grapevine moth	Tortricidae	Grape	Louis and Schirra (2001) and Gordon *et al.* (2005)
Lymantria dispar	Gypsy moth	Lymantriidae	Trees, shrubs, and landscapes	Sharov *et al.* (2002), Tcheslavskaia *et al.* (2005), and Onufrieva *et al.* (2008)
Mamestra brassicae	Cabbage moth	Noctuidae	Cabbage	Kakizaki (2002)
Paralobesia viteana	Grape berry moth	Tortricidae	Vineyards	Jenkins and Isaacs (2008)
Orgyia pseudotsugata	Douglas-fir tussock moth	Lymantriidae	Douglas-fir and true firs	Cook *et al.* (2005)
Ostrinia nubilalis	European corn borer	Crambidae	Corn/Maize	Eizaguirre *et al.* (2002)
Palpita unionalis	Jasmine moth	Pyralidae	Olive	Hegazi *et al.* (2005)

(continued)

Table 20.1 (*continued*)

Scientific name	Common name	Family	Host plants	References
Pectinophora gossypiella	Pink bollworm	Gelechiidae	Cotton	Lykouressis *et al.* (2004, 2005) and Koch *et al.* (2009)
Phyllocnistis citrella	Citrus leafminer	Gracillariidae	Citrus	Mafi *et al.* (2005) and Stelinski *et al.* (2009)
Phyllonorycter ringoniella	Apple leafminer	Gracillariidae	Apple	Trimble and Tyndall (2000)
Platynota idaeusalis	Tufted apple bud moth	Tortricidae	Apple	Meissner *et al.* (2001) and Borchert and Walgenbach (2000)
Platynota stultana	Omnivorous leafroller	Tortricidae	Vineyards	Welter *et al.* (2005)
Plodia interpunctella	Indian meal moth	Pyralidae	Stored products	Svensson *et al.* (2003) and Camilla *et al.* (2007)
Plutella xylostella	Diamondback moth	Plutellidae	Vegetables	Schroeder *et al.* (2000) and Zeng *et al.* (2007)
Prays oleae	Olive moth	Yponomeutidae	Olive	Mazomenos *et al.* (2002)
Rhopobota naevana	Blackheaded fireworm	Tortricidae	Cranberry	Fitzpatrick *et al.* (2004), Fitzpatrick (2006), and Gillette *et al.* (2006)
Rhyacionia zozana	Ponderosa pine tip moth	Tortricidae	Pine	Gillette *et al.* (2006)
Scirpophaga incertulas	Rice yellow stem borer	Pyralidae	Rice	Varma *et al.* (2002)
Sesamia nonagrioides	Corn stalk borer	Noctuidae	Corn	Albajes *et al.* (2002), and Eizaguirre *et al.* (2002)
Sitotroga cerealella	Angoumois grain moth	Gelechiidae	Stored products	Fadamiro and Baker (2002)
Sparganothis sulfureana	Blueberry leafroller	Tortricidae	Cranberries	Polavarapu *et al.* (2001)
Spilonota ocellana	Eye-spotted budmoth	Apple	Grape	Mcbrien *et al.* (1998)
Spodoptera exigua	Beet armyworm	Noctuidae	Cotton	Mitchell and Mayer (2001)

Synanthedon tipuliformis	Currant clearwing	Sesiidae	Currant and Ribes crops	Grassi *et al.* (2002) and Suckling *et al.* (2005)
Tecia (Scrobipalpopsis) solanivora	Guatemalan potato moth	Gelechiidae	Potato	Bosa *et al.* (2005)
Trichoplusia ni	Cabbage looper	Noctuidae	Cabbage	Spohn *et al.* (2003)
Tuta absoluta	Tomato leafminer	Gelechiidae	Tomato	Filhoa *et al.* (2000), and Ferrara *et al.* (2004)
Vitacea polistiformis	Grape root borer	Sesiidae	Grape	Weihman and Liburd (2006)

approaches to increase moth captures has been to increase the amount of pheromone in the lures. For example, catches of codling moth males in disrupted orchards increased considerably when traps were baited with 10–20 mg of pheromone or by placing traps in the upper canopy (Gut *et al.*, 2004). However, deployment of high-load pheromone traps alone is not enough to assess the effectiveness of the disruption treatment and should be complementary to regular visual inspection of the fruit for possible damage.

A variety of pheromone-dispensing technologies in mating disruption has been developed over the years, and many of them have shown promise and success in the market. They include microencapsulation, in which small droplets of pheromone are enclosed within a polymer matrix; hand applied dispensers in the form of laminate systems; polymer spirals and ropes, for instance, the traditional hollow fibers employed in the 1970s; and the most recent high-emission dispensers, which have been developed to emit larger quantities of pheromone in fewer numbers of dispensers per hectares to cut down labor costs (Shorey and Gerber, 1996). These high-load release devices consist of a pressurized aerosol can ("puffer") containing a solution of pheromone in ethanol, a valving mechanism periodically triggered by a timing device, and a power source. The primary advantages of these devices are higher chemical stability of the pheromone while in the reservoir, high release of pheromone in a unique deployment, possibility of releasing pheromone blends of several pests simultaneously, and substantial labor savings. A commercially available puffer by Suterra Co. releases the pheromone of the codling moth for up to 180 days, and in low to moderate pest populations the puffer can provide control of the pest to a level equivalent to conventional insecticides (Steinmann *et al.*, 2008). New devices in the form of large polymer bags loaded with large amounts of pheromones have been developed to avoid the use of batteries and other moving parts of the puffers (Welter *et al.*, 2005).

In highly mobile pests, such as *Plutella xylostella*, mating disruption may be difficult to evaluate because pheromone and insects may move freely between plots, which often limits the ability to have experimental replications and untreated controls (Schroeder *et al.*, 2000). The use of screened field cages infested with *P. xylostella* pupae, prior to emergence, prevented immigration or emigration of the pest, but even under these highly controlled conditions the authors did not detect any mating suppression or decrease in the population of the subsequent generation (Schroeder *et al.*, 2000). These results provide evidence of the difficulty in conducting successful disruption experiments in highly mobile pests.

Undoubtedly, additional work is needed to develop mating disruption as a reliable tool for managing insect population on crops and nonagricultural ecosystems. Research on pheromone release rates and different dispenser types would help in showing if the control failures observed were caused by inadequate amounts of pheromone, dispenser placement, or by excessively high population densities. Additionally, information on the dispersal and movement of insects into the ecosystem is required to determine the minimum trapping area for mating disruption, and to know whether spraying orchard borders with insecticide is necessary. Nevertheless, it is a general feeling among the scientific community that mating disruption, if effective, is an excellent technique to consider in IPM approaches.

III. Pheromone Antagonists as Chemical Communication Inhibitors

Mating disruption failures may be mainly caused by two reasons: a very high population and a wrong pheromone formulation. In this case, impurities present in the pheromone, minor pheromone components added in wrong proportions or interspecific pheromone components can act as pheromone antagonists inhibiting upwind flight to the lure (Fadamiro *et al.*, 1999). The possibility of interfering the chemical communication channels of insect pests by semiochemicals represents another approach with potential use in pest management programs. These compounds, generally called *parapheromones* (Renou and Guerrero, 2000), are chemicals of anthropogenic origin unknown to exist in nature but structurally related to natural pheromone components that in some way affect physiologically or behaviorally the insect pheromone communication system. Many disruption experiments have used analogues of natural pheromones, such as alcohols when the natural pheromone compounds are acetates, synthetic geometric isomers of the pheromone, formate esters instead of the parent pheromone aldehydes, etc. Although the complete blend of the natural pheromone components is generally the best formulation for mating disruption, mixtures of these components and attraction antagonists have been efficient for mating disruption of *Synanthedon pictipes*, *Eupoecilia ambiguella*, and *Planotortrix octo* (Renou and Guerrero, 2000). Remarkably, in *C. pomonella* pheromone antagonists have resulted in more potent communication disruptants than the pheromone itself (McDonough *et al.*, 1996). Communication disruption trials have been applied also for *Ostrinia nubilalis* with the acetylenic analogue of the pheromone 11-tetradecynyl acetate at a rate of 66.4 g/ha. Also, the 2-fluoro analogue of the pheromone caused mating suppression at concentrations equivalent to that needed with the pheromone (Klun *et al.*, 1997). It should be noted that pheromone antagonists inhibit upwind flight only when they are completely mixed with the pheromone because males have been found to discern pheromone and antagonist plumes when they are separated 1 mm and 1 ms apart (Fadamiro *et al.*, 1999) (Table 20.2).

Pheromone inhibitors should be active at concentrations similar to the pheromone and they should inhibit specific components of the peripheral

Table 20.2 Recent compounds described as communication inhibitors on various insect pests

Compound inhibitor	Organism	Order: Family	References
3-Octylthio-1,1,1-trifluoro-2-propanone	*Sesamia nonagrioides*	Lepidoptera: Noctuidae	Reddy *et al.* (2002b) and Riba *et al.* (2001)
	Spodoptera littoralis	Lepidoptera: Noctuidae	
(*Z*)-11-Hexadecenyl trifluoromethyl ketone	*Sesamia nonagrioides*	Lepidoptera: Noctuidae	Bau *et al.* (1999), Riba *et al.* (2001), and Quero *et al.* (2004)
n-Dodecyl trifluoromethyl ketone	*Sesamia nonagrioides*	Lepidoptera: Noctuidae	Riba *et al.* (2001)
n-Hexadecyl trifluoromethyl ketone	*Sesamia nonagrioides*	Lepidoptera: Noctuidae	Riba *et al.* (2001)
(*Z*)-1,1,1-Trifluoro-15-octadecen-13-yn-2-one and (*Z*)-1,1,1-trifluoro-16-nonadecen-14-yn-2-one	*Thaumetopoea pityocampa*	Lepidoptera: Thaumetopoeidae	Parrilla and Guerrero (1994)
(*Z*)-11-Hexadecenyl trifluoromethyl ketone	*Ostrinia nubilalis*	Lepidoptera: Pyralidae	Solé *et al.* (2008)
n-Decylthiotrifluoropropanone	*Bombyx mori*	Lepidoptera: Bombycidae	Pophof *et al.* (2000)
(*E*,*E*)-8,10-Dodecadienyl trifluoromethyl ketone	*Cydia pomonella*	Lepidoptera: Tortricidae	Giner *et al.* (2009)
(*Z*)-11-Tetradecenyl acetate, (*E*)-11-tetradecenyl acetate, (Z)-11-tetradecenol, (Z)-11-tetradecenal, and (Z)-9-tetradecenyl acetate	*Pandemis pyrusana*	Lepidoptera: Tortricidae	Curkovic and Brunner (2007)
	Choristoneura rosaceana		
2-(1-Phenylethylamino)-2-oxazoline, 2-(2-ethyl-6-ethylanilino)oxazolidine, 2-(2-methylbenzylamino)-2-thiazoline, and 2-(2,6-diethylanilino)thiazolidine	*Plodia interpunctella*	Lepidoptera: Pyralidae	Hirashima *et al.* (2003)
(*Z*)-5-Decenyl acetate and (*Z*)-9-tetradecenyl acetate	*Autographa gamma*	Lepidoptera: Noctuidae	Subchev *et al.* (2009)
(*Z*)-3-Hexen-1-ol	*Pityogenes chalcographus*	Coleoptera: Scolytidae	Byers *et al.* (1998)
1-Hexanol	*Ips typographus*		
(*Z*)-11-Tetradecenyl acetate and (*E*)-11-tetradecenyl acetate	*Sesamia nonagrioides*	Lepidoptera: Noctuidae	Eizaguirre *et al.* (2007)
(*Z*)-11-Hexadecenal	*Ostrinia nubilalis*	Lepidoptera: Pyralidae	Gemeno *et al.* (2006) and Linn *et al.* (2007)

olfactory system so that the insect response threshold to the pheromone is increased (Plettner, 2002). To reach the sensory cells, pheromone inhibitors should be bound to and be transported by pheromone binding proteins (PBPs). In this context, trifluoromethylketones (TFMKs) and their β-thio derivatives (β-thiotrifluoropropanones) are good disruptants of pheromone perception and their inhibitory activity has been established in a number of moth species, *S. littoralis* (Durán *et al.*, 1993; Rosell *et al.*, 1996), *P. xylostella* (Prestwich and Streinz, 1988), *Thaumetopoea pityocampa* (Parrilla and Guerrero, 1994), *Sesamia nonagrioides* (Bau *et al.*, 1999; Riba *et al.*, 2001), *Mamestra brassicae* (Renou *et al.*, 1997), *O. nubilalis* (Riba *et al.*, 2005), *Antheraea polyphemus* (Vogt *et al.*, 1985), *Bombyx mori* (Pophof *et al.*, 2000), and *C. pomonella* (Giner *et al.*, 2009) (Fig. 20.1). These compounds have been reported to be bound to the PBPs and transported to the sensillum lymph in competition with pheromone molecules, facilitating interaction with the pheromone catabolic enzymes (Campanacci *et al.*, 1999; Feixas *et al.*, 1995; Pophof *et al.*, 2000). Also, TFMKs reversibly inhibit *in vitro* the antennal esterases responsible for the pheromone catabolism (pheromone degrading enzymes, PDEs) in male olfactory tissues with IC_{50} values in the range 0.3–10 μM, being particularly effective 3-octylthiotrifluoropropanone (OTFP) and structurally-close TFMK analogues of the pheromone (Durán *et al.*, 1993; Riba *et al.*, 2005; Rosell *et al.*, 1996). These chemicals act as transition-state analogues of the enzyme, the inhibition activity arising by formation of a stable hemiacetal of tetrahedral geometry between the serine residue of the esterase with the highly electrophilic carbonyl. OTFP has been found also as an oviposition deterrent on second instar larvae of *S. littoralis* and

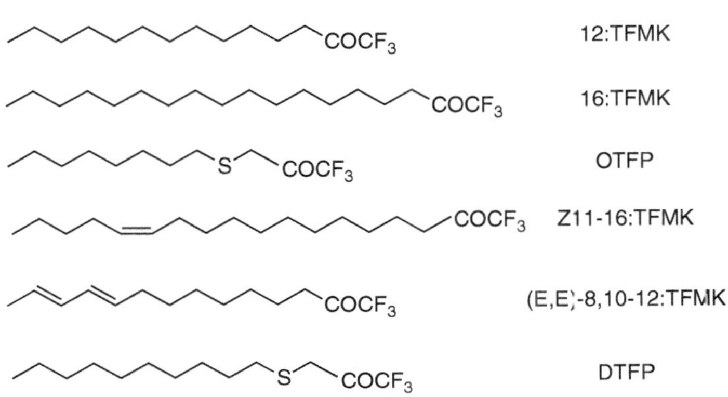

Figure 20.1 Structures of *n*-dodecyl trifluoromethyl ketone (12:TFMK), *n*-hexadecyl trifluoromethyl ketone (16:TFMK), 3-octylthio-1,1,1-trifluoro-2-propanone (OTFP), (*Z*)-11-hexadecenyl trifluoromethyl ketone (*Z*11-16:TFMK), (*E*,*E*)-8,10-dodecadienyl trifluoromethyl ketone ((*E*,*E*)-8,10-12:TFMK), and 3-decylthio-1,1,1-trifluoro-2-propanone (DTFP) as communication inhibitors of some insect pests (see Table 20.2).

S. nonagrioides reducing food consumption and growth, pupation and adult emergence (Reddy *et al.*, 2002b). In addition, adult males, previously treated with this chemical at the larval stage, were less attracted to the pheromone or virgin females than untreated males (Reddy *et al.*, 2002b).

In wind tunnel, TFMKs elicited a disruptive effect when males were allowed to fly toward a source baited with mixtures of the pheromone and TFMK analogues particularly in the source contact behavior (Bau *et al.*, 1999; Giner *et al.*, 2009; Renou *et al.*, 1997; Riba *et al.*, 2001, 2005). Presence of these analogues at the lure induced a highly erratic flight in males in contrast to the much more oriented flight onto the plume shown by control insects. In the field, these chemicals displayed a significant decrease in the number of males caught in traps baited with mixtures of the pheromone and the antagonist compared to the pheromone alone (Giner *et al.*, 2009; Riba *et al.*, 2001, 2005). In large scale treatments on maize fields, a remarkable reduction in damage (86–90% reduction in the number of plants attacked and 67–98% reduction in the number of larvae per plant in treated fields) caused by *S. nonagrioides* and *O. nubilalis* using (*Z*)-11-hexadecenyl trifluoromethyl ketone, an analogue of the major component of *S. nonagrioides* pheromone, has been noticed (Solé *et al.*, 2008). The low toxicity on mice shown by this chemical (LD_{50} of 1 g/kg body weight), in comparison to that of the supposedly innocuous pheromone (LD_{50} of 5 g/kg body weight), in addition to good stability in the field and easy preparation on multigram scale, makes this compound an attractive choice to consider in future alternative approaches to control the pest (Solé *et al.*, 2008).

IV. Use of Pheromones with Plant-Based Volatiles

Some plant volatiles are considered an integral part of the pheromone system of many coleopteran species investigated so far. How mixtures of pheromone components and plant volatiles are integrated into the insects olfactory systems so that they can discriminate pheromone molecules alone and pheromone plus odor plume strands, and respond behaviorally to these signals is a question of increasing importance (Baker and Heath, 2004). As a matter of fact, a number of field-trapping experiments have demonstrated that the attractiveness of pheromone blends may be enhanced by specific host plant volatiles (Light *et al.*, 1993). However, it is not clear whether enhancement of the male attraction to the traps is due to separate increased responses of the insects to the pheromone or the plant volatiles or to a response of the global mixture as an entirely unique odor (Table 20.3).

Table 20.3 Recent examples of synergism of host volatiles and pheromone

Host	Insect	Plant volatiles	Pheromone compounds	References
Brassica oleracea subsp. *capitata*	*Plutella xylostella*	(*Z*)-3-Hexenyl acetate, (*E*)-2-hexenal, (*Z*)-3-hexenol, hexanal, 1-hexanol, 1-hexen-3-ol, and hexyl acetate	(*Z*)-11-Hexadecenal, (*Z*)-11-hexadecenyl acetate, and (*Z*)-11-hexadecenol	Reddy and Guerrero (2000)
Plutella xylostella	*Trichogramma chilonis*, *Cotesia plutellae*, and *Chrysoperla carnea*	(*Z*)-3-Hexenyl acetate, (*E*)-2-hexenal, (*Z*)-3-hexenol, hexanal, 1-hexanol, 1-hexen-3-ol, and hexyl acetate	(*Z*)-11-hexadecenal, (*Z*)-11-hexadecenyl acetate, and (*Z*)-11-hexadecenol	Reddy *et al.* (2002a)
Pinus sylvestris	*Hylotrupes bajulus*	(+)-α-Pinene, (−)-verbenone, (−)-*trans*-pinocarveol, and (+)-terpinen-4-ol	(3*R*)-3-Hydroxy-2-hexanone (3*R*)-ketol) and 1-butanol	Fettköther *et al.* (2000) and Reddy *et al.* (2005b,c)
Pinus sylvestris	*Hylotrupes bajulus*	Ethyl acetate	(3*R*)-3-Hydroxy-2-hexanone (3*R*)-ketol) and 1-butanol	Reddy (2007)
Cocos nucifera, *Areca catechu*, *Saccharum officinarum*, and ornamental palms	*Rhabdoscelus obscurus*	Ethyl acetate	2-Methyl-4-octanol, (*E*)-6-methyl-2-hepten-4-ol (rhynchophorol), and 2-methyl-4-heptanol	Muniappan *et al.* (2004) and Reddy *et al.* (2005a)
Malus domestica and other tree fruits	*Cydia pomonella*	(*Z*)-3-Hexenol	(*E*,*E*)-8,10-Dodecadienol (codlemone)	Yang *et al.* (2004)
Prunus spp.	*Rhopalosiphum padi* and *Phorodon humuli*	Benzaldehyde and methyl salicylate	(1*R*,4a*S*,7*S*,7a*R*)- and (1*RS*,4a*R*,7*S*,7a*S*)-nepetalactol	Pope *et al.* (2007)

(*continued*)

Table 20.3 (*continued*)

Host	Insect	Plant volatiles	Pheromone compounds	References
Many different plants (i.e., polyphagous)	*Helicoverpa zea*	Linalool and (*Z*)-3-hexenol	(*Z*)-11-Hexadecenal	Ochieng *et al.* (2002)
Crops and ornamental plants	*Spodoptera exigua*	Benzaldehyde, phenylacetaldehyde, (*Z*)-3-hexenyl acetate, and linalool	Tetradecanol, (*Z*)-9-tetradecenol, (*E*)-9-tetradecenol, (*Z*,*E*)-9,12-tetradecadienol, and (*Z*,*Z*)-9,12-tetradecadienol	Deng *et al.* (2004a)
Many different plants (i.e., polyphagous)	*Helicoverpa armigera*	Phenyl acetaldehyde, benzyl alcohol, phenylethanol, methylsalicylate, linalool, benzaldehyde, (*Z*)-3-hexenol, (*Z*)-3-hexenyl acetate, (*Z*)-6-nonenol, cineole, (*E*)-2-hexenal, and geraniol	(*Z*)-11-Hexadecenal and (*Z*)-9-hexadecenal	Deng *et al.* (2004b)
Many different plants (i.e., polyphagous)	*Gnathotrichus sulcatus*	(*E*)-2-Hexenol	(*R*)-Sulcatol	Deglow and Borden (1998)
Many different plants (i.e., polyphagous)	*Spodoptera littoralis*	Linalool	(*Z*,*E*)-9,11-Tetradecadienyl acetate	Party *et al.* (2009)
Morus spp.	*Bombyx mori*	A mulberry leaf volatile	Bombykol and (*Z*)-3-hexenol	Namiki *et al.* (2008)

Green leaf volatiles (GLVs), a short chain (six carbon atoms) group of alcohols, acetates, and aldehydes, can enhance or interrupt the behavioral responses of insects to their pheromones depending on the species and the context in which they are encountered. For example, release of the GLV (*E*)-2-hexenol with the boll weevil aggregation pheromone resulted in more than twice as many weevils caught in traps compared to the pheromone alone (Aldrich *et al.*, 2003). Pheromones of other insects associated with deciduous plants, such as the corn earworm and the codling moth, were also enhanced by GLVs (Light *et al.*, 1993). By contrast, the GLVs *n*-hexanol and hexanal promoted a decrease of the pheromone response in bark beetle *Ips avulsus* infesting southern pines. More recently, disruption of pheromone responses by GLVs in the red pine cone beetle *Conophthorus resinosae*, the Douglas-fir beetle *Dendroctonus pseudotsugae*, the spruce bark beetle *Ips typographus,* and the pine shoot beetle *Tomicus piniperda* have been reported (Aldrich *et al.*, 2003). The diamondback moth *P. xylostella* uses (*Z*)-3-hexenyl acetate, one of the ubiquitous components in many GLVs, as a key chemical to locate its host (Reddy and Guerrero, 2000). The compound combined with the synthetic pheromone evoked the highest response of male moths of any other single GLV of the host. Single cell recordings from antennal receptors have revealed that not only some olfactory receptor neurons (ORNs) responded selectively to GLVs but also that these chemicals synergized responses of pheromone-specific ORNs (Ochieng *et al.*, 2002).

Plants under aphid attack release volatile compounds that trigger chemical defense mechanisms in neighboring plants. The emitted volatiles attract aphid predators, methyl salicylate being particularly active in these interactions (Norin, 2001). In the presence of this compound, the colonization density of aphids in the crop is remarkably reduced. Methyl salicylate acts as an antiaphrodisiac and males of the butterfly *Pieris napi* refrain from mating virgin females to whom extremely small amounts (20 ng per female) of the compound have been applied.

Many coniferophagous Scolytidae detect and respond to volatiles from nonhost angiosperm trees. These volatiles were tested for their ability to disrupt the attraction of sawyer beetles, *Monochamus* spp. (Coleoptera, Cerambycidae) to traps baited with host volatiles and pheromones. Of the compounds tested, only conophthorin disrupted the attraction of the beetles to the bark beetle pheromones ipsenol and ipsdienol (Morewood *et al.*, 2003). Conophthorin, as other GLVs such as (*Z*)-3-hexenol, elicited strong Electroantennogram (EAG) responses on antennae of *Monochamus spp*. The chemical was also previously reported to inhibit attraction to aggregation pheromones or host kairomones in many species of Scolytidae (Morewood *et al.*, 2003), with the exception of *Pityophthorus carmeli* for which conophthorin was highly attractive in combination with the pheromone pityol (Dallara *et al.*, 2000). In summary, the effect displayed of the GLVs at the insect receptor level along with the different responses induced when mixed with pheromones make these chemicals an interesting subject to consider in future IPM strategies.

V. Attract-and-Kill

The attracticide ("attract-and-kill") concept-based method consists of using pheromone or other attractant semiochemicals to lure insects to a specific point source or area containing a conventional insecticide. This method is similar to mass trapping but many more insects are affected because the attracticide is spread over a larger area and the killing effect is not limited to individual traps (Trematerra, 2002). Despite considerable research, there are few successfully commercialized attracticides. For example, attract-and-kill has been reported to work efficiently against codling moth and a commercial product ("Sirene" by Novartis) has been registered in Switzerland (Charmillot and Hofer, 1997). Other successful examples include control of the Japanese beetle *Popillia japonica*, in which the lure is a dual-scented trap, one scent is a floral lure to attract females and the other is the sex pheromone that lures males, and for the pink bollworm, *P. gossypiella*, in which the pheromone (*Z*,*Z*)- and (*Z*,*E*)-7,11-hexadecadienyl acetate is dispensed in a variety of formulations, some of them containing an insecticide (permethrin). An alternative to conventional pesticides could be the use of insect pathogens as biopesticides if they can kill the attracted insects before mating occurs. The aim of this tactic is not to kill the insects right away but rather to use them as vector of the disease into the population. A major advantage of this approach is that it can generate disease outbreaks that can multiply in the area greatly affecting the pest population. This approach has been explored with a nucleopolyhydrosis virus against tobacco budworm, a granulosis virus against codling moth and *Plodia interpunctella*, and a fungus against *P. xylostella* and *P. japonica*, among others (Suckling and Karg, 1998).

In stored-products protection, use of attracticides has been promising in flour mills and confectionary industries for control of *Ephestia kuehniella* and *Ephestia cautella*. Thus, in Italian mills, *E. kuehniella* males were successfully lured to laminar dispensers containing (*Z*,*E*)-9,12-tetradecadienyl acetate, the major component of the pheromone, and then treated with cypermethrin. This caused a marked decrease in moth population at the mill with the consequent reduction in chemical treatments (Trematerra, 2002).

In addition to pheromones, olfactory attractants have been also used to lure insects to traps, which often contain an insecticide. For example, tsetse flies have been the target of extensive trapping trials in Africa. Analysis of volatiles from cattle and their urine allowed discovery of attractive compounds, including acetone, 1-octen-3-ol, 3-propylphenol, and 4-methylphenol, that have been used in certain blends in conjunction with visual cues to attract tsetse flies to insecticide-laden screens (Leak, 1999). One of the most serious fruit and vegetable insect pests worldwide is the Mediterranean fruit fly, *Ceratitis capitata*. A notably effective commercially available lure for this insect, which has been effective for monitoring and mass trapping programs, is based on compounds of protein degradation, such as putrescine and trimethylamine, in combination with ammonium acetate (Baker and Heath, 2004).

VI. Push–Pull Strategies

Push–pull strategies involve a combination of repellent and attractive stimuli, which are usually deployed simultaneously, to control distribution and abundance of a pest. The pests are repelled or deterred away from the resource (crop or farm) ("push") using stimuli that mask host apparency or are just repellent or deterrent (Cook *et al.*, 2007). The insects are simultaneously attracted ("pull") using attractive stimuli to other areas, such as traps or crops, where they can be eliminated. Stimuli for push components include visual cues, repellents, host and nonhost volatiles, antiaggregation pheromones, alarm pheromones, antifeedants, and oviposition-deterrent pheromones. Pull components include visual stimuli, host volatiles, sex and aggregation pheromones, and oviposition and gustatory stimulants (Cook *et al.*, 2007).

Development of push–pull strategies has been mainly directed to agricultural systems to manage insecticide resistance threats or diminish the use of insecticides. Examples of push–pull strategies using pheromones include control of the pea leaf weevil, *Sitona lineatus*, in peas or beans. The male-produced aggregation pheromone "pull" weevils away from a pea or bean crop, whereas an antifeedant, such as neem oil from the neem tree *Azadirachta indica*, "push" weevils away from the crop. The attracted weevils to the trap crop were treated with insecticide to reduce weevil populations (Smart *et al.*, 1994). Neem oil effectively deters feeding on *fava* beans and significantly reduced weevil damage and larval populations relative to control plants.

Natural control of aphids by their parasitoids can be achieved by using the aphid sex pheromone component *nepetalactone* and the plant volatile (*Z*)-jasmone, to which aphid parasitoids are attracted. To push the parasitoids from surrounding areas to the treatment crop, it used the recently discovered lady beetle pheromone, tricosane and pentacosane, used by the aphid parasitoid *Aphidius ervi* to avoid predation by the sevenspotted lady beetle (Powell and Pickett, 2003).

In the forest, push–pull strategies have shown remarkable promise to control bark beetles (Scolytidae) using aggregation and antiaggregation pheromones. For instance, the antiaggregation pheromone 3-methylcyclohex-2-

en-1-one (push) and traps baited with aggregation pheromones (frontalin, seudenol, 1-methylcyclohex-2-enol and ethanol) (pull) reduced populations of the Douglas-fir beetle *D. pseudotsugae* (Ross and Daterman, 1994). Populations of other forest pests, such as the mountain pine beetle *Dendroctonus ponderosae*, the southern pine beetle *Dendroctonus frontalis*, and the spruce bark beetle *I. paraconfusus* have also been successfully reduced with push–pull strategies using aggregation and antiaggregation pheromones (Cook *et al.*, 2007), pointing out that this strategy is a useful tool for IPM programs to reduce pesticide use.

VII. Conclusions and Outlook

Many efforts have been made along the years to control insect pests, but their efficacy has been limited. In addition, the great concern over human and environmental health has led to ban some highly effective broad spectrum pesticides. Therefore, new environmentally friendly alternative approaches have been developed. Pheromones have been demonstrated to be highly useful in a number of cases, particularly with Lepidoptera, over the past 20 years with mating disruption formulations leading the way. There is no doubt that this trend will continue in the future. One factor of concern is the relatively high cost of the semiochemicals and formulations containing them in the three areas of application: mass trapping, attract-and-kill, and mating disruption, in comparison to insecticide treatments. Therefore, a combined effort of scientists, farmers, and producers is required to reduce the cost of application of semiochemicals to acceptable thresholds.

Basic studies on the biology of insect olfaction offer new opportunities for the development of new strategies for pest control. For example, identification of odorant receptor genes allows discovery of compounds that can excite or block these receptors. Odorants that could excite the receptors could be used as trapping agents whereas odorants that inhibit them might be useful as insect repellents (Van Naters and Carlson, 2006). Further research of compounds able to inhibit enzymes involved in the degradation of pheromones and odorants (Guerrero and Rosell, 2005; Maibêche-Coisné *et al.*, 2004) should also be of interest since these chemicals interfere the chemical communication in insects and might also play a relevant role in plant–insect interactions.

ACKNOWLEDGMENTS

This material is based upon work supported by federal funds from the grant #98-34135-6786 from the Tropical and Subtropical Agricultural Research (TSTAR), special grants, National

Institute of Food and Agriculture (NIFA), USDA, and CICYT (projects AGL2006-13489-C02-01 and AGL2009-13452-C02-01).

REFERENCES

Albajes, R., Konstantopoulou, M., Etchepare, O., Eizaguirre, M., Frérot, B., Sans, A., Krokos, F., Ameline, A., and Mazomenos, B. (2002). Mating disruption of the corn borer *Sesamia nonagrioides* (Lepidoptera: Noctuidae) using sprayable formulations of pheromone. *Crop Protect.* **21,** 217–225.

Aldrich, J. R., Bartelt, R. J., Dickens, J. C., Knight, A. L., Light, D. M., and Tumlinson, J. H. (2003). Insect chemical ecology research in the United States Department of Agriculture–Agricultural Research Service. *Pest Manag. Sci.* **59,** 777–787.

Alfaro, C., Navarro-Llopis, V., and Primo, J. (2009). Optimization of pheromone dispenser density for managing the rice striped stem borer, *Chilo suppressalis* (Walker), by mating disruption. *Crop Protect.* **28,** 547–628.

Ambrogi, B. G., Lima, E. R., and Sousa-Souto, L. (2006). Efficacy of mating disruption for control of the coffee leaf miner *Leucoptera coffeella* (Guérin-Méneville) (Lepidoptera: Lyonetiidae). *BioAssay* **1,** 1–5.

Antonaroli, R. (2000). Control of two tortricid chestnut pests by mating disruption. *Inf. Agrar* **56,** 89–91.

Atanasov, A., Shearer, P. W., Hamilton, G., and Polk, D. (2002). Development and implementation of a reduced risk peach arthropod management program in New Jersey. *J. Econ. Entomol.* **95,** 803–812.

Baker, T. C., and Heath, J. J. (2004). Pheromones—Function and use in insect control. *In* "Molecular Insect Science," (L. I. Gilbert, K. Iatro, and S. S. Gill, Eds.), pp. 407–460. Elsevier, Amsterdam, The Netherlands.

Bau, J., Martínez, D., Renou, M., and Guerrero, A. (1999). Pheromone-triggered orientation flight of male moths can be disrupted by trifluoromethyl ketones. *Chem. Senses* **24,** 473–480.

Borchert, D. M., and Walgenbach, J. F. (2000). Comparison of pheromone-mediated mating disruption and conventional insecticides for management of tufted apple bud moth (Lepidoptera: Tortricidae). *J. Econ. Entomol.* **93,** 769–776.

Bosa, E., Cotes, A., Fukumoto, T., Bengtsson, M., and Witzgall, P. (2005). Pheromone-mediated communication disruption in Guatemalan potato moth *Tecia solanivora* Povolny (Lepidoptera: Gelechiidae). *Entomol. Exp. Appl.* **114,** 137–142.

Brunner, J., Welter, S., Calkins, C., Hilton, R., Beers, E., Dunley, J., Unruh, T., Knight, A., Van Steenwyk, R., and Van Buskirk, P. (2002). Mating disruption of codling moth: A perspective from the Western United States. *IOBC WPRS Bull.* **25,** 1–11.

Byers, J. A., Zhang, Q.-H., and Schlyter, F. (1998). Volatiles from nonhost birch trees inhibit pheromone response in spruce bark beetles. *Naturwissenschaften* **85,** 557–561.

Camilla, R., Svensson, G. P., Anderbrant, O., and Löfstedt, C. (2007). Evaluation of long-term mating disruption of *Ephestia kuehniella* and *Plodia interpunctella* (Lepidoptera: Pyralidae) in indoor storage facilities by pheromone traps and monitoring of relative aerial concentrations of pheromone. *J. Econ. Entomol.* **100,** 1017–1025.

Campanacci, V., Longhi, S., Nagnan-Le Meillour, P., Cambillau, C., and Tegoni, M. (1999). Recombinant pheromone binding protein 1 from *Mamestra brassicae* (MbraPBP1). Functional and structural characterization. *Eur. J. Biochem.* **264,** 707–716.

Charmillot, P. J., and Hofer, D. (1997). Control of codling moth, *Cydia pomonella* L., by an attract and kill formulation. *IOBC WPRS Bull.* **20,** 139–140.

Ciglar, I., Baric, B., Tomsic, T., and Subic, M. (2002). Control of grape berry moths (*Eupoecilia ambiguella* Hb., *Lobesia botrana* Den. & Schiff; Lepidoptera: Tortricidae) by mating disruption technique. *Frag. Phytomed. Herb.* **27,** 31–37.

Cook, S., Wenz, J., Ragenovich, I., Reardon, R., and Randall, C. (2005). Impact of mating disruption pheromone treatments to control Douglas-fir tussock moth, *Orgyia pseudotsugata* (McDonough) (Lepidoptera: Lymantriidae) on egg parasitoids. *Pan-Pacific Entomol.* **81,** 41–46.

Cook, S. M., Khan, Z. R., and Pickett, J. A. (2007). The use of push–pull strategies in integrated pest management. *Annu. Rev. Entomol.* **52,** 375–400.

Coracini, M. D. A., Bengtsson, M., Reckziegel, A., Löfqvist, J., Francke, W., Vilela, E. F., Eiras, A. E., Kovaleski, A., and Witzgall, P. (2001). Identification of a four-component sex pheromone blend in *Bonagota cranaodes* (Lepidoptera: Tortricidae). *J. Econ. Entomol.* **94,** 911–914.

Curkovic, T., and Brunner, J. F. (2007). Pheromone inhibitors for *Pandemis pyrusana* males (Lepidoptera: Tortricidae). *Spanish J. Agric. Res.* **5,** 385–388.

Dallara, P. L., Seybold, S. J., Meyer, H., Tolasch, T., Francke, W., and Wood, D. L. (2000). Semiochemicals from three species of *Pityophthorus* (Coleoptera: Scolytidae): Identification and field response. *Can. Entomol.* **132,** 889–906.

Debarr, G. L., Hanula, J. L., Niwa, C. G., and Nord, J. C. (2000). Synthetic pheromones disrupt male *Dioryctria* spp. moths in a loblolly pine seed orchard. *Can. Entomol.* **132,** 345–351.

Deglow, E. K., and Borden, J. H. (1998). Green leaf volatiles disrupt and enhance response to aggregation pheromones by the ambrosia beetle, *Gnathotrichus sulcatus* (Coleoptera: Scolytidae). *Can. J. Forest Res.* **28,** 1697–1705.

Deng, J. Y., Wei, H. Y., Huang, Y. P., and Du, J. W. (2004a). Enhancement of attraction to sex pheromones of *Spodoptera exigua* by volatile compounds produced by host plants. *J. Chem. Ecol.* **30,** 2037–2045.

Deng, J. Y., Huang, Y. P., Wei, H. Y., and Du, J. W. (2004b). EAG and behavioral responses of *Helicoverpa armigera* males to volatiles from poplar leaves and their combinations with sex pheromone. *J. Zhejiang Univ. Sci.* **5,** 1577–1582.

Durán, I., Parrilla, A., Feixas, J., and Guerrero, A. (1993). Inhibition of antennal esterases of the Egyptian armyworm *Spodoptera littoralis* by trifluoromethyl ketones. *Bioorg. Med. Chem. Lett.* **3,** 2593–2598.

Eizaguirre, M., Sans, A., López, C., and Albajes, R. (2002). Effects of mating disruption against the Mediterranean corn borer, *Sesamia nonagrioides*, on the European corn borer *Ostrinia nubilalis*. *IOBC WPRS Bull.* **25,** 1–10.

Eizaguirre, M., Albajes, R., López, C., Sans, A., and Gemeno, C. (2007). Inhibition of pheromone response in *Sesamia nonagrioides* by the pheromone of the sympatric corn borer, *Ostrinia nubilalis*. *Pest Manag. Sci.* **63,** 608–614.

Fadamiro, H. Y., and Baker, T. C. (2002). Pheromone puffs suppress mating by *Plodia interpunctella* and *Sitotroga cerealella* in an infested corn store. *Entomol. Exp. Appl.* **102,** 239–251.

Fadamiro, H. Y., Cossé, A. A., and Baker, T. C. (1999). Fine-scale resolution of closely spaced pheromone and antagonist filaments by flying male *Helicoverpa zea*. *J. Comp. Physiol. A* **185,** 131–141.

Feixas, J., Prestwich, G. D., and Guerrero, A. (1995). Ligand specificity of pheromone-binding proteins of the processionary moth. *Eur. J. Biochem.* **234,** 521–526.

Femenia-Ferreri, B., Bosch, D., Moya, P., Avilla, J., and Primo, J. (2007). Field assays of a new biodegradable controlled-release pheromone dispensers for mating disruption of *Cydia pomonella* (L.). *IOBC WPRS Bull.* **30,** 107–114.

Ferrara, F. A. A., Vilela, E. F., Jham, G. N., Eiras, Á. E., Picanço, M. C., Attygalle, A. B., Svatos, A., Frighetto, R. T. S., and Meinwald, J. (2004). Evaluation of the synthetic major component of the sex pheromone of *Tuta absoluta* (Meyrick) (Lepidoptera: Gelechiidae). *J. Chem. Ecol.* **27,** 907–917.

Fettköther, R., Reddy, G. V. P., Noldt, U., and Dettner, K. (2000). Effect of host and larval frass volatiles on behavioral response of the old house borer *Hylotrupes bajulus* (L.) (Coleoptera: Cerambycidae), in a wind tunnel bioassay. *Chemoecology* **10,** 1–10.

Filhoa, M. M., Vilela, E. F., Jhamb, G. N., Attygalle, A., Svatos, A., and Meinwald, J. (2000). Initial studies of mating disruption of the tomato moth, *Tuta absoluta* (Lepidoptera: Gelechiidae) using synthetic sex pheromone. *J. Braz. Chem. Soc* **11,** 621–628.

Fitzpatrick, S. M. (2006). Delayed mating reduces fecundity of blackheaded fireworm, *Rhopobota naevana* (Lepidoptera: Tortricidae), on cranberry. *Entomol. Exp. Appl.* **120,** 245–250.

Fitzpatrick, S. M., Troubridge, J. T., and Maurice, C. (2004). Pheromone released from polyvinyl chloride dispensers disrupts mate-finding and pheromone-source location by *Rhopobota naevana* (Lepidoptera: Tortricidae) in cranberries. *Can. Entomol.* **136,** 91–108.

Gemeno, C., Sans, A., López, C., Albajes, R., and Eizaguirre, M. (2006). Pheromone antagonism in the European corn borer moth *Ostrinia nubilalis*. *J. Chem. Ecol.* **32,** 1071–1084.

Gillette, N. E., Stein, J. D., Owen, D. R., Webster, J. N., and Mori, S. R. (2006). Pheromone-based disruption of *Eucosma sonomana* and *Rhyacionia zozana* (Lepidoptera: Tortricidae) using aerially applied microencapsulated pheromone. *Can. J. Forest Res.* **36,** 361.

Giner, M., Sans, A., Riba, M., Bosch, D., Gago, R., Rayo, J., Rosell, G., and Guerrero, A. (2009). Development and biological activity of a new antagonist of the pheromone of the codling moth *Cydia pomonella*. *J. Agric. Food Chem.* **57,** 8514–8519.

Gordon, D., Anshelevich, L., Zahavi, T., Ovadia, S., Dunkelblum, E., Harari, A., and Lozzia, C. (2003). Integrating mating disruption techniques against the honeydew moth and the European grapevine moth in vineyards. *IOBC WPRS Bull.* **26,** 131–134.

Gordon, D., Zahavi, T., Anshelevich, L., Harel, M., Ovadia, S., Dunkelblum, E., and Harari, A. R. (2005). Mating disruption of *Lobesia botrana* (Lepidoptera: Tortricidae): Effect of pheromone formulations and concentrations. *J. Econ. Entomol.* **98,** 135–142.

Grassi, A., Zini, M., and Forno, F. (2002). Mating disruption field trials to control the currant clearwing moth, *Synanthedon tipuliformis* Clerck: A three-year study. *IOBC WPRS Bull.* **25,** 69–76.

Grodner, J., Jabłoński, T., Kolk, A., Przybysz, E., and Ślusarski, S. (2008). Possibilities to monitoring/control of the horse-chestnut leafminer (Cameraria ohridella) with some acetal derivatives of (8E, 10Z)-tetradeca-8,10-dienal. *Pesticides* **3/4,** 5–13.

Guerrero, A., and Rosell, G. (2005). Biorational approaches for insect control by enzymatic inhibition. *Curr. Med. Chem.* **12,** 461–469.

Gut, L. J., Stelinski, L. L., Thomson, D. R., and Miller, J. R. (2004). Behaviour-modifying chemicals: Prospects and constraints in IPM. *In* "Integrated Pest Management: Potential Constraints and Challenges," (O. Koul, G. S. Dhaliwal, and G. W. Cuperus, Eds.), pp. 73–121. CABI, New York.

Hegazi, E. M., Herz, A., Hassan, S., Agamy, E., Khafagi, W., Shweil, S., Zaitoun, A., Mostafa, S., Hafez, M., El-Shazly, A., El-Said, S., Abo-Abdala, L., Khamis, N., and El-Kemny, S. (2005). Naturally occurring *Trichogramma* species in olive farms in Egypt. *Insect Sci.* **12,** 185–192.

Hirashima, A., Shigeta, Y., Eiraku, T., and Kuwano, E. (2003). Inhibitors of calling behavior of *Plodia interpunctella*. *J. Insect Sci.* **4,** 1–9.

Howse, P., Stevens, I., and Jones, O. (Eds.) (1998). Insect Pheromones and their use in Pest Management. Chapman & Hill, London, UK, p. 639.

Il'ichev, A. L. (2006). Area-wide application of pheromone mediated mating disruption in sustainable IPM. *IOBC WPRS Bull.* **29,** 95–104.

Il'ichev, A. L., Stelinski, L. L., Williams, D. G., and Gut, L. J. (2006). Sprayable microencapsulated sex pheromone formulation for mating disruption of Oriental fruit moth (Lepidoptera: Tortricidae) in Australian peach and pear orchards. *J. Econ. Entomol.* **99,** 2048–2054.

Jenkins, P. E., and Isaacs, R. (2008). Mating disruption of *Paralobesia viteana* in vineyards using pheromone deployed in SPLAT-GBM™ wax droplets. *J. Chem. Ecol.* **34,** 1089–1095.

Jones, V. P., and Aihara-Sasaki, M. (2001). Demographic analysis of delayed mating in mating disruption: A case study with *Cryptophlebia illepida* (Butler) (Lepidoptera: Tortricidae). *J. Econ. Entomol.* **94,** 785–792.

Kakizaki, M. (2002). Suppression effects on populations of the cabbage armyworm, *Mamestra brassicae*, and the flax budworm, *Heliothis maritima adaucta* (Lepidoptera: Noctuidae), by mating disruption using the sex pheromone. *Annu. Rep. Soc. Plant Protect. N. Jpn.* **53,** 213–215.

Kehat, M., and Dunkelblum, E. (1990). Behavioral response male *Heliothis armigera* (Lepidoptera: Noctuidae) moths in a flight tunnel to combinations of components identified from female sex pheromome glands. J. *Insect Behav.* **3,** 75–84.

Klun, J. A., Oliver, J. E., Khrimian, A. P., Dickens, J. C., and Potts, W. J. E. (1997). Behavioral and electrophysiological activity of the racemate and enantiomers of a monofluorinated analog of European corn borer (Lepidoptera: Pyralidae) sex pheromone. *J. Entomol. Sci.* **32,** 37–49.

Koch, U. T., Lüder, W., Andrick, U., Staten, R. T., and Cardé, R. T. (2009). Measurement by electroantennogram of airborne pheromone in cotton treated for mating disruption of *Pectinophora gossypiella* following removal of pheromone dispensers. *Entomol. Exp. Appl.* **130,** 1–9.

Kovanci, O. B., Walgenbach, J. F., and Kennedy, G. G. (2004). Evaluation of extended-season mating disruption of the Oriental fruit moth *Grapholita molesta* (Busck) (Lep., Tortricidae) in apples. *J. Appl. Entomol.* **128,** 664–669.

Leak, S. G. A. (Ed.) (1999). Tsetse Biology and Ecology: Their Role in the Epidemiology and Control of *Trypanosomosis*. CABI, Wallingford, p. 568.

Light, D. M., Flath, R. A., Buttery, R. G., Zalom, F. G., Rice, R. E., and Jung, E. B. (1993). Host plant green leaf volatiles synergize the synthetic sex pheromones of the corn ear worm and codling moth (Lepidoptera). *Chemoecology* **4,** 145–152.

Linn, C. E., Domingue, M. J., Musto, C. J., Baker, T. C., and Roelofs, W. L. (2007). Support for (*Z*)-11-hexadecanal as a pheromone antagonist in *Ostrinia nubilalis*: Flight tunnel and single sensillum studies with a New York population. *J. Chem. Ecol.* **33,** 909–921.

Louis, F., and Schirra, K.-J. (2001). Mating disruption of *Lobesia botrana* (Lepidoptera: Tortricidae) in vineyards with very high population densities. *IOBC WPRS Bull.* **24,** 75–79.

Lykouressis, D., Perdikis, D., Michalis, C., and Fantinou, A. (2004). Mating disruption of the pink bollworm *Pectinophora gossypiella* (Saund.) (Lepidoptera: Gelechiidae) using gossyplure PB-rope dispensers in cotton fields. *J. Pest Sci.* **77,** 205–210.

Lykouressis, D., Perdikis, D., Samartzis, D., Frantinou, A., and Toutouzas, S. (2005). Management of the pink bollworm *Pectinophora gossypiella* (Saunders) (Lepidoptera: Gelechiidae) by mating disruption in cotton fields. *Crop Protect.* **24,** 177–183.

Mafi, S. A., Vang, L. V., Nakata, Y., Ohbayashi, N., Yamamoto, M., and Ando, T. (2005). Identification of the sex pheromone of the citrus leafminer (*Phyllocnistis citrella* Stainton, Lepidoptera: Gracillariidae) with a trial of control by the communication disruption method. *J. Pest Sci.* **30,** 361–367.

Maibêche-Coisné, M., Nikonov, A. A., Ishida, Y., Jacquin-Joly, E., and Leal, W. S. (2004). Pheromone anosmia in a scarab beetle induced by in vivo inhibition of a pheromone-degrading enzyme. *Proc. Natl. Acad. Sci. USA* **101,** 11459–11464.
Mazomenos, B. E., Pantazi-Mazomenou, A., and Stefanou, D. (2002). Attract and kill of the olive fruit fly *Bactrocera oleae* in Greece as a part of an integrated control system. *IOBC WPRS Bull.* **25,** 137–146.
McBrien, H. L., Judd, G. J. R., and Borden, J. H. (1998). Development of pheromone-based mating disruption for control of the eye-spotted bud moth, *Spilonota ocellana*. *Entomol. Exp. Appl.* **88,** 101–107.
McDonough, L. M., Chapman, P. S., Weissling, T. J., and Smithhisler, C. L. (1996). Efficacy of nonpheromone communication disruptants of codling moth (*Cydia pomonella*): Effect of pheromone isomers and of distance between calling females and dispensers. *J. Chem. Ecol.* **22,** 415–423.
Meissner, H. E., Walgenbach, J. F., and Kennedy, G. G. (2001). Effects of mating disruption and conventional pesticide treatments on populations of the tufted apple bud moth, *Platynota idaeusalis*, in North Carolina apple orchards. *Crop Protect.* **20,** 373–378.
Mitchell, E. R., and Mayer, M. S. (2001). *Spodoptera exigua*: Mating disruption, measurement of airborne concentration of pheromone, and use of specialist receptor cell responses for comparison to female pheromone emission. *J. Environ. Sci. Health* **36,** 467–488.
Mo, J., Glover, M., Munro, S., and Beattie, G. A. C. (2006). Evaluation of mating disruption for control of lightbrown apple moth (Lepidoptera: Tortricidae) in citrus. *J. Econ. Entomol.* **99,** 421–426.
Mochizuki, F., Fukumoto, T., Noguchi, H., Sugie, H., Morimoto, T., and Ohtani, K. (2002). Resistance to a mating disruptant composed of (*Z*)-11-tetradecenyl acetate in the smaller tea tortrix, *Adoxophyes honmai* (Yasuda) (Lepidoptera: Tortricidae). *Appl. Entomol. Zool.* **37,** 299–304.
Morewood, W. D., Simmonds, K. E., Gries, G., Allison, J. D., and Borden, J. H. (2003). Disruption by conophthorin of the kairomonal response of sawyer beetles to bark beetle pheromones. *J. Chem. Ecol.* **29,** 2115–2129.
Muniappan, R., Bamba, J., Cruz, J., and Reddy, G. V. P. (2004). Field response of Guam populations of the New Guinea sugarcane weevil, *Rhabdoscelus obscurus* (Boisduval) (Coleoptera: Curculionidae), to aggregation pheromones and food volatiles. *Micronesica* **37,** 57–68.
Namiki, S., Iwabuchi, S., and Kanzaki, R. (2008). Representation of a mixture of pheromone and host plant odor by antennal lobe projection neurons of the silkmoth *Bombyx mori*. *J. Comp. Physiol. A* **194,** 501–515.
Navrozidis, E., Thomidis, T., Tsipouridis, C., Xatzicharisis, I., Fotiadis, I., and Servis, D. (2005). Pheromone-based communication disruption of *Adoxophyes orana* on peach using the new RAK 3+4 dispensers and their effect on development of fruit rot diseases. *Phytoparasitica* **33,** 149–153.
Norin, T. (2001). Pheromones and kairomones for control of pest insects. Some current results from a Swedish research program. *Pure Appl. Chem.* **73,** 607–612.
Ochieng, S. A., Park, K. C., and Baker, T. C. (2002). Host plant volatiles synergize responses of sex pheromone-specific olfactory receptor neurons in male *Helicoverpa zea*. *J. Comp. Physiol. A* **188,** 325–333.
Ohtani, K., Witjaksono, T., Fukumoto, T., Mochizuki, F., Yamamoto, M., and Ando, T. (2001). Mating disruption of the Japanese giant looper in tea gardens permeated with synthetic pheromone and related compounds. *Entomol. Exp. Appl.* **100,** 203–209.
Okazaki, K., Arakawa, A., Noguchi, H., and Mochizuki, F. (2001). Further studies on mating disruptants for the summerfruit tortrix moth, *Adoxophyes orana fasciata*. *Jpn. J. Appl. Entomol. Zool.* **45,** 137–141.

Onufrieva, K. S., Thorpe, K. W., Hickman, A. D., Leonard, D. S., Mastro, V. C., and Roberts, E. A. (2008). Gypsy moth mating disruption in open landscapes. *J. Agric. Forest Entomol.* **10,** 175–179.

Ortiz, A., Perabá, A., and Sánchez, A. Q. (2007). Mating disruption of the olive pyralid moth, *Euzophera pinguis*. *IOBC WPRS Bull.* **30,** 179–180.

Parrilla, A., and Guerrero, A. (1994). Trifluoromethyl ketones as inhibitors of the processionary moth sex pheromone. *Chem. Senses* **19,** 1–10.

Party, V., Hanot, C., Said, I., Rochat, D., and Renou, M. (2009). Plant terpenes affect intensity and temporal parameters of pheromone detection in a moth. *Chem. Senses* **34,** 763–774.

Plettner, E. (2002). Insect pheromone olfaction: New targets for the design of species-selective pest control agents. *Curr. Med. Chem.* **9,** 1075–1085.

Polavarapu, S., Lonergan, G., Peng, H., and Neilsen, K. (2001). Potential for mating disruption of *Sparganothis sulfureana* (Lepidoptera: Tortricidae) in cranberries. *J. Econ. Entomol.* **94,** 658–665.

Pope, T. W., Campbell, C. A. M., Hardie, J., Pickett, J. A., and Wadhams, L. J. (2007). Interactions between host-plant volatiles and the sex pheromone of the bird cherry-oat aphid, *Rhopalosiphum padi* and the damson-hop aphid, *Phorodon humuli*. *J. Chem. Ecol.* **33,** 157–165.

Pophof, B., Gebauer, T., and Ziegelberger, A. (2000). Decyl-thio-trifluoropropanone, a competitive inhibitor of moth pheromone receptors. *J. Comp. Physiol. A* **186,** 315–323.

Powell, W., and Pickett, J. A. (2003). Manipulation of parasitoids for aphid pest management: Progress and prospects. *Pest Manag. Sci.* **59,** 149–155.

Prestwich, G. D., and Streinz, L. (1988). Haloacetate analogs of pheromones: Effects on catabolism and electrophysiology in *Plutella xylostella*. *J. Chem. Ecol.* **14,** 1003–1021.

Quero, C., Bau, J., Guerrero, A., and Renou, M. (2004). Responses of the olfactory receptor neurons of the corn stalk borer *Sesamia nonagrioides* to components of the pheromone blend and their inhibition by a trifluoromethyl ketone analogue of the main component. *Pest Manag. Sci.* **60,** 719–726.

Reddy, G. V. P. (2007). Improved semiochemical-based trapping method for old-house borer, *Hylotrupes bajulus* (Coleoptera: Cerambycidae). *Environ. Entomol.* **36,** 281–286.

Reddy, G. V. P., and Guerrero, A. (2000). Pheromone-based integrated pest management to control the diamondback moth *Plutella xylostella* in cabbage fields. *Pest Manag. Sci.* **56,** 882–888.

Reddy, G. V. P., and Guerrero, A. (2004). Interactions of insect pheromones and plant semiochemicals. *Trends Plant Sci.* **9,** 253–261.

Reddy, G. V. P., Holopainen, J. K., and Guerrero, A. (2002a). Olfactory responses of *Plutella xylostella* natural enemies to host pheromone, larval frass, and green leaf cabbage volatiles. *J. Chem. Ecol.* **28,** 131–143.

Reddy, G. V. P., Quero, C., and Guerrero, A. (2002b). Activity of octylthiotrifluoropropan-2-one, a potent esterase inhibitor, on growth, development and intraspecific communication in *Spodoptera littoralis* and *Sesamia nonagrioides*. *J. Agric. Food Chem.* **50,** 7062–7068.

Reddy, G. V. P., Cruz, Z. T., Bamba, J., and Muniappan, R. (2005a). Development of a semiochemical-based trapping method for the New Guinea sugarcane weevil, *Rhabdoscelus obscurus*. *J. Appl. Entomol.* **129,** 65–69.

Reddy, G. V. P., Fettköther, R., Noldt, U., and Dettner, K. (2005b). Capture of female *Hylotrupes bajulus* as influenced by trap type and pheromone blend. *J. Chem. Ecol.* **31,** 2169–2177.

Reddy, G. V. P., Fettköther, R., Noldt, U., and Dettner, K. (2005c). Enhancement of the attraction and trap catches of the old-house borer, *Hylotrupes bajulus* (Coleoptera:

Cerambycidae), by combination of male sex pheromone and monoterpenes. *Pest Manag. Sci.* **61,** 699–704.

Renou, M., and Guerrero, A. (2000). Insect parapheromones in olfaction research and semiochemical-based pest control strategies. *Annu. Rev. Entomol.* **48,** 605–630.

Renou, M., Lucas, P., Malo, E., Quero, C., and Guerrero, A. (1997). Effects of trifluoromethyl ketones and related compounds on the EAG and behavioural responses to pheromones in male moths. *Chem. Senses* **22,** 407–416.

Riba, M., Sans, A., Bau, P., Grolleau, G., Renou, M., and Guerrero, A. (2001). Pheromone response inhibitors of the corn stalk borer *Sesamia nonagrioides*. Biological evaluation and toxicology. *J. Chem. Ecol.* **27,** 1879–1897.

Riba, M., Sans, A., Solé, J., Muñoz, L., Bosch, M. P., Rosell, G., and Guerrero, A. (2005). Antagonism of pheromone response of *Ostrinia nubilalis* males and implications on behavior in the laboratory and in the field. *J. Agric. Food Chem.* **53,** 1158–1165.

Rosell, G., Herrero, S., and Guerrero, A. (1996). New trifluoromethyl ketones as potent inhibitors of esterases: ^{19}F NMR spectroscopy of transition state analog complexes and structure-activity relationships. *Biochem. Biophys. Res. Comm.* **226,** 287–292.

Ross, D. W., and Daterman, G. E. (1994). Reduction of Douglas-fir beetle infestation of high-risk stands by antiaggregation and aggregation pheromones. *Can. J. Forest Res.* **24,** 2184–2190.

Ryne, C., Ekeberg, M., Jonzen, N., Oehlschlager, C., Löfstedt, C., and Anderbrant, O. (2006). Reduction in an almond moth *Ephestia cautella* (Lepidoptera: Pyralidae) population by means of mating disruption. *Pest Manag. Sci.* **62,** 912–918.

Schroeder, P. C., Shelton, A. M., Ferguson, C. S., Hoffmann, M. P., and Petzoldt, C. H. (2000). Application of synthetic sex pheromone for management of diamondback moth, *Plutella xylostella*, in cabbage. *Entomol. Exp. Appl.* **94,** 243–248.

Shani, A., and Clearwater, J. (2001). Evasion of mating disruption in *Ephestia cautella* (Walker) by increased pheromone production relative to that of undisrupted populations. *J. Stored Prod. Res.* **37,** 237–252.

Sharov, A. A., Leonard, D., Liebhold, A. M., and Clemens, N. S. (2002). Evaluation of preventive treatments in low-density gypsy moth populations using pheromone traps. *J. Econ. Entomol.* **95,** 1205–1215.

Sheng, C. F., Yang, F. A., Wei, Y. B., Zhu, C. Q., and Xiong, Y. W. (2000). Field tests of the effects of the mass trapping with synthetic sex pheromone on rice stem borer. *Plant Prot.* **26,** 4–5.

Shorey, H. H., and Gerber, R. G. (1996). Disruption of pheromone communication through the use of puffers for control of beet armyworm (Lepidoptera: Noctuidae) in tomatoes. *Environ. Entomol.* **25,** 1401–1405.

Siekmann, G., Meyerhofer, R., and Hommes, M. (2009). Testing mating disruption of the horse chestnut leafminer *Cameraria ohridella* (Lepidoptera: Gracillariidae) in field tents. *J. Pest Sci.* **82,** 129–136.

Sieminska, E., Ryne, C., Löfstedt, C., and Anderbrant, O. (2009). Long-term pheromone-mediated mating disruption of the Mediterranean flour moth, *Ephestia kuehniella*, in a flourmill. *Entomol. Exp. Appl.* **131,** 294–299.

Smart, L. E., Blight, M. M., Pickett, J. A., and Pye, B. J. (1994). Develoopment of field strategies incorporating semiochemicals for the control of pea and bean weevil, *Sitona lineatus* L. *Crop Protect.* **13,** 127–135.

Solé, J., Sans, A., Riba, M., Rosa, E., Bosch, M. P., Barrot, M., Palència, J., Castellà, J., and Guerrero, A. (2008). Reduction of damage by the Mediterranean corn borer, *Sesamia nonagrioides*, and the European corn borer, *Ostrinia nubilalis*, in maize fields by a trifluoromethyl ketone pheromone analog. *Entomol. Exp. Appl.* **126,** 28–39.

Spohn, B. G., Zhu, J., Chastain, B. B., and Haynes, K. F. (2003). Influence of mating success of two strains of cabbage loopers, *Trichoplusia ni* (Hübner) (Lepidoptera: Noctuidae). *Environ. Entomol.* **32,** 736–741.

Steinmann, K. P., Zhang, M. H., Grant, J. A., Pickel, C., and Goodhue, R. E. (2008). Pheromone-based pest management can be cost-effective for walnut growers. *Calif. Agric.* **62,** 105–110.

Stelinski, L. L., Gut, L. J., Pierzchala, A. V., and Miller, J. R. (2004). Field observations quantifying attraction of four tortricid moth species to high-dosage, polyethylene-tube pheromone dispensers in untreated and pheromone-treated orchards. *Entomol. Exp. Appl.* **113,** 187–196.

Stelinski, L. L., Zhang, A., Onagbola, E. O., and Meyer, W. L. (2009). Recognition of foreign oviposition marking pheromones is context dependent and determined by preimaginal conditioning. *Commun. Integr. Biol.* **2,** 391–393.

Subchev, M. A., Voerman, S., and Milkova, T. S. (2009). Inhibitors for *Autographa gamma* L. (Lep., Noctuidae) sex pheromone. *J. Appl. Entomol.* **104,** 425–429.

Suckling, D. M., and Karg, G. (1998). Pheromones and other semiochemicals. *In* "Biological and biotechnological control of insect pests," (J. E. Rechcigl and A. A. Rechcigl, Eds.), pp. 63–99. CRC Press, Boca Raton, FL.

Suckling, D. M., Gibb, A. R., Burnip, G. M., Snelling, C., Ruiter, J. D., Langford, G., and El-Sayed, A. M. (2005). Optimization of pheromone lure and trap characteristics for currant clearwing, *Synanthedon tipuliformis*. *J. Chem. Ecol.* **31,** 393–406.

Svensson, G. P., Skals, N., and Löfstedt, C. (2003). Disruption of the odour-mediated mating behaviour of *Plodia interpunctella* using high-frequency sound. *Entomol. Exp. Appl.* **106,** 187–192.

Tcheslavskaia, K. S., Thorpe, K. W., Sharov, A. A., Leonard, D. S., Reardon, R. C., Mastro, V. C., Sellers, P., Brewster, C. C., and Roberts, E. A. (2005). Optimization of pheromone dosage for gypsy moth (Lepidoptera: Lymantriidae) mating disruption. *Entomol. Exp. Appl.* **115,** 355–361.

Toyoshima, G., Kobayashi, S., and Yoshihama, T. (2001). Control of *Helicoverpa armigera* (Hübner) by mating disruption using diamolure in lettuce fields. *Jpn. J. Appl. Entomol. Zool.* **45,** 183–188.

Trematerra, P. (2002). Pheromones and integrated pest management in stored products. *IOBC WPRS Bull.* **25,** 9–14.

Trematerra, P., Sciarretta, A., and Gentile, P. (2000). Trials on combined mating disruption in *Anarsia lineatella* (Zeller) and *Cydia molesta* (Busck) using CheckMate (R) SF dispenser. *Atti. Gior. Fitopatol.* **1,** 349–354.

Trimble, R. M., and Appleby, M. E. (2004). Comparison of efficacy of programs using insecticide and insecticide plus mating disruption for controlling the obliquebanded leafroller in apple (Lepidoptera: Tortricidae). *J. Econ. Entomol.* **97,** 518–524.

Trimble, R. M., and Tyndall, C. A. (2000). Disruption of mating in the spotted tentiform leafminer (Lepidoptera: Gracillariidae) using synthetic sex pheromone. *Can. Entomol.* **132,** 107–117.

Trimble, R. M., Vickers, P. M., Nielsen, K. E., and Barinshteyn, G. (2003). Sprayable pheromone for controlling the North American grape berry moth by mating disruption. *J. Agric. Forest Entomol.* **5,** 263–268.

Trudel, R., Guertin, C., and Grant, G. G. (2006). Potential for mating disruption to reduce cone damage by the spruce seed moth, *Cydia strobilella*, in spruce seed orchards. *J. Appl. Entomol.* **130,** 245–250.

Van Naters, W. v. d. G., and Carlson, J. R. (2006). Insects as chemosensors of humans and crops. *Nature* **444,** 302–307.

Varma, N. R. G., Krishnaiah, K., Pasalu, I. C., and Katti, G. R. (2002). Synergizing rice yellow stem borer pheromone with addition of plant extracts and vitamin E. *Indian J. Plant Prot.* **30,** 161–163.

Vetter, R. S., Millar, J. G., Vickers, N. J., and Baker, T. C. (2006). Mating disruption of carob moth *Ectomyelois ceratoniae* (Lepidoptera: Pyralidae), with a sex pheromone analog. *Southwest Entomol.* **31,** 33–48.

Vickers, R. A. (2002). Control of *Ichneumonoptera chrysophanes* (Meyrick) (Lepidoptera: Sesiidae) by mating disruption in persimmons. *Aust. J. Entomol.* **41,** 316–320.

Vickers, R. A., Thwaite, W. G., Williams, D. G., and Nicholas, A. H. (1998). Control of codling moth in small plots by mating disruption: Alone and with limited insecticide. *Entomol. Exp. Appl.* **86,** 229–239.

Vogt, R. G., Riddiford, L. M., and Prestwich, G. D. (1985). Kinetic properties of a pheromone-degrading enzyme: The sensillar esterase of *Antheraea polyphemus*. *Proc. Natl Acad. Sci. USA* **82,** 8827–8831.

Wang, Y., Feng, G., Liu, X., Feng, F., and Wang, L. (2005). Evaluation of mass-trapping for control of tea tussock moth *Euproctis pseudoconspersa* (Strand) (Lepidoptera: Lymantriidae) with synthetic sex pheromone in South China. *Int. J. Pest Manag.* **51,** 289–295.

Weihman, S. W., and Liburd, O. E. (2006). Mating disruption and attract-and-kill as reduced-risk strategies for control of grape root borer *Vitacea polistiformis* (Lepidoptera: Sesiidae) in Florida vineyards. *Fla. Entomol.* **89,** 245–250.

Welter, S., and Cave, F. (2007). Pheromone mating disruption of *Cydia pomonella* (L.) in California pears: Balancing dispenser emission rates and program performance. *IOBC WPRS Bull.* **30,** 123–124.

Welter, S. C., Pickel, C., Millar, J., Cave, F., Van Steenwyk, R. A., and Dunley, J. (2005). Pheromone mating disruption offers selective management options for key pests. *Calif. Agric.* **59,** 16–22.

Witzgall, P., Bengtsson, M., Karg, G., Backman, A. C., Streinz, L., Kirsch, P. A., Blum, Z., and Lofqvist, J. (1996). Behavioral observations and measurements of aerial pheromone concentrations in a mating disruption trial against pea moth *Cydia nigricana* F. (Lepidoptera, Tortricidae). *J. Chem. Ecol.* **22,** 191–206.

Witzgall, P., Lindblom, T., Bengtsson, M., and Tóth, M. (2004). The Pherolist, http://www-pherolist.slu.se./pherolist.php.

Witzgall, P., Stelinski, L. L., Gut, L. J., and Thomson, D. (2008). Codling moth management and chemical ecology. *Annu. Rev. Entomol.* **53,** 503–522.

Yang, F. A., Sheng, C. F., Wei, Y. B., Zhu, C. Q., and Xiong, Y. W. (2001). Study on mating disruption with synthetic sex pheromone for controlling rice stem borer. *Plant Protect.* **27,** 4–6.

Yang, Z. H., Bengtsson, M., and Witzgall, P. (2004). Host plant volatiles synergize response to sex pheromone in codling moth, *Cydia pomonella*. *J. Chem. Ecol.* **30,** 619–629.

Zeng, L., Chen, F. Y., and Zhang, Z. N. (2007). Synthesis and assessment of attractiveness and mating disruption efficacy of sex pheromone microcapsules for the diamondback moth, *Plutella xylostella* (L.). *Chin. Sci. Bull.* **52,** 1365–1371.

Zhang, G. F., Sheng, C. F., Han, Y., and Meng, X. Z. (2003). Interference with the mate-finding communication system of the Chinese tortrix *Cydia trasias* (Lep., Olethreutidae) using synthetic sex pheromones. *J. Appl. Entomol.* **127,** 282–287.

CHAPTER TWENTY-ONE

Pheromones and Exocrine Glands in Isoptera

Ana Maria Costa-Leonardo *and* Ives Haifig

Contents

Departamento de Biologia, Instituto de Biociências, Unesp—Univ Estadual Paulista, CEP 13506-900, Rio Claro—SP, Brasil

Vitamins and Hormones, Volume 83
ISSN 0083-6729, DOI: 10.1016/S0083-6729(10)83021-3

Abstract

Termites are eusocial insects that have a peculiar and intriguing system of communication using pheromones. The termite pheromones are composed of a blend of chemical substances and they coordinate different social interactions or activities, including foraging, building, mating, defense, and nestmate recognition. Some of these sociochemicals are volatile, spreading in the air, and others are contact pheromones, which are transmitted by trophallaxis and grooming. Among the termite semiochemicals, the most known are alarm, trail, sex pheromones, and hydrocarbons responsible for the recognition of nestmates. The sources of the pheromones are exocrine glands located all over the termite body. The principal exocrine structures considered pheromone-producing glands in Isoptera are the frontal, mandibular, salivary or labial, sternal, and tergal glands. The frontal gland is the source of alarm pheromone and defensive chemicals, but the mandibular secretions have been little studied and their function is not well established in Isoptera. The secretion of salivary glands involves numerous chemical compounds, some of them without pheromonal function. The worker saliva contains a phagostimulating pheromone and probably a building pheromone, while the salivary reservoir of some soldiers contains defensive chemicals. The sternal gland is the only source of trail-following pheromone, whereas sex pheromones are secreted by two glandular sources, the sternal and tergal glands. To date, the termite semiochemicals have indicated that few molecules are involved in their chemical communication, that is, the same compound may be secreted by different glands, different castes and species, and for different functions, depending on the concentration. In addition to the pheromonal parsimony, recent studies also indicate the occurrence of a synergic effect among the compounds involved in the chemical communication of Isoptera.

I. Introduction

The order Isoptera comprises seven families (Table 21.1), which include 280 genera and about 3000 species (Inward *et al.*, 2007). Termites are eusocial insects and their colonies present a structure of castes composed by different individuals: workers, soldiers, and reproductives. The workers are responsible for the maintenance of the termite colony, while soldiers are specialized for its defense. The reproductives are represented by the royal couple (the king and queen) and the imagoes or alates, which are the individuals responsible for colony dispersion. Secondary or neotenic reproductives may also occur in the termite colony, mainly when the primary royal pair dies or is removed (Noirot, 1990).

Table 21.1 Classification of Isoptera with 7 families and 17 subfamilies (after Inward *et al.*, 2007)

Family	Subfamily
1. Mastotermitidae	
2. Hodotermitidae	
3. Termopsidae	Porotermitinae
	Stolotermitinae
	Termopsinae
4. Serritermitidae	
5. Kalotermitidae	
6. Rhinotermitidae	Coptotermitinae
	Heterotermitinae
	Prorhinotermitinae
	Psammotermitinae
	Rhinotermitinae
	Stylotermitinae
	Termitogetoninae
7. Termitidae	Macrotermitinae
	Sphaerotermitinae
	Foraminitermitinae
	Apicotermitinae
	Syntermitinae
	Termitinae
	Nasutitermitinae

II. Pheromonal Communication

Termites developed a peculiar and intriguing system of communication through chemical substances or pheromones. The social life involves precise interactions among the nestmates, and chemical communication requires a specificity of chemical signals. The majority of the members of termite societies are blind, and communication through pheromones is very important for the transmission of information inside the colony (Costa-Leonardo *et al.*, 2009a). Pheromones are chemical substances produced by one individual of the colony that elicit a change of behavior in the others (Karlson and Lüscher, 1959). Generally, the pheromones are mixtures of many chemical substances, including some volatiles. Chemical communication requires a source of pheromone, which is an exocrine gland that produces semiochemicals and opens in the surface of the termite body. The specificity of the pheromone is provided by their basic molecular structure and specific mixture of compounds (Chapman, 1998). The majority of these chemicals are releaser pheromones because they cause immediate behavioral changes in the receiving individuals of the termite colony (Pasteels and Bordereau, 1998). Few chemicals are primer pheromones, which cause physiological changes in the receiving individuals, such as alterations of the reproductive or endocrine systems (Henderson, 1998). Social interactions or activities, such as foraging, building, mating, defense, egg, and nestmate recognition, and others, involve specific pheromones that are produced by determined exocrine glands. A specific behavior may be elicited by different concentrations of pheromones. Some pheromones are very volatile, as is the case for terpenoids. They are spread in the air and then detected by the other individuals of the colony. Other pheromones are transmitted by contact and may be deposited on the surface of a solid substrate, such as the soil or food (Ali and Morgan, 1990). In this way, the pheromones coordinate many social activities and are spread through the colony by two behavioral processes: trophallaxis and grooming, both primordial in the communication (Kaib, 1999). Trophallaxis involves the exchange of food among the individuals of the colony. Grooming always occurs before the request of food by one termite, and sensory receptors are involved in this process. In the termite colony, the queen is constantly groomed by the workers, and multiple grooming, with the participation of many individuals at the same time, also occurs. The grooming of mandibles and palps provides sensory contact, involving the mechanoreceptors and chemoreceptors of the individuals (Pearce, 1997). Through the sensory organs, the termites detect environmental changes and recognize chemical signals, which enable them to carry out all of the communication in their societies. The body of a termite is covered with sensorial sensilla, which vary in function, number, and distribution. The termites may distinguish odors using peg sensilla, which are small sensorial structures that contain numerous orifices along their wall and enable the exchange of air via diffusion. These sensilla are found in the antennae, palps, and other mouth parts and are utilized in the detection of pheromones, such as the sex and trail pheromones (Pearce, 1997).

III. Principal Exocrine Glands: Source of Pheromones

The exocrine glands of termites have ectodermal origin and are mostly pluricellular. They are spread all over the insect body and generally consist of epidermal cells with large secretory capacities (Blum, 1985). Morphologically, the simplest glands are those that develop through an increase in the size of epidermal cells, such as the sternal and tergal glands. In some cases, a more structured gland may appear as an invagination of the tegument and the differentiation of a cavity that works as a reservoir to accumulate the secretion (Billen and Morgan, 1998). This is the case for the frontal gland in termites, in which such modification enables storage of the glandular secretion, which may then be released in larger quantities (Costa-Leonardo, 1998a, 2001; Costa-Leonardo and De Salvo, 1987; Santos and Costa-Leonardo, 2006).

The principal exocrine structures considered pheromone-producing glands in Isoptera are the frontal, mandibular, salivary or labial, sternal and tergal glands. A general schema of these glands in different castes of Isoptera is shown in the Fig. 21.1. Ultrastructural data demonstrate that exocrine glands are composed of three types of glandular cells, according to the localization of these cells in relation to the insect cuticle and to the way the secretion is produced and discharged (Noirot and Quennedey, 1974, 1991). In class 1 cells, epidermal cells become secretory and the glandular secretion needs to cross the cuticle to be released. This class is frequently associated with others (Blum, 1985). Class 2 cells are surrounded by epidermal cells and are not in contact with the cuticle. In this class, the secretion must pass through class 1 cells before crossing the cuticle via pore canals. Class 3 cells are isolated from the cuticle and possess a chitinous canal, which connects the glandular cell with the insect cuticle and drains the secretion outside the insect body. The tegumental cuticle that covers the exocrine glands of the termites has some structural modifications to facilitate the discharge of secretions outside the insect body. Perfurations in the epicuticle with the formation of pores are common, as is a great variation in the number of epicuticular filaments

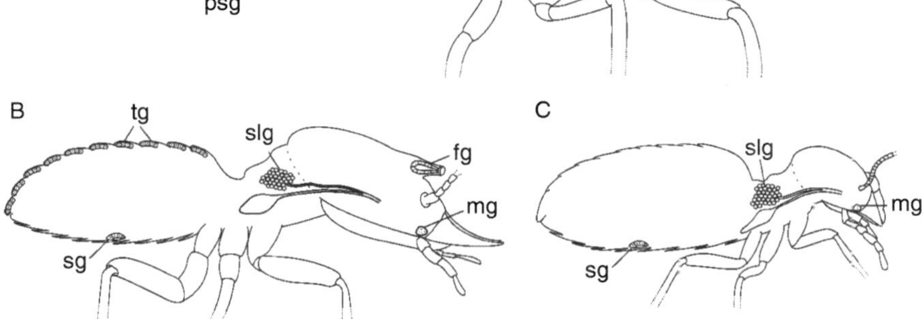

Figure 21.1 General schema of pheromone-producing glands in different castes of Isoptera. (A) Generalized imago with all pheromonal glands, although they do not occur simultaneously in the same termite. (B) Nasute mandibulate soldier of Termitidae. (C) Worker of Termitidae. fg, frontal gland; mg, mandibular gland; psg, posterior sternal gland; sg, sternal gland; slg,= salivary gland; tg, tergal gland.

(Quennedey, 1998). Another type of modification that occurs in termite exocrine glands, especially in the frontal, tergal, and sternal glands, is the development of extracellular spaces, generally constituting subcuticular cavities located between the cuticle and the class 1 cells. These spaces may be also observed among the cuticle layers and they are sometimes filled with secretions, working as storage sites for glandular products.

IV. Frontal Gland

A. Occurrence and morphology

The frontal gland is a tegumental and unpaired exocrine gland, specific of termites. It is differentiated in soldiers of the families Termitidae, Rhinotermitidae, and Serritermitidae and in some imagoes of the families Termitidae and Rhinotermitidae. In the reproductive caste, the frontal gland is always smaller in size and presents a structure similar to soldiers, although it is restricted to the head. In imagoes of *Prorhinotermes*, this gland is active only at the swarming period, although it remains in queens and kings of incipient colonies (Piskorski *et al.*, 2009). The frontal gland is a sac-like organ and, in the soldiers, may be limited to the head or it may be hypertrophied, occupying a large part of the abdomen. The pheromones produced by the frontal gland may be eliminated by the frontal pore present in the termite head or by autothysis, that is, glandular rupture. This is the case for soldiers of the species *Serritermes serrifer* (Costa-Leonardo, 1998b; Costa-Leonardo and Kitayama, 1991), *Globitermes sulphureus* (Bordereau *et al.*, 1997), *Apilitermes longiceps* (Deligne and DeConinck, 2006), *Glossotermes oculatus*, and *Dentispicotermes brevicarinatus* (Šobotník *et al.*, 2010). In nasute soldiers, the frontal pore is localized in the extremity of a tube known as the nasus (Fig. 21.2) and the frontal gland is restricted to the head. According to the cellular structure, the frontal gland in Isoptera may be of two types: one constituted only by class 1 cells and other constituted of class 1 and class 3 cells together. In both cases, there is a cuticular layer that internally covers the gland. The organization of the cuticle overlying class 1 cells varies among different species. A reduction or the complete disappearance of the cuticular layer has been observed in frontal glands of termites in which autothysis occurs (Costa-Leonardo, 1998b; Šobotník *et al.*, 2010). The frontal gland cells present special cytological characteristics, such as apical and basal differentiations of the plasma membrane, septate junctions, abundant smooth endoplasmic reticulum, Golgi apparatuses, and mitochondria (Costa-Leonardo, 2001). The secretion granules have an enormous variety in shape and electron density, and the occurrence of lipids and proteinaceous material is common (Quennedey, 1998).

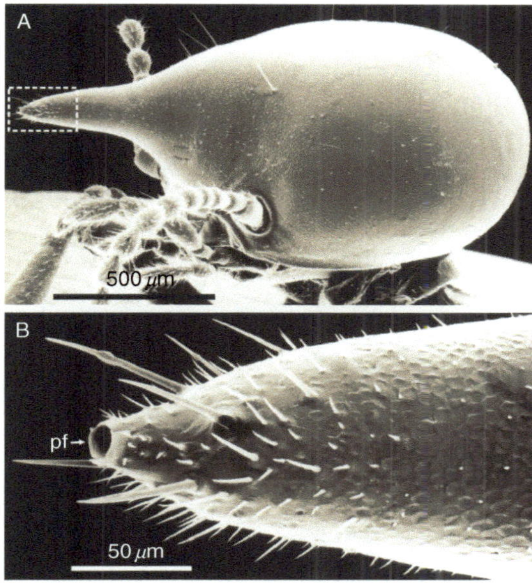

Figure 21.2 (A) Scanning electron micrograph of the soldier head of *Nasutitermes jaraguae*. (B) Detail of the nasus with the frontal gland opening. pf, frontal pore.

B. Frontal secretion chemicals

The chemicals of the soldier frontal gland represent a vast biodiversity of natural products and strategies of synthesis, storage, and ejection of substances that may be toxic, repellent, or sticky for the termite enemies (Prestwich, 1979a, 1984). These products have different molecular structures and physical properties as well as a diverse biochemical origin. They can be classified in three main groups: terpenoids; compounds derived from fatty acid metabolism, such as quinones, lactones, alkanes; compounds derived from carbohydrate and/or amino acid metabolism (Costa-Leonardo, 1989; Prestwich, 1984). Some compounds have mixed origin, such as nitroalkenes, which originate from fatty acid metabolism and an amino acid (Prestwich, 1983). Chemical analyses of the frontal gland secretion of Rhinotermitidae and Termitidae have revealed monoterpenes, diterpenes, sesquiterpenes, quinones, macrocyclic lactones, alkanes, alkenes, nitroalkenes, vinyl ketones, aldehydes, proteins, and mucopolysaccharides (Prestwich, 1979b, 1983). Alarm pheromones are volatile components, often monoterpenes, found in the defensive secretions from the soldier frontal gland (Pasteels and Bordereau, 1998). In the soldier of *Prorhinotermes*, the frontal secretion is composed of high amounts of toxic nitropentadecene with smaller amounts of other nitroalkenes, sesquiterpenes, and α-farnesene

(Piskorski *et al.*, 2009). The last of these substances has been shown to act as an alarm pheromone in *Prorhinotermes canalifrons* (Šobotník *et al.*, 2008). Table 21.2 shows some examples of alarm pheromones, including terpenoids and other components of defensive secretions from the frontal glands of termite soldiers. Differences among the chemical substances from the frontal gland secretions of different species may be seen within the same subfamily (Table 21.3). Data concerning frontal gland secretions of reproductives are available only for imagoes of *Prorhinotermes*, which synthesize a mixture of sesquiterpene hydrocarbons and nitroalkenes during the swarming period (Piskorski *et al.*, 2009).

Table 21.2 Some components of defense secretion from the frontal gland of termite soldiers

	Genus	References
Terpenoids		
Monoterpenes	*Syntermes*	Baker *et al.* (1981)
	Amitermes	Moore (1968)
	Nasutitermes	Prestwich (1983)
	Curvitermes	Baker *et al.* (1981)
	Reticulitermes	Parton *et al.* (1981)
Diterpenes	*Nasutitermes*	Prestwich (1984)
	Cubitermes	Prestwich (1984)
Sesquiterpenes	*Cornitermes*	Prestwich (1983)
	Curvitermes	Prestwich (1983)
	Prorhinotermes	Pirskorski *et al.* (2007); Šobotník *et al.* (2008)
	Reticulitermes	Zalkow *et al.* (1981)
Compounds derived from fatty acid		
Macrocyclic lactones	*Armitermes*	Prestwich (1983)
Alkanes	*Macrotermes*	Prestwich (1983)
	Reticulitermes	Baker *et al.* (1982)
	Macrotermes	Prestwich (1984)
Alkenes	*Reticulitermes*	Baker *et al.* (1982)
Ketones	*Schedorhinotermes*	Quennedey *et al.* (1973)
	Rhinotermes	Prestwich and Collins (1982)
Other compounds		
Nitroalkenes	*Prorhinotermes*	Prestwich (1983)
Mucopolysaccharides	*Coptotermes*	Moore (1968)
Protein-rich aqueous quinone	*Odontotermes*	Wood *et al.* (1975)
Aldehydes	*Reticulitermes*	Zalkow *et al.* (1981)

Table 21.3 Chemical components of frontal gland secretions in the subfamily Coptotermitinae

Species	Chemicals of the frontal secretion	References
Coptotermes lacteus	*n*-Alkanes	Moore (1969)
	Mucopolysacharides	Moore (1968)
	n-Tricosane	
Coptotermes testaceus	Hexadecanal	Blum *et al.* (1982)
	Heptadecanal	
Coptotermes formosanus	Mucopolysaccharides	Prestwich (1984)
	Hydrocarbons	
	Free fatty acids	Chen *et al.* (1999)
	Lignoceric acid	
	Hexacosanoic acid	
	Lysozyme	Hardt *et al.* (2003)
	Free ceramides	Ohta *et al.* (2007)

C. Function

The frontal gland of the soldiers produces and stores substances that act as alarm pheromones and defensive chemicals. Alarm pheromones are one constituent of the defensive and offensive warfare of termite species (Pasteels and Bordereau, 1998). According to Ali and Morgan (1990), alarm and defensive behavior occur side by side in social insects. Actions such as accelerate movement and attack precede the liberation of chemical releasers of alarm behavior, which are composed of volatile compounds (Brown, 1960). In the soldier caste, the frontal gland is primordially involved with colony defense, synthesizing toxic products or alarm pheromones, which attract soldiers and repel workers (Eisner *et al.*, 1976). The substances secreted by this gland may be glues, contact poisons, and irritating compounds that can act as repellents, cause deterrence and disorientation in the termite enemies, principally ants. The secretions of the frontal glands of soldiers of the subfamily Nasutitermitinae may act as repellents to invertebrates and vertebrates, such as anteaters (Howse, 1984). The frontal secretion of the nasute mandibulate *Armitermes euamignathus* has a slightly toxic effect on ants and contains tri-, tetra-, and pentadecene, substances that interfere in the communication of ants, because they act as allomones, which are interspecific semiochemicals (Howse, 1984). There are also soldiers that injure enemies with their mandibles and simultaneously apply an oily substance to the wound that is anticoagulant or toxic and originates from the frontal gland. The secretion of *Coptotermes formosanus* has several roles, including immobilization, acting like glue, and as an irritant against predators (Ohta *et al.*, 2007). Behavioral studies with *Coptotermes gestroi* have demonstrated alarm behavior mediated by semiochemicals from the frontal gland of soldiers (Costa-Leonardo *et al.*, 2005). The frontal gland of soldiers is also involved with the production of primer pheromones, and this is the case of *Nasutitermes lujae*, which produces a primer pheromone that inhibits the differentiation of new soldiers (Lefeuve and Bordereau, 1984). According to Mao *et al.* (2005), chemicals from the frontal secretion of *C. formosanus* soldiers may stimulate workers to morph into soldiers in their next two molts. The function of the frontal gland secretion is not clear in reproductives, although Piskorski *et al.* (2009) have suggested a defensive role in imagoes of *Prorhinotermes* during colony foundation. Additionally, nitroalkenes present in the frontal gland secretions of Isoptera soldiers and imagoes seem to function as bactericidal or fungicidal agents (Fuller, 2007; Rosengaus *et al.*, 2000).

V. Mandibular Glands

A. Occurrence and morphology

The mandibular glands are paired cephalic glands and are present in all castes and species of termites. A mandibular complex composed of the mandibular glands and accessory glands was described only in the termite *Zootermopsis angusticollis* (Greenberg and Plavcan, 1986). In forager nymphs of *C. gestroi* these glands are already differentiated and their size is similar to those present in female imagoes (Costa-Leonardo *et al.*, 2009b). These glands are composed of class 3 secretory cells, which have small canals that discharge the secretion in a cuticle fold that forms a collector duct. This duct opens in the exterior of the body of these insects between the mandible and the maxilla (Costa-Leonardo and Shields, 1990). The mandibular glands are small oval-shaped structures in sagittal histological sections and occupy only a limited space on the termite head (Fig. 21.1). However, a variation in size may occur in some castes and species of Isoptera, as is the case for nasute soldiers of the subfamily Nasutitermitinae, in which the mandibular gland is greatly reduced (Noirot, 1969). In workers of *Constrictotermes cyphergaster*, *Constrictotermes rupestris*, and *Constrictotermes cavifrons*, the mandibular glands reach a considerable size and sometimes penetrate the upper part of the mandibles (Constantino and Costa-Leonardo, 1997; Costa-Leonardo and Shields, 1990, Costa-Leonardo, unpublished data).

B. Mandibular secretion chemicals

The chemical composition of the mandibular gland secretion is unknown for the majority of Isoptera. The ultrastructure of the mandibular glands of 3- and 4-year-old queens of *C. gestroi* showed a lamellar secretion, and the histochemical periodic acid-schiff (PAS) test was positive, indicating the presence of glycol radicals, probably glycoproteins (Costa-Leonardo *et al.*, 2009b). In soldiers of *Hodotermopsis japonica*, this gland is well developed and secretes a specific protein (Miura *et al.*, 1999). A chemical analysis of the mandibular gland secretion from workers of *C. formosanus* identified a range of different compounds, including 32 alkanes, 9 aromatics, 2 ketones, 1 ether, 1 ester, 1 alcohol, 1 hydroxybenzene, and 1 carboxylic acid (Mo *et al.*, 2006). The major components of the secretion of the accessory mandibular glands of *Z. angusticollis* were identified as the hydrocarbons *n*-heneicosane and *n*-tricosane (Greenberg and Plavcan, 1986).

C. Function

The function of the mandibular glands in Isoptera is not well established. Lebrun (1972) suggested the involvement of these glands in caste regulation in *Kalotermes flavicollis*. As these glands open to the exterior of the body of the insect, it has been assumed that their function is related to pheromone production. The great development of these glands in workers of *Constrictotermes* and the aggressive behavior of this caste suggest that the mandibular glands participate in the defense of the referred genus (Constantino and Costa-Leonardo, 1997; Costa-Leonardo and Shields, 1990). According to Greenberg and Plavcan (1986), the secretion of the accessory mandibular glands may function as a recognition pheromone and/or as a spreading agent for the secretion of the mandibular glands in the termite *Z. angusticollis*.

VI. Salivary or Labial Glands

A. Occurrence and morphology

The salivary glands are present in all castes of Isoptera (Fig. 21.1). They are paired glands and are composed of groups of acini and two reservoirs, both connected to a duct system that opens in the head, precisely at the basis of the termite labium (Costa-Leonardo, 1987; Noirot, 1969). In termites, the salivary acini are restricted to the thorax and do not occur in the head, a common occurrence in other social insects, such as bees. Small collector ducts emerge from the salivary acini and fuse to originate the efferent ducts, which end in a final duct. The salivary reservoirs are located in the distal part of a final duct, of which the diameter is larger than that of the efferent ducts. The reservoirs are transparent and are bag shaped. In some African soldiers of the subfamily Macrotermitinae, such as *Macrotermes carbonarius*, the salivary reservoirs are hypertrophied and penetrate deep into the abdomen (Deligne *et al.*, 1981; Howse, 1975).

There is an intracinar duct in the central region of the salivary acinous that is continuous with the collector duct and presents similar morphology. In addition to intracinar duct cells, the salivary acini are generally composed of central cells and parietal cells (Billen *et al.*, 1989; Costa-Leonardo, 1997; Costa-Leonardo and Cruz-Landim, 1991; Šobotník and Weyda, 2003). The parietal cells are small and occur in the periphery of the acinous, frequently in pairs. The central cells have many secretory vesicles, and in general, the acinous of termite workers is composed of type I and type II central cells (Fig. 21.3). Type I vesicular cells are abundant and present several electron-lucid vesicles of various sizes. The type II vesicular cells are narrow and possess small electron-lucid secretory vesicles with similar size. These two cellular types contain numerous Golgi apparatuses and abundant rough endoplasmic reticulum. Secretory vesicles have been named secretory vacuoles in several bibliographies about termite salivary glands. The salivary acini of the termite workers may have another central cellular type, as is the case for *S. serrifer*, in which there is an extra central type with a great quantity of electron dense secretion, sometimes in the shape of concentric spirals (Costa-Leonardo, 1997). The ultrastructure of the salivary reservoirs demonstrates that they are constituted by a delicate squamous epithelium, lined internally by a thin cuticular layer involving the lumen of these organs (Billen *et al.*, 1989; Grube *et al.*, 1997). Recent studies have described structures between the duct and water sac that seem to control the opening and closing of the salivary reservoir (Šobotník and Weyda, 2003, Šobotník *et al.*, 2010).

B. Salivary secretion chemicals

Thin-layer chromatography of the salivary acini of *Reticulitermes santonensis* displayed different chemical compounds, including sugars, alcohols, amino acids, peptides, enzymes, carboxylic acids, and salts (Reinhard and Kaib, 2001).

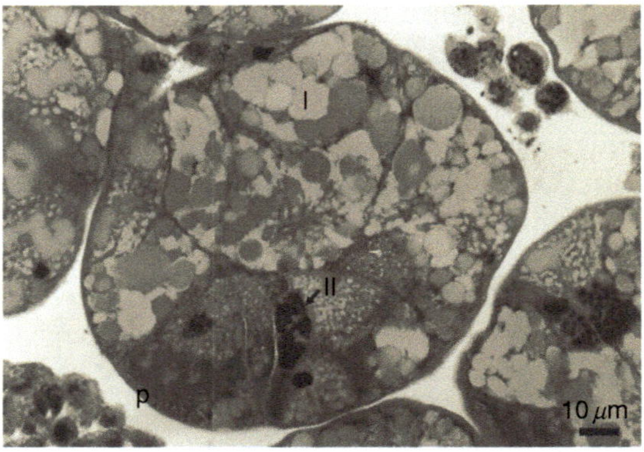

Figure 21.3 Histological section of the salivary acini in worker of *Cornitermes cumulans*. p, parietal cell; I, type I central cell; II, type II central cell.

Subsequent chemical analyses with gas chromatograph coupled to mass spectrometer and feeding bioassays identified hydroquinone as the general phagostimulating pheromone in worker labial glands (Reinhard *et al.*, 2002). However, hydroquinone alone does not act as a phagostimulant for *C. formosanus*, and the explanation for this occurrence relies on the multiple-component pheromones (Raina *et al.*, 2005a).

The secretory products from the salivary reservoirs that act as defensive chemicals were identified as benzoquinones in soldiers of *Macrotermes bellicosus* and *Odontotermes badius* (Howse, 1975, Wood *et al.*, 1975) and toluquinone in soldiers of *M. carbonarius* (Maschwitz *et al.*, 1972).

C. Function

According to Reinhard *et al.* (2002), the salivary secretion contains numerous compounds and has diverse nonpheromonal functions. The salivary secretion contributes to the digestive process through enzymes and has a primordial role in the trophallaxis process, which occurs among the individuals of the termite colony (Grassé, 1982; Noirot, 1969; Veivers *et al.*, 1991). The queens, kings, and immatures receive saliva from workers as food. The soldiers do not feed alone and receive a food composed of a mixture of saliva and crop content of workers. The saliva is also used in nest building and in mycostatic and bacterial control (Grassé, 1982; Matsuura *et al.*, 2007; Noirot, 1969). The salivary reservoirs function as water storage for building activities or regulation of the nest microclimate. Generally, a colorless liquid is stored in the lumen of the salivary reservoirs, which has been shown to be water taken directly from the insect mouth and used in humidity control for some subterranean termites (Grube and Rudolph, 1999; Grube *et al.*, 1997). The hypertrophied salivary reservoirs of some soldiers of Macrotermitinae produce chemicals involved in defense. The brownish salivary secretion of these African soldiers contains quinones and acts as contact poison in wounds caused by their mandibles on the enemies (Maschwitz and Tho, 1974; Moore, 1968).

In the nest building of the termite *Macrotermes subhyalinus*, the workers use soil pellets moistened with saliva and liquid feces. Bruinsma (1979) showed that the saliva of this termite contains an attractive "cement" pheromone that helps coordinate building activity inside the colony. This "cement" pheromone seems to lose its biological activity within a few minutes of deposition and orients workers 1–2 cm from the deposition site inducing them to pick up soil pellets and deposit them. The building and movement behaviors of the termite workers are controlled locally by pheromone concentration. The salivary glands also produce pheromones that participate in intraspecific communication of subterranean termites during foraging and building activities (Kaib and Ziesmann, 1992; Reinhard and Kaib, 1995; Reinhard *et al.*, 1997). Studies indicate that a generic pheromone that works as phagostimulant is present in the saliva of Isoptera (Casarin *et al.*, 2003; Reinhard *et al.*, 1997, 2002). During food source exploration, the termite workers aggregate at specific sites of the food, named chew zones due to the chemical signals at these areas with the saliva. The communally chewed areas of the food are marked by the workers that moisten the food and reinforce the chemical signal of the salivary phagostimulant (Reinhard *et al.*, 1997).

VII. Sternal Gland

A. Occurrence and morphology

The sternal gland is unpaired, occurs in all termite castes, and is present as an epidermal thickening of the sternite (Fig. 21.1). A single gland located under the 5th sternite is present in the families Kalotermitidae, Rhinotermitidae, Serritermitidae, and Termitidae (Fig. 21.4), while in the Hodotermitidae and Termopsidae this gland is placed under the 4th sternite. The termite *Mastotermes darwiniensis*, the unique still-living representative of the family Mastotermitidae, has three sternal glands, located under the 3rd, 4th, and 5th sternites (Ampion and Quennedey, 1981; Noirot, 1969). Campaniform sensilla are always associated with the sternal gland and have been observed in the middle of the glandular mass. The ultrastructure of the sternal gland showed that this gland may be composed of classes 1, 2, and 3 cells (Ampion and Quennedey, 1981; Quennedey *et al.*, 2008). In addition to sternal glands, other abdominal glands, such as posterior sternal glands and

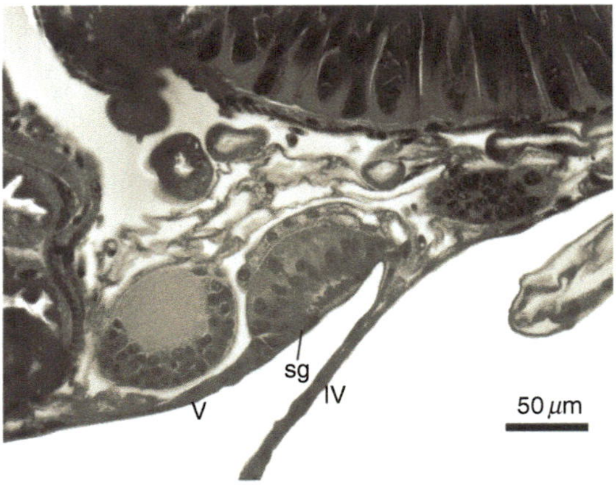

Figure 21.4 Sternal gland of *Cornitermes cumulans* worker in sagittal histological section. sg, sternal gland; IV, 4th sternite; V, 5th sternite.

pleural glands, have also been described in termites. The posterior sternal glands occur in both sexes of *M. darwiniensis* (at sternites 6–9 in males and 6–7 in females), in males of *Porotermes*, *Stolotermes*, and *Prorhinotermes simplex* (8 and 9 sternites), and in females of *Macrotermes annandalei* and *Macrotermes barneyi* occur at the anterior margin of sternites 6 and 7 (Ampion and Quennedey, 1981; Peppuy *et al.*, 2004; Quennedey *et al.*, 2004; Šobotník *et al.*, 2005). The ultrastructure of the posterior sternal glands showed class 1 and class 3 cells arranged together or comprised of only class 3 cells. The pleural glands occur in female imagoes of *Cubitermes fungifaber* and are comprised of a thickening of the pleural epidermis made up of class 3 cells associated with chemoreceptor sensilla (Grassé, 1982).

B. Sternal secretion chemicals

Termite trail pheromones are a multicomponent blend with a common component eliciting movement and specific secondary compounds that determine the specificity of trails among species (Arab *et al.*, 2004; Kaib, 1999). Studies with different species showed different biological activity between trail pheromones and sternal gland extract, suggesting synergy with minor components (Sillam-Dussès *et al.*, 2005). Chemical analyses of these minor components are lacking in the majority of termite species. The sternal gland is the only termite gland responsible for the production of the trail pheromone, and only a few molecules have been identified as worker semiochemicals to date, including decadienol, dodecanal, dodecenol, dodecadienol, dodecatrienol, C18 aldehyde, neocembrene, and some mixtures, including dodecatrienol + neocembrene, dodecatrienol + neocembrene + trinervitatriene (Bordereau and Pasteels, 2010; Sillam-Dussès *et al.*, 2006, 2007, 2009a,b, 2010). Some termite genera and their respective trail pheromones are listed in Table 21.4.

Chemical analyses of secretions from the sternal glands of Isoptera reproductives have identified the following semiochemicals: decadienal, dodecanal, dodecadienol, dodecatrienol, neocembrene, and tetradecyl propionate, which function as sex pheromones (Table 21.5) (Bordereau and Pasteels, 2010; Costa-Leonardo *et al.*, 2009a; Pasteels and Bordereau, 1998).

C. Function

The sternal glands of workers produce trail pheromones, but these glands are involved with courtship behavior in imagoes. The odoriferous trails that guide termite foraging are produced by the sternal gland, which is pressured against the substrate. Sternal gland secretions are produced by the glandular cells and drain to a cavity that is between these cells and the cuticle of the insect body. When the glandular region is pressed against the soil, the secretion is released. The sternal gland is not functional in larval instars

Table 21.4 Trail pheromones in some termite genera

Family	Genus	Trail pheromone	References
Mastotermitidae	*Mastotermes*	Decadienol	Sillam-Dussès *et al.* (2007)
Hodotermitidae	*Hodotermes*	C18 aldehyde	Bordereau and Pasteels (2010)
Termopsidae	*Zootermopsis*	Dodecanal	Bordereau *et al.* (2006)
	Stolotermes	Decadienol	Sillam-Dussès *et al.* (2007)
	Porotermes	Decadienol	Sillam-Dussès *et al.* (2007)
Kalotermitidae	*Kalotermes*, *Cryptotermes*	Dodecenol	Sillam-Dussès *et al.* (2009b)
Rhinotermitidae	*Prorhinotermes*	Neocembrene + Dodecatrienol	Sillam-Dussès *et al.* (2009a)
	Heterotermes	Dodecatrienol	Sillam-Dussès *et al.* (2006)
	Coptotermes	Dodecatrienol	Sillam-Dussès *et al.* (2006)
	Rhinotermes	Dodecatrienol	Sillam-Dussès *et al.* (2006)
Termitidae	*Constrictotermes*	Dodecatrienol + Neocembrene	Sillam-Dussès *et al.* (2010)
	Nasutitermes	Dodecatrienol + Neocembrene + Trinervitatriene	Sillam-Dussès *et al.* (2010)
	Cubitermes	Dodecatrienol	Sillam-Dussès *et al.* (2006)
	Cornitermes	Dodecatrienol	Sillam-Dussès *et al.* (2006)
	Syntermes	Dodecatrienol	Sillam-Dussès *et al.* (2006)
	Macrotermes	Dodecenol	Peppuy *et al.* (2001)
	Pseudacanthotermes	Dedocatrienol	Bordereau *et al.* (1993)

and is less developed in young workers. The trails are used to recruit individuals to the food source and to galleries and nest repair sites. The trail concentration increases with the worker number, and this affects the locomotion ratio and the direction followed by the insects. The soldiers

Table 21.5 Sex pheromones and their exocrine gland source in some termite reproductives

Pheromones	Reproductives	Species	Exocrine glands	References
Decadienal, Dodecanal	Female, male	*Zootermopsis nevadensis*	SG	Bordereau *et al.* (2006)
Dodecatrienol	Female	*Prorhinotermes simplex*	TG	Hanus *et al.* (2009)
Dodecatrienol	Female	*Reticulitermes santonensis*	SG	Laduguie *et al.* (1994)
Dodecatrienol	Female	*Cornitermes bequaerti*	TG	Bordereau *et al.* (2002)
Neocembrene	Female	*Trinervitermes bettonianus*	SG	McDowell and Oloo (1984)
NI	Female	*Macrotermes annandalei*	PSG/TG	Quennedey *et al.* (2004) Peppuy *et al.* (2004)
NI	Female	*Macrotermes barneyi*	PSG/TG	Quennedey *et al.* (2004) Peppuy *et al.* (2004)
Dodecatrienol	Female	*Pseudacanthotermes spiniger*	SG	Bordereau *et al.* (1993)
Dodecatrienol	Female	*Pseudacanthotermes militares*	SG	Bordereau *et al.* (1993)
Dodecadienol	Female	*Ancistrotermes pakistanicus*	SG	Robert *et al.* (2004)

SG, sternal gland; PSG, posterior sternal gland; TG, tergal glands; NI, not identified.

participate in foraging activities, and they are the individuals initially attracted by trails in nasute termites of the subfamily Nasutitermitinae (Costa-Leonardo and Kitayama, 1990; Traniello, 1981). Later, when the trail concentration increases, the workers also participate in foraging. The different castes may have different quantities of trail pheromones. However, termites may individually regulate the quantity and composition of the trail.

In some species, courtship behavior begins with an appeal of the female imago or calling position, in which the reproductive lifts the abdomen and exposes the sternal gland. The liberated pheromone calls to the male and attracts it to the female. The two then begin the tandem or nuptial dancing phase, in which the male generally follows the female (Howse, 1984). The posterior sternal glands also have a role in the sexual behavior of the imagoes and the termites *M. annandalei* and *M. barneyi*, in which these glands are involved in calling and tandem behaviors, that is, short- and long-range attractants, while the sternal gland of the 5th sternite is connected with the production of trail pheromone (Peppuy *et al.*, 2004).

VIII. Tergal Gland

A. Occurrence and morphology

The occurrence of tergal glands in the abdomen of the reproductives is well documented in Isoptera (Ampion and Quennedey, 1981; Bordereau *et al.*, 2002; Raina *et al.*, 2005b). These glands appear as epidermal thickenings under some tergites of the imagoes and can occur only in females or in both sexes (Fig. 21.1). They have been observed in neotenic nonfunctional reproductives of *K. flavicollis* (Lebrun, 1971), but regress in the functional reproductives and may be absent in physogastric queens, for example, the queen of *Cornitermes cumulans* (Ignatti and Costa-Leonardo, 2001). These glands may be absent in the male and female imagoes, as they are in *Zootermopsis nevadensis* and *R. santonensis*. Nevertheless, there are species in which these glands are present in both sexes of imagoes, as in *K. flavicollis*, or only in the female, as in *C. cumulans*. The number of glands is variable as *M. darwiniensis* has eight (from the 3rd to the 10th tergite) while *Apicotermes trägårdhi* has one (10th tergite). Variation inside the same genus can also occur, as in the case for *Macrotermes*, in which *M. bellicosus* possesses five (from the 6th to the 10th tergite), and *M. subhyalinus*, *Macrotermes natalensis*, and *Macrotermes ukuzii* possess eight (from the 3rd to the 10th tergite). The tergal glands are not present in all Hodotermitidae, among the Heterotermitinae of the genus *Reticulitermes*, among the Macrotermitinae of the genera *Megaprotermes*, *Protermes*, *Odontotermes*, *Ancistrotermes*, *Pseudacanthotermes*, among the Apicotermitinae of the genera *Firmitermes*, *Skatitermes*, among the Termitinae of the genera *Euchilotermes*, *Procubitermes*, *Cubitermes*, *Lepidotermes*, *Thoracotermes*, *Basidentitermes*, *Ovambotermes*, and among the Nasutitermitinae of the genera *Spatulitermes* and *Eutermellus* (Ampion and Quennedey, 1981; Grassé, 1982). The tergal glands are principally composed of class 1 and class 2 cells (Ampion and Quennedey, 1981), although class 3 cells have been described in the tergal glands of *Cornitermes bequaerti* (Bordereau *et al.*, 2002) and *P. simplex* (Šobotník *et al.*, 2005). The tergal gland secretory cells of some female imagoes present an extensive smooth endoplasmic reticulum, numerous mitochondria, and lipid droplets (Fig. 21.5).

To date, tergal glands have been described only in the reproductive caste, although these glands also occur in some soldiers of Syntermitinae, including *Syntermes nanus*, *C. cumulans*, and *Procornitermes araujoi* (Costa-Leonardo *et al.*, unpublished data). In these soldiers, the tergal glands appear

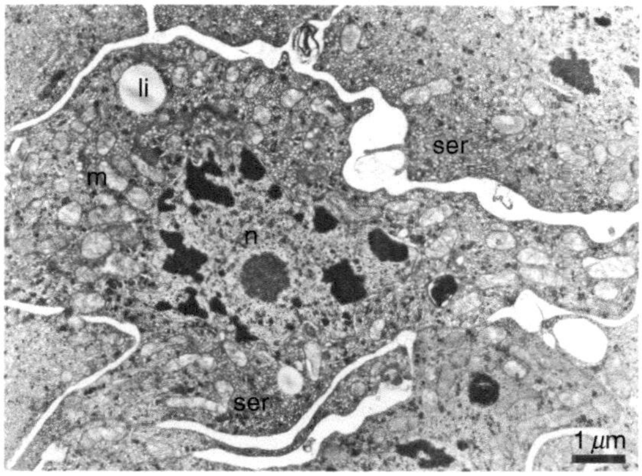

Figure 21.5 Electron micrograph of tergal gland secretory cells of *Cornitermes cumulans* female imago showing the well-developed smooth endoplasmic reticulum (ser). li, lipid droplet; n, nucleus; m, mitochondria.

as cellular thickenings under all tergites and are composed of classes 2 and 3 glandular cells (Fig. 21.1).

B. Tergal secretion chemicals

Chemical analyses of the reproductive tergal gland secretions have identified the following semiochemicals: dodecenol, dodecadienol, dodecatrienol, neocembrene, nerolidol, and trinervitatriene, which function as sex pheromones (Bordereau and Pasteels, 2010; Hanus *et al.*, 2009; Pasteels and Bordereau, 1998). The chemical composition of this type of glandular secretion in the soldier caste is unknown, but in cockroaches, where its role is in defense, the secretion is composed of cyclohexanone, heptanone, and undecene (Brossut, 1983).

C. Function

The role of tergal glands in imagoes seems to be connected to reproductive activity and especially to the formation of the sexual pair after swarming. According to some authors, the tergal glands are responsible for the tandem behavior or short-range attraction in some species of termites (Barth, 1955; Bordereau *et al.*, 2002). Nevertheless, this function is not clear for some researchers because reproductives that do not possess tergal glands also show tandem behavior and others, which present these structures, do not have this behavior (Bordereau and Pasteels, 2010; Leuthold, 1975; Raina *et al.*, 2003). In addition, other glands may be involved in tandem behavior. In the Neotropical termite *C. cumulans*, the male approaches after the calling behavior of the female and begins the tandem behavior, at which point its antennae are put in the last female tergites, the location of the tergal and tegumental glands, which open in the intersegmental membranes (Costa-Leonardo, unpublished data). In a few species, the tergal glands are also involved in long-range attraction or calling, as is the case for *M. annandalei*, *M. barneyi*, and *Trinervitermes bettonianus* (Leuthold, 1975; Peppuy *et al.*, 2004).

In the soldier caste, morphological evidence obtained for the tergal glands suggests that these structures may be involved in pheromone production, because their glandular cells have well developed smooth endoplasmic reticulum and Golgi apparatus (Costa-Leonardo *et al.*, unpublished data). This cytological morphology is consistent with the elaboration of low molecular weight compounds, which are characteristic of many pheromone-producing glands (Billen, 1991). In addition, the tergal gland in this caste may be connected to the production of defensive chemicals, which occurs in the tergal glands of some roaches (Brossut, 1983; Masson and Brossut, 1981).

IX. Termite Recognition Pheromones

Hydrocarbons are chemical compounds used by several insects as intra- and interspecific signals, and numerous studies indicate their role in the nestmate recognition of social insects (Howard and Blomquist, 2005). The composition of cuticular hydrocarbons differs among termite colonies of the same species, and the differences might be correlated with intercolonial aggression (Jmhasly *et al.*, 1998; Kaib *et al.*, 2002, 2004). Some studies have indicated that there is a genetic mechanism for the production of cuticular hydrocarbons, while others have suggested that there is an environmental effect (Dronnet *et al.*, 2006; Florane *et al.*, 2004; Matsuura, 2001). Large colonies, such as those found for some termite species, require the sharing of individual chemical profiles to produce an average colony profile (Crozier and Dix, 1979). The cuticle may be the source of these chemical compounds, which are spread to the colony during the grooming behavior. Among the social insects, an exocrine gland may also be the source of these hydrocarbons, which are spread to the colony through trophallaxis. This occurs with the postpharyngeal gland of ants (Vander Meer and Morel, 1998). Interactions between semiochemicals from the cuticle and from the exocrine glands may occur, creating a specific hydrocarbon profile that characterizes colony recognition. To date, no termite glands are known to contain cuticular lipids, and these substances may be spread to the Isoptera colony only by grooming (Clément and Bagnères, 1998, Howard and Blomquist, 2005). According to Kaib (1999), the termite cuticle functions as a large exocrine gland that produces a blend of chemical compounds, including hydrocarbons. In the Neotropical termite *Heterotermes tenuis*, the composition of the cuticular extract was determined using gas chromatography–mass spectrometry and electrophysiological studies. The hydrocarbons identified were restricted to linear alkanes (Batista-Pereira *et al.*, 2004). Termite research with hydrocarbons shows differences among species (Clément and Bagnères, 1998; Sevala *et al.*, 2000), and few authors discuss that semiochemicals other than cuticular hydrocarbons are important in the production of nestmate recognition cues (Howard and Blomquist, 2005). According to Keller and Nonacs (1993), the stability of eusocial colonies depends on communication between reproductive and nonreproductive individuals through pheromones to maintain the central division of labor. Pheromonal inhibition has been implicated in the reproductive division of labor within termite colonies (Vieau, 1990). Differences in the specificity of termite hydrocarbons also occur among castes and sexes (Bagnères *et al.*, 1991; Pasteels and Bordereau, 1998). Present data show that cuticular hydrocarbon profiles may indicate the reproductive status inside the termite colony, and specific reproductive hydrocarbons may promote tending behavior in workers or act as primer pheromones, inhibiting gonad development in immatures (Liebig *et al.*, 2009). Weil *et al.* (2009) found qualitative differences in the cuticular hydrocarbon profiles between workers and neotenic queens in *Cryptotermes secundus*. Four polyunsaturated alkenes occur as hydrocarbon profiles in *Z. nevadensis*, but higher concentrations of these compounds have been found only in functional reproductives and not in soldiers, worker-like larvae, or secondary reproductives with inactive gonads, in which these alkenes occur in small amounts or are absent (Liebig *et al.*, 2009).

Recent studies with termites of the genus *Reticulitermes* have demonstrated that proteins produced by the salivary glands, including lysozyme and the enzyme *β*-glucosidase, which are respectively responsible for antibacterial activity and cellulose digestion, are also present on the termite egg surface and function together as a pheromone for egg recognition. This was the first identification of proteinaceous pheromones in social insects, and bioassays demonstrated perfect pheromonal activity when both enzymes were present together, also suggesting a synergic interaction between the lysozyme and *β*-glucosidase (Matsuura *et al.*, 2007, 2009). In addition to this pheromone, termite egg recognition is also based on egg morphology, including size, shape, and surface texture (Matsuura, 2006).

X. Concluding Remarks

The recent discovery of new Isoptera semiochemicals is principally due to the method of solid-phase microextraction which allowed for the selective extraction of products secreted at the surface of pheromone glands (Sillam-Dussès *et al.*, 2010). Present data confirm that trail and sex pheromones appear to be very conservative in their chemical evolution, that is, many termite species use only a few substances (Bordereau and Pasteels, 2010). Additionally, many species of termites may use the same molecule as a pheromone, but this is dependent on the chemical concentration and on the caste involved. The remarkable simplicity of termite trail pheromones is probably due to the unique glandular source, the sternal gland, and the simplicity of their food (Noirot, 1969; Sillam-Dussès *et al.*, 2010). Additionally, the termites present a pheromonal parsimony in which the same chemical compound is produced by different glands and different species and is used for different functions (Bordereau and Pasteels, 2010; Costa-Leonardo *et al.*, 2009a). The termite pheromones suggest that a great economy exists in the strategies of chemical communication for this group. In *C. bequaerti*, the same compound (dodecatrienol) is used both as a sex and a trail pheromone (Bordereau *et al.*, 2002). Dodecatrienol is also present in the blend of sex pheromones of many species of Termitidae and Rhinotermitidae, demonstrating that the same molecule is present in different families. Pheromone compounds might have originally evolved from other contexts and only later developed the role on chemical communication. This seems to be the case of the egg recognition pheromone, for which the components were probably produced for other primary functions in the past (Matsuura *et al.*, 2007, 2009). The glandular sources of the pheromones are the exocrine glands, but in Isoptera, some of these glands are still little known, including the mandibular glands, because most of their products have not been identified and characterized as pheromones. Despite the ecological and economical roles of termites, little is known about their exocrine glands and semiochemicals when compared to what is already known for other social insects. Studies using bioassays, quantitative gas chromatography–mass spectrometry, and electroantennography will contribute to a better understanding of the chemical communication inside the termite colony and the involvement of other exocrine glands with secretion of pheromones. Knowledge of the pheromonal regulation of reproduction in termites and the elucidation of their chemical communication system will enhance our understanding about the evolution and social organization of Isoptera.

ACKNOWLEDGMENT

The authors thank CNPq (Conselho Nacional de Pesquisa e Desenvolvimento) for financial support during their termite research.

REFERENCES

Ali, M. F., and Morgan, D. (1990). Chemical communication in insect communities: A guide to insect pheromones with special emphasis on social insects. *Biol. Rev.* **65,** 227–247.

Ampion, M., and Quennedey, A. (1981). The abdominal epidermal glands of termites and their phylogenetic significance. *In* "Biosystematics of Social Insects," (P. E. Howse and J. L. Clément, Eds.), Vol. 19, pp. 249–261. Academic Press, London.

Arab, A., Costa-Leonardo, A. M., Batista-Pereira, L. G., Santos, M. G., Corrêa, A. G., and Blanco, Y. C. (2004). Trail-pheromone specificity of two sympatric termites (Rhinotermitidae) from Southeastern Brazil. *Sociobiology* **43,** 377–387.

Backer, R., Coles, H. R., Edwards, M., Evans, D. A., Howse, P. E., and Walmsley, S. (1981). Chemical composition of the frontal gland secretion of *Syntermes* soldiers (Isoptera: Termitidae). *J. Chem. Ecol.* **7,** 135–146.

Bagnères, A. G., Killian, A., Clément, J. L., and Lange, C. (1991). Interspecific recognition among termites of the genus *Reticulitermes*: Evidence for a role for the cuticular hydrocarbons. *J. Chem. Ecol.* **17,** 2397–2420.

Baker, R., Parton, A. H., and Howse, P. E. (1982). Identification of an acyclic diterpene alcohol in the defense secretion of soldiers of *Reticulitermes lucifugus*. *Experientia* **38,** 297–298.

Barth, R. (1955). Über die tergitalen druesenfelder von *Syntermes dirus* (Isoptera). *Rev. Bras. Entomol.* **15,** 257–263.

Batista-Pereira, L. G., Santos, M. G., Corrêa, A. G., Fernandes, J. B., Arab, A., Costa-Leonardo, A. M., Camargo-Dietrich, C. R. R., Pereira, D. A., and Bueno, O. C. (2004). Cuticular hydrocarbons of *Heterotermes tenuis* (Isoptera: Rhinotermitidae): Analyses and electrophysiological studies. *Z. Naturforsch.* **59,** 135–139.

Billen, J. (1991). Ultrastructural organization of the exocrine glands in ants. *Ethol. Ecol. Evol.* **1,** 67–73.

Billen, J., and Morgan, E. D. (1998). Pheromone communication in social insects: Sources and secretions. *In* "Pheromone communication in social insects: Ants, wasps, bees, and termites," (R. K. Vander Meer, M. D. Breed, K. E. Espelie, and M. L. Winston, Eds.), pp. 3–33. Westview Press, Boulder.

Billen, J., Joye, L., and Leuthold, R. H. (1989). Fine structure of the labial gland in *Macrotermes bellicosus* (Isoptera, Termitidae). *Acta Zool.* **70,** 37–45.

Blum, M. S., Jones, T. H., Howard, D. F., and Overal, W. L. (1982). Biochemistry of termite defenses: *Coptotermes*, *Rhinotermes*, and *Cornitermes* species. *Comp. Biochem. Physiol. B* **71,** 731–733.

Blum, M. S. (1985). Exocrine systems. *In* "Fundamentals of Insect Physiology," (M. S. Blum, Ed.), pp. 535–579. Wiley, New York.

Bordereau, C., and Pasteels, J. M. (2010). Pheromones and chemical ecology of dispersal and foraging in termites. *In* "Biology of Termites: A Modern Synthesis," (D. E. Bignell, Y. Roisin, and N. Lo, Eds.). Springer, Heidelberg in press.

Bordereau, C., Robert, A., Laduguie, N., Bonnard, O., Le Quére, J. L., and Yamaoka, R. (1993). Détection du (Z,Z,E)-3,6,8-dodecatrien-1-ol par les ouvriers et les essaimants de deux espèces de termites champignonnistes: *Pseudacanthotermes spiniger* et *P. militaris* (Termitidae, Macrotermitinae). *Actes. Coll. Ins. Soc.* **8,** 145–149.

Bordereau, C., Robert, A., Tuyen, V. V., and Peppuy, A. (1997). Suicidal defensive behaviour by frontal gland dehiscence in *Globitermes sulphureus* Haviland soldiers (Isoptera). *Insectes Soc.* **44,** 289–296.

Bordereau, C., Cancello, E. M., Sémon, E., Courrent, A., and Quennedey, A. (2002). Sex pheromone identified after solid phase microextraction from tergal glands of female alates in *Cornitermes bequaerti* (Isoptera, Nasutitermitinae). *Insectes Soc.* **49,** 209–215.

Bordereau, C., Lacey, M., Ghostin, J. C., Braekman, J. C., Sillam-Dussès, D., Robert, A., Shellman, J. S., and Sémon, E. (2006). Sex pheromones and trail-following pheromones in *Zootermopsis nevadensis* and *Z. angusticollis* (Isoptera, Termopsidae). *Proc. XV Congr. IUSSI*, Washington, DC, USA.

Brossut, R. (1983). Allomonal secretions in cockroaches. *J. Chem. Ecol.* **9,** 143–158.

Brown, W. L. J. (1960). The release of alarm and attack behavior in some New World army ants. *Psyche* **66,** 25–27.

Bruinsma, O. M. (1979). An analysis of building behaviour of the termite *Macrotermes subhyalinus*. Doctoral thesis, Agricultural University, Wageningen, Holland.

Casarin, F. E., Arab, A., and Costa-Leonardo, A. M. (2003). Influence of the labial gland's semiochemicals on the feeding behavior of *Coptotermes havilandi* (Isoptera: Rhinotermitidae). *Sociobiology* **42,** 485–493.
Chapman, R. F. (1998). The Insects: Structure and Function. 4th edn. Cambridge University Press, United Kingdom.
Chen, J., Henderson, G., and Laine, R. A. (1999). Lignoceric acid and hexacosanoic acid: major components of soldier frontal gland secretions of the Formosan subterranean termite (*Coptotermes formosanus*). *J. Chem. Ecol.* **25,** 817–824.
Clément, J. L., and Bagnères, A. G. (1998). Nestmate recognition in termites. *In* "Pheromone Communication in Social Insects: Ants, Wasps, Bees, and Termites," (R. K. Vander Meer, M. Breed, M. Winston, and K. Espelie, Eds.), pp. 126–155. Westview Press, Boulder.
Constantino, R., and Costa-Leonardo, A. M. (1997). A new species of *Constrictotermes* from Central Brazil with notes on the mandibular glands of workers (Isoptera, Termitidae, Nasutitermitinae). *Sociobiology* **30,** 213–223.
Costa-Leonardo, A. M. (1987). Morfologia das glândulas salivares de *Cornitermes cumulans* e *Armitermes euamignathus* (Isoptera, Termitidae, Nasutitermitinae). *Naturalia* **11**(12), 71–76.
Costa-Leonardo, A. M. (1989). A guerra química dos cupins. *Ciência Hoje* **56,** 26–34.
Costa-Leonardo, A. M. (1997). Secretion of salivary glands of the Brazilian termite *Serritermes serrifer* Hagen & Bates (Isoptera, Serritermitidae). *Ann. Soc. Entomol. Fr.* **33,** 29–37.
Costa-Leonardo, A. M. (1998a). Morphology of the frontal weapon in the soldier caste of *Cornitermes cumulans* (Isoptera, Termitidae). *Rev. Bras. Entomol.* **41,** 195–197.
Costa-Leonardo, A. M. (1998b). The frontal weapon of the termite soldier *Serritermes serrifer* (Isoptera, Serritermitidae). *Ciênc. Cult.* **50,** 65–67.
Costa-Leonardo, A. M. (2001). The frontal weapon of the termite *Armitermes euamignathus* Silvestri (Isoptera, Termitidae, Nasutitermitinae). *Rev. Bras. Zool.* **18,** 411–419.
Costa-Leonardo, A. M., and Cruz-Landim, C. (1991). Morphology of the salivary gland acini in *Grigiotermes bequaerti* (Isoptera: Termitidae: Apicotermitinae). *Entomol. Gen.* **16,** 13–21.
Costa-Leonardo, A. M., and De Salvo, C. R. A. (1987). A comparative study of the frontal glands in three species of Brazilian termite soldiers (Isoptera, Termitidae). *Rev. Bras. Entomol.* **31,** 465–471.
Costa-Leonardo, A. M., and Kitayama, K. (1990). Sternal gland size related to polyetism in the termite *Constrictotermes cyphergaster* soldiers (Termitidae, Nasutitermitinae). *Ciênc. Cult.* **42,** 975–977.
Costa-Leonardo, A. M., and Kitayama, K. (1991). Frontal gland dehiscence in the Brazilian termite *Serritermes serrifer* (Isoptera: Serritermitidae). *Sociobiology* **19,** 333–338.
Costa-Leonardo, A. M., and Shields, K. S. (1990). Morphology of the mandibular glands in workers of *Constrictotermes cyphergaster* soldiers (Termitidae, Nasutermitinae). *Int. J. Insect Morphol. Embryol.* **19,** 61–64.
Costa-Leonardo, A. M., Lima, J. T., Casarin, F. E., Marchetti, F. F., Haifig, I., and Chaves, R. C. S. (2005). Comportamento de alarme mediado por semioquímicos da glândula frontal do soldado de *Coptotermes gestroi* (Isoptera, Rhinotermitidae). Anais do IV Encontro Brasileiro de Ecologia Química FEALQ—Fundação de Estudos Agrários Luiz de Queiroz, Piracicaba. p. 67.
Costa-Leonardo, A. M., Casarin, F. E., and Lima, J. T. (2009a). Chemical communication in Isoptera. *Neotrop. Entomol.* **38,** 1–6.
Costa-Leonardo, A. M., Gonçalves, F. C., and Laranjo, L. T. (2009b). Mandibular glands in reproductives of Asian termite *Coptotermes gestroi* (Isoptera: Rhinotermitidae). *Acta Microsc.* **18,** 220–231.
Crozier, R. H., and Dix, M. W. (1979). Analysis of two genetic models for the innate components of colony odour in social Hymenoptera. *Behav. Ecol. Sociobiol.* **4,** 217–224.

Deligne, J., and DeConinck, E. (2006). Suicidal defence through a dehiscent frontal weapon in *Apilitermes longiceps* soldiers (Isoptera: Termitidae). *Belg. J. Entomol.* **8,** 3–10.
Deligne, J., Quennedey, A., and Blum, M. S. (1981). The enemies and defense mechanisms of termites. *In* "Social Insects, Vol. 2," (H. R. Hermann, Ed.), pp. 1–76. Academic Press, New York.
Dronnet, S., Lohou, C., Christides, J. P., and Bagnères, A. G. (2006). Cuticular hydrocarbon composition reflects genetic relationship among colonies of the introduced termite *Reticulitermes santonensis* Feytaud. *J. Chem. Ecol.* **32,** 1027–1042.
Eisner, T., Kriston, I., and Aneshansley, D. J. (1976). Defensive behavior of a termite (*Nasutitermes exitiosus*). *Behav. Ecol. Sociobiol.* **1,** 83–125.
Florane, C. B., Bland, J. M., Husseneder, C., and Raina, A. K (2004). Diet-mediated inter-colonial aggression in the Formosan subterranean termite *Coptotermes formosanus*. *J. Chem. Ecol.* **30,** 2259–2574.
Fuller, C. A. (2007). Fungistatic activity of freshly killed termite, *Nasutitermes acajutlae*, soldiers in the Caribbean. *J. Insect Sci.* **7,** 1–8.
Grassé, P. P. (1982). Termitologia: Anatomie-Physiologie-Reproduction des Termites. 1st edn. Masson, Paris.
Greenberg, S. L., and Plavcan, K. A. (1986). Morphology and chemistry of the mandibular gland complex in the primitive termite, *Zootermopsis angusticollis* (Hagen) (Isoptera: Hodotermitidae). *Int. J. Insect Morphol. Embryol.* **15,** 283–292.
Grube, S., and Rudolph, D. (1999). The labial gland reservoirs (water sacs) in *Reticulitermes santonensis* (Isoptera: Rhinotermitidae): studies of the functional aspects during microclimatic moisture regulation and individual water balance. *Sociobiology* **33,** 307–323.
Grube, S., Rudolph, D., and Zerbst-Boroffka, I. (1997). Morphology, fine structure, and functional aspects of the labial gland reservoirs of the subterranean termite *Reticulitermes santonensis* De Feytaud (Isoptera: Rhinotermitidae). *Int. J. Insect Morphol. Embryol.* **26,** 49–53.
Hanus, R., Luxová, A., Šobotník, J., Kalinová, B., Jiroš, P., Křeček, J., Bourguignon, T., and Bordereau, C. (2009). Sexual communication in the *Prorhinotermes simplex* (Isoptera, Rhinotermitidae) mediated by a pheromone from female tergal glands. *Insectes Soc.* **56,** 111–118.
Hardt, M., Guo, Y., Henderson, G., and Laine, R. A. (2003). Zymogram with Remazol brilliant blue-labeled *Micrococcus lysodeikticus* cells for the detection of lysozymes: example of a new lysozyme activity in Formosan termite defense secretions. *Anal. Biochem.* **312,** 73–76.
Henderson, G. (1998). Primer pheromones and possible soldier caste influence on the evolution of sociality in lower termites. *In* "Pheromone Communication in Social Insects: Ants, Wasps, Bees, and Termites," (R. K. VanderMeer, M. D. Winston, and K. E. Espelie, Eds.), pp. 314–330. Westview Press, Oxford.
Howard, R. W., and Blomquist, G. J. (2005). Ecological, behavioral, and biochemical aspects of insect hydrocarbons. *Annu. Rev. Entomol.* **50,** 371–393.
Howse, P. E. (1975). Chemical defence of ants, termites and other insects: some outstanding questions. *In* "Pheromones and Defensive Secretions in Social Insects," (C. Noirot, P. E. Howse, and G. Le Masne, Eds.), pp. 23–40. Université de Dijon, Dijon.
Howse, P. E. (1984). Sociochemicals of termites. *In* "Chemical Ecology of Insects," (W. J. Bell and R. T. Cardé, Eds.), pp. 475–519. Chapman and Hall, London.
Ignatti, A. C., and Costa-Leonardo, A. M. (2001). The exocrine glands of swarming females and physogastric queens of *Cornitermes cumulans* (Kollar) (Isoptera, Termitidae, Nasutitermitinae). *Revta Bras. Zool.* **18,** 1089–1096.
Inward, D. J. G., Vogler, A. P., and Eggleton, P. (2007). A comprehensive phylogenetic analysis of termites (Isoptera) illuminates key aspects of their evolutionary biology. *Mol. Phylogenet. Evol.* **44,** 953–967.

Jmhasly, P., Brandl, R., Leuthold, R. H., and Kaib, M. (1998). Aggression and cuticular hydrocarbon profiles in a termite. *Zoology* **101,** 11.

Kaib, M. (1999). Termites. *In* "Pheromones of Non-Lepidopteran Insects Associated with Agricultural Plants," (J. Hardie and A. K. Minks, Eds.), pp. 329–353. CABI, Wallingford Oxon.

Kaib, M., and Ziesmann, J. (1992). The labial gland in the termite *Schedorhinotermes lamanianus* (Isoptera: Rhinotermitidae): Morphology and function during communal food exploitation. *Insectes Soc.* **39,** 373–384.

Kaib, M., Franke, S., Francke, W., and Brandl, R. (2002). Cuticular hydrocarbons in a termite: Phenotypes and a neighbour-stranger effect. *Physiol. Entomol.* **27,** 189–198.

Kaib, M., Jmhasly, P., Wilfert, L., Durka, W., Franke, S., Francke, W., Leuthold, R. H., and Brandl, R. (2004). Cuticular hydrocarbons and aggression in the termite *Macrotermes subhyalinus*. *J. Chem. Ecol.* **30,** 365–385.

Karlson, P., and Lüscher, M. (1959). Pheromones, a new term for a class of biologically active substances. *Nature* **183,** 55–56.

Keller, L., and Nonacs, P. (1993). The role of queen pheromones in social insects: Queen control or queen signal? *Anim. Behav.* **45,** 787–794.

Laduguie, N., Robert, A., Bonnard, O., Vieau, F., Le Quéré, J. L., Sémon, E., and Bordereau, C. (1994). Isolation and identification of (3Z,6Z,8E)-3,6,8-dodecatrien-1-ol in *Reticulitermes santonensis* Feytaud (Isoptera, Rhinotermitidae): roles in worker trail-following and in alate sex-attraction behavior. *J. Insect Physiol.* **40,** 781–787.

Lebrun, D. (1971). Glandes tergales et surfaces cuticulaires correspondantes chez le termite à cou jaune, *Calotermes flavicollis*. *C. R. Acad. Sci. Paris* **272D,** 3162–3164.

Lebrun, D. (1972). Effets de l'implantation de glandes mandibulaires sur la differenciation imaginable de *Calotermes flavicollis* Fabr. *C. R. Acad. Sci. Paris* **274D,** 2077–2079.

Lefeuve, P., and Bordereau, C. (1984). Soldier formation regulated by a primer pheromone from the soldier frontal gland in a higher termite, *Nasutitermes lujae*. *Proc. Natl. Acad. Sci.* **81,** 7665–7668.

Leuthold, R. H. (1975). Orientation mediated by pheromones in social insects. *In* "Pheromone and Defensive Secretions in Social Insects," (C. Noirot, P. E. Howse, and G. Le Masne, Eds.). Imprimerie Université de Dijon, Dijon.

Liebig, J., Eliyahu, D., and Brent, C. S. (2009). Cuticular hydrocarbon profiles indicate reproductive status in the termite *Zootermopsis nevadensis*. *Behav. Ecol. Sociobiol.* **63,** 1799–1807.

Mao, L. G., Henderson, G., Liu, Y., and Laine, R. A. (2005). Formosan subterranean termite (Isoptera: Rhinotermitidae) soldiers regulate juvenile hormone levels and caste differentiation in workers. *Ann. Entomol. Soc.* **98,** 340–345.

Maschwitz, U., and Tho, Y. P. (1974). Chinone als Wehrsubstanzen bei einiger orientalischen Macrotermitinen. *Insectes Soc.* **21,** 231–233.

Maschwitz, U., Jander, R., and Burkhard, D. (1972). Wehrsubstanzen und Wehrverhalten der termite *Macrotermes carbonarius*. *J. Insect Physiol.* **18,** 1715–1720.

Masson, C., and Brossut, R. (1981). La communication chimique chez les insectes. *Recherche* **121,** 406–416.

Matsuura, K. (2001). Nestmate recognition mediated by intestinal bacteria in a termite, *Reticulitermes speratus*. *Oikos* **92,** 20–26.

Matsuura, K. (2006). Termite-egg mimicry by a sclerotium-forming fungus. *Proc. R. Soc. Lond. B. Biol. Sci.* **273,** 1203–1209.

Matsuura, K., Tamura, T., Kobayashi, N., Yashiro, T., and Tatsumi, S. (2007). The antibacterial protein lysozyme identified as the termite egg recognition pheromone. *PLoS One* **8,** 1–9.

Matsuura, K., Yashiro, T., Shimizi, K., Tatsumi, S., and Tamura, T. (2009). Cuckoo fungus mimics termite eggs by producing the cellulose-digesting enzyme β-glucosidase. *Curr. Biol.* **19,** 30–36.

McDowell, P. G., and Ollo, G. W. (1984). Isolation, identification, and biological activity of trail-following pheromone of termite *Trinervitermes bettonianus* (Sjöstedt) (Termitidae: Nasutitermitinae). *J. Chem. Ecol.* **10,** 835–851.
Miura, T., Kamikouchi, A., Sawata, M., Takeuchi, H., Natori, S., Kubo, T., and Matsumoto, T. (1999). Soldier caste-specific gene expression in the mandibular glands of *Hodotermopsis japonica* (Isoptera: Termopsidae). *PNAS* **96,** 13874–13879.
Mo, J., Chen, C., Pan, C., Cheng, J., and Teng, L. (2006). Mandibular gland chemistry of *Coptotermes formosanus* (Isoptera: Rhinotermitidae). *Sociobiology* **48,** 543–552.
Moore, B. P. (1968). Studies on the chemical composition and function of the cephalic gland secretion in Australian termites. *J. Insect Physiol.* **14,** 33–39.
Moore, B. P. (1969). Biochemical studies in termites. *In* "Biology of Termites," (K. Krishna and F. M. Weesner, Eds.), Vol. 1, pp. 407–432. Academic Press, New York.
Noirot, C. (1969). Glands and secretions. *In* "Biology of Termites" (K. Krishna and F. M. Weesner, Eds.), Vol. 1, pp. 89–123. Academic Press, New York.
Noirot, C. (1990). Sexual castes and reproductive strategies in termites. *In* "Social Insects—An Evolutionary Approach to Castes and Reproduction," (W. Engels, Ed.), pp. 5–35. Springer-Verlag, New York.
Noirot, C., and Quennedey, A. (1974). Fine structure of insect epidermal glands. *Ann. Rev. Entomol.* **19,** 61–80.
Noirot, C., and Quennedey, A. (1991). Glands, gland cells, glandular units: Some comments on terminology and classification. *Ann. Soc. Entomol. Fr.* **27,** 123–128.
Ohta, M., Matsuura, F., Henderson, G., and Laine, R. A. (2007). Novel free ceramides as components of the soldier defense gland of the Formosan subterranean termite (*Coptotermes formosanus*). *J. Lipid Res.* 1–21.
Parton, A. H., Howse, P. E., Baker, R., and Clément, J. L. (1981). Variation in the chemistry of the frontal gland secretion of European *Reticulitermes* species. *In* "Biosystematics of Social Insects," (P. E. Howse and J. L. Clément, Eds.), pp. 193–209. Academic Press, New York and London.
Pasteels, J. M., and Bordereau, C. (1998). Releaser pheromones in termites. *In* "Pheromone Communication in Social Insects: Ants, Wasps, Bees, and Termites," (R. K. VanderMeer, M. D. Winston, and K. E. Espelie, Eds.), pp. 193–215. Westview Press, Oxford.
Pearce, M. J. (1997). Termites: Biology and Pest Management. 1st edn. CABI, Wallingford, Oxon.
Peppuy, A., Robert, A., Sémon, E., Bonnard, O., Son, N. T., and Bordereau, C. (2001). Species specificity of trail pheromones of fungus-growing termites from northern Vietnam. *Insectes Soc.* **48,** 245–250.
Peppuy, A., Robert, A., and Bordereau, C. (2004). Species-specific sex pheromones secreted from new sexual glands in two sympatric fungus-growing termites from Northern Vietnam, *Macrotermes annandalei* and *M. barney*. *Insectes Soc.* **51,** 91–98.
Piskorski, R., Hanus, R., Vašíčková, S., Cvačka, J., Šobotník, J., Svatoš, A., and Valterová, I. (2007). Nitroalkenes and sesquiterpene hydrocarbons from the frontal gland of three *Prorhinotermes* termite species. *J. Chem. Ecol.* **33,** 1787–1794.
Piskorski, R., Hanus, R., Kalinová, B., Valterová, I., Křeček, J., Bourguignon, T., Roisin, Y., and Šobotník, J. (2009). Temporal and geographic variations in the morphology and chemical composition of the frontal gland in imagoes of *Prorhinotermes* species (Isoptera: Rhinotermitidae). *Biol. J. Linn. Soc.* **98,** 384–392.
Prestwich, G. D. (1979a). Termite chemical defense: New natural products and chemosystematics. *Sociobiology* **4,** 127–140.
Prestwich, G. D. (1979b). Chemical defense by termite soldiers. *J. Chem. Ecol.* **5,** 459–480.
Prestwich, G. D., and Collins, M. S. (1982). Chemical defense secretions of the termite soldiers of *Acorhinotermes* and *Rhinotermes* (Isoptera, Rhinotermitidae): ketones, vinyl ketones and β-ketoaldehydes derived from fatty acids. *J. Chem. Ecol.* **8,** 147–161.

Prestwich, G. D. (1983). Chemical systematics of termite exocrine secretions. *Ann. Rev. Ecol. Syst.* **14,** 287–311.
Prestwich, G. D. (1984). Defense mechanisms of termites. *Ann. Rev. Entomol.* **29,** 201–232.
Quennedey, A., Baulé, G., Rigaud, J., Dubois, P., and Brossut, R. (1973). La glande frontale des soldats de *Schedorhinotermes putorius* (Isoptera): analyse chemique et fonctionnement. *Insect. Biochem.* **3,** 61–67.
Quennedey, A. (1998). Insect epidermal gland cells: Ultrastructure and morphogenesis. *In* "Microscopic Anatomy of Invertebrates," (F. W. Harrison and M. Locke, Eds.), Vol. 11A, pp. 177–207. Wiley-Liss, New York.
Quennedey, A., Peppuy, A., Courrent, A., Robert, A., Everaerts, C., and Bordereau, C. (2004). Ultrastructure of posterior sternal glands of *Macrotermes annandalei* (Silvestri): New members of the sexual glandular set found in termites (Insecta). *J. Morphol.* **262,** 683–691.
Quennedey, A., Sillam-Dussès, D., Robert, A., and Bordereau, C. (2008). The fine structural organization of sternal glands of pseudergates and workers in termites (Isoptera): A comparative survey. *Arthropod Struct. Dev.* **37,** 168–185.
Raina, A. K., Bland, J. M., Dickens, J. C., Park, Y. I., and Hollister, B. (2003). Premating behavior of dealates of the Formosan subterranean termite and evidence for the presence of a contact sex pheromone. *J. Insect Behav.* **16,** 233–245.
Raina, A. K., Bland, J. M., and Osbrink, W. (2005a). Hydroquinone is not a phagostimulant for the Formosan subterranean termite. *J. Chem. Ecol.* **31,** 509–517.
Raina, A. K., Park, Y. I., Ingber, B. F., and Murphy, C. (2005b). Structure and developmental changes in the tergal glands of adult females of *Coptotermes formosanus* (Isoptera, Rhinotermitidae). *Arthropod Struct. Dev.* **34,** 117–124.
Reinhard, J., and Kaib, M. (1995). Interaction of pheromones during food exploitation by the termite *Schedorhinotermes lamanianus*. *Physiol. Entomol.* **20,** 266–272.
Reinhard, J., and Kaib, M. (2001). Thin-layer chromatography assessing feeding stimulation by labial gland secretion compared to synthetic chemicals in the subterranean termite *Reticulitermes santonensis*. *J. Chem. Ecol.* **27,** 175–187.
Reinhard, J., Hertel, H., and Kaib, M. (1997). Feeding stimulating signal in labial gland secretion of the subterranean termite *Reticulitermes santonensis*. *J. Chem. Ecol.* **23,** 2371–2381.
Reinhard, J., Lacey, M. J., Ibarra, F., Schroeder, F. C., Kaib, M., and Lenz, M. (2002). Hydroquinone: A general phagostimulating pheromone in termites. *J. Chem. Ecol.* **28,** 1–14.
Robert, A., Peppuy, A., Sémon, E., Boyer, F. D., Lacey, M. J., and Bordereau, C. (2004). A new C12 alcohol identified as a sex pheromone and a trail-following pheromone in termites: The diene (Z,Z)-dodeca-3,6-dien-1-ol. *Naturwiss.* **91,** 34–39.
Rosengaus, R. B., Lefebvre, M. L., and Traniello, J. F. A. (2000). Inhibition of fungal spore germination by *Nasutitermes*: Evidence for a possible antiseptic role of soldier defensive secretions. *J. Chem. Ecol.* **26,** 21–39.
Santos, C. A., and Costa-Leonardo, A. M. (2006). Anatomy of the frontal gland and ultramorphology of the frontal tube in the soldier caste of species of Nasutitermitinae (Isoptera, Termitidae). *Microsc. Res. Tech.* **69,** 913–918.
Sevala, V., Bagnères, A. G., Kuenzli, M., Blomquist, G. J., and Schal, C. (2000). Cuticular hydrocarbons of the termite *Zootermopsis nevadensis* (Hagen): Caste differences and role of lipophorin in transport of hydrocarbons and hydrocarbon metabolites. *J. Chem. Ecol.* **26,** 765–789.
Sillam-Dussès, D., Sémon, E., Moreau, C., Valterová, I., Šobotník, J., Robert, A., and Bordereau, C. (2005). *Chemoecology* **15,** 1–6.
Sillam-Dussès, D., Robert, A., Sémon, E., Lacey, M., and Bordereau, C. (2006). Trail-following pheromones and phylogeny in termites. Proc. 15th Congr IUSSI, Washington, DC.
Sillam-Dussès, D., Sémon, E., Lacey, M. J., Robert, A., Lenz, M., and Bordereau, C. (2007). Trail-following pheromones in basal termites, with special reference to *Mastotermes darwiniensis*. *J. Chem. Ecol.* **33,** 1960–1977.

Sillam-Dussès, D., Kalinová, B., Jiroš, P., Březinová, A., Cvačka, J., Hanus, R., Šobotník, J., Bordereau, C., and Valterová, I. (2009a). Identification by GC-EAD of the two-component trail-following pheromone of *Prorhinotermes simplex* (Isoptera, Rhinotermitidae, Prorhinotermitinae). *J. Insect Physiol.* **55,** 751–757.

Sillam-Dussès, D., Sémon, E., Robert, A., and Bordereau, C. (2009b). (Z)-Dodec-3-en-1-ol, a common major component of the trail-following pheromone in the termites Kalotermitidae. *Chemoecology* **19,** 103–108.

Sillam-Dussès, D., Sémon, E., Robert, A., Cancello, E., Lenz, M., Valterová, I., and Bordereau, C. (2010). Identification of multi-component trail pheromones in the most evolutionarily derived termites, the Nasutitermitinae (Termitidae). *Biol. J. Linn. Soc.* **99,** 20–27.

Šobotník, J., and Weyda, F. (2003). Ultrastructural ontogeny of the labial gland apparatus in termite *Prorhinotermes simplex* (Isoptera, Rhinotermitidae). *Arthropod Struct. Dev.* **31,** 255–270.

Šobotník, J., Weyda, F., and Hanus, R. (2005). Ultrastructural study of tergal and posterior sternal glands in *Prorhinotermes simplex* (Isoptera: Rhinotermitidae). *Eur. J. Entomol.* **102,** 81–88.

Šobotník, J., Hanus, R., Kalinová, B., Pirskorski, R., Cvačka, J., Bourguignon, T., and Roisin, Y. (2008). (E, E)-α-Fanersene, an alarm pheromone of the termite *Prorhinotermes canalifrons*. *J. Chem. Ecol.* **34,** 478–486.

Šobotník, J., Bourguignon, T., Hanus, R., Wyeda, F., and Roisin, Y. (2010). Structure and function of defensive glands in soldiers of *Glossotermes oculatus* (Isoptera: Serritermitidae). *Biol. J. Linn. Soc.* **99,** 839–848.

Traniello, J. F. A. (1981). Enemy deterrence in the recruitment strategy of a termite: Soldier-organized foraging in *Nasutitermes costalis*. *Proc. Natl. Acad. Sci.* **78,** 1976–1979.

Vander Meer, R. K., and Morel, L. (1998). Nestmate recognition in ants. *In* "Pheromone Communication in Social Insects: Ants, Wasps, Bees, and Termites," (R. K. Vander Meer, M. Breed, M. Winston, and K. Espelie, Eds.), pp. 79–103. West View Press, Boulder.

Veivers, P. C., Mühlemann, R., Slaytor, M., Leuthold, R. H., and Bignell, D. E. (1991). Digestion, diet and polyethism in two fungus-growing termites: *Macrotermes subhyalinus* Rambur and *M. michaelseni* Sjödtedt. *J. Insect Physiol.* **37,** 675682.

Vieau, F. (1990). The male effect upon the female reproductive potency in the incipient laboratory colonies of *Kalotermes flavicollis* Fabr. *Insectes Soc.* **37,** 169–180.

Weil, T., Hoffmann, K., Kroiss, J., Strohm, E., and Korb, J. (2009). Scent of a queen-cuticular hydrocarbons specific for female reproductives in lower termites. *Naturwissenschaften* **96,** 315–319.

Wood, W. F., Truckenbrodt, W., and Meinwald, J. (1975). Chemistry of the defensive secretion from the African termite *Odontotermes badius*. *Ann. Entomol. Soc. Am.* **68,** 359–360.

Zalkow, L. H., Howard, R. W., Gelbaum, L. T., Gordon, M. M., Deutsch, H. M., and Blum, M. S. (1981). Chemical ecology of *Reticulitermes flavipes* (Kollar) and *R. virginicus* (Banks) (Rhinotermitidae): Chemistry of the soldier cephalic secretions. *J. Chem. Ecol.* **7,** 717–732.

CHAPTER TWENTY-TWO

Aphid Pheromones

Sarah Y. Dewhirst,* John A. Pickett,* *and* Jim Hardie†

Contents

Abstract

Aphids are the main insect pests of agricultural crops in temperate regions causing major economic losses. Although broad-spectrum insecticides are available for control, alternative and more targeted methods are needed due to insecticide resistance and increasing environmental pressures. An alternative control method for aphids is to exploit their pheromones, which have been extensively studied in recent years. For example, aphids release alarm pheromones in response to natural enemy attack and these could be used to deter aphids from the crops. Sex pheromones have also been identified which could be used to interfere males locating conspecific females (oviparae), as well as for manipulating natural enemies. Several hypotheses relating to how species integrity is maintained via the

* Biological Chemistry Department, Rothamsted Research, Harpenden, Herts, United Kingdom
† Department of Life Sciences, Imperial College London, Silwood Park campus, Ascot, Berkshire, United Kingdom

Vitamins and Hormones, Volume 83
ISSN 0083-6729, DOI: 10.1016/S0083-6729(10)83022-5

aphid sex pheromone have been proposed. The composition and behavioral activity of these pheromones, and how their use could be implemented in integrated pest management systems to control aphids, is discussed.

I. Introduction

Aphids (Sternorrhyncha: Hemiptera: Aphidoidea) occur throughout the world. Polyphenism and complex life cycles enable them to exploit their often ephemeral host plants (Blackman and Eastop, 2000). The greatest numbers of species occur in the temperate regions where they are the main economic insect pests of agricultural crops (Pickett *et al.*, 2003). In this review, aphids belonging only to the largest family Aphididae are considered as this contains the majority pest aphid species (Birkett and Pickett, 2003; Kennedy and Stroyan, 1959; Powell and Hardie, 2001).

Aphids are small (1.5–3.5 mm), soft-bodied insects (Blackman and Eastop, 2000) that feed exclusively on sap from the vascular tissues of plants, mainly the phloem. They can damage plants by imbibing sap causing wilting of the plant, injection of toxic saliva, and the production of honeydew (encouraging sooty moulds to colonize leaf surfaces and decreasing photosynthesis in the plant) (Blackman, 1974). More importantly, their biology and feeding behavior make them ideally suited to transmitting plant viruses. Aphids transmit more plant viruses than any other sap-feeding insects. Approximately, 200 aphid species are known to transmit 275 viruses in 19 plant virus genera (Nault, 1997). *Myzus persicae* (the peach-potato aphid) is the most important vector of viral disease, shown to transmit over 100 plant viruses (Blackman and Eastop, 2000). An aphid infestation in crop plants results in a reduction of biomass production, yield, and crop quality.

Aphid control is mainly via the use of broad-spectrum insecticides, specifically organophosphates, carbamates, pyrethroids, and more recently the neonicotinoids. In 2004, in Great Britain, wheat and ware potato crops on average received two insecticide treatments which approached 90% and 70% of insecticidal applications, respectively, for control of aphids. Pirimicarb, a selective carbamate aphicide, and cypermethrin, a pyrethroid insecticide, accounted for over 40% of insecticide-treated area in potato and wheat crops, respectively (Garthwaite *et al.*, 2004). The future of insecticide usage looks compromised due to resistance (Barber *et al.*, 1998; Devonshire *et al.*, 1998; Wedge *et al.*, 1998) and increasing political and public pressures relating to perceptions of a safe environment (Jones, 1998; Luijk *et al.*, 1998; Pimentel, 2005; Pretty *et al.*, 2000). *M. persicae* has already developed resistance against most organophosphates, carbonates (Devonshire and Moores, 1982) including pirimicarb (Moores *et al.*, 1994), and pyrethroids (Martinez-Torres *et al.*, 1999). Thus, there is a continuous search for new ways of controlling aphids. One option is to interfere with the aphid's biology and behavior with the use of semiochemicals (behavior and development modifying chemicals) (Pickett, 1991).

II. SEMIOCHEMICALS

Specific chemical compounds or mixtures of chemical compounds that function in communication between the same (pheromones) and among different species (allelochemicals) are called semiochemicals [simeon (Gr.) = a mark or signal]. Pheromones [pherein (Gr.) = to transfer + hormone (Gr.) = to excite] are chemicals that exclusively convey information between members of the same species. Products of the insects' primary metabolism are converted by one or a few tissue-specific enzymes to make these mostly stereochemically specific compounds (Tillman *et al.*, 1999). It has been reported that aphids release sex pheromones (Marsh, 1972; Pettersson, 1970), alarm pheromones (Kislow and Edwards, 1972; Nault *et al.*, 1973), spacing pheromones (Pettersson *et al.*, 1995), and aggregation pheromones (Pettersson and Stephansson, 1991).

There are various approaches by which to identify and investigate volatile semiochemicals from insects. In order to collect volatile from insects, as the first stage in identification, there are three main methods. The first involves the collection from intact insects (headspace collection), the second involves collection from disrupted insect tissues, for example, solvent washings (Golub and Weatherston, 1984), and the third to capture directly exocrine secretions. Headspace collection can be static, no air-flow, or dynamic, a continuous airflow across the insect. The volatiles are trapped on a porous polymer, which can then be eluted from the polymer with a solvent (solvent desorption). Headspace analysis allows samples to be collected that contain chemicals in the ratios similar to those found in nature due to the insects being kept alive throughout the experiment. Also, only the volatile chemicals produced by the insect are collected and how the volatiles change over time can be studied (Agelopoulos *et al.*, 1999). Solvent extractions have a number of disadvantages (Millar and Sims, 1998). These include, that every chemical present on the surface of the insect when the solvent washing occurred is collected which may not be a true representation of the volatile profile over time and postisolation, or after tissue homogenization extraction modification of the chemicals due to enzymatic degradation may occur. The direct collection of exocrine secretions gives a product close to what is produced naturally without other contaminants, but has only been employed so far with the alarm pheromone (Pickett and Griffiths, 1980).

After volatile collection, the sample can be examined by high-resolution gas chromatography (GC) coupled with electrophysiological preparations of the aphid to locate neurophysiological active compounds. Either electroantennogram (EAG), comprising the whole antenna, or single cell recording (SCR), comprising recordings of single or a few, neurone(s) from individual olfactory sensilla in the antennae (Wadhams, 1984), can be conducted. The active compounds are then identified tentatively by GC coupled with mass spectrometry (GC–MS) with identification confirmed by peak enhancement with authentic compounds on GC columns of different polarities (Pickett, 1990). Biological activity is then assessed in behavioral bioassays.

III. Aphid Alarm Pheromones

Nault *et al.* (1973) provided evidence that aphids release an alarm pheromone when attacked or disturbed by parasitoids or predators, promoting defense or escape behavior by neighbors. When aphids are attacked, a sticky droplet is secreted from their cornicles or siphunculi that rapidly hardens (Hottes, 1928). These droplets principally contain triglycerides (Greenway and Griffiths, 1973; Strong, 1967) and were thought to have a defense function by "fixing" predators on contact (Goff and Nault, 1974; Hottes, 1928). They were also found to contain an alarm pheromone (Kislow and Edwards, 1972). The response to the pheromone by the receiving aphid varies—some jump or fall from their host plants, some disperse by walking, while others show a mixture of responses (Montgomery and Nault, 1977). The majority of aphids have been shown to produce the sesquiterpene hydrocarbon (*E*)-*β*-farnesene (EBF) as their alarm pheromone (Edwards *et al.*, 1973; Francis *et al.*, 2005; Pickett and Griffiths, 1980) but exceptions have been found, for example, the spotted alfalfa aphid, *Therioaphis maculata*, produces a related sesquiterpene (−)-germacrene A (Bowers *et al.*, 1977; Nishino *et al.*, 1977).

A. Applications of the aphid alarm pheromone for aphid control

The aphid alarm pheromone could be used in direct application treatments to crops in order to reduce aphid colonization. For example, when slow release point sources containing essential oil from mountain sage, *Hemizygia petiolata* Ashby (Lamiaceae), which contains high levels of EBF, were placed in small plots of spring sown field beans, *Vicia faba* L. var Quattro, a significant reduction in *Acyrthosiphon pisum* (the pea aphid) was observed (Bruce *et al.*, 2005). The alarm pheromone could also be used in combination with insecticidal sprays, increasing aphid mobility thereby increasing contact and effectiveness of the insecticide (Ester *et al.*, 1993; Griffiths and

Pickett, 1980). EBF is a common secondary plant metabolite, and therefore it is possible to express heterologous genes encoding enzymes for the production of EBF in crop plants. The gene for EBF in black peppermint (*Mentha* × *piperita*) has recently been successfully expressed in *Arabidopsis thaliana* (Beale *et al.*, 2006; Prosser *et al.*, 2006). In laboratory bioassays, a significant alarm and repellent response by *M. persicae* was elicited by the volatiles of transformed plants due to the increase in the emissions of EBF (Beale *et al.*, 2006).

IV. Aphid Sex Pheromone

The annual life cycle of an aphid often includes many female parthenogenetic (asexual) generations, followed by one sexual generation (males and oviparae) that is concluded by the laying of over-wintering eggs (Blackman, 1974). Mature sexual female aphids (oviparae) release a sex pheromone from scent plaques on their hind tibiae which attracts conspecific males (Marsh, 1972, 1975; Pettersson, 1970). In 1987, Dawson *et al.* (1987) collected components of the sex pheromone by washing excised hind tibiae from *Megoura viciae* (the vetch aphid) oviparae using a solvent (pentane). Two major compounds were collected. Identification of the first compound was achieved by GC–MS by comparison with authenticated compounds isolated from catmint plants, *Nepeta cataria* (Lamiaceae = Labiatae) and *N. mussinii* (Eisenbraun *et al.*, 1980). One of the chemicals, (4a*S*,7*S*,7a*R*)-nepetalactone (**I,** Fig. 22.1) from *N. cataria*, coeluted with the first compound in the sample. (4a*S*,7*S*,7a*R*)-Nepetalactone (**I**) was electrophysiologically active with males antennae, whereas its enantiomer (4a*R*,7*R*,7a*S*)-nepetalactone (**II,** Fig. 22.1) was electrophysiologically inactive when tested at the same level. It was concluded that *M. viciae* oviparae released (4a*S*,7*S*,7a*R*)-nepetalactone (**I**) as a component of the sex pheromone.

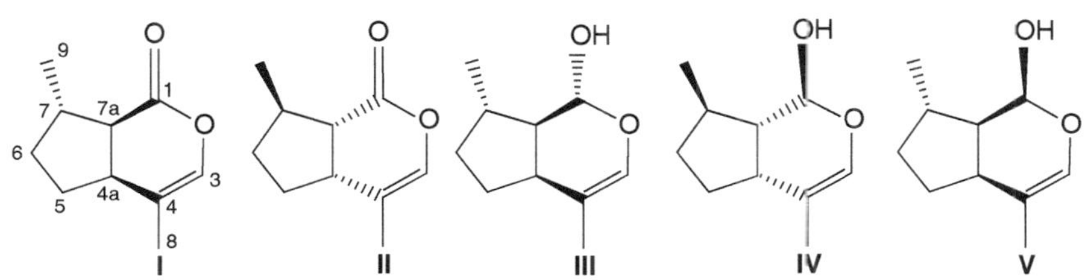

Figure 22.1 **I**: (4a*S*,7*S*,7a*R*)-nepetalactone, **II**: (4a*R*,7*R*,7a*S*)-nepetalactone, **III**: (1*R*,4a*S*,7*S*,7a*R*)-nepetalactol, **IV**: (1*S*,4a*R*,7*R*,7a*S*)-nepetalactol, **V**: (1*S*,4a*S*,7*S*,7a*R*)-nepetalactol.

The hydride reduction of (4a*S*,7*S*,7a*R*)-nepetalactone (**I**), obtained from *N. cataria*, produced two diastereoisomers, a major component (1*R*,4a*S*,7*S*,7a*R*)-nepetalactol (**III,** Fig. 22.1) and a minor component (1*S*,4a*S*,7*S*,7a*R*)-nepetalactol (**V,** Fig. 22.1). By using nuclear magnetic resonance (NMR), GC, GC–MS, and X-ray diffraction on a crystalline derivative, it was confirmed that the diastereoisomer produced by *M. viciae* oviparae was identical to the major component (1*R*,4a*S*,7*S*,7a*R*)-nepetalactol (**III**) (Dawson *et al.*, 1989). The enantiomer (1*S*,4a*R*,7*R*,7a*S*)-nepetalactol (**IV,** Fig. 22.1) was thought not to be present as it was concluded that oviparae produce (4a*S*,7*S*,7a*R*)-nepetalactone (**I**) and the inversion of three chiral centers would be unlikely. This, together with data from behavioral bioassays, led to the conclusion that *M. viciae* ovipara sex pheromone comprised a synergistic mixture of two compounds, (4a*S*,7*S*,7a*R*)-nepetalactone (**I**) and (1*R*,4a*S*,7*S*,7a*R*)-nepetalactol (**III**).

The sex pheromone of the greenbug, *Schizaphis graminium*, was then investigated, but this time solvent washings of the hind tibiae contained neither these chemicals nor structurally related chemicals (Dawson *et al.*, 1988). Volatiles were then collected from oviparae by air entrainment (dynamic headspace analysis). The same two chemicals, (4a*S*,7*S*,7a*R*)-nepetalactone (**I**) and (1*R*,4a*S*,7*S*,7a*R*)-nepetalactol (**III**), were identified in the air entrainment sample by GC and GC–MS though which enantiomer was present was not studied (Dawson *et al.*, 1988). This provided evidence suggesting that the pheromonal components were being released as soon as they were formed. How oviparae produce (4a*S*,7*S*,7a*R*)-nepetalactone (**I**) and (1*R*,4a*S*,7*S*,7a*R*)-nepetalactol (**III**) is unknown but it has been suggested that the nepetalactol is produced from a glycoside precursor and a proportion of this is sequentially oxidized to the nepetalactone (Dawson *et al.*, 1990).

To date, and with one exception (see Section IV.B), the sex pheromone of many aphid species from the subfamily Aphididae have been shown to comprise of a mixture of the iridoids (cyclopentanoids) (4a*SR*,7*SR*,7a*RS*)-nepetalactone and (1*RS*,4a*SR*,7*SR*,7a*RS*)-nepetalactol. If (4a*SR*,7*SR*,7a*RS*)-nepetalactone and (1*RS*,4a*SR*,7*SR*,7a*RS*)-nepetalactol are ubiquitous aphid sex pheromone components, how is species integrity maintained? A number of different hypotheses have been investigated. These include hypotheses relating to the aphid's biology and morphology: differences in oviparae color, species-specific movements, genitalia incompatibility, spatial and seasonal separation of populations, and diel separation of pheromone release (Hardie, 1991; Hardie *et al.*, 1990; Steffan, 1990; Thieme and Dixon, 1996), as well as hypotheses relating the pheromone components: species-specific ratio and blends of diastereoisomers or enantiomers (Campbell *et al.*, 1990; Hardie *et al.*, 1997), the presence of additional constituents (Guldemond *et al.*, 1993; Lilley and Hardie, 1996), and interactions with host-plant volatiles (Campbell *et al.*, 1990; Hardie *et al.*, 1994; Lösel *et al.*, 1996a; Pettersson, 1970). The hypotheses relating to pheromone components are discussed below.

A. Ratio of the aphid sex pheromone components

The ratio of the iridoids released by oviparae is thought to convey species integrity. Volatile collections from 17 species of oviparae have been shown to contain (4a*SR*,7*SR*,7a*RS*)-nepetalactone and (1*RS*,4a*SR*,7*SR*,7a*RS*)-nepetalactol in different ratios (Table 22.1). Bioassays and field trials show that males from these species do respond to a range of ratios of (4a*S*,7*S*,7a*R*)-nepetalactone (**I**) and (1*R*,4a*S*,7*S*,7a*R*)-nepetalactol (**III**) but the behavioral response was increased toward the ratio identified from conspecific oviparae (Boo *et al.*, 2000; Dawson *et al.*, 1990; Hardie *et al.*,

Table 22.1 Ratios of (1*RS*,4a*SR*,7*SR*,7a*RS*)-nepetalactol:(4a*SR*,7*SR*,7a*RS*)-nepetalactone released by oviparae of different species

Common name	Species	Average ratio (ol:one)	Reference
Black-bean aphid	*Aphis fabae*	1:29	Dawson *et al.* (1990)
Spiraea aphid	*Aphis spiraecola*	1:7	Jeon *et al.* (2003)
Vetch aphid	*Megoura viciae*	1:5 and 1:12	Dawson *et al.* (1990), Hardie *et al.* (1990)
Peach aphid	*Tuberocephalus momonis*	1:4	Boo *et al.* (2000)
	Ovatus insitus	1:2	Dewhirst (2007)
Grain aphid	*Sitobion avenae*	0:1	Lilley *et al.* (1994/1995)
Black-berry cereal aphid	*Sitobion fragariae*	0:1	Hardie *et al.* (1992)
Cabbage aphid	*Brevicoryne brassicae*	0:1	Gabrys *et al.* (1997)
Bird-cherry oat aphid	*Rhopalosiphum padi*	1:0	Hardie *et al.* (1994)
Pea Aphid	*Acyrthosiphon pisum*	1:1	Dawson *et al.* (1990)
Lettuce aphid	*Nasonovia ribis-nigri*	1:1.5	Dewhirst (2007)
Peach-potato aphid	*Myzus persicae*	1.5:1	Dawson *et al.* (1990)
Potato aphid	*Macrosiphum euphorbiae*	3:1	Goldansaz *et al.* (2004)
Rosy apple aphid	*Dysaphis plantaginea*	4:1	Stewart-Jones *et al.* (2007)
Greenbug	*Schizaphis graminium*	8:1	Dawson *et al.* (1988)
Apple grass aphid	*Rhopalosiphum insertum*	21:1	Dewhirst (2007)
Currant aphids	*Cryptomyzus* spp.	25:1 to 50:1 depending on species	Guldemond *et al.* (1993)

1990; Lilley and Hardie, 1996). The behavior response of males over a range of ratios may be due to the age effect on the ratio stability of the pheromone components. Hardie *et al.* (1990) first showed that the ratio between the two iridoids released by *M. viciae* oviparae was age dependent. From the second day after adult molt to day 6, a 1:5 ratio (ol:one) was recorded. This ratio increases to 1:12 for days 7–8 and then returned to 1:5 on day 10. More recently, *Dysaphis plantaginea* (the rosy apple aphid) oviparae have been shown to release a constant ratio of 3.7:1 until day 14, when the percentage of nepetalactol decreased (Stewart-Jones *et al.*, 2007). A decrease in relative levels of the nepetalactol as oviparae aged was also recorded for *Macrosiphum euphorbiae* (the potato aphid) (Goldansaz *et al.*, 2004). It has been hypothesized that the decrease in nepetalactol with age maybe a symptom of senescence in the glandular pheromone-producing cells, that the oxidation of the nepetalactol to nepetalactone may be less synchronized in older aphids, or that the amounts of nepetalactone optimizes attraction of the pheromone in line with the physiological status of the aphid.

The specificity of sex pheromones is extremely important when different species of aphid occur on the same primary host. *Malus* spp. are the primary host of *D. plantaginea* as well as *Rhopalosiphum insertum* (the apple grass aphid) and sometimes *Ovatus insitus*. Very different ratios of (1*RS*,4a*SR*,7*SR*,7a*RS*)-nepetalactol:(4a*SR*,7*SR*,7a*RS*)-nepetalactone have been collected from these three species. *O. insitus* releases twice as much (4a*S*,7*S*,7a*R*)-nepetalactone (**I**) as (1*RS*,4a*SR*,7*SR*,7a*RS*)-nepetalactol but the other two species release more (1*RS*,4a*SR*,7*SR*,7a*RS*)-nepetalactol than (4a*SR*,7*SR*,7a*RS*)-nepetalactone. *R. insertum* releases 20 times more (1*RS*,4a*SR*,7*SR*,7a*RS*)-nepetalactol than (4a*SR*,7*SR*,7a*RS*)-nepetalactone where as *D. plantaginea* releases only four times more. Again this provides evidence to support the hypothesis that ratios play an important role in species specificity.

B. Role of stereochemistry of the aphid sex pheromone components

Stereochemistry could also play an important role in male aphids identifying sex pheromones released by the same species in the field. *Phorodon humuli* (the damson-hop aphid) oviparae release a mixture of two diastereoisomers, (1*S*,4a*R*,7*S*,7a*S*)-nepetalactol (**VI,** Fig. 22.2) and (1*R*,4a*R*,7*S*,7a*S*)-nepetalactol (**VII**, Fig. 22.2) (Campbell *et al.*, 1990). These compounds have an alternative stereochemistry at C-4a and C-7a compared to the nepetalactol identified from other species. Male *P. humuli* responded electrophysiologically to a mixture of these two diastereoisomers as well as the two compounds identified in other species sex pheromone [(4a*S*,7*S*,7a*R*)-nepetalactone (**I**) and (1*R*,4a*S*,7*S*,7a*R*)-nepetalactol (**III**)] (Campbell *et al.*, 2003). In the field, male *P. humuli* were caught in significantly higher

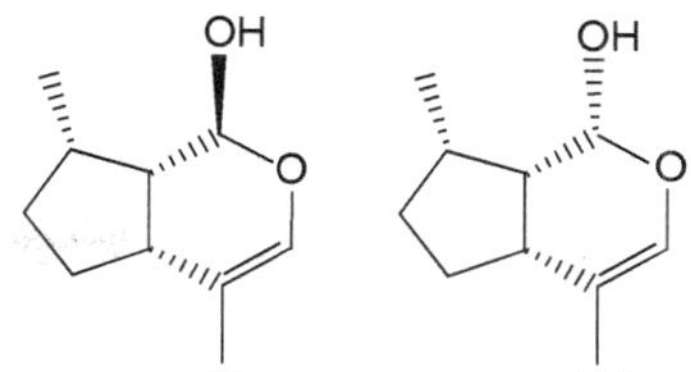

VI VII

Figure 22.2 VI: (1*S*,4a*R*,7*S*,7a*S*)-nepetalactol, VII: (1*R*,4a*R*,7*S*,7a*S*)-nepetalactol.

amounts in traps containing the mixture of diastereoisomers, (1*S*,4a*R*,7*S*,7a*S*)-nepetalactol (**VI**) and (1*R*,4a*R*,7*S*,7a*S*)-nepetalactol (**VII**), compared to traps containing the two other compounds [(4a*S*,7*S*,7a*R*)-nepetalactone (**I**) and (1*R*,4a*S*,7*S*,7a*R*)-nepetalactol (**III**)] (Pope *et al.*, 2007). The detection of the chemicals released by oviparae of other species may assist in discrimination of the sex pheromone released by conspecifics and other species.

As Mori (1989) summarized, different enantiomers can also induce a different behavioral response by different insects and this is likely to be true for aphids. The ability of aphids to distinguish between different enantiomers or mixtures of enantiomers has already been demonstrated. For example, the two enantiomers (*R*)-6-methyl-5-hepten-2-ol and (*S*)-6-methyl-5-hepten-2-ol are released from aphid-infested wheat seedlings. No behavioral response by *Rhopalosiphum padi* (the bird-cherry oat aphid) was recorded when the single enantiomers were tested in a four-way olfactometer but *R. padi* spent less time in the area where mixtures of the enantiomers were present (Quiroz and Niemeyer, 1998). It was concluded that a synergism between the enantiomers occurred.

To date, there is only one study on the behavioral responses of male aphids to the enantiomers of the aphid sex pheromone components. In 1997, Hardie *et al.* conducted a field trial to test if catches of *R. padi* were altered due to the enantiomers of the sex pheromone components. Different purities of the (4a*SR*,7*SR*,7a*RS*)-nepetalactone enantiomers [99% and 95% (4a*S*,7*S*,7a*R*)-nepetalactone (**I**), 98% (4a*R*,7*R*,7a*S*)-nepetalactone (**II**) and racemic (50% **I** and 50% **II**)] were synthesized from citronellol. The nepetalactones were then reduced to the corresponding enantiomers (1*R*,4a*S*,7*S*,7a*R*)-nepetalactol (**III**) and (1*S*,4a*R*,7*R*,7a*S*)-nepetalactol (**IV**), and placed in glass vials which were suspended in water traps. In previous field studies, water traps containing (1*R*,4a*S*,7*S*,7a*R*)-nepetalactol (**III**) alone caught significantly higher numbers of *R. padi* compared to other ratios of (4a*S*,7*S*,7a*R*)-nepetalactone (**I**) and (1*R*,4a*S*,7*S*,7a*R*)-nepetalactol (**III**) (Hardie *et al.*, 1994). *R. padi* were caught in significantly higher amounts in water traps releasing synthetic 99% (1*R*,4a*S*,7*S*,7a*R*)-nepetalactol (**III**) compared to traps releasing 98% (1*S*,4a*R*,7*R*,7a*S*)-nepetalactol (**IV**). It was concluded that the presence of the (1*S*,4a*R*,7*R*,7a*S*)-nepetalactol (**IV**) reduced the male response to (1*R*,4a*S*,7*S*,7a*R*)-nepetalactol (**III**).

The absolute stereochemistry of the sex pheromone for many aphid species has not yet been established, only the relative structural stereochemistry has been determined. Goldansaz *et al.* (2004) developed a protocol to determine which enantiomer of nepetalactol was released by *M. euphorbiae*. The nepetalactol was collected from *M. euphorbiae* oviparae by air entrainment and was reacted with a chiral reagent (a Moshers' acid chloride). Analysis of the esters by NMR from natural and synthetic standards showed conclusively that the nepetalactol enantiomer released by *M. euphorbiae* was (1*R*,4a*S*,7*S*,7a*R*)-nepetalactol (**III**). It is unusual to use NMR to determine the structure of components in complex mixtures and even more unusual at this microscale level. The chemical shift of the derivative allowed NMR analysis in a readily analyzable region of the spectrum. The procedure was successfully repeated with volatiles collected from *D. plantaginea* oviparae (Stewart-Jones *et al.*, 2007), which were also shown to release the enantiomer (1*R*,4a*S*,7*S*,7a*R*)-nepetalactol (**III**).

To date, no conclusive evidence has been obtained, with the exception of *P. humuli*, to support the hypothesis that different species of oviparae released different enantiomers therefore suggesting the absolute stereochemistry of the components may not play an important role in males locating conspecific oviparae. Laboratory behavioral studies should be conducted before the stereochemistry–pheromone activity relationship (Mori, 1989) is determined.

C. Additional sex pheromone components

The ratio of the two iridoids, nepetalactone and nepetalactol, released by oviparae is thought to play an important role in the identification of sex pheromones, released by conspecific oviparae, by males (Boo *et al.*, 2000; Dawson *et al.*, 1990; Lilley and Hardie, 1996). However, a few experiments have suggested that the two iridoids do not always convey species integrity. For example, the ratio of (4a*SR*,7*SR*,7a*RS*)-nepetalactone:(1*RS*,4a*SR*,7*SR*,7a*RS*)-nepetalactol released from different species of *Cryptomyzus* oviparae were found to be similar. However, *C. galesopsidis* (the European blackcurrant aphid) males could distinguish between the sex pheromone released by conspecific oviparae and the sex pheromone from other species of *Cryptomyzus* oviparae (Guldemond *et al.*, 1992). Male *C. galesopsidis* could also discriminate between a synthetic pheromone blend (30:1 (1*RS*,4a*SR*,7*SR*,7a*RS*)-nepetalactol:(4a*SR*,7*SR*,7a*RS*)-nepetalactone) and volatiles from conspecific oviparae (Guldemond *et al.*, 1993). A stronger positive behavioral response to the conspecific oviparae occurred, suggesting that the sex pheromone of aphids is likely to consist of more than two components.

Dewhirst *et al.* (2008) investigated whether chemicals additional to (1*R*,4a*S*,7*S*,7a*R*)-nepetalactol (**III**) and (4a*S*,7*S*,7a*R*)-nepetalactone (**I**) were released from the *D. plantaginea* oviparae as part of its sex pheromone blend. Electrophysiological responses of male *D. plantaginea* antennae to two chemicals, in addition to (1*R*,4a*S*,7*S*,7a*R*)-nepetalactol (**III**) and (4a*S*,7*S*,7a*R*)-nepetalactone (**I**), present in an air entrainment sample collected from *D. plantaginea* oviparae were recorded. By GC and GC–MS, these were identified as phenylacetonitrile and (1*SR*,2*RS*,3*SR*)-dolichodial. The relative stereochemistry of the dolichodial collected from the oviparae was the same as the dolichodial present as the major constituent [9:1 (1*S*,2*R*,3*S*)-dolichodial (**VIII**):(1*S*,2*S*,3*S*)-dolichodial (**IX**)] in the essential oil from *Teucrium marum* (cat thyme, Lamiaceae) (Bellesia *et al.*, 1983b; Pagnoni *et al.*, 1976), but the absolute stereochemistry present in the air entrainment samples collected from oviparae was not determined (Fig. 22.3).

Previous reports suggested that phenylacetonitrile was a plant volatile, identified as a major volatile from apple fruit (Boeve *et al.*, 1996), whereas (1*SR*,2*RS*,3*SR*)-dolichodial may originate from the oviparae and be an additional component of the aphid sex pheromone. (1*S*,2*R*,3*S*)-Dolichodial (**VIII**) was originally identified as a defense or trail pheromone released from various *Dolichoderus* (*D. acanthoclinea clarki*, *D. denta*, *D. scabridus*, and *D. diceratoclinea*) and *Iridomyrmex* (*I. rufoniger*, *I. humilis*, *I. nitidiceps*, *I. detectus*, and *I. myrmecodiae*) species of ants (Cavill and Hinterberger, 1960; Cavill and Houghton, 1974; Cavill *et al.*, 1982). Also, (1*S*,2*R*,3*S*)-dolichodial is both structurally and biosynthetically related to a known component of the aphid sex pheromone, (4a*S*,7*S*,7a*R*)-nepetalactone. Both compounds are thought to originate biosynthetically from citronellol and are methylcyclopentanoid terpenes (Bellesia *et al.*, 1983a, 1984).

Indeed when tested in a behavioral bioassay, the four-way olfactometer, male *D. plantaginea* spent significantly more time in the arm containing the (1*S*,2*R*,3*S*)-dolichodial alone compared to the control arms. When tested as part of a three component mixture, with (1*R*,4a*S*,7*S*,7a*R*)-nepetalactol and

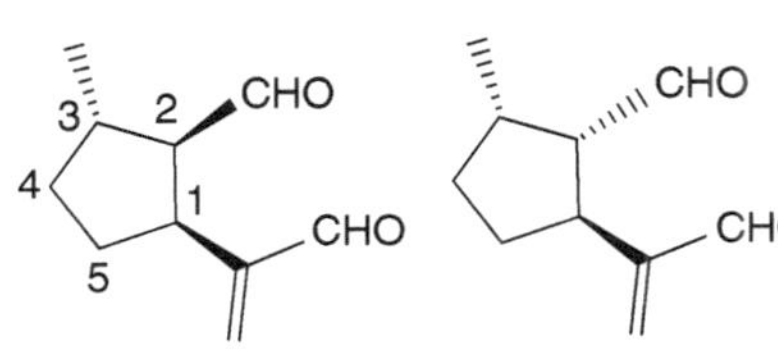

Figure 22.3 **VIII**: (1*S*,2*R*,3*S*)-dolichodial, **IX**: (1*S*,2*S*,3*S*)-dolichodial (XI).

(4a*S*,7*S*,7a*R*)-nepetalactone, with a ratio equivalent to the ratio in the air entrainment sample, male *D. plantaginea* preferred this arm to the control arms. No significant difference was seen when the two-component mixture of the two known sex pheromone components were present. These results suggest that (1*S*,2*R*,3*S*)-dolichodial (**VIII**) may cause an attraction/arrestant response by male *D. plantaginea* and adds weight to the possibility that (1*S*,2*R*,3*S*)-dolichodial (**VIII**) is a component of the sex pheromone.

As discussed above, biological evidence suggested that the sex pheromone of the *Cryptomyzus* species is likely to consist of more than (4a*SR*,7*SR*,7a*RS*)-nepetalactone and (1*RS*,4a*SR*,7*SR*,7a*RS*)-nepetalactol. MS analysis on air entrainment samples collected from *R. padi*, *Aphis fabae* (the black-bean aphid), *Cryptomyzus maudamanti*, and *Cryptomyzus ribis* (the redcurrent blister aphid) oviparae all contain a chemical with the same mass spectra as (1*S*,2*R*,3*S*)-dolichodial (**VIII**) (Dewhirst *et al.*, 2008). As (1*S*,2*R*,3*S*)-dolichodial (**VIII**) has been shown to elicit a behavioral response in male *D. plantaginea*, this chemical may also be a component of the sex pheromone of *Cryptomyzus* species and may play a role in species integrity, thus adding a new dimension to the ratios of the sex pheromone components. (1*SR*,2*RS*,3*SR*)-Dolichodial has also been identified in air entrainment samples collected from *R. insertum*, *N. ribis-nigri*, and *O. insitus* oviparae (Dewhirst, 2007).

D. Synergism between plant volatiles and the aphid sex pheromone components

It has also been considered likely that volatiles from the primary host plants may have a role in males locating conspecific oviparae (Powell and Hardie, 2001). In the field, the number of male *R. padi* caught in water traps containing (1*RS*,4a*SR*,7*SR*,7a*RS*)-nepetalactol was increased by the addition of an extract from the winter host *Prunus padus* (the bird-cherry tree, Rosaceae) (Hardie *et al.*, 1994). Similarly, the number of male *P. humuli* caught in water traps containing (1*S*,4a*R*,7*S*,7a*S*)-nepetalactol (**VI**) and (1*R*,4a*R*,7*S*,7a*S*)-nepetalactol (**VII**) was increased by the addition of a steam distillation extract of *Prunus domestica* (plum tree) leaves or *Prunus spinosa* (blackthorn or sloe) drupes (Lösel *et al.*, 1996a,b). Catches of *R. padi* increased in water traps containing (1*RS*,4a*SR*,7*SR*,7a*RS*)-nepetalactol with methyl salicylate and benzaldehyde (two volatile components from *Prunus* spp., (Pettersson, 1994)) compared with water traps containing (1*RS*,4a*SR*,7*SR*,7a*RS*)-nepetalactol alone (Pope *et al.*, 2007). However, when methyl salicylate and benzaldehyde were added to (1*S*,4a*R*,7*S*,7a*S*)-nepetalactol (**VI**) and (1*R*,4a*R*,7*S*,7a*S*)-nepetalactol (**VII**), catches of male *P. humuli* decreased compared to the two iridoids alone (Pope *et al.*, 2007). In both studies, the winter host components alone did not increase numbers of *R. padi* or *P. humuli* caught in the water traps above control levels. This suggested that specific plant volatiles synergize the response of males to their sex pheromone. However, it appears that host volatiles do not have a role in the attraction of male *C. galesopsidis* (Guldemond *et al.*, 1993), *A. fabae* (Thieme and Dixon, 1996), and *Sitobion fragariae* (the black-berry cereal aphid) (Lilley and Hardie, 1996) to the sex pheromone from conspecific females.

Recently, van Tol *et al.* (2009) suggested that oviparae may manipulate host-plant volatiles and when the aphid sex pheromone is present with these conspecific-induced plant volatiles a synergistic effect on male behavior occurs. Headspace collection of apple plants infested with *D. plantaginea* oviparae was collected and an increase in hexyl butyrate, (*E*)-2-hexenyl butyrate, (*Z*)-3-hexenyl 3-methylbutyrate, and hexyl 2-methylbutyrate compared to uninfested plants was recorded. When presented in a mixture these chemicals did not significantly affect *D. plantaginea* trap catch in the orchard, but when the mixture was presented with the major aphid sex pheromone components, (1*R*,4a*S*,7*S*,7a*R*)-nepetalactol and (4a*S*,7*S*,7a*R*)-nepetalactone, a significant increase in trap catch was recorded in comparison to the catch in traps containing only the major sex pheromone components. In addition, a significant decrease in trap catch of other aphid species in comparison to the catch in traps containing the major sex pheromone components was observed. Thus suggesting that oviparae-induced host-plant volatiles play an important role in males locating conspecific oviparae.

E. Applications of the aphid sex pheromone for control and monitoring systems

Sex pheromones could be implemented in direct pest control programs, that is, mating disruption and mass trapping. Mating disruption is where large amounts of sex pheromone is released into the crop in order to prevent males locating the females, whereas mass trapping involves insect pests being attracted to a site where they can be removed (Foster and Harris, 1997). The physiological mechanism behind mating disruption is unknown but many theories have been suggested (Foster and Harris, 1997). Both mating disruption and mass trapping incorporating the use of sex pheromones have been successfully implemented within pest management programs for many species of pest, especially Lepidoptera. For example, a pheromone-based mating disruption system has become an important component in pest management programs for the control of the codling moth (*Cydia pomonella*) in apple, pear, and walnut orchards (Calkins, 1998; Cardé and Minks, 1995; Thomson *et al.*, 2001). Large amounts of the synthetic sex pheromone, (*E*,*E*)-8,10-dodecadien-1-ol (codlemone) (McDonough and Moffitt, 1974), can be introduced into the crop by the use of several different pheromone-delivery systems, that is, isomate polyethylene-tube dispensers (Thomson *et al.*, 2001), puffers (Shorey and Gerber, 1996), and microcapsules

(Stelinski *et al.*, 2005). This prevents the males from locating the females. Examples of successful mass trapping of pests with sex pheromones include *Prays citri* (the citrus flower moth) on lemons in Israel (Sternlicht *et al.*, 1990) and *Lymantria dispar* (the gypsy moth) in the United States (Kolodny-Hirsch and Schwalbe, 1990).

The aphid sex pheromone has potential to be used in pest management systems. Nepetalactone and nepetalactol are commercially available. A commercial system has been developed where 30 kg of essential oil, comprising 85–97.5% enantiomeric pure (4a*S*,7*S*,7a*R*)-nepetalactone (**I**), is extracted from 35 t of *N. cataria* (Birkett and Pickett, 2003). Compared to conventional synthesis from citronellol, this has dramatically reduced the cost of (4a*S*,7*S*,7a*R*)-nepetalactone (**I**) by 1000-fold, from £1000 g^{-1} to £1 g^{-1} (Birkett and Pickett, 2003). The (4a*S*,7*S*,7a*R*)-nepetalactone (**I**) is then readily reduced to (1*R*,4a*S*,7*S*,7a*R*)-nepetalactol (**III**). In addition, (4a*S*,7*S*,7a*R*)-nepetalactone (**I**) and (1*R*,4a*S*,7*S*,7a*R*)-nepetalactol (**III**) have been formulated using polymer extrusion technology to produce a flexible PVC rope. This formulation maintains a slow and consistent release rate of the active ingredients as well as preventing UV degradation and oxidation (Birkett and Pickett, 2003). The use of essential oils from renewable stocks is not only cheaper and sustainable compared to synthesis using fine chemicals from mineral oil stocks, but would also be more readily accepted by organic growers. If further research shows that dolichodial is an important component of the aphid sex pheromone, a similar system could be used to extract (1*S*,2*R*,3*S*)-dolichodial (**VIII**) from *T. marum*.

Although the components of the aphid sex pheromone are readily available, the use of the aphid sex pheromone in direct aphid control programs has not been commercially developed. One limiting factor is the biology of the aphid pest. Aphids which alternate between hosts are generally an agricultural pest on the summer secondary host. It is in the autumn on the primary host where the sexual morphs occur (Blackman and Eastop, 2000) and where the farmers generally cannot implement control measures. Also, the opportunity to exploit the aphid sex pheromone for control purposes is limited to a 2-month period. In addition, when conditions in winter permit the survival of an aphid, and a suitable food quality is found, the aphid may continue to produce parthenogenetic generations (Blackman, 1974).

Direct control measures using the sex pheromone can generally only be implemented where the aphid is a pest on the primary host, that is, in fruit orchards. For example, *D. plantaginea*, the second most important pest of apple in Europe and North America (Blommers *et al.*, 2004). In the autumn, gynoparous (winged females that produce oviparae on the winter host) and male *D. plantaginea* migrate to apple trees where over-wintering eggs are laid. It is in the following spring, when the fundatrices hatch, that the new population of *D. plantaginea* causes the most economic damage. Substantial damage to the fruits occurs even when aphid densities are so low as to defy visual monitoring (Blommers *et al.*, 2004). Currently, the application of insecticides occurs when a single fundatrix per 100 buds is found (Graf, 1999; Miñarro *et al.*, 2005; Wyss *et al.*, 1999). This selection pressure has lead to the development of insecticide resistance (Delorme *et al.*, 1997). The spring population could be reduced by controlling the autumn population by utilizing the sex pheromone and therefore less damage will occur. Only one investigation into the use of direct control measures using the aphid sex pheromone has been reported. *R. padi* is a main pest of cereal crops in the summer but in the autumn sexual forms migrate to *P. padus* trees (Pettersson *et al.*, 1994). The sex pheromone of *R. padi* has been reported to consist of (1*RS*,4a*SR*,7*SR*,7a*RS*)-nepetalactol (Hardie *et al.*, 1994). Donato (2001) attached vials containing (1*R*,4a*S*,7*S*,7a*R*)-nepetalactol (**III**) to *P. padus* trees to assess if mating could be disrupted. A significant increase in the number of males landing on the trees was observed but whether the behavior exhibited by the males locating conspecific oviparae was affected was not conclusive.

The use of the aphid sex pheromone could also be part of an integrated pest management (IPM) scheme. In IPM, the sex pheromone could be used to monitor male or gynoparous (see below) populations, used together with the exploitation of biological control agents (Hockland *et al.*, 1986) or used to manipulate insects as part of a push–pull system (Cook *et al.*, 2007; Pickett *et al.*, 1994, 1997). Currently, the most common strategy to control *D. plantaginaea* is to apply insecticides in early spring when fundatrices hatch, but aphid populations could also be reduced by spraying insecticides in autumn. Kehrli and Wyss (2001) reported that insecticide applications against the oviparae in autumn strongly inhibited the threat of an outbreak the next spring. As the window of opportunity is small, aphid monitoring systems using the sex pheromone components of *D. plantaginea* could be developed to gather information allowing accurate timing of insecticide treatment, that is, when the gynoparae are present but no mating has occurred. Gynoparae appear first in the crop with the males following approximately 2 weeks later (Blommers *et al.*, 2004). The sex pheromone components have been shown to attract gynoparae as well as male aphids (Gabrys *et al.*, 1997; Hardie *et al.*, 1996; Lösel *et al.*, 1996a,b) thus additionally acting as aggregation pheromones. Thus information on when the gynoparae are present and when the first males start to appear in the crop can be collated. Spraying insecticides in the autumn will reduce the number of sexual females; therefore, as a consequence less or no eggs are laid thus lowering the damage the following spring.

Hartfield *et al.* (2001) investigated the potential of lure and infect traps in the control of *P. humuli* in hop and plum orchards. The lure and infect mechanism involves the insect being lured into a trap where it is infected with a pathogen, then allowed to escape. When it is released, the insect locates other conspecific aphids which it then infects with the pathogen. Male *P. humuli* entered traps containing the sex pheromone component

(1*RS*,4a*R*,7*S*,7a*S*)-nepetalactol (**VII**) and an inoculum of the pathogen *Verticillium lecanii* but the effectiveness of this control mechanism in the field was questioned.

Finally, the aphid sex pheromone has been shown to elicit a positive behavioral response by aphid parasitoids (Glinwood *et al.*, 1998; Hardie *et al.*, 1991; Lilley et al., 1994; Powell *et al.*, 1993). The response of *Aphidius ervi* to (4a*S*,7*S*,7a*R*)-nepetalactone (**I**) was found to be innate, thus not easily modified by learning experiences (Vet and Dicke, 1992). Therefore, the aphid sex pheromone could be used to manipulate natural populations of parasitoids to control aphid populations. In order for parasitoids to be used as an effective control system it is necessary to achieve early-season synchrony between the aphid and parasitoid populations (Powell *et al.*, 1998). Unfortunately synchronization tends not to occur in the field, consequently large aphid colonies develop before the parasitoids arrive into the crop. To combat this problem, a parasitoid management system using the aphid sex pheromone has been developed. In the autumn when the parasitoids are forced to leave the harvested crop, sex pheromone lures are placed around the field in order to attract the parasitoid into the field margins where they overwinter as pupae. The following spring, the parasitoids emerge and rapidly recolonize the crops, therefore better synchrony occurs with the invading aphids (Powell *et al.*, 1998). Field studies have been conducted which demonstrate the feasibility of this approach (Pickett *et al.*, 1998).

V. Other Aphid Pheromones

Behavioral evidence has suggested that some aphids produce an aggregation pheromone, but the identification of the chemical composition has not been successful (Pettersson and Stephansson, 1991). An aggregation pheromone may be produced when an aphid has recently landed on a new host plant, signaling to others that aphid density is low on an unlimited supply of food or to attract others to reduce the probability of the individual aphid being attacked by natural enemies. At the other end of the scale, when aphid densities become too large, food supply will be limited and therefore the aphid may produce a spacing pheromone allowing better exploitation of host plant and decreasing intraspecific competition. Pettersson *et al.* (1995) investigated the possibility of cereal aphids producing a spacing pheromone in a four-way olfactometer. A negative linear relationship was found between the number of *R. padi* apterae on excised oat leaves and number of visits apterae *R. padi* made into the arm containing the infested oat leaf volatiles. As aphid density increased above four aphids per square centimeter, restlessness in the aphid cohort increased. This work did not distinguish whether the effect was due to pheromones released by the aphids or a change in the volatile profile of the plant. They suggested that it was unlikely to be due to a change in plant chemistry as a change would have to occur within 15 min, the time period between the aphids being placed on the plant and the experiment occurring.

VI. Conclusion

Aphid pheromones have been extensively studied over the last 40 years. Important discoveries have resulted in the identification of alarm and sex pheromones. Significant progress has been made toward an understanding of how the identified chemical blends and ratios play an important role in mediating behavior, and how this might be exploited in control/monitoring technologies. There are several challenges involved in the development of control methods that utilize aphid pheromones, not least including their volatile nature. However, this can be overcome by using essential oils from renewable plant sources which contain the relevant components and through the development of transgenic plants. For example, the recent identification and expression of genes encoding enzymes for the production of the alarm pheromone in *A. thaliana* has led to current efforts to transform crop plants, particularly to effect expression of the alarm pheromone synthesis gene under control of a natural product plant elicitor (Bruce *et al.*, 2008). Also, the essential oil from *N. cataria*, which contains the aphid sex pheromone components can be utilized to monitor *D. plantaginea* in orchards and to manipulate aphid natural enemies in summer crops, are looking like viable control/monitoring tools. However, for a sex pheromone-based control strategy to be successfully implemented, complete characterization of all factors involved in each agricultural system is required. For example, the involvement of host-plant volatiles and aphid-induced plant volatiles, as well as the way in which males locate conspecific oviparae has yet to be fully understood. Nevertheless, technologies based on the aphid alarm and sex pheromone are progressing well and could be utilized in future pest management programs to control aphids as an alternative to broad-spectrum insecticides or to optimize the application and effectiveness of broad-spectrum insecticides.

REFERENCES

Agelopoulos, N. G., Hooper, A. M., Maniar, S. P., Pickett, J. A., and Wadhams, L. J. (1999). A novel approach for isolation of volatile chemicals released by individual leaves of a plant *in situ*. *J. Chem. Ecol.* **25**, 1411–1425.

Barber, M. D., Moores, G. D., Denholm, I., Tachell, G. M., and Vice, W. E. (1998). Confirmation of insecticide resistance in UK populations of the currant-lettuce aphid,

Nasonovia ribis-nigri. The 1998 Brighton Conference Proceedings: Pests and Diseases, Vol. 2 pp. 485–490. The British Crop Protection Council, Brighton.

Beale, M. H., Birkett, M. A., Bruce, T. J. A., Chamberlain, K., Field, L. M., Huttly, A. K., Martin, J. L., Parker, R., Phillips, A. L., Pickett, J. A., Prosser, I. M., Shewry, P. R., *et al.* (2006). Aphid alarm pheromone produced by transgenic plants affects aphid and parasitoid behavior. *Proc. Natl. Acad. Sci. USA* **103,** 10509–10513.

Bellesia, F., Pagnoni, U. M., Pinetti, A., and Trave, R. (1983a). The biosynthesis of dolichodial in *Teucrium marum*. *Phytochemistry* **22,** 2197–2201.

Bellesia, F., Pagnoni, U. M., Pinetti, A., and Trave, R. (1983b). Teucrein, a new iridolactol from *Teucrium marum*, and its biosynthetic relationship with dolichodial. *J. Chem. Res.-S* **12,** 328–329.

Bellesia, F., Grandi, R., Pagnoni, U. M., Pinetti, A., and Trave, R. (1984). Biosynthesis of nepetalactone in *Nepeta cataria*. *Phytochemistry* **23,** 83–87.

Birkett, M. A., and Pickett, J. A. (2003). Aphid sex pheromones: From discovery to commercial production. *Phytochemistry* **62,** 651–656.

Blackman, R. L. (1974). Aphids. Ginn & Company Limited, London.

Blackman, R. L., and Eastop, V. F. (2000). Aphids on the Worlds Crops. Wiley, Chichester.

Blommers, L. H. M., Helsen, H. H. M., and Vaal, F. W. N. M. (2004). Life history data of the rosy apple aphid *Dysaphis plantaginea* (Pass.) (Homoptera: Aphididae) on plantain and as migrant to apple. *J. Pest Sci.* **77,** 155–163.

Boeve, J. L., Lengwiler, U. B., Tollsten, L., Dorn, S., and Turlings, T. C. J. (1996). Volatiles emitted by apple fruitlets infested by larvae of the European apple sawfly. *Phytochemistry* **42,** 373–381.

Boo, K. S., Choi, M. Y., Chung, I. B., Eastop, V. F., Pickett, J. A., Wadhams, L. J., and Woodcock, C. M. (2000). Sex pheromone of the peach aphid, *Tuberocephalus momonis* and optimal blends for trapping males and females in the field. *J. Chem. Ecol.* **26,** 601–609.

Bowers, W. S., Nishino, C., Montgomery, M. E., Nault, L. R., and Nielson, M. W. (1977). Sesquiterpene progenitor, germacrene A: An alarm pheromone in aphids. *Nature* **196,** 680.

Bruce, T. J. A., Birkett, M. A., Blande, J., Hooper, A. M., Martin, J. L., Khambay, B., Prosser, I. M., Smart, L. E., and Wadhams, L. J. (2005). Response of economically important aphids to components of *Hemizygia petiolata* essential oil. *Pest Manag. Sci.* **61,** 1115–1121.

Bruce, T. J. A., Matthes, M. C., Chamberlain, K., Woodcock, C. M., Mohib, A., Webster, B., Smart, L. E., Birkett, M. A., Pickett, J. A., and Napier, J. A. (2008). *cis*-Jasmone induces *Arabidopsis* genes that affect the chemical ecology of multitrophic interactions with aphids and their parasitoids. *Proc. Natl. Acad. Sci. USA* **105,** 4553–4558.

Calkins, C. O. (1998). Review of the codling moth area-wide suppression program in the western United States. *J. Agric. Entomol.* **15,** 327–333.

Campbell, C. A. M., Dawson, G. W., Griffiths, D. C., Pettersson, J., Pickett, J. A., Wadhams, L. J., and Woodcock, C. M. (1990). Sex attractant pheromone of damson-hop aphid *Phorodon humuli* (Homoptera: Aphididae). *J. Chem. Ecol.* **16,** 3455–3465.

Campbell, C. A. M., Cook, F. J., Pickett, J. A., Pope, T. W., Wadhams, L. J., and Woodcock, C. M. (2003). Responses of the aphids *Phorodon humuli* and *Rhopalosiphum padi* to sex pheromone stereochemistry in the field. *J. Chem. Ecol.* **29,** 2225–2234.

Cardé, R. T., and Minks, A. K. (1995). Control of moth pests by mating disruptions: Successes and constraints. *Annu. Rev. Entomol.* **40,** 559–585.

Cavill, G. W. K., and Hinterberger, H. (1960). The chemistry of ants. IV. Terpenoid constituents of some *Dolichoderus* and *Iridomyrmex* species. *Aust. J. Chem.* **13,** 514–519.

Cavill, G. W. K., and Houghton, E. (1974). Volatile constituents of argentine ant, *Iridomyrmex humilis*. *J. Insect Physiol.* **20,** 2049–2059.

Cavill, G. W. K., Robertson, P. L., Brophy, J. J., Clark, D. V., Duke, R., Orton, C. J., and Plant, W. D. (1982). Defensive and other secretions of the Australian cocktail ant, *Iridomyrmex nitidiceps*. *Tetrahedron* **38,** 1931–1938.

Cook, S. M., Khan, Z. R., and Pickett, J. A. (2007). The use of push–pull strategies in integrated pest management. *Annu. Rev. Entomol.* **52,** 375–400.

Dawson, G. W., Griffiths, D. C., Janes, N. F., Mudd, A., Pickett, J. A., Wadhams, L. J., and Woodcock, C. M. (1987). Identification of an aphid sex-pheromone. *Nature* **325,** 614–616.

Dawson, G. W., Griffiths, D. C., Merritt, L. A., Mudd, A., Pickett, J. A., Wadhams, L. J., and Woodcock, C. M. (1988). The sex-pheromone of the greenbug, *Schizaphis graminum*. *Entomol. Exp. Appl.* **48,** 91–93.

Dawson, G. W., Janes, N. F., Mudd, A., Pickett, J. A., Slawin, A. M. Z., Wadhams, L. J., and Williams, D. J. (1989). The aphid sex-pheromone. *Pure Appl. Chem.* **61,** 555–558.

Dawson, G. W., Griffiths, D. C., Merritt, L. A., Mudd, A., Pickett, J. A., Wadhams, L. J., and Woodcock, C. M. (1990). Aphid semiochemicals: A review and recent advances on the sex-pheromone. *J. Chem. Ecol.* **16,** 3019–3030.

Delorme, R., Auge, D., Touton, P., and Villatte, F. (1997). Insecticide resistance in *Dysaphis plantaginea* in France. Fourth International Conference on Pests in Agriculture, Vol. 1, Montpellier, pp. 45–52.

Devonshire, A. L., and Moores, G. D. (1982). A carboxylesterase with broad substrate-specificity causes organo-phosphorus, carbamate and pyrethroid resistance in peach-potato aphids (*Myzus persicae*). *Pestic. Biochem. Physiol.* **18,** 235–246.

Devonshire, A. L., Field, L. M., Foster, S. P., Moores, G. D., Williamson, M. S., and Blackman, R. L. (1998). The evolution of insecticide resistance in the peach-potato aphid, *Myzus persicae*. *Philos. Trans. R. Soc. Lond. Ser. B-Biol. Sci.* **353,** 1677–1684.

Dewhirst, S. Y. (2007). Aspects of aphid chemical ecology: Sex pheromones and induced plant defences. Ph.D. Thesis. Imperial College, London.

Dewhirst, S. Y., Birkett, M. A., Fitzgerald, J. D., Stewart-Jones, A., Wadhams, L. J., Woodcock, C. M., Hardie, J., and Pickett, J. A. (2008). Dolichodial: A new aphid sex pheromone component? *J. Chem. Ecol.* **34,** 1575–1583.

Donato, B. J. (2001). Chemical ecology studies on autumn migrant aphids and their natural enemies. Ph.D. Thesis. London University.

Edwards, L. J., Siddall, J. B., Dunham, L. L., Uden, P., and Kislow, C. (1973). *Trans-β-*farnesene, alarm pheromone of the green peach aphid, *Myzus persicae* (sulzer). *Nature* **241,** 126–127.

Eisenbraun, E. J., Browne, C. E., Irvin-Willis, R. L., McGurk, D. J., Eliel, E. L., and Harris, D. L. (1980). Structure and stereochemistry of 4aβ-7α-7aβ-nepetalactone from *Nepeta mussini* and its relationship to 4aα-7α-7aα and 4aα-7α-7aβ-nepetalactones from *N. cataria*. *J. Org. Chem.* **45,** 3811–3814.

Ester, A., Gut, J., Vanoosten, A. M., and Pijnenburg, H. C. H (1993). Controlling aphids in iceberg lettuce by alarm pheromone in combination with an insecticide. *J. Appl. Entomol.* **115,** 432–440.

Foster, S. P., and Harris, M. O. (1997). Behavioral manipulation methods for insect pest-management. *Annu. Rev. Entomol.* **42,** 123–146.

Francis, F., van der Moten, S., Verheggen, F., Lognay, G., and Haubruge, E. (2005). Is (*E*)-*β*-farnesene the only volatile terpenoid in aphids? *J. Appl. Entomol.* **129,** 6–11.

Gabrys, B. J., Gadomski, H. J., Klukowski, Z., Pickett, J. A., Sobota, G. T., Wadhams, L. J., and Woodcock, C. M. (1997). Sex pheromone of cabbage aphid *Brevicoryne brassicae*: Identification and field trapping of male aphids and parasitoids. *J. Chem. Ecol.* **23,** 1881–1890.

Garthwaite, D. G., Thomas, M. R., Anderson, H., and Stoddart, H. (2004). Pesticide Usage Survey Report 202: Arable Crops in Great Britain 2004. Pesticide Usage Survey Team, Central Science Laboratory, Yorkp. 111.

Glinwood, R. T., Powell, W., and Tripathi, C. P. M. (1998). Increased parasitation of aphid parasitoids (Hymenoptera: Aphidiinae) on trap plants baited with aphid sex pheromone, and effective range of aphid sex pheromone lures. *Biocontrol Sci. Technol.* **8,** 607–614.

Goff, A. M., and Nault, L. R. (1974). Aphid cornicle secretions ineffective against attack by parasitoid wasps. *Environ. Entomol.* **3,** 565–566.

Goldansaz, S. H., Dewhirst, S. Y., Birkett, M. A., Hooper, A. M., Smiley, D. W. M., Pickett, J. A., Wadhams, L. J., and McNeil, J. N. (2004). Identification of two sex pheromone components of the potato aphid, *Macrosiphum euphorbiae* (Thomas). *J. Chem. Ecol.* **30,** 819–834.

Golub, M. A., and Weatherston, I. (1984). Techniques for extracting and collecting sex pheromones from live insects and from artificial sources. *In* "Techniques in Pheromone Research," (H. E. Hummel and T. A. Miller, Eds.), pp. 222–286. Springer-Verlag, New York.

Graf, B. (1999). Optimising the control of rosy apple aphid *Dysaphis plantaginea* (Pass.) (Homoptera: Aphididae). *IOBC/WPRS Bull.* **22,** 71–76.

Greenway, A. R., and Griffiths, D. C. (1973). A comparison of triglycerides from aphids and their cornicle secretions. *J. Insect Physiol.* **19,** 1649–1655.

Griffiths, D. C., and Pickett, J. A. (1980). A potential application of aphid alarm pheromones. *Entomol. Exp. Appl.* **27,** 199–201.

Guldemond, J. A., Dixon, A. F. G., Pickett, J. A., Wadhams, L. J., and Woodcock, C. M. (1992). The role of host plant odour and sex pheromones in mate recognition in the aphid *Cryptomyzus*. *In* "Proceedings of the 8th International Symposium of Insect–Plant Relationships," (S. B. J. Menken, J. H. Visser, and P. Harrewijn, Eds.), pp. 119–121. Kluwer, Dordrecht.

Guldemond, J. A., Dixon, A. F. G., Pickett, J. A., Wadhams, L. J., and Woodcock, C. M. (1993). Specificity of sex-pheromones, the role of host-plant odor in the olfactory attraction of males, and mate recognition in the aphid *Cryptomyzus*. *Physiol. Entomol.* **18,** 137–143.

Hardie, J. (1991). Contribution of sex-pheromone to mate location and reproductive isolation in aphid species (Homopter, Aphidinea). *Entomol. Gen.* **16,** 249–256.

Hardie, J., Holyoak, M., Nicholas, J., Nottingham, S. F., Pickett, J. A., Wadhams, L. J., and Woodcock, C. M. (1990). Aphid sex pheromone components: Age-dependent release by females and species-specific male response. *Chemoecology* **1,** 63–68.

Hardie, J., Nottingham, S. F., Powell, W., and Wadhams, L. J. (1991). Synthetic aphid sex-pheromone lures female parasitoids. *Entomol. Exp. Appl.* **61,** 97–99.

Hardie, J., Nottingham, S. F., Dawson, G. W., Harrington, R., Pickett, J. A., and Wadhams, L. J. (1992). Attraction of field-flying aphid males to synthetic sex pheromone. *Chemoecology* **3,** 3–4.

Hardie, J., Storer, J. R., Nottingham, S. F., Peace, L., Harrington, R., Merritt, L. A., Wadhams, L. J., and Wood, D. K. (1994). The interaction of sex pheromone and plant volatiles for field attraction of male bird-cherry aphid, *Rhopalosiphum padi*. The 1994 Brighton Crop Protection Conference: Pests and Diseases, Vol. 3, Brighton, England, pp. 1223–1230.

Hardie, J., Storer, J. R., Cook, F. J., Campbell, C. A. M., Wadhams, L. J., Lilley, R., and Peace, L. (1996). Sex pheromone and visual trap interactions in mate location strategies and aggregation by host-alternating aphids in the field. *Physiol. Entomol.* **21,** 97–106.

Hardie, J., Peace, L., Pickett, J. A., Smiley, D. W. M., Storer, J. R., and Wadhams, L. J. (1997). Sex pheromone stereochemistry and purity affect field catches of male aphids. *J. Chem. Ecol.* **23,** 2547–2554.

Hartfield, C. M., Campbell, C. A. M., Hardie, J., Pickett, J. A., and Wadhams, L. J. (2001). Pheromone traps for the dissemination of an entomopathogen by the damson hop aphid *Phorodon humuli*. *Biocontrol Sci. Technol.* **11,** 401–410.

Hockland, S. H., Dawson, G. W., Griffiths, D. C., Marples, B., Pickett, J. A., and Woodcock, C. M. (1986). The use of aphid alarm pheromone (*E*)-*β*-farnesene to increase effectiveness of the entomophilic fungus *Verticillium lecanii* in controlling aphids on chrysanthemums under glass. *In* "Fundamental and Applied Aspects of Invertebrate Pathology," (R. A. Samson, J. M. Vlak, and D. Peters, Eds.), p. 252. Foundation of the Fourth International Colloquium on Invertebrate Pathology. Society of Invertebrate Pathology, Veldhoven.

Hottes, F. C. (1928). Concerning the structure, function and origin of the cornicles of the family Aphididae. *Proc. Biol. Soc. Wash.* **41,** 71–84.

Jeon, H., Han, K. S., and Boo, K. S. (2003). Sex pheromone of *Aphis spiraecola* (Homoptera: Aphididae): Composition and circadian rhythm in release. *J. Asia-Pac. Entomol.* **6,** 159–165.

Jones, O. T. (1998). Practical applications of pheromones and other semiochemicals. *In* "Insect Pheromones and Their Use in Pest Management," (P. E. Howse, R. Stevens, and O. T. Jones, Eds.), pp. 263–355. Chapman & Hall, London.

Kehrli, P., and Wyss, E. (2001). Effects of augmentative releases of the coccinellid, *Adalia bipunctata*, and of insecticide treatments in autumn on the spring population of aphids of the genus *Dysaphis* in apple orchards. *Entomol. Exp. Appl.* **99,** 245–252.

Kennedy, J. S., and Stroyan, H. L. G. (1959). Biology of aphids. *Annu. Rev. Entomol.* **4,** 139–160.

Kislow, C., and Edwards, L. J. (1972). Repellent odour in aphids. *Nature* **235,** 108–109.

Kolodny-Hirsch, D. M., and Schwalbe, C. P. (1990). Use of disparlure in the management of the gypsy moth. *In* "Behaviour-Modifying Chemicals for Insect Management: Application of Pheromones and Other Attractants," (R. L. Ridgway and R. M. Silvestein, Eds.), pp. 363–385. Marcel Dekker, New York.

Lilley, R., and Hardie, J. (1996). Cereal aphid responses to sex pheromones and host-plant odours in the laboratory. *Physiol. Entomol.* **21,** 304–308.

Lilley, R., Hardie, J., and Wadhams, L. J. (1994a). Field manipulation of *Praon* populations using semiochemicals. *Norwegian J. Agric. Sci.* **16,** 221–226.

Lilley, R., Hardie, J., Merritt, L. A., Pickett, J. A., Wadhams, L. J., and Woodcock, C. M. (1994b). The sex pheromone of the grain aphid, *Sitobion avenae* (Fab.) (Homoptera: Aphididae). *Chemoecology* **5/6,** 43–46.

Lösel, P. M., Lindemann, M., Scherkenbeck, J., Campbell, C. A. M., Hardie, J., Pickett, J. A., and Wadhams, L. J. (1996a). Effect of primary-host kairomones on the attractiveness of the hop-aphid sex pheromone to *Phorodon humuli* males and gynoparae. *Entomol. Exp. Appl.* **80,** 79–82.

Lösel, P. M., Lindemann, M., Scherkenbeck, J., Maier, J., Engelhard, B., Campbell, C. A. M., Hardie, J., Pickett, J. A., Wadhams, L. J., Elbert, A., and Thielking, G. (1996b). The potential of semiochemicals for control of *Phorodon humuli* (Homoptera: Aphididae). *Pestic. Sci.* **48,** 293–303.

Luijk, R., Lefferts, L. Y., and Groth, III, E. (1998). The importance of food safety issues from the public perspective. Public perception and the consumer's interest in pesticide residues. *In* The 1998 Brighton Conference Proceedings: Pests and Diseases, Vol. 2, pp. 475–482. The British Crop Protection Council, Brighton.

Marsh, D. (1972). Sex pheromone in the aphid *Megoura viciae*. *Nat.—New Biol.* **238,** 31–32.

Marsh, D. (1975). Responses of male aphids to female sex pheromone in *Megoura viciae* Buckton. *J. Entomol. Ser. A-Physiol. Behav.* **50,** 43–64.

Martinez-Torres, D., Foster, S. P., Field, L. M., Devonshire, A. L., and Williamson, M. S. (1999). A sodium channel point mutation is associated with resistance to DDT and pyrethroid insecticides in the peach-potato aphid, *Myzus persicae* (Sulzer) (Hemiptera: Aphididae). *Insect Mol. Biol.* **8,** 339–346.

McDonough, L. M., and Moffitt, H. R. (1974). Sex pheromone of the codling moth. *Science* **183,** 978.
Millar, J. G., and Sims, J. J. (1998). Preparation, clean up and preliminary fractionation of extracts. *In* "Methods in Chemical Ecology: Chemical Methods," (J. G. Millar and K. F. Haynes, Eds.), Vol. 1, pp. 1–32. Kluwer, Norwell.
Miñarro, M., Hemptinne, J. L., and Dapena, E. (2005). Colonization of apple orchards by predators of *Dysaphis plantaginea*: Sequential arrival, response to prey abundance and consequences for biological control. *Biocontrol* **50,** 403–414.
Montgomery, M. E., and Nault, L. R. (1977). Comparative response of aphids to the alarm pheromone, (*E*)-beta-farnesene. *Entomol. Exp. Appl.* **22,** 236–242.
Moores, G. D., Devine, G. J., and Devonshire, A. L. (1994). Insecticide-insensitive acetylcholinesterase can enhance esterase-based resistance in *Myzus persicae* and *Myzus nicotianae*. *Pestic. Biochem. Physiol.* **49,** 114–120.
Mori, K. (1989). Synthesis of optically-active pheromones. *Tetrahedron* **45,** 3233–3298.
Nault, L. R. (1997). Arthropod transmission of plant viruses: A new synthesis. *Ann. Entomol. Soc. Am.* **90,** 521–541.
Nault, L. R., Edwards, L. J., and Styer, W. E. (1973). Aphid alarm pheromones: Secretion and reception. *Environ. Entomol.* **2,** 101–105.
Nishino, C., Bowers, W. S., Montgomery, M. E., Nault, L. R., and Nielson, M. W. (1977). Alarm pheromone of the spotted alfalfa aphid, *Therioaphis maculata* Buckton (Homoptera: Aphididae). *J. Chem. Ecol.* **3,** 349–357.
Pagnoni, U. M., Pinetti, A., Trave, R., and Garanti, L. (1976). Monoterpenes of *Teucrium marum*. *Aust. J. Chem.* **29,** 1375–1381.
Pettersson, J. (1970). An aphid sex attractant I. Biological studies. *Entomol. Scand.* **1,** 63–73.
Pettersson, J. (1994). The bird cherry-oat aphid, *Rhopalosiphum padi* (L.) (Homoptera: Aphididae) and odours. *In* "Individuals, Populations and Patterns in Ecology," (S. R. Leather, A. D. Watt, N. J. Mills, and K. F. A. Walters, Eds.). Intercept, Hampshire.
Pettersson, J., and Stephansson, D. (1991). Odor communication in two brassica feeding aphid species (Homoptera: Aphidinea: Aphididae). *Entomol. Gen.* **16,** 241–247.
Pettersson, J., Pickett, J. A., Pye, B. J., Quiroz, A., Smart, L. E., Wadhams, L. J., and Woodcock, C. M. (1994). Winter host component reduces colonization by bird-cherry oat aphid, *Rhopalosiphum padi* (L) (Homoptera: Aphididae), and other aphids in cereal fields. *J. Chem. Ecol.* **20,** 2565–2574.
Pettersson, J., Quiroz, A., Stephansson, D., and Niemeyer, H. M. (1995). Odor communication of *Rhopalosiphum padi* on grasses. *Entomol. Exp. Appl.* **76,** 325–328.
Pickett, J. A. (1990). Gas chromatography–mass spectrometry in insect pheromone identification: Three extreme case histories. *In* "Chromatography and Isolation of Insect Hormones and Pheromones," (A. R. McCaffery and I. D. Wilson, Eds.), pp. 299–309. Plenum Press, New York and London.
Pickett, J. A. (1991). Novel approaches to crop protection. Proceedings Symposium on Poverty Alleviation through Chemistry for Improved Food Production, Columbo, Sri Lanka, pp. 57–62.
Pickett, J. A., and Griffiths, D. C. (1980). Composition of aphid alarm pheromones. *J. Chem. Ecol.* **6,** 349–360.
Pickett, J. A., Wadhams, L. J., and Woodcock, C. M. (1994). Attempts to control aphid pests by integrated use of semiochemicals. *In* The 1994 Brighton Conference Proceedings: Pests and Diseases, Vol. 1 pp. 1239–1246. The British Crop Protection Council, Brighton.
Pickett, J. A., Wadhams, L. J., and Woodcock, C. M. (1997). First steps in the use of aphid sex pheromones. *In* "Insect Pheromone Research: New Directions," (R. T. Cardé and A. K. Minks, Eds.), pp. 439–444. Chapman & Hall, New York.

Pickett, J. A., Wadhams, L. J., and Woodcock, C. M. (1998). Insect supersence: Mate and host location by insects as model systems for exploiting olfactory interactions. *The Biochemist* August, 8–13.

Pickett, J. A., Rasmussen, H. B., Woodcock, C. M., Matthes, W., and Napier, J. A. (2003). Plant stress signalling: Understanding and exploiting plant–plant interactions. *Biochem. Soc. Trans.* **31,** 123–127.

Pimentel, D. (2005). Environmental and economic costs of the application of pesticides primarily in the United States. *Environ. Dev. Sustainability* **7,** 229–252.

Pope, T. W., Campbell, C. A. M., Hardie, J., Pickett, J. A., and Wadhams, L. J. (2007). Interactions between host-plant volatiles and the sex pheromones of the bird cherry-oat aphid, *Rhopalosiphum padi* and the damson-hop aphid, *Phorodon humuli. J. Chem. Ecol.* **33,** 157–165.

Powell, G., and Hardie, J. (2001). The chemical ecology of aphid host alternation: How do return migrants find the primary host plant? *Appl. Entomol. Zool.* **36,** 259–267.

Powell, W., Hardie, J., Hick, A. J., Holler, C., Mann, J., Merritt, L. A., Nottingham, S. F., Wadhams, L. J., Witthinrich, J., and Wright, A. F. (1993). Responses of the parasitoid *Praon volucre* (Hymenoptera, Braconidae) to aphid sex-pheromone lures in cereal fields in autumn: Implications for parasitoid manipulation. *Eur. J. Entomol.* **90,** 435–438.

Powell, W., Pennacchio, F., Poppy, G. M., and Tremblay, E. (1998). Strategies involved in the location of hosts by the parasitoid *Aphidius ervi* Haliday (Hymenoptera: Braconidae: Aphidiinae). *Biol. Control* **11,** 104–112.

Pretty, J. N., Brett, C., Gee, D., Hine, R. E., Mason, C. F., Morison, J. I. L., Raven, H., Rayment, M. D., and van der Bijl, G. (2000). An assessment of the total external costs of UK agriculture. *Agric. Syst.* **65,** 113–136.

Prosser, I. M., Adams, R. J., Beale, M. H., Hawkins, N. D., Phillips, A. L., Pickett, J. A., and Field, L. M. (2006). Cloning and functional characterisation of a *cis*-muuroladiene synthase from black peppermint (*Mentha* × *piperita*) and direct evidence for a chemotype unable to synthesise farnesene. *Phytochemistry* **67,** 1564–1571.

Quiroz, A., and Niemeyer, H. M. (1998). Activity of enantiomers of sulcatol on apterae of *Rhopalosiphum padi. J. Chem. Ecol.* **24,** 361–370.

Shorey, H. H., and Gerber, R. G. (1996). Use of puffers for disruption of sex pheromone communication of codling moths (Lepidoptera: Torticidae) in walnut orchards. *Environ. Entomol.* **25,** 1398–1400.

Steffan, A. W. (1990). Courtship behaviour and possible pheromone spread by hindleg raising in sexual females in aphids (Homoptera: Aphidinea). *Entomol. Gen.* **15,** 33–49.

Stelinski, L. L., Gut, L. J., Ketner, K. C., and Miller, J. R. (2005). Orientational disruption of codling moth, *Cydia pomonella (L.)* (Lep., Tortricidae), by concentrated formulations of microencapsulated pheromone in flight tunnel assays. *J. Appl. Entomol.* **129,** 481–488.

Sternlicht, M., Barzakay, I., and Tamim, M. (1990). Management of *Prays citri* in lemon orchards by mass trapping of males. *Entomol. Exp. Appl.* **55,** 59–67.

Stewart-Jones, A., Dewhirst, S. Y., Durrant, L., Fitzgerald, J. D., Hardie, J., Hooper, A. M., Pickett, J. A., and Poppy, G. M. (2007). Structure, ratios and patterns of release in the sex pheromone of an aphid, *Dysaphis plantaginea. J. Exp. Biol.* **210,** 4335–4344.

Strong, F. E. (1967). Observations on aphid cornicle secretions. *Ann. Entomol. Soc. Am.* **60,** 668–673.

Thieme, T., and Dixon, A. F. G. (1996). Mate recognition in the *Aphis fabae* complex: Daily rhythm of release and specificity of sex pheromones. *Entomol. Exp. Appl.* **79,** 85–89.

Thomson, D. R., Brunner, J. F., Gut, L. J., Judd, G. J. R., and Knight, A. L. (2001). Ten years implementing codling moth mating disruption in orchards of Washington and British Columbia: Starting right and managing for success. *Bull. IOBC/WPRS* **24,** 23–30.

Tillman, J. A., Seybold, S. J., Jurenka, R. A., and Blomquist, G. J. (1999). Insect pheromones: An overview of biosynthesis and endocrine regulation. *Insect Biochem. Mol. Biol.* **29,** 481–514.

van Tol, R. W. H. M., Helsen, H. H. M., Griepink, F. C., and de Kogel, W. J. (2009). Female-induced increase of host-plant volatiles enhance specific attraction of aphid male *Dysaphis plantaginea* (Homoptera: Aphididae) to the sex pheromone. *Bull. Entomol. Res.* **99,** 593–602.

Vet, L. E. M., and Dicke, M. (1992). Ecology of infochemical use by natural enemies in a tritrophic context. *Annu. Rev. Entomol.* **37,** 141–172.

Wadhams, L. J. (1984). The coupled gas chromatography-single cell recording technique. *In* "Techniques in Pheromone Research," (H. E. Hummel and T. A. Miller, Eds.), pp. 179–190. Springer-Verlag, New York.

Wedge, P. J., Parker, W. E., and Denholm, I. (1998). Resistance in *Myzus persicae*: Current status in Europe and future prospects. The 1998 Brighton Conference Proceedings: Pests and Diseases, Vol. 2, pp. 497–502. The British Crop Protection Council, Brighton.

Wyss, E., Villiger, M., Hemptinne, J. L., and Scharer, H. M. (1999). Effects of augumentative release of eggs and larvae of the ladybird beetle, *Adalia bipuncata,* on the abundance of the rosy apple aphid, *Dysaphis plantaginea,* in organic apple orchards. *Entomol. Exp. Appl.* **90,** 167–173.

CHAPTER TWENTY-THREE

Recent Advances in Methyl Eugenol and Cue-Lure Technologies for Fruit Fly Detection, Monitoring, and Control in Hawaii☆

Roger I. Vargas,* Todd E. Shelly,† Luc Leblanc,‡ *and* Jaime C. Piñero‡,§

Contents

Abstract

Worldwide, an important aspect of invasive insect pest management is more effective, safer detection and control systems. Phenyl propanoids are attractive to numerous species of Dacinae fruit flies. Methyl eugenol (ME) (4-allyl-1, 2-

* U.S. Pacific Basin Agricultural Research Center, USDA, ARS, Hilo, Hawaii USA
† USDA-APHIS, Waimanalo, Hawaii, USA
‡ Department of Plant Environmental Protection Science, University of Hawaii, Honolulu, Hawaii, USA
§ Cooperative Research and Extension, Lincoln University of Missouri, Jefferson City, Missouri, USA

☆ This chapter reports the results of research only. Mention of proprietary product does not constitute an endorsement or recommendation by the USDA

Vitamins and Hormones, Volume 83
ISSN 0083-6729, DOI: 10.1016/S0083-6729(10)83023-7

dimethoxybenzene-carboxylate), cue-lure (C-L) (4-(*p*-acetoxyphenyl)-2-butanone), and raspberry ketone (RK) (4-(*p*-hydroxyphenyl)-2-butanone) are powerful male-specific lures. Most evidence suggests a role of ME and C-L/RK in pheromone synthesis and mate attraction. ME and C-L/RK are used in current fruit fly programs for detection, monitoring, and control. During the Hawaii Area-Wide Pest Management Program in the interest of worker safety and convenience, liquid C-L/ME and insecticide (i.e., naled and malathion) mixtures were replaced with solid lures and insecticides. Similarly, Male Annihilation Technique (MAT) with a sprayable Specialized Pheromone and Lure Application Technology (SPLAT), in combination with ME (against *Bactrocera dorsalis*, oriental fruit fly) or C-L/RK (against *B. cucurbitae*, melon fly), and the reduced-risk insecticide, spinosad, was developed for area-wide suppression of fruit flies. The nontarget effects of ME and C-L/RK to native invertebrates were examined. Although weak attractiveness was recorded to flower-visiting insects, including bees and syrphid flies, by ME, effects to native *Drosophila* and other Hawaiian endemics were found to be minimal. These results suggested that the majority of previously published records, including those of endemic Drosophilidae, were actually for attraction to dead flies inside fruit fly traps. Endemic insect attraction was not an issue with C-L/RK, because *B. cucurbitae* were rarely found in endemic environments.

I. Introduction

Methyl eugenol (ME) (4-allyl-1, 2-dimethoxybenzene-carboxylate) is a widely distributed natural plant product and occurs in >200 plant species in 32 families found mainly in the tropics (Tan and Nishida, 1996). It is consumed by humans and animals in many plants and fruits (e.g., anise, nutmeg, basil, blackberry essence, bananas, and citrus; De Vincenzi *et al.*, 2000). ME is also used as a flavoring in ice cream, cookies, pies, puddings, candy, cola soft drinks, and chewing gum (De Vincenzi *et al.*, 2000). For example, clove oil contains approximately 15% ME and is generally recognized as a safe (GRAS) compound by the U.S. Food and Drug Administration as a food additive (http://www.epa.gov).

Cue-lure (C-L) (4-(*p*-acetoxyphenyl)-2-butanone) has not been isolated as a natural product but is rapidly hydrolyzed to form 4-(*p*-hydroxyphenyl)-2-butanone, rheosimin, or raspberry ketone (RK), which is a natural plant constituent (Metcalf and Metcalf, 1992). C-L is a colorless to pale yellow liquid with a raspberry-like odor (http://www.epa.gov). RK was originally isolated from an orchid, *Dendrobium superbum* Rchb. F (Nishida *et al.*, 1993), and is found in raspberries (*Rubus idaeus* L. and *R. strigosus* Michx.) (Schinz and Seidel, 1961) and in the juice of cranberries, *Vaccinium oxycoccos* L. and *V. macrocarpon* Aiton (Ericaceae) (Lin and Chen, 1984). Apparently, the name C-L is derived from the scientific name of the target species, the melon fly, *Bactrocera cucurbitae* (Coquillett).

Both ME and C-L belong to the class of organic compounds based on a C6–C3 skeleton referred to as phenyl propanoids (Friedrich, 1976). The shikimic acid/shikimate pathway is the main biosynthetic route by which these aromatic compounds are produced from carbohydrates. Phenyl propanoids are attractive to numerous species of Dacinae fruit flies (Diptera: Tephritidae), which are among the most economically important pests attacking soft fruits worldwide. In this chapter, we review past and recent developments with ME and C-L as fruit fly attractants and highlight the importance of early detection and eradication of invasive fruit-infesting fruit flies. In addition, we describe the key elements of the Hawaii Area-Wide Pest Management (HAWPM) Program which provided the basis for elimination of liquid lures and highly toxic organophosphate insecticides and discuss the relationship between fruit fly male behavior (with a focus on *Bactrocera* species) and ME and C-L/RK, as well as the environmental impacts (i.e., nontarget effects to invertebrates) of male lures used for Male Annihilation Technique (MAT) in Hawaii.

II. Insect Pheromones and Parapheromones

Pheromones (from the Greek word *pherein* (to transport) and *hormone* (to stimulate)) are chemical compounds secreted by an animal which mediate behavior of another animal belonging to the same species (Karlson and Butenandt, 1959). Many types of animals, including insects, are known to produce and naturally respond to pheromones. Pheromones are subdivided into several types based on the nature of the interaction. Examples include sex pheromones (released by members of one sex to attract the opposite sex), aggregation pheromones (attract both males and females to a small area), alarm pheromones (alert individuals to danger), and trail pheromones (deposited on a substrate by one member of a species and followed by another member of the same species) (Gordh and Headrick, 2001). The first insect sex pheromone identified was bombykol, (*E*, *Z*)-10,12-hexadecadien-1-ol, (Butenandt *et al.*, 1959), which is released by the female silkworm moth, *Bombyx mori* (L.), to attract mates.

Parapheromones can be defined as chemical compounds of anthropogenic origin, not known to exist in nature but structurally related to natural pheromone components, that in some way affect physiologically or behaviorally the insect pheromone communication system, eliciting a similar response to that of a true pheromone (Renou and Guerrero, 2000). Males of many tephritid species (see below) are strongly attracted to specific chemical compounds, which either occur naturally in plants (e.g., ME) or are synthetic analogues of plant-borne substances (e.g., C-L) (Cunningham, 1989; Fletcher, 1987).

These powerful male lures are commonly referred to as parapheromones, even though the chemical structure of the male lures is very different from that of the natural fruit fly pheromone (Renou and Guerrero, 2000). Parapheromones are used in current control programs of tephritid pests for detection and monitoring of populations and control with MAT (Vargas *et al.*, 2008a).

III. Fruit Flies and Economic Importance

The family Tephritidae, the true fruit flies, includes over 4000 species, which are among the most economically important pests attacking soft fruits worldwide (White and Elson-Harris, 1992). From an economic perspective, fruit flies (1) inflict extensive direct damage to fruits and vegetables, (2) cause quarantine restrictions on infested areas, (3) require that commercial fruits undergo quarantine treatment prior to export, and (4) provide a breeding reservoir for their introduction into other parts of the world due to current unprecedented levels of travel and trade between countries. The complex behavior of fruit flies is mediated by a variety of chemical cues. Those involved with feeding, host location, mating, and oviposition have been used in control.

Lists of the most important agricultural pests have been prepared by many researchers (Carey and Dowell, 1989; Metcalf and Metcalf, 1992). Among the most notorious members of the family are the Mediterranean fruit fly, *Ceratitis capitata* (Wiedemann), oriental fruit fly, *Bactrocera dorsalis* (Hendel), Queensland fruit fly, *B. tryoni* (Froggatt), peach fruit fly, *B. zonata* (Saunders), melon fly, *B. cucurbitae*, olive fly, *Bactrocera oleae* (Gmelin), South American fruit fly, *Anastrepha fraterculus* (Wiedemann), the Mexican fruit fly, *A. ludens* (Loew), West Indian fruit fly, *A. obliqua* (Macquart), and apple maggot fly, *Rhagoletis pomonella* (Walsh). With expanding international trade in fresh fruits and vegetables and human travel, fruit flies as major quarantine pests of fruits and vegetables have taken on added importance, triggering the need for improved detection and control systems. For example, every year exotic fruit flies are accidentally introduced from various parts of the world into California and require expensive eradication treatments. Due to continuous introductions, current annual costs to exclude *C. capitata* from California total over $15 million (http://www.cdfa.ca.gov). If *C. capitata* became permanently established in California, projected losses could exceed $1 billion per year due to lost revenues, export treatment costs, trade and crop damage (Faust, 2004).

A. *Bactrocera* species

Bactrocera is a tephritid fly genus of at least 440 species distributed primarily in tropical Asia, the south Pacific, and Australia (White and Elson-Harris, 1992). Relatively few species have existed in Africa, except for those recently introduced (e.g., *B. cucurbitae*, *B. zonata*, and *B. invadens* (*Drew, Tsutsura, and White*)) (White and Elson-Harris, 1992). At least 176 species of the male Dacinae (comprised of the two major genera *Bactrocera* Macquart and *Dacus* Fabricius) are attracted to C-L/RK, and 58 species to ME (Metcalf, 1990). Of the 54 Dacinae species that are agricultural pests, 26 respond to C-L/RK and 16 to ME (compiled from Clarke *et al.*, 2005; Drew, 1989; Drew *et al.*, 1978; White and Elson-Harris, 1992).

B. Discovery of ME and C-L/RK attraction to fruit flies

ME, the most powerful of the male lures and the first structure (Figure 23.1) that was identified, was discovered serendipitously by Howlett (1912) while working in Pusa, India. Howlett first discovered that citronella oil was attractive to fruit flies and subsequently determined that the most attractive component was ME (Howlett, 1915). Barthel *et al.* (1957) reported that anisyl acetone was attractive to male *B. cucurbitae*. However, Beroza *et al.* (1960)discovered that C-L (4-(*p*-acetoxyphenyl)-2-butanone) was a more effective lure for male *B. cucurbitae*. In 1959, RK was developed as an attractant for male *B. tryoni* in Australia and called Willison's lure (Drew, 1974). C-L has never been isolated as a natural product, but quickly

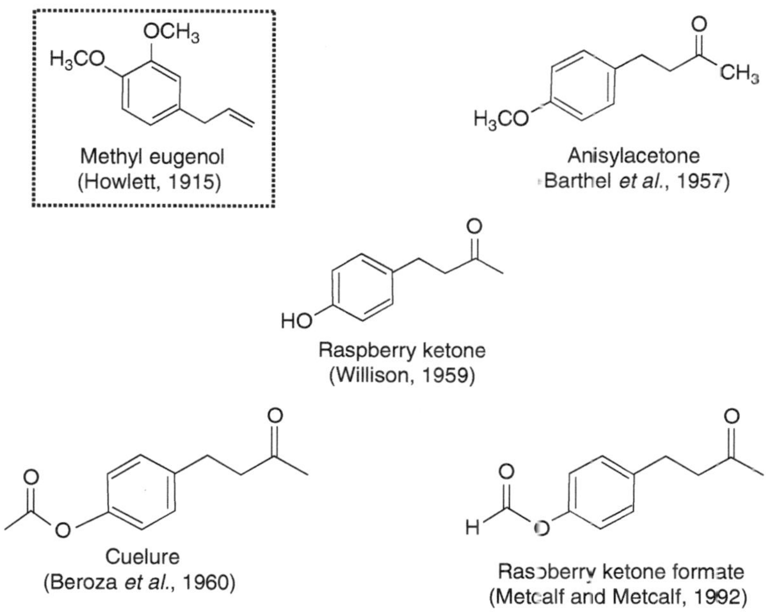

Figure 23.1 Chemical structure of methyl eugenol and cue-lure/raspberry ketone compounds, and date of attractiveness to fruit flies discovered.

hydrolyzes to form RK, a very effective lure for *B. cucurbitae*, more persistent but with a lower release rate, hence less efficient than C-L for long-range attraction. A closely related, more volatile compound, RK formate, was reported to be twice as attractive as C-L in 2-day laboratory tests (Metcalf and Metcalf, 1992) and was subsequently found to be 1.7 times more attractive to wild flies in the field in Hawaii, consistently outperforming C-L for periods exceeding 1 month (Casaña-Giner *et al.*, 2003; Jang *et al.*, 2007). Nonetheless, virtually all of the lures for *B. cucurbitae* and related species are based on lure hydrolysis leading back to RK (Metcalf and Metcalf, 1992), and of these, C-L (the acetate of RK) has been the most widely used over the past 50 years (Oliver *et al.*, 2002).

C. Implications of fruit fly attraction to ME and C-L/RK

No fruit fly species have been identified that respond to both ME and C-L, and response is associated with specific antennal receptor sites (Metcalf and Metcalf, 1992). Host plant odors acting as kairomones are particularly significant in the ecology of fruit flies, naturally attracting them to plants scattered throughout dense tropical forests (Metcalf and Metcalf, 1992). Some of these kairomone responses have taxonomic, evolutionary, zoogeographical, and behavioral implications. The two categories of dacine lure responses to ME and to C-L/RK are correlated with systematic classification based on morphological characteristics (Drew, 1974; Drew and Hooper, 1981). Specific kairomonal responses are associated with closely related complexes of morphologically similar species (Drew, 1989). There is evidence that the two groups of Dacinae distinguished by male lure responses to ME or C-L/RK represent divergent evolution from a common ancestral association with plants (Metcalf, 1990). Analyses of lure responses have even raised questions about the zoogeographic origin of the Dacinae. Munro (1984) believes dacine fruit flies to be native to Africa, whereas Drew (1989) believes them to be native to New Guinea.

IV. Relationship Between Male Behavior and ME and C-L/RK

Raghu (2004) provided an insightful review of the two main explanations regarding the biological function of male lures in dacine fruit flies, namely the ancestral host hypothesis, which posits that the lures originated as plant kairomones serving as rendezvous stimulants to promote mating, and the sexual selection hypothesis, which suggests that the lures serve as male pheromone precursors and play an important role in affecting female choice of mates. Ample evidence exists to support the latter explanation, including male-biased attraction to (Fitt, 1981a; Raghu and Clarke, 2003a; Steiner *et al.*, 1965) and feeding on (Khoo and Tan, 2005) the lures, post-feeding detection of ME metabolites in the hemolymph (Hee and Tan, 2004) and rectal gland (Nishida *et al.*, 1988, 1997), post-feeding detection of RK in the rectal gland (Nishida *et al.*, 1993; Tan and Nishida, 1995), detection of ME metabolites (Nishida and Fukami, 1990) in emitted volatiles, and female attraction to ME metabolites (Tan and Nishida, 1996). Tan and Nishida (2007) have described the pollination-sex pheromone precursor relationship between certain plants and fruit flies, respectively, as being a synomone interaction. Here, we briefly review behavioral aspects in the male *Bactrocera*–parapheromone association, focusing on feeding behavior, mate attraction, and mating success.

Despite the conclusion by Steiner, 1952 that newly emerged males feed on parapheromones, various studies clearly show that male response to ME (Wee and Tan, 2000) or C-L (Wong *et al.*, 1991) increases with age and does so most rapidly with the onset of sexual maturation. Attraction of immature males to lures is perplexing given the observation, for *B. dorsalis*, that ME feeding by such males confers no mating advantage when sexual maturity is later attained (Shelly *et al.*, 2008). ME feeding by immature *B. dorsalis* males may serve in predator deterrence (Tan and Nishida, 1998). Among mature males, responsiveness to lures varies among species. ME is generally recognized as a more powerful lure than C-L. For example, Shelly *et al.* (2010a) released marked males of *B. dorsalis* and *B. cucurbitae* 50 m from ME- and C-L-baited traps placed in the same trees in Anaheim, CA, and recaptured nearly 50% of the *B. dorsalis* males compared to only 5% of the *B. cucurbitae* males. Wee *et al.* (2002) also documented interspecific differences in male responsiveness and consumption among ME-sensitive species. Contrary to the observation that *B. dorsalis* males feed on ME until "they kill themselves with over indulgence" (Steiner, 1952), males offered ME freely did not feed continuously (Shelly, 1994) and did not suffer higher mortality than males deprived of ME (Shelly *et al.*, 2010b). Ingestion of ME likewise had no apparent effect on male mortality in *B. cacuminata* (Hering) (Raghu *et al.*, 2002).

The effect of lure feeding on subsequent responsiveness to the lure has serious implications for management of *Bactrocera* species. For example, MAT programs may be hindered if males visit natural lure sources and thus are less responsive to lure-baited traps. However, for *B. dorsalis* at least, it appears that feeding on ME-bearing flowers does not reduce subsequent capture probability, presumably because the traps contain much higher amounts of ME than available naturally (Shelly, 2000a). Regarding SIT, the prerelease exposure to lures may increase control efforts if such males are less likely to be captured in lure-baited traps, as found by Chambers *et al.* (1972), Fitt (1981b), and Shelly (1994), operating to monitor population levels or in a simultaneous program of MAT.

A link between lure-feeding and heightened mating success has been demonstrated for males of both ME- (Wee *et al.*, 2007) and C-L/RK- (Shelly, 2000b) responding species, though the effect appears more pronounced and long lasting for the former group. Males of *B. dorsalis* permitted to feed for 30 s on a cotton wick containing ME enjoyed a mating advantage over ME-deprived males as long as 35 days after feeding (Shelly and Dewire, 1994). In contrast, *B. cucurbitae* males that fed on RK had a short-term mating advantage, lasting only 1 day post-feeding (Shelly, 2000b). Mating enhancement has also been described when males feed on natural sources of ME (Shelly, 2000c), but comparable data are lacking for RK/C-L sensitive species. Larval feeding on ME-enriched diet had no effect on the mating success of the subsequently emerged adult males (Shelly and Nishida, 2004). Interestingly, adult males of *B. cacuminata* fed ME enjoyed no mating advantage (Raghu and Clarke, 2003b), revealing interspecific variation in the importance of ME in influencing the sexual behavior of ME-responding species.

In *B. dorsalis*, the enhanced mating success appears to result from increased signal production as well as increased signal attractiveness to females. In a laboratory study (Shelly and Dewire, 1994), ME-fed and ME-deprived males were placed individually in small mini-cages (placed within a larger cage), and wing-fanning activity and female visitation were monitored. Treated males were observed wing-fanning during approximately 50% of the trial compared to only 30% for control males. In addition, among individuals that signaled during at least 30% of the trial, 5–10 times as many females were sighted on the mini-cages of ME-fed males than on the mini-cages of ME-deprived males. Similar results were found in a field experiment in which groups (leks) of ME-fed or ME-deprived males were placed in host trees (one group per tree) in a circular array, and females released from the center were free to disperse in any direction (Shelly, 2001). While the above studies largely involved artificial sources of ME, feeding on ME-bearing flowers was also found to boost both the output and attractiveness of the male pheromone (Shelly, 2000c). Working with *B. cucurbitae* in a wind tunnel, Khoo and Tan (2000) similarly reported that females showed higher attraction to C-L–fed males than C-L–deprived males. To date, no studies have confirmed greater female attraction to males following male feeding at a natural RK source.

While growing evidence clearly indicates a role of ME and C-L/RK in pheromone synthesis and mate attraction, the adaptive basis of female preference for lure-fed males remains unknown. In *B. dorsalis*, mating with ME-fed males did not result in significant increase in egg hatch rate, total fecundity, or female longevity (Shelly, 2000d). It is possible that female preference for ME-fed males represents a case of runaway selection, whereby the presence of ME metabolites in the male signal may indicate a superior ability to locate natural sources of ME in the wild. As such, by selecting males whose pheromone contains ME metabolites, females may increase the odds that their sons will have high ability to locate ME sources and hence enjoy high mating success. Alternatively, pheromone containing ME metabolites may be more attractive because they more closely resemble other resources, such as food or oviposition substrate, critical to females. In this case, ME-bearing pheromone may represent a "sensory trap" and function by triggering a strong, preexisting sensory bias that evolved in a nonsexual context.

V. Technology Development and Transfer Through the Hawaii Area-Wide Pest Management Program

In Hawaii, fruit flies infest over 400 different host fruits and represent one of the greatest obstacles to expansion or development of diversified agriculture. Although scientists in Hawaii have developed various technologies (i.e., Sterile Insect Technique (SIT) and MAT) over the years to combat accidental fruit fly outbreaks on the U.S. mainland (e.g., California and Florida) and other parts of the world, the technologies were never made readily available to Hawaiian farmers. During the past decade (2000–2009) the HAWPM program effectively researched, developed, and registered novel fruit fly monitoring and control technologies. Previous fruit fly control measures in Hawaii relied heavily on the application of organophosphate insecticides to crops. The HAWPM program developed a comprehensive IPM package that was economically viable, environmentally acceptable, and sustainable. Components included (1) monitoring, (2) field sanitation, (3) protein bait sprays, (4) MAT, (5) augmentative parasitoid releases, and (6) sterile insect releases (Mau *et al.*, 2007; Vargas *et al.*, 2008a). The program resulted in area-wide suppression of fruit flies; a reduction in the use of organophosphate insecticides; and the rapid development, testing, and deployment of new technologies. An important activity of the program was creation of partnerships with industry and the development and transfer of novel technologies immediately to farmers for on-farm testing. Among the technologies developed were (1) reduced-risk bait sprays (i.e., GF-120 NF Naturalyte™ Fruit Fly Bait, Dow AgroSciences, Indianapolis, IN), (2) novel monitoring and detection methods, and (3) reduced-risk MAT. These technologies represent some of the most environmentally safe and technologically advanced fruit fly detection and control products developed to date. The use of spinosad-based GF-120 NF Naturalyte™ Fruit Fly Bait as a substitute for malathion protein bait spray has been reviewed elsewhere (Piñero *et al.*, 2009, Prokopy *et al.*, 2003). Here we briefly review the novel ME/C-L technologies researched, developed, and transferred to farmers through the HAWPM program in the areas of monitoring and MAT. After 25 years of effort, manufacturing use permits were finally obtained not only for ME and C-L/RK to be used for fruit fly survey applications but also for control programs. Table 23.1 chronologically lists Environmental Protection Agency (EPA) and Hawaii registration numbers and companies for ME/C-L products researched and developed through industry partnerships with the Hawaii AWPM program. Since *B. cucurbitae* and *B. dorsalis* are the major pests impacting Hawaiian agriculture, registration focused on products developed to control these species, but can effectively be used against other *Bactrocera* species.

A. Traps for detection of invasive fruit flies

Rapid expansion of world trade and human travel has increased introductions of fruit flies worldwide. For example, in 1996, *B. dorsalis* became established in Tahiti and has since spread throughout French Polynesia. Two species in the *B. dorsalis* complex were established on two new continents: *B. carambolae* Drew and Hancock, the carambola fruit fly, in South America (Suriname) and *B. invadens* in Africa (Kenya) (Drew *et al.*, 2005; Rousse *et al.*, 2005). Early detection of incipient outbreaks is one of the most crucial aspects of fruit fly eradication. Some of the common traps used for detection with ME and C-L are Steiner, Jackson, ChamP, and bucket traps (IAEA, 2003; Vargas *et al.*, 2003). The standard lure has been a mixture of ME or C-L and naled or malathion placed on a cotton wick.

Recently, in the interests of convenience and worker safety, there has been progress toward replacement of liquid ME and C-L and insecticides with solid formulations (e.g., Scentry ME cones or C-L plugs, Boseman, MT; Farma Tech (FT) ME wafers, North Bend, WA) (Hiramoto *et al.*, 2006; Mau *et al.*, 2007; Suckling *et al.*, 2008; Vargas *et al.*, 2008a) and with solid lure/insecticide (e.g., 2, 2-dichlorovinyl dimethyl phosphate, DDVP) combinations (Vargas *et al.*, 2010). In the most recent tests with solid lure/insecticide wafers, Vargas *et al.* (2010a) demonstrated that standard Jackson traps or AWPM bucket traps with FT-Mallet-ME wafers impregnated with DDVP and the HAWPM trap with Scentry ME cones and vapor tape, which contains DDVP, performed as well as the standard Jackson trap with liquid ME and naled against *B. dorsalis*. Similarly, Jackson traps or HAWPM traps with FT-Mallet-C-L wafers impregnated with DDVP or the HAWPM trap with Scentry C-L plugs with vapor tape performed as well as a standard Jackson trap with liquid C-L and naled against *B. cucurbitae*. The dispensers without an embedded insecticide have the advantage of being deployed without an insecticide if placed in a relatively escape-proof trap (Hiramoto *et al.*, 2006). Captures of *B. dorsalis* and *B. cucurbitae* with wafers containing both ME and RK (FT-Mallet MC) were equivalent to those containing separate lures. From a worker safety and convenience

Table 23.1 Registration of agricultural chemicals through the Hawaii area-wide pest management fruit fly program for use against tephritid fruit flies in Hawaii[a]

Date of registration	EPA registration no.	Hawaii licensing no.	Product	Source
August 1, 2002	8730-50	9628.6	Vaportape II™	Hercon Environmental Inc.
September 20, 2007	7969-253	9131.131	Amulet™ C-L w/fipronil stations	BASF Corp.
October 3, 2007	36638-42	9721.4	Cue-lure in plastic matrix w/o toxicant	Scentry Biologicals Inc.
December 11, 2007	36638-40	9721.3	Methyl eugenol in plastic matrix w/o toxicant	Scentry Biologicals Inc.
October 26, 2007	81325-3	8637.1	Methyl eugenol in plastic matrix	Farma Tech International Corp.
January 2008	62719-592	9786.282	Sprayable SPLAT-MAT with methyl eugenol and spinosad	Dow Agro Sciences LLC/ ISCA Technologies
January 2011	Final label approval projected by Farma Tech in 2011	NA	Mallet ME, C-L, MC wafers with DDVP	Farma Tech International Corp.

[a] This does not imply endorsement of specific commercial products.

standpoint, FT Mallet ME and C-L wafers with DDVP or Scentry plugs, with or without DVVP strips, are more convenient and safer to handle than standard liquid insecticide formulations (e.g., naled) used previously for monitoring and male annihilation programs in Hawaii and for detection traps used on the U.S. mainland. Furthermore, the FT Mallet MC wafer offers the potential of being used in a single trap in place of two separate traps for detection of ME- and C-L-responding fruit flies.

B. History of MAT

Suppression and even eradication of fruit flies has been achieved through area-wide application of ME or C-L (+ toxicant). MAT carriers commonly used throughout the Pacific include fiberboard blocks, cotton wicks, Min-U-Gel, and molded paper fiber (Vargas *et al.*, 2000, 2005). Fiberboard blocks impregnated with ME and various organophosphate insecticides (e.g., naled and malathion) were used to eradicate *B. dorsalis* from Rota (Steiner *et al.*, 1965), Saipan (Steiner *et al.*, 1970), Okinawa (Koyama *et al.*, 1984), and papaya fruit fly, *Bactrocera papayae* Drew and Hancock from Australia (Cantrell *et al.*, 2002). Min-U-Gel with naled has been used as a sprayable application to telephone poles and tree trunks in California and Florida, for the eradication of *B. dorsalis* (Chambers *et al.*, 1974; Cunningham and Suda, 1985). Results of MAT programs with C-L have not been as spectacular as with ME and often had to be used in combination with other techniques. Queensland fruit fly (*B. tryoni*) was eradicated from Rapa Nui (Easter Island) in the southern Pacific using a combined treatment of 2 g each of C-L and malathion on pieces of cotton string and spot spraying with protein–malathion bait spray (Bateman *et al.*, 1973). A *B. cucurbitae* population was reduced by 99% throughout 5.2 km^2 plot for over 7 months in Hawaii with C-L (+ naled) on fiberboard blocks (Cunningham and Steiner, 1972). *C. curcurbitae* was successfully suppressed for 5 months in Okinawa with cotton rope soaked in a solution of C-L and naled (Taniguchi *et al.*, 1988), and eradicated from Nauru Island using MAT and protein bait sprays (Allwood *et al.*, 2002).

C. More environmentally friendly MAT developments

Mixtures of liquid ME or C-L on cotton wicks inside bucket traps (Vargas *et al.*, 2000) have been used for suppression of *B. dorsalis* and *B. cucurbitae.* Enclosing wicks inside bucket traps not only provided protection from the weather (lasting up to 20 weeks) but also made the device visible, retrievable, and reusable with limited environmental contamination and exposure to humans and pets. Vargas *et al.* (2003) found that spinosad, although not as persistent as naled or malathion, is safer to handle and a more environmentally friendly substitute for organophosphate insecticides in ME and C-L traps for use in male annihilation for *B. dorsalis* and *B. cucurbitae* in the HAWPM program. Newly developed solid lure and insecticide formulations replaced liquid formulations. In the Hawaii program, a solid formulation with DDVP (Hercon® Vaportape™ II (DDVP), Emigsville, PA) strips in place of liquid naled was an improvement from a worker safety viewpoint. An HAWPM program that included MAT with C-L in bucket traps reduced a *B. cucurbitae* population to near zero for 1 year throughout a 40 km^2 area (Jang *et al.*, 2008, Vargas *et al.*, 2008a). Amulet C-L (BASF, Australia) molded paper fiber stations (Vargas *et al.*, 2005) with C-L and fipronil have been registered for control of *B. tryoni* in Australia and *B. cucurbitae* in Hawaii. However, placement of many traps or paper stations in the field can be time consuming and is not always ideal for eradication programs. Recent research, development, and registration has focused on SPLAT-MAT-Spinosad-ME (Dow AgroSciences, Indianapolis, IN and ISCA Technologies, Riverside, CA) (Vargas *et al.*, 2008b, 2009) as a replacement for Min-U-Gel ME with naled. SPLAT (Specialized Pheromone and Lure Application Technology) has a waxy outer coating that acts as a reservoir with time release properties, which allows the lure to last longer when applied to surfaces than Min-U-Gel. SPLAT, like Min-U-Gel, can be sprayed from small sprayers, trucks, and aircraft making the technology convenient and flexible. Current work is focusing on research and development of a SPLAT-spinosad-C-L/RK product for use against C-L/RK responding species such as *B. cucurbitae* and *B. tryoni* (Vargas *et al.*, 2010b).

VI. Environmental Impact of ME and C-L/RK

The use of male lures for fruit fly control may impact nontarget insects or risk possible extinction of small endemic populations in large-scale fruit fly eradication programs (Asquith and Messing, 1993). To address these risks, research in Hawaii has focused on determining the diversity of nontarget invertebrates attracted to male lures (Asquith and Burny, 1998; Asquith and Kido, 1994; Conant, 1978; Kido and Asquith, 1995; Kido *et al.*, 1996, Loope and Medeiros, 1992; Uchida *et al.*, 2003, 2006, 2007). Results from these studies indicate that 36 insect species, in 16 families of Diptera, Coleoptera, Hemiptera, and Hymenoptera, were captured in significantly larger numbers in traps baited with ME than unbaited control traps. These included 11 species of endemic Hawaiian Drosophilidae, a very diverse group with 559 described species (O'Grady *et al.*, 2010), of which 12 are listed as endangered by US Fish and Wildlife (2007). However, at least 26 of the 36 species, including drosophilids, are scavengers and may have been attracted to the accumulation of decaying flies, rather than the lure itself, because the traps could not exclude the entry of *B. dorsalis*. Nonetheless, honeybees were clearly attracted to ME (Asquith and Burny, 1998).

More recently in Hawaii, captures of male lure traps were compared to captures of unbaited controls and traps artificially baited with decaying *B. dorsalis* in a diversity of environments ranging from endemic forest to agricultural land (Leblanc *et al.*, 2009). Over 56 species, in 21 families of saprophagous flies, including numerous drosophilids, saprophagous beetles (Nitidulidae), predatory beetles (Staphylinidae), and hymenopterous parasitoids of house flies, were attracted to the decaying flies, but not to male lures. These results suggested that the majority of previously published records, including those of endemic Drosophilidae, were actually for attraction to dead flies.

Whereas C-L never attracted any insect other than the target melon flies, at least 17 species of nontarget insects, in 8 families and 6 orders, were confirmed to be attracted to ME. A wide diversity of the species belong to unrelated groups associated with flowers, including honeybees (*Apis mellifera* L.) (Asquith and Burny, 1998; Leblanc *et al.*, 2009), the flower fly *Allograpta obliqua* (Say) (Syrphidae) (Leblanc *et al.*, 2009), three species of green lacewings (Chrysopidae) whose adults feed on flower pollen and nectar (Pai *et al.*, 2004; Suda and Cunningham, 1970; Umeya and Hirao, 1975), two endemic Hawaiian moths (Crambidae) commonly observed on flowers in farmlands on Maui (Leblanc *et al.*, 2009), and the nitidulid beetle *Carpophilus marginellus* Motsch., attracted to both ME and decaying fruit flies (Leblanc *et al.*, 2009). Similarly, euglossine bees were reported to be attracted to ME in South America (Vayssières *et al.*, 2007; Williams and Whitten, 1983). Asquith and Burny (1998) hypothesized that the response is due to the natural presence of ME in flower blossoms of a number of plants.

Other ME-attracted plant-feeding insects, not associated with flowers, include three endemic Hawaiian species of beetles (Anobiidae) (Asquith and Kido, 1994) that feed on dry wood and four species of endemic plant bugs (Miridae) in the genera *Orthotylus* and *Sarona* (Miridae) (Asquith and Kido, 1994; Leblanc *et al.*, 2009). At least one species of *Orthotylus* feeds on a host plant known to contain ME (Scheuer and Hudgins, 1964). Females of an endemic Sciaridae (*Bradysia setigera* (Hardy)) are attracted to ME, when traps are set in endemic forest habitats (Leblanc *et al.*, 2009). The attraction is highly specific because conspecific males and other sciarids are not attracted.

The negative nontarget impact of male lures, at least in agricultural environments, is likely to be minimal. The capture of flower insects in modest numbers in ME traps (Asquith and Burny, 1998; Leblanc *et al.*, 2009) suggests that attraction is likely short ranged and is further minimized if one avoids applying ME to trees during the flowering stage (Leblanc *et al.*, 2009). Because attraction of endemic Diptera to decaying fruit flies can be important in native habitats (Leblanc *et al.*, 2009), traps should not be used within a minimum safe distance of 300 m from native forest to minimize such undesirable attraction (Leblanc *et al.*, 2009). The use of mineral oil to kill and retain fruit flies and slow their decomposition is recommended by Uchida *et al.* (2007) if traps must be maintained in endemic forest.

VII. CONCLUSIONS AND FUTURE APPLICATIONS

Phenyl propanoids are attractive to numerous species of Dacinae fruit flies (Diptera: Tephritidae), including species members of the genera *Bactrocera* and *Dacus*. Both ME and C-L/RK are very powerful male-specific lures, and these lures are used in current control programs of pestiferous fruit flies for detection and monitoring of populations as well as for MAT through mass trapping. The HAWPM program provided the basis for elimination of liquid lures and highly toxic organophosphate insecticides. These IPM technologies (i.e., reduced-risk monitoring dispensers, protein bait sprays, and MAT dispensers) represent some of the most environmentally safe and advanced fruit fly detection and control products developed to date, and have important applications for area-wide suppression of fruit flies not only in Hawaii but also throughout south and western Pacific Island Nations, Australia, and tropical Asia where *Bactrocera* spp. are serious economic pests. Furthermore, development of environmentally friendly area-wide tools has important applications for detection and eradication of accidental introductions of fruit flies into the U.S. mainland and the rest of the world. For example, over 30,000 detection traps with liquid ME or C-L and the highly toxic organophosphate naled mixtures are deployed in California and Florida for rapid detection of accidental introductions of fruit flies.

Dacine flies have been spreading throughout the world at an alarming rate over the past 10 years. (i.e., *B. dorsalis* throughout French Polynesia, *B. carambolae* throughout areas of South America, *B. invadens* and melon fly in Africa, and *B. zonata* in Africa and the Mediterranean region). Future work needs to address more widespread testing of the types of the novel detection and control products outlined in this chapter in different environments. Of high priority would be the total elimination of organophosphate (i.e., DDVP) in detection traps with substitution of reduced-risk insecticides or development of traps not requiring insecticides. Finally, effectiveness of the novel SPLAT MAT products needs to be tested more in large area-wide tests.

ACKNOWLEDGMENTS

We thank Steven Souder (Agricultural Research Center, USDA-ARS, Hilo, HI) for assistance in summarizing the different types of data included in this chapter. IR-4 (Michael Braverman, IR-4) and CDFA funds provided by Bob Dowell (CDFA, Sacramento, CA) and Kevin Hoffman (CDFA, Sacramento, CA) were essential in conducting research and completing this work. The HAWPM program, a partnership among USDA, the University of Hawaii (Ron Mau, UH, Honolulu, HI), and the Hawaii Department of Agriculture (Lyle Wong, HDOA, Honolulu, HI), provided the research and development platform for rapid technology transfer to farmers who validated the technologies. Opinions, findings, conclusions, or recommendations expressed in this publication are those of the authors and do not necessarily reflect the views of the USDA. Finally, we thank Rui Pereira (IAEA, Vienna, Austria), Nikos Papadopoulos (University of Thessaly, Greece), and Victoria Yokoyama (USDA-ARS, Parlier, CA) for comments on an earlier draft of this chapter.

REFERENCES

Allwood, A. J., Vueti, E. T., Leblanc, L., and Bull, R. (2002). Eradication of introduced *Bactrocera* species (Diptera: Tephritidae) in Nauru using male annihilation and protein bait application techniques. *In* "Turning the Tide: The Eradication of Invasive Species. Proceedings of the International Conference on Eradication of Island Invasives," (C. R. Veitch and M. N. Clout, Eds.), pp. 19–25. IUCN Publications Services Unit, Cambridge, UK.

Asquith, A., and Burny, D. (1998). Honeybees attracted to the semiochemical methyl eugenol, used for male annihilation of the Oriental fruit fly (Diptera: Tephritidae). *Proc. Hawaii. Entomol. Soc.* **33,** 57–66.

Asquith, A., and Kido, M. (1994). Native Hawaiian insects attracted to the semiochemical methyl eugenol, used for male annihilation of the Oriental fruit fly (Diptera: Tephritidae). *Environ. Entomol.* **23,** 1397–1408.

Asquith, A., and Messing, R. H. (1993). Contemporary Hawaiian insect fauna of a lowland agricultural area on Kaua'i: Implications for local and island-wide fruit fly eradication programs. *Pac. Sci.* **47,** 1–16.

Barthel, W. F., Green, N., Keiser, I., and Steiner, L. F. (1957). Anisyl acetone, synthetic attractant for male melon fly. *Science* **126,** 654.

Bateman, M. A., Insungza, V., and Arreta, P. (1973). The eradication of Queensland fruit fly from Easter Island. *FAO Plant Prot. Bull.* **21,** 114.

Beroza, M., Alexander, B. H., Steiner, L. F., Mitchell, W. C., and Miyashita, D. H. (1960). New synthetic lures for the male melon fly. *Science* **131,** 1044–1045.

Butenandt, A., Beckmann, R., Stamm, D., and Hecker, E. (1959). Uber den Sexual-Lockstoff des Seidenspinners Bombyx mori. Reindarstellung und Konstitution. *Zeitschrift fur Naturforschung B Chemie Biochemie Biophysik Biologie und Verwandten Gebiete* **14,** 283.

Cantrell, B. K., Chadwick, B., and Cahill, A. (2002). Fruit fly fighters: Eradication of papaya fruit fly. Commonwealth Scientific and Industrial Research Organization Publishing, Collingwood, VIC, Australia.

Carey, J. R., and Dowell, R. V. (1989). Exotic fruit fly pests and California agriculture. *Calif. Agric.* **43**(3), 38–40.

Casaña-Giner, V., Oliver, J. E., Jang, E. B., Carvalho, L., Khrimian, A., DeMilo, A. B., and McQuate, G. T. (2003). Raspberry ketone formate as an attractant for melon fly (Diptera: Tephritidae). *J. Entomol. Sci.* **38,** 120–126.

CDFA. California Department of Food and Agriculture. http://www.cdfa.ca.gov.

Chambers, D. L., Ohinata, K., Fujimoto, M., and Kashiwai, S. (1974). Treating tephritids with attractants to enhance their effectiveness in sterile-release programs. *J. Econ. Entomol.* **65,** 279–282.

Clarke, A. R., Armstrong, K. F., Carmichael, A. E., Milne, J. R., Raghu, S., Roderick, G. K., and Yeates, D. K. (2005). Invasive phytophagous pests arising through a recent tropical evolutionary radiation: The *Bactrocera dorsalis* complex of fruit flies. *Annu. Rev. Entomol.* **50,** 293–319.

Conant, P. (1978). A test of the attraction of non-target flying insects to a poison fruit fly lure composed of methyl eugenol and malathion. Technical report for USDA-ARS.

Cunningham, R. T. (1989). Parapheromones. *In* "World Crop Pests, Volume 3A, Fruit Flies, Their Biology, Natural Enemies and Control," (A. S. Robinson and G. Hooper, Eds.), pp. 221–230. Elsevier Science Publishers, Amsterdam.

Cunningham, R. T., and Steiner, L. F. (1972). Field trial of cue-lure + naled on saturated fiberboard blocks for control of the melon fly by the male-annihilation technique. *J. Econ. Entomol.* **65,** 505–507.

Cunningham, R. T., and Suda, D. Y. (1985). Male annihilation of the oriental fruit fly, *Dacus dorsalis* Hendel (Diptera: Tephritidae): A new thickener and extender for methyl eugenol formulations. *J. Econ. Entomol.* **75,** 503–504.

De Vincenzi, M., Silano, M., Stacchini, P., and Scazzocchio, B. (2000). Constituents of aromatic plants: I. Methyl Eugenol. *Fitoterapia* **71,** 216–221.

Drew, R. A. I. (1974). The responses of fruit fly species (Diptera: Tephritidae) in the South Pacific area to male attractants. *J. Aust. Entomol. Soc.* **13,** 267–270.

Drew, R. A. I. (1989). The tropical fruit flies (Diptera: Tephritidae: Dacinae) of the Australasian and Oceanean region. *Mem. Queensl. Mus.* **26,** 521.

Drew, R. A. I., and Hooper, G. H. S. (1981). The response of fruit fly species (Diptera: Tephritidae) to various attactants. *J. Aust. Entomol. Soc.* **20,** 201–208.

Drew, R. A. I., Hooper, G. H. S., and Bateman, M. A. (1978). Economic Fruit Flies of the South Pacific region Misc. Publ. Queensland Dept of Primary Industries, Brisbane. 139pp.

Drew, R. A. I., Tsuruta, K., and White, I. M. (2005). A new species of pest fruit fly (Diptera: Tephritidae:Dacinae) from Sri Lanka and Africa. *Afr. Entomol.* **13,** 149–154.

EPA. Environmental Protection Agency. http://www.epa.gov.

Faust, R. M. (2004). Local research, but everyone's watching. (Forum, Hawaii Area Wide Fruit Fly Control Program, Pacific Basin Agricultural Research Center). *Agric. Res.* **52**(2), 2.

Fitt, G. P. (1981a). Responses by female Dacinae to "male" lures and their relationship to patterns of mating behaviour and pheromone response. *Entomol. Exp. Appl.* **29,** 87–97.

Fitt, G. P. (1981b). The influence of age, nutrition and time of day on the responsiveness of male *Dacus opiliae* to the synthetic lure, methyl eugenol. *Entomol. Exp. Appl.* **30,** 83–90.

Fletcher, B. S. (1987). The biology of dacine fruit flies. *Annu. Rev. Entomol.* **32,** 115–144.

Friedrich, H. (1976). Phenylpropanoid constituents of essential oils. *Lloydia* **39,** 1–7.

Gordh, G., and Headrick, D. H. (2001). A Dictionary of Entomology. CABI Publishing, New York. 1032pp.

Hee, A. K. W., and Tan, K. H. (2004). Male sex pheromonal components derived from methyl eugenol in the hemolymph of the fruit fly *Bactrocera papayae*. *J. Chem. Ecol.* **30,** 2127–2138.

Hiramoto, M. K., Arita-Tsutsumi, L., and Jang, E. B. (2006). Test of effectiveness of newly formulated plastic matrix with methyl eugenol for monitoring *Bactrocera dorsalis* (Hendel) populations. *Proc. Hawaii Entomol. Soc.* **38,** 103–110.

Howlett, F. M. (1912). The effect of oil of citronella on two species of *Dacus*. *Entomol. Soc. London Trans.* **60,** 412–418.

Howlett, F. M. (1915). Chemical reactions of fruit flies. *Bull. Entomol. Res.* **6,** 297–305.

IAEA, (2003). Trapping guidelines for area-wide fruit fly programmes. International Atomic Energy Agency, Vienna.47pp.

Jang, E. B., Casaña-Giner, V., and Oliver, J. E. (2007). Field captures of wild melon fly (Diptera:Tephritidae) with an improved male attractant, raspberry ketone formate. *J. Econ. Entomol.* **100,** 1124–1128.

Jang, E. B., McQuate, G. T., McInnis, D. O., Harris, E. J., Vargas, R. I., Bautista, R. C., and Mau, R. F. L. (2008). Targeted trapping, bait-spray, sanitation, sterile-male, and parasitoid releases in an area wide integrated melon fly (Diptera:Tephritidae) control program in Hawaii. *Am. Entomol.* **54,** 240–250.

Karlson, P., and Butenandt, A. (1959). Pheromones (ectohormones) in insects. *Annu. Rev. Entomol.* **4,** 49–58.

Khoo, C. C. H., and Tan, K. H. (2000). Attraction of both sexes of melon fly, *Bactrocera cucurbitae*, to conspecific males—A comparison after pharmacophagy of cue-lure and a new attractant—Zingerone. *Entomol. Exp. Appl.* **97,** 317–320.

Khoo, C. C. H., and Tan, K. H. (2005). Rectal gland of *Bactrocera papayae*: Ultrastructure, anatomy, and sequestration of autofluorescent compounds upon methyl eugenol consumption by the male fruit fly. *Microsc. Res. Tech.* **67,** 219–226.

Kido, M. H., and Asquith, A. (1995). Attraction of Hawaiian aquatic insects to pest tephritid parakairomone lures. *Environ. Entomol.* **24,** 810–816.

Kido, M. H., Asquith, A., and Vargas, R. I. (1996). Nontarget insect attraction to methyl eugenol traps used in male annihilation of the Oriental fruit fly (Diptera: Tephritidae) in riparian Hawaiian stream habitat. *Environ. Entomol.* **25,** 1279–1289.

Koyama, J., Teruya, T., and Tanaka, K. (1984). Eradication of the oriental fruit fly (Diptera: Tephritidae) from the Okinawa Islands by a male annihilation method. *J. Econ. Entomol.* **77,** 468–472.

Leblanc, L., Rubinoff, D., and Vargas, R. I. (2009). Attraction of nontarget species to fruit fly (Diptera: Tephritidae) male lures and decaying fruit flies in traps in Hawaii. *Environ. Entomol.* **38,** 1446–1461.

Lin, Y.-L., and Chen, C.-J. (1984). Studies on the constituents of aerial parts of *Scutellaria rivularis* Wall. *Chem. Abs.* **102,** 92951m.

Loope, L. L., and Medeiros, A. C. (1992). Potential effects of alien fruit fly eradication on natural areas of Hawaii: An exploratory investigation in Haleakala National Park. *Elepaio* **52,** 71–75.

Mau, R. F. L., Jang, E. B., and Vargas, R. I. (2007). The Hawaii fruit fly area-wide fruit fly pest management programme: Influence of partnership and a good education programme. *In* "Area-Wide Control of Insect Pests: From Research to Field Implementation," (M. J. B. Vreysen, A. S. Robinson, and J. Hendrichs, Eds.), pp. 671–683. Springer, Dordrect, The Netherlands.

Metcalf, R. L. (1990). Chemical ecology of Dacinae fruit flies (Diptera: Tephritidae). *Ann. Entomol. Soc. Am.* **83,** 1017–1030.

Metcalf, R. L., and Metcalf, E. R. (1992). Fruit flies of the family Tephritidae. 139-142. *In* "Plant Kairomones in Insect Ecology and Control," (R. L. Metcalf, E. R. Metcalf, R. L. Metcalf, and E. R. Metcalf, Eds.), pp. 109–152. Routledge, Chapman & Hall Inc, New York.

Munro, H. K. (1984). A taxonomic treatise on the Dacinae (Diptera: Tephritidae) of Africa. *Entomol. Mem. S. Afr. Dep. Agric. Dev.* **61,** 313.

Nishida, R., and Fukami, H. (1990). Sequestration of distasteful compounds by some pharmacophagous insects. *J. Chem. Ecol.* **16,** 151–164.

Nishida, R., Tan, K. H., Serit, M., Lajis, N. H., Sukari, A. M., Takahashi, S., and Fukami, H. (1988). Accumulation of phenylpropanoids in the rectal glands of males of the oriental fruit fly, *Dacus dorsalis*. *Experientia* **44,** 534–536.

Nishida, R., Iwahashi, O., and Tan, K. H. (1993). Accumulation of *Dendrobium superbum* (Orchidaceae) fragrance in the rectal glands by males of the melon fly, *Dacus cucurbitae*. *J. Chem. Ecol.* **19,** 713–722.

Nishida, R., Shelly, T. E., and Kaneshiro, K. Y. (1997). Acquisition of female-attracting fragrance by males of oriental fruit fly from a Hawaiian lei flower, *Fagraea berteriana*. *J. Chem. Ecol.* **23,** 2275–2285.

O'Grady, P. M., Magnacca, K. N., and Lapoint, R. T. (2010). Taxonomic relationships within the endemic Hawaiian Drosophilidae. *Bishop Mus. Occas. Pap.* **108,** 1–34.

Oliver, J. E., Casaña-Giner, V., Jang, E. B., McQuate, G. T., and Carvalho, L. (2002). Improved attractants for the melon fly, *B. cucurbitae*. *In* "Proceedings of 6th International Fruit Fly Symposium," (B. N. Barnes, Ed.), pp. 283–290. Stellenbosch, South Africa.
Pai, K. F., Chen, C. J., Yang, J. T., and Chen, C. C. (2004). Green lacewing *Ankylopteryx exquisite* attracted to methyl eugenol. *Plant Protect. Bull.* **46,** 93–97.
Piñero, J. C., Mau, R. F. L., and Vargas, R. I. (2009). Managing oriental fruit fly, *Bactrocera dorsalis* (Diptera: Tephritidae), using spinosad-based protein bait sprays in papaya orchards in Hawaii. *J. Econ. Entomol.* **102,** 1123–1132.
Prokopy, R. J., Miller, N. W., Piñero, J. C., Barry, J. D., Tran, L. C., Oride, L. K., and Vargas, R. I. (2003). Effectiveness of GF-120 fruit fly bait spray applied to border area plants for control of melon flies (Diptera: Tephritidae). *J. Econ. Entomol.* **96,** 1485–1493.
Raghu, S. (2004). Functional significance of phytochemical lures to dacine fruit flies (Diptera: Tephritidae): An ecological and evolutionary synthesis. *Bull. Entomol. Res.* **94,** 385–399.
Raghu, S., and Clarke, A. R. (2003a). Spatial and temporal partitioning of behaviour by adult dacines: Direct evidence for methyl eugenol as a mate rendezvous cue for *Bactrocera cacuminata*. *Physiol. Entomol.* **28,** 175–184.
Raghu, S., and Clarke, A. R. (2003b). Sexual selection in a tropical fruit fly: Role of a plant derived chemical in mate choice. *Entomol. Exp. Appl.* **108,** 53–58.
Raghu, S., Clarke, A. R., and Yuval, B. (2002). Investigation of the physiological consequences of feeding on methyl eugenol by *Bactrocera cacuminata* (Diptera: Tephritidae). *Environ. Entomol.* **31,** 941–946.
Renou, M., and Guerrero, A. (2000). Insect parapheromones in olfaction research and semiochemical-based pest control strategies. *Annu. Rev. Entomol.* **45,** 605–630.
Rousse, P., Harris, E. J., and Quilici, S. (2005). *Fopius arisanus*, an egg-pupal parasitoid of Tephritidae. Overview. *Biocontrol News Inf.* **26**(2), 59N–69N.
Scheuer, P. J., and Hudgins, W. R. (1964). Major constituents of the essential oil of *Pelea christophersenii* St. John & Hume. *Perfum. Ess. Oil Rec.* **55,** 723–724.
Schinz, H., and Seidel, C. F. (1961). Nachtrag zu der Arbeit Nr. 194 im. *Helv Chim Acta* **40,** 1829, (1937, *Helv. Chim. Acta* 44, 278).
Shelly, T. E. (1994). Consumption of methyl eugenol by male *Bactrocera dorsalis* (Diptera: Tephritidae): Low incidence of repeat feeding. *Fla. Entomol.* **77,** 201–208.
Shelly, T. E. (2000a). Trapping male oriental fruit flies (Diptera: Tephritidae): Does feeding on a natural source of methyl eugenol reduce capture probability? *Fla. Fla. Entomol.* **83,** 109–111.
Shelly, T. E. (2000b). Effects of raspberry ketone on the mating success of male melon flies (Diptera: Tephritidae). *Proc. Hawaii Entomol. Soc.* **34,** 163–167.
Shelly, T. E. (2000c). Flower-feeding affects mating performance in male oriental fruit flies *Bactrocera dorsalis*. *Ecol. Entomol.* **25,** 109–114.
Shelly, T. E. (2000d). Fecundity of female oriental fruit flies (Diptera: Tephritidae): Effects of methyl eugenol-fed and multiple mates. *Ann. Entomol. Soc. Am.* **93,** 559–564.
Shelly, T. E. (2001). Feeding on methyl eugenol and *Fagraea berteriana* flowers increases long-range female attraction by males of the oriental fruit fly (Diptera: Tephritidae). *Fla. Entomol.* **84,** 634–640.
Shelly, T. E., and Dewire, A. L. M. (1994). Chemically mediated mating success in male oriental fruit flies (Diptera: Tephritidae). *Ann. Entomol. Soc. Am.* **87,** 375–382.
Shelly, T. E., and Nishida, R. (2004). Larval and adult feeding on methyl eugenol and the mating success of male oriental fruit flies, *Bactrocera dorsalis*. *Entomol. Exp. Appl.* **112,** 155–158.
Shelly, T. E., Edu, J., Pahio, E., Wee, S. L., and Nishida, R. (2008). Re-examining the relationship between sexual maturation and age of response to methyl eugenol in males of the oriental fruit fly. *Entomol. Exp. Appl.* **128,** 380–388.

Shelly, T.E., Nishimoto, J., Diaz, A., Leathers, J., War, M., Shoemaker, R., Al-Zubaidy, M., Joseph, D. (2010a). Capture probability of released males of two *Bactrocera* species (Diptera: Tephritidae) in detection traps in California. *J. Econ. Entomol.* (in review).

Shelly, T. E., Edu, J., and McInnis, D. O. (2010b). Pre-release consumption of methyl eugenol increases the mating competitiveness of sterile males of the oriental fruit fly, *Bactrocera dorsalis*, in large field enclosures. *J. Insect Sci.* (insectscience.org/10.8).

Steiner, L. F. (1952). Methyl eugenol as an attractant for oriental fruit fly. *J. Econ. Entomol.* **45,** 241–248.

Steiner, L. F., Mitchell, W. C., Harris, E. J., Kozuma, T. T., and Fujimoto, M. S. (1965). Oriental fruit fly eradication by male annihilation. *J. Econ. Entomol.* **58,** 961–964.

Steiner, L. F., Hart, W. G., Harris, E. J., Cunningham, R. T., Ohinata, K., and Kamakahi, D. C. (1970). Eradication of the oriental fruit fly from the Mariana Islands by the methods of male annihilation and sterile insect release. *J. Econ. Entomol.* **63,** 131–1351.

Suckling, D. M., Jang, E. B., Holder, P., Carvalho, L., and Stephens, A. E. A. (2008). Evaluation of lure dispensers for fruit fly surveillance in New Zealand. *Pest. Manag. Sci.* **64,** 848–856.

Suda, D. Y., and Cunningham, R. T. (1970). *Chrysopa basalis* captured in plastic traps containing methyl eugenol. *J. Econ. Entomol.* **63,** 1706.

Tan, K. H., and Nishida, R. (1995). Incorporation of raspberry ketone in the rectal glands of males of the Queensland fruit fly, *Bactrocera tryoni* Froggatt (Diptera: Tephritidae). *Appl. Entomol. Zool.* **30,** 494–497.

Tan, K. H., and Nishida, R. (1996). Sex pheromone and mating competition after methyl eugenol consumption in the *Bactrocera dorsalis* complex. *In* "Fruit Fly Pests," (B. A. McPheron and G. J. Steck, Eds.), pp. 147–153. St. Lucie Press, Delray Beach, FL.

Tan, K. H., and Nishida, R. (1998). Ecological significance of male attractant in the defence and mating strategies of the fruit fly, *Bactrocera papayae*. *Entomol. Exp. Appl.* **89,** 155–158.

Tan, K. H., and Nishida, R. (2007). Zingerone in the floral synomone of *Bulbophyllum baileyi* (Orchidaceae) attracts Bactrocera fruit flies during pollination. *Biochem. Syst.Ecol.* **35,** 334–341.

Taniguchi, M., Nakamori, H., Kakinohana, H., Yogi, Y., and Zukeyama, H. (1988). Suppression of male melon fly *Dacus cucurbitae* Coquillett (Diptera; Tephritidae) populations using cotton ropes infiltrated with a lure-toxicant. *Appl. Entomol. Zool.* **32,** 126–128.

Uchida, G. K., McInnis, D. O., Vargas, R. I., Kumashiro, B. R., Klungness, L. M., and Jang, E. (2003). Nontarget arthropods captured in cue-lure-baited bucket traps at area-wide pest management implementation sites at Kamuela and Kula, Hawaiian Islands. *Proc. Hawaii Entomol. Soc.* **36,** 135–143.

Uchida, G. K., Mackey, B. E., Vargas, R. I., Beardsley, J. W., Hardy, D. E., Goff, M. L., and Stark, J. D. (2006). Response of nontarget insects to methyl eugenol, cue-lure, trimedlure, and protein bait bucket traps on Kauai island, Hawaii, USA. *Proc. Hawaii Entomol. Soc.* **38,** 61–72.

Uchida, G. K., Mackey, B. E., McInnis, D. O., and Vargas, R. I. (2007). Attraction of *Bactrocera dorsalis* (Diptera: Tephritidae) and nontarget insects to methyl eugenol bucket traps with different preservative fluids on Oahu island, Hawaiian Islands. *J. Econ. Entomol.* **100,** 723–729.

Umeya, K., and Hirao, J. (1975). Attraction of the jackfruit fly, *Dacus umbrosus* F. (Diptera: Tephritidae) and lacewing, *Chrysopa* sp. (Neuroptera: Chrysopidae) by lure traps baited with methyl eugenol and cue-lure in the Philippines. *Appl. Entomol. Zool.* **10,** 60–62.

US Fish and Wildlife Service, (2007). Endangered and threatened wildlife and plants: Revised proposed designation of critical habitats for 12 species of picture-wing flies from the Hawaiian Islands: Proposed rule. *Fed. Regis.* **72,** 67427–67522.

Vargas, R. I., Stark, J. D., Kido, M. H., Ketter, H. M., and Whitehand, L. C. (2000). Methyl eugenol and cue-lure traps for suppression of male oriental fruit flies and melon flies (Diptera: Tephritidae) in Hawaii: Effects of lure mixtures and weathering. *J. Econ. Entomol.* **93,** 81–87.

Vargas, R. I., Miller, N. W., and Stark, J. D. (2003). Field trials of spinosad as a replacement for naled ddvp, and malathion in methyl eugenol and cue-lure bucket traps to attract and kill male oriental fruit flies and melon flies (Diptera: Tephritidae) in Hawaii. *J. Econ. Entomol.* **96,** 1780–1785.

Vargas, R. I., Stark, J. D., Mackey, B., and Bull, R. (2005). Weathering trials of Amulet Cue-lure and methyl eugenol "attract and kill" stations with male melon flies and oriental fruit flies (Diptera: Tephritidae) in Hawaii. *J. Econ. Entomol.* **98,** 1551–1559.

Vargas, R. I., Mau, R. F. L., Jang, E. B., Faust, R. M., and Wong, L. (2008a). The Hawaii fruit fly area-wide pest management program. *In* "Area wide Pest Management: Theory to Implementation," (O. Koul, G. W. Cuperus, and N. C. Elliott, Eds.), pp. 300–325. CABI Books, London.

Vargas, R. I., Stark, J. D., Hertlein, M., Mafra Neto, A., Coler, R., and Piñero, J. C. (2008b). Evaluation of SPLAT with spinosad and methyl eugenol or cue-lure for "attract-and-kill" of oriental and melon fruit flies (Diptera: Tephritidae) in Hawaii. *J. Econ. Entomol.* **101,** 750–768.

Vargas, R. I., Piñero, J. C., Mau, R. F. L., Stark, J. D., Hertlein, M., Mafra-Neto, A., Coler, R., and Getchell, A. (2009). Attraction and mortality of oriental fruit flies (Diptera: Tephritidae) to SPLAT-MAT-methyl eugenol with spinosad. *Entomol. Exp. Appl.* **131,** 286–293.

Vargas, R. I., Mau, R. F. L., Stark, J. D., and Piñero, J. C. (2010a). Evaluation of methyl eugenol and cue-lure traps with solid lure and insecticide dispensers for monitoring and male annihilation in Hawaii. *J. Econ. Entomol.* **103,** 409–415.

Vargas, R. I., Piñero, J. C., Jang, E. B., Mau, R. F. L., Stark, J. D., Gomez, L., and Stoltman, Mafra-Neto (2010b). Response of melon fly (Diptera: Tephritidae) to weathered SPLAT-spinosad-C-L. *J. Econ. Entomol.* (in press).

Vayssières, J. F., Cayol, J. P., and Perrier, X. (2007). Impact of methyl eugenol and malathion bait stations on non-target insect populations in French Guiana during an eradication program for *Bactrocera carambolae*. *Entomol. Exp. Appl.* **125,** 55–62.

Wee, S. L., and Tan, K. H. (2000). Sexual maturity and intraspecific mating success of two sibling species of the *Bactrocera dorsalis* complex. *Entomol. Exp. Appl.* **94,** 133–139.

Wee, S. L., Hee, A. K. W., and Tan, K. H. (2002). Comparative sensitivity to and consumption of methyl eugenol in three *Bactrocera dorsalis* (Diptera: Tephritidae) complex sibling species. *Chemoecology* **12,** 193–197.

Wee, S. L., Tan, K. H., and Nishida, R. (2007). Pharmacophagy of methyl eugenol by males enhances sexual selection of *Bactrocera carambolae*. *J. Chem. Ecol.* **33,** 1272–1282.

White, I. M., and Elson-Harris, M. M. (1992). Fruit flies of economic significance: Their identification and bionomics. CAB International, Wallingford, UK.

Williams, N. H., and Whitten, W. M. (1983). Orchid floral fragrances and male euglossine bees: Methods and advances in the last sesquidecade. *Biol. Bull.* **164,** 355–395.

Wong, T. T. Y., McInnis, D. O., Ramadan, M. M., and Nishimoto, J. I. (1991). Age-related response of male melon flies *Dacus cucurbitae* (Diptera: Tephritidae) to cue-lure. *J. Chem. Ecol.* **17,** 2481–2487.

CHAPTER TWENTY-FOUR

Oviposition Pheromones in Haematophagous Insects

T. Seenivasagan *and* R. Vijayaraghavan

Contents

Abstract

Pheromones influencing oviposition behavior in females of haematophagous insects have been the interest of recent past by many group of scientists working on oviposition pheromones. Finding and choosing a good site for oviposition is a challenging task for females of haematophagous insects, especially in those insects which does not have the parental care. Their decisions have far-reaching

Defence Research & Development Establishment, Ministry of Defence, Government of India, Jhansi Road, Gwalior-474 002, MP, India

Vitamins and Hormones, Volume 83
ISSN 0083-6729, DOI: 10.1016/S0083-6729(10)83024-9

and profound consequences for the life history of the offspring. In such blood feeding insects, the choice of oviposition site is affected by pheromones, which may function either as deterrents or stimulants in short range, while they may also act as repellents or attractants in long range perception. During the location of a suitable oviposition site for egg laying or a potential host for blood feeding, haematophagous insects mainly use olfactory and visual cues. These pheromones are produced by the ovipositing female or by conspecific larvae co-occurring with gravid females. Adult females detect oviposition pheromones by odor receptors on the antennae, as well as by contact chemoreceptors on tarsi, mouthparts and antennae. Different cues exploited by gravid females from a diversified arena include egg, larva, habitat, microbes, infusions and plant produced volatiles influence the oviposition behavior. Traps baited with pheromones, infusions, and insecticides shall be promising tools for monitoring and control of target insect using integrated vector management strategies.

I. Introduction

The ability of some insects to transmit pathogens that cause infectious diseases is of great medical and veterinary importance owing to their ability during the feeding process to vector (transmit) pathogens to both human beings and livestock. Haematophagous insects have a highly developed olfactory system and mainly use their antennae and, in some cases maxillary palps, to detect semiochemicals. Semiochemicals can provide information about the location suitability or physiological state of conspecifics, host, or breeding sites (McIver, 1982; Pickett *et al.*, 1998). Pheromones which mediate interactions between members of the same species can be divided into different categories, depending upon the type of behavior that is mediated, for example, mating, aggregation, oviposition (egg laying) and invitation behavior, and each class of pheromone has the potential to be utilized in traps. Pheromones, although not always directly related to the vectoring component of the life cycle, represent essentially potent means of vector detection through the deployment of pheromone baits in trapping systems (Logan and Birkett, 2007).

The research on semiochemicals especially on the oviposition pheromones involved in the behavior mediation of haematophagous insects has been growing fast, providing a number of valuable answers as well as leaving a number of new questions. This chapter primarily deals with pheromones and certain chemical substances mediating the oviposition behavior of blood sucking insects, which are also vectors of many deadly diseases to human beings and animals. Oviposition in any insect is particularly very important, that one has to focus upon. Because, once the oviposition is effected by a female haematophagous insect in a suitable aquatic or terrestrial habitat, the subsequent life stages develop to produce adults, which are mostly vectors of deadly microorganisms that cause various diseases. Mosquitoes are very important vectors of deadly diseases. They use various cues from the environment for oviposition (Bentley and Day, 1989).

Upon egg laying, the female of a particular genera/species provides cue for their conspecifics to oviposit in the same location leading to population buildup of that insect species. Subsequent life stages, that is, larva and pupa also release/emit certain odorant molecules into the water/breeding environment that influence the gravid females to oviposit in conspecific larval habitats. However, overcrowding sites repel the females from further oviposition. Oviposition pheromones in vectors by McCall and Cameron (1995) present details on various aspects on this subject with a wider scope for further research. This review focuses on literatures related to pheromones/parapheromones/semiochemicals identified in various haematophagous insects. McCall (2002) extensively reviewed the ecological aspects of oviposition by insects of medical and veterinary importance. Earlier reviews suggested the importance of pheromone based pest management. Literatures on arthropod semiochemicals (Mordue (Luntz), 2003), ecology of biting midges (Mordue (Luntz) and Mordue, 2003), ecology of Triatomine bugs (Cruz-López *et al.*, 2001), cattle flies (Birkett *et al.*, 2004), various traps for mosquito management (Kline, 2007), influence of semiochemicals on group behavior of insects (Kabeh, 2007), semiochemicals to manage Culicidae (Navarro-Silva *et al.*, 2009) postulated the use of semiochemicals in the control of insect pests. Some compounds that were not shown to be present in an insect may elicit behavior very similar to that elicited by pheromones are called parapheromones. The use of such parapheromones has been reviewed by Renou and Guerrero (2000). Different behaviors such as aggregation, lekking (Cabrera and Jaffe, 2007), and swarming which are mediated by pheromone like substances, lead to oviposition in few haematophagous insects have also got mention in this review. It is not surprising, that the volume of literatures published on haematophagous insects with respect to oviposition is slightly biased, that not all insects have been studied with equal importance to evolve a strategy for the control of deadly vector insects.

II. Origin of Oviposition Pheromones

A. Pheromones of egg origin

Females of many *Culex* species lay their eggs in clusters on the water surface called rafts. Osgood (1971) reported an oviposition pheromone associated with the egg rafts of *Culex tarsalis* Coquillett. Olfactometer tests with this material showed significantly greater mosquito attraction to the pheromone than to distilled water. Further, previous investigations focusing on the rafts as a potential source of attraction for gravid female *Culex* spp. showed that

1,3-diacylglycerols washed from the eggs elicited preferential oviposition (Starratt and Osgood, 1972, 1973). This pheromone is genus- rather than species-specific, eliciting similar responses from *Cx. tarsalis* and *Culex pipiens molestus* Forskal as well as *Culex quinquefasciatus* Say (Bruno and Laurence, 1979). The active substance, subsequently identified, synthesized, and shown to have biological activity comprised a single compound, erythro-6-acetoxy-5-hexadecanolide (Laurence and Pickett, 1982, 1985). The oviposition aggregation pheromone in *Cx. quinquefasciatus* the vector of human filariasis was the first pheromone identified in any species of medical or veterinary importance.

Blackflies lay their eggs in or close to running water. Females have been observed laying eggs communally in a manner, which over a period of a few hours can lead to deposits of thousands of eggs on a single substrate. In the Afro-tropical species complex, *Simulium damnosum* Theobald s.l., this behavior is mediated by a volatile pheromone emitted from freshly laid eggs (McCall, 1995a). The volatile compounds emitted by *S. damnosum* eggs were trapped using a closed collection system and their attractiveness to gravid flies was studied in a two-choice behavioral bioassay, in which significantly more female blackflies oviposited on substrates baited with freshly laid eggs, or with the volatiles collected from freshly laid eggs, in preference to the relevant control substrates. Substrates baited with volatiles from 12-h-old eggs were not significantly more attractive than controls (McCall, 1995b). The fractionated hexane extracts of gravid ovaries prepared by gas chromatography in a two-choice bioassay attracted ca. 66% of ovipositing blackflies to the substrate baited with a mixture of the four recombined fractions and it was observed that fraction 3, though mainly responsible for mediating aggregated oviposition by wild-caught *Simulium yahense* Vajime & Dunbar, was acting in tandem with additional cues (McCall *et al.*, 1997). The gas chromatographic analysis of hexane extracts of the ovaries from wild-caught flies, blood-fed and maintained until gravid in the laboratory showed that the composition of the aggregation pheromone is similar throughout the *S. damnosum* species complex. Also the analysis of *Simulium leonense* Boakye, Post & Mosha adults of different age groups and physiological states showed that the compounds are detectable only in gravid ovaries at two or more days following the blood meal, suggesting that production of the pheromone occurs during egg development (McCall *et al.*, 1997). The pheromone has both attractant and stimulant properties (McCall *et al.*, 1994; Wilson *et al.*, 2000) and comprises two methyl-branched saturated hydrocarbons.

The immature stages of two families of medically important Diptera, the sandflies (Psychodidae), and the tsetse flies (Glossinidae), develop in terrestrial environments. Both families include species that produce oviposition (sandflies) or larviposition (tsetse) aggregation pheromones. El Naiem and Ward (1990) reported an oviposition pheromone on the eggs of sandflies. Females of *Lutzomyia longipalpis* (Lutz & Neiva) produce a pheromone in the accessory glands that is passed on to the eggs as they are laid (El Naiem and Ward, 1991), and that the nonpolar extracts of both eggs and accessory glands attracts and stimulates other gravid females to oviposit at the same site (Dougherty *et al.*, 1992). In choice chambers, El Naiem *et al.* (1991) studied the chemical factors controlling oviposition of *L. longipalpis* where the females were attracted and/or stimulated to lay eggs on sites containing hexane extracts of conspecific eggs. Gas chromatography analysis of hexane extracts of the eggs demonstrated the presence of several compounds, of which cholesterol and squalene were identified. Further, Dougherty *et al.* (1994) separated the semiochemical components of eggs of *L. longipalpis* by high performance liquid chromatography and examined the HPLC fractions quantitatively and qualitatively by gas chromatography. A chemical substance/pheromone of egg origin was reported by Srinivasan *et al.* (1995) which stimulated the oviposition rate, where a significantly larger number of eggs were laid at the site treated with a di-ethyl ether extract of egg compared to water extract indicating that the oviposition attractant associated with the eggs dissolves in the organic solvent, but not in water. Dougherty and Hamilton (1997) identified dodecanoic acid as the oviposition pheromone of *L. longipalpis* using gas chromatography–mass spectrometry and chemical derivatizations. The synthetic analog induced the same behavioral response in gravid sandflies as the whole egg extract when present in biologically relevant quantities. There was a strong additive interaction upon the behavior of *L. longipalpis* when dodecanoic acid was tested along with hexanal and 2-methyl-2-butanol. The results suggested that sandflies acquired hexadecanoic acid (palmitic acid) from the blood meal and over a period of 4 days this was converted to dodecanoic acid. Alves *et al.* (2003) have reported that the hexane extract of 1000 eggs of conspecific *Lutzomyia renei* (Martins, Falcao, & Silva) showed slight attractancy to females in laboratory assays.

B. Pheromones of larval origin

The urge for isolation and identification of a chemical substance from the larva/immature stages of haematophagous insect yielded many promising lead molecules that can be exploited as pheromone to influence the oviposition behavior of the target insect. Early literatures suggested that at least some chemical factors produced by immature stages of mosquitoes influenced the oviposition. Kalpage and Brust (1973) reported an oviposition attractant produced by immature *Aedes atropalpus* (Coquillett). The holding waters of fourth instar larvae of *Aedes triseriatus* (Say) and *Ae. atropalpus* contain an oviposition attractant for *Ae. triseriatus* adults (Bentley *et al.*, 1976). Similarly, the tree hole water and laboratory rearing water were attractive to females of western tree hole mosquito, *Aedes sirrensis* (Ludlow) (Ahmadi and McClelland, 1983), but the emergence water, larval holding water, and water exposed to newly laid eggs did not influence the oviposition by the females.

McCrae (1984) studied the effects of site tone, water type, and conspecific immatures on target selection and oviposition by freshwater *Anopheles gambiae* Giles and reported that significantly more eggs were laid overnight in water over black than over paler tones, and this difference increased as contrast with the surrounding floor was increased. Turbid water from a development site thus seemed to possess an arrestant property which overrode selection favoring darker targets, and which was not derived from prior presence of conspecific immatures.

Studies such as, the effect of axenic larvae on the oviposition site selection by *Ae. atropalpus* revealed that the tested waters were significantly preferred by the *Ae. atropalpus* females. Sterile, distilled water was also significantly attractive after only 48-h immersion of axenic fourth-instar larvae (Maire, 1985). However, axenic larval rearing water with higher larval density was repulsive to ovipositing females. Interestingly, *Toxorhynchites splendens* Wiedemann exhibited a cross-preference for cups containing *Aedes aegypti* Linnaeus larval rearing water (Benzon *et al.*, 1988), but not for cups containing liquid cultures of bacteria, live *Ae. aegypti* in distilled water, *Ae. aegypti* larval holding water with reduced bacterial contamination, or methyl propionate.

The effect of larval rearing water and existing eggs on the oviposition responses by gravid female *Ae. aegypti* and *Aedes albopictus* (Skuse) in two-choice laboratory bioassays revealed a differential oviposition response by the females (Allan and Kline, 1998). Starved larvae also rendered water unattractive to gravid female *Ae. aegypti* (Zahiri *et al.*, 1997b), suggesting that an attractant was produced in the larval environment only under optimal conditions. When the biomass of *Ae. aegypti* larvae increased in relation to the volume of rearing waters, oviposition attraction of these waters to conspecific, gravid females first rose to a peak and then declined. Further increase in biomass rendered waters strongly repellent. Titration of repellent waters revealed that infection with the digenean *Plagiorchis elegans* (Rudolphi) generated the most powerful repellent effect, whereas crowding or starvation induced significantly weaker responses in the same study (Zahiri and Rau, 1998). Comparable responses occurred as the volume of water decreased or the number of larvae increased, suggesting a feedback mechanism that results in the maintenance of larval populations at an optimal level.

An oviposition attraction pheromone, heneicosane has been identified in both larval conditioned water and larval cuticle extracts of *Ae. aegypti* (Mendki *et al.*, 2000). When a question of how the females of *Ae. aegypti* were influenced by heneicosane for oviposition remained unrevealed for many years, Seenivasagan *et al.* (2009) confirmed the behavioral response of gravid *Ae. aegypti* mosquitoes to heneicosane odor using electrophysiology and flight orientation experiments and reported that the oviposition response was dose dependent, but reversed at higher doses.

To identify a potential oviposition attractant for *Anopheles gambiae* s.s. Blackwell and Johnson (2000) conducted electrophysiological investigation of larval water. The ether extracts of the water samples, were active in electroantennogram (EAG) studies with *An. (Cellia) gambiae* KWA. The regulation of oviposition in *An. gambiae* is by volatile pheromone emitted by conspecific larvae (Sumba *et al.*, 2008), which augment the effect of volatile signals emitted by preferred habitats and a non-olfactory cue associated with high densities of larvae that deters oviposition.

Larva produced pheromones influencing the oviposition behavior of certain blood feeding insect of terrestrial habitat had also been well documented. For example, the tsetse females deposit their large single larva in soil at the base of vegetation. The fully mature larva burrows into the soil and pupates within about 2 h. In *Glossina morsitans morsitans* Westwood and *Glossina morsitans centralis* Machado, aggregation is mediated by a pheromone in the anal exudate of the larva (Leonard and Saini, 1993; Nash *et al.*, 1976). The major components of the pheromone are *n*-pentadecane and *n*-dodecane in *G. m. morsitans* and *G. m. centralis*, respectively (Saini *et al.*, 1996).

III. Habitat Associated Kairomones

Oviposition response of a haematophagous insect is influenced by certain chemical substances as well as the odors associated with their habitat. Odors emanating from submerged organic infusions act as oviposition attractants and/or repellents to *Culex* mosquitoes (Kramer and Mulla, 1979). Significantly, more oviposition by *Toxorhynchites moctezuma* (Dyar and Knab) mosquitoes occurred in seasonal-deciduous forest than in either montane or evergreen-seasonal forest in the ovitraps (O'Malley *et al.*, 1989). While, Jordan and Hubbard (1991) in the field found that more eggs were laid by *Tx. moctezuma* into ovitraps situated either within or directly adjacent to trees or bamboo stools than those not associated with trees or bamboo. From the ether extract of the aqueous infusion of fermented Bermuda grass, Millar *et al.* (1992) isolated and identified compounds which attract and stimulate oviposition by gravid *Cx. quinquefasciatus*. Similarly, Trexler *et al.* (1998) reported that the organic infusions created by fermenting white oak, *Quercus alba* leaves in water attracted *Ae. Albopictus* and *Ae. triseriatus*. Various types of organic infusions at 1% and 10% dilutions elicited differential ovipositonal responses (Allan *et al.*, 2005) from *Cx. quinquefasciatus* and *Culex nigripalpus* Theobald in two-choice bioassays.

Interestingly, females of African malaria mosquito, *An. gambiae*, laid four times more eggs on bare, wet soil than soil populated with grasses (Huang *et al.*, 2006b), than the soil populated with short grass than medium or tall grass. Whereas, Achee *et al.* (2006) reported the enclosures containing the overhanging bamboo with detritus, function as a barrier to surface water flow causing the lodging of debris, the preferred habitat for *Anopheles darlingi* Root, and attracted gravid females for oviposition.

IV. Microbial Volatiles Eliciting Oviposition

Protein hydrolysates (egg albumin, lactalbumin hydrolysate, casein hydrolysate, and yeast hydrolysate) and associated bacterial contaminants attracted gravid females of *Cx. quinquefasciatus* for oviposition (Beehler *et al.*, 1994). Ovipositing *Anopheles albimanus* Wiedemann females exhibited a strong preference for cyanobacterial mats in a field experiment, because of higher temperatures and higher CO_2 emissions from cyanobacterial mats acting as possible ovipositional cues in marshes (Rejmankova *et al.*, 1996). Volatile substances from larval habitats extracted by freeze-drying and trapping the volatiles on a titanium condenser mediated species-specific oviposition in *An. albimanus* and *Anopheles vestitipennis* Dyar & Knab (Rejmankova *et al.*, 2005). For both species, volatile materials in low concentrations increased oviposition, whereas there was a shift to reduced oviposition at higher concentrations. Cultured bacterial volatiles on a 0.5% agarose media attracted *An. gambiae* for oviposition (Huang *et al.*, 2006a).

Romero *et al.* (2006) studied the role of certain bacteria in the oviposition behavior and larval development of stable flies and found that *Citrobacter freundii* stimulated the oviposition to great extent, and sustained stable fly development but to a lesser degree than *Serratia fanticola*. *Serratia marcescens* and *Aeromonas* spp. neither stimulated oviposition nor supported stable fly development which depends on a live microbial community in the natural habitat.

Water treated with aqueous fungal infusion (AFI) prepared from a wood inhabiting fungus (*Polyporus* spp.) at 4 ppm received significantly more egg rafts/eggs of vector mosquitoes (Sivagnaname *et al.*, 2001), than other substrates like rearing water, natural breeding water, and tap water. Poonam *et al.* (2002) reported that the culture filtrates of *Bacillus cereus* and *Pseudomonas fluorescens* exhibited oviposition attractancy at 100 ppm to the gravid females of *Cx. quinquefasciatus*, whereas, the culture filtrates of *Bacillus thuringiensis* var. *israelensis* (wild type), *B. t.* var. *israelensis* (mutant), and *Bacillus sphaericus* showed attractancy at 2000 ppm. Similarly, a significantly increased oviposition response of *Cx. quinquefasciatus* to the secondary metabolite(s) of a deuteromycetes fungus, *Trichoderma viride* under submerged culture condition (Geetha *et al.*, 2003) at 10 μg/mL compared with a known oviposition attractant, *p*-cresol has been observed. Gravid females of *Anopheles pseudopunctipennis* Theobald deposited significantly more eggs in cups containing natural algae *Spirogyra majuscula* in water from breeding sites than in cups containing artificial life-like algae in water from the corresponding natural breeding site, or in cups containing natural algae in distilled water (Torres-Estrada *et al.*, 2007). Gas chromatography and mass spectrometry analysis of algae organic extracts revealed a mixture of ethyl acetate and hydrocarbons compounds.

Navarro *et al.* (2003) reported that *Ae. aegypti* deposited more eggs in a water contaminated with bacteria than in distilled water. Similarly,

(Ponnusamy *et al.,* 2008) identified some bacteria and bacteria-associated chemical cues that mediate oviposition site preferences by *Ae. aegypti.* In binary choice assays the microorganisms in leaf infusions produced oviposition-stimulating kairomones, and using a combination of bacterial culturing approaches, bioassay-guided fractionation of bacterial extracts, and chemical analyses they have reported specific bacteria-associated carboxylic acids and methyl esters served as potent oviposition stimulants for gravid *Ae. aegypti.*

V. Parapheromones Mediating Oviposition

The role of habitat related and synthetic chemicals mediating the oviposition responses of various mosquito species has been well documented. A wide range of compounds, encompassing saturated and unsaturated carboxylic acids, ketones, phenols, and indoles, have all been shown to elicit oviposition and/or olfactory responses either by bioassay or electroantennography. Perry and Fay (1967) reported certain short chain fatty acid esters to influence the oviposition responses of *Ae. aegypti.* The tree hole mosquito, *Ae. triseriatus* has been found to oviposit in large numbers to *p*-cresol treated sites (Bentley *et al.*, 1979), to both *Cis*- and *trans* 4-methylcyclohexanol (Bentley *et al.*, 1982). It is likely that many volatile compounds will be common to fermentations of different media. Dark or colored waters, presumably indicative of such high organic content, are more attractive (Beehler *et al.*, 1993; Dhileepan, 1997). The allelochemicals known to attract gravid mosquitoes (Clements, 1999, pp. 569–570) have been presented.

George *et al.* (1986) reported oviposition attractancy of some substituted esters at 15 ppm concentration against control, while against the egg raft pheromone *Cx. quinquefasciatus* oviposited more in pheromone treated bowls compared to ester treatment. Certain compounds, like skatole and *p*-cresol, are indicators of site quality to a range of mosquito species with differing breeding site preferences. A number of attractants have been isolated from fermented grass infusions and of which, skatole (3-methyl-indole) has consistently proven to be the most attractive in laboratory studies (Beehler *et al.*, 1994; Blackwell *et al.*, 1993; Millar *et al.*, 1992). Gravid *Cx. quinquefasciatus* mosquitoes were strongly attracted and/or stimulated to oviposit by a habitat-derived chemical cue, 3-methylindole, at several concentrations ranging from 0.01 to 1 μg/L in water under laboratory conditions. In *Cx. quinquefasciatus*, the interaction of oviposition aggregation pheromone with site-derived odors had an additive effect (Millar *et al.*, 1994; Mordue *et al.*, 1992). Extracts of water from *An. gambiae* breeding sites contained skatole, indole, *m*-cresol, and 4-methylcyclohexanol (Blackwell and Johnson, 2000), all of which elicited electroantennographic responses in *An. gambiae.*

Predatory mosquito *Toxorhynchites brevipalpis* Theobald, *Toxorhynchites amboinensis* (Doleschall), and *Tx. splendens* laid significantly more eggs in cups containing *p*-cresol (Linley, 1989), whereas only *Tx. brevipalpis* and *Tx. amboinensis* responded similarly to 4-methylcycohexonol and to the mixture of both chemicals which indicated that the chemicals were acting as attractants, causing more females to fly to treated cups. Collins and Blackwell (1998) showed that ether extracts of water samples taken from tire sections were active in EAG studies with female *Tx. moctezuma* and *Tx. amboinensis* and recorded EAGs from both species for seven compounds viz., 4-methylcyclohexanol, phenol, indole, 3-methylindole, *m*-cresol, *o*-cresol, and *p*-cresol found commonly in water containing decaying leaves and known to be oviposition attractants for other mosquito species. Tyre water extract and the test compounds 4-methylcyclohexanol, 3-methylindole, 2-methylphenol, 3-methylphenol, and 4-methylphenol acted as oviposition attractants and stimulants for *Tx. moctezuma* and *Tx. amboinensis* (Collins and Blackwell, 2002), with the threshold amounts required to elicit these behaviors varying between the species and among the compounds tested.

Dimethyl disulfide, indole, 4-methylphenol, 3-methylindole, and trimethylamine loaded into controlled-release packets induced oviposition by *Ae. albopictus* in field and laboratory experiments (Trexler *et al.*, 2003); however, they exhibited no oviposition preference for any of the baited traps to the adjacent traps containing only water. Gravid females of *Ae. aegypti* were found to be sensitive to certain compounds present in egg extracts identified by GC–MS. Among them, dodecanoic and (Z)-9-hexadecenoic acids showed significant positive ovipositional response at different concentrations (Ganesan *et al.*, 2006), whereas, all the esters showed deterrent/repellent ovipositional effect. A series of C_{21} fatty acid esters have been found to influence the oviposition responses from *Ae. aegypti* and *Ae. albopictus* (Sharma *et al.*, 2008) and from *Anopheles stephensi* Liston (Sharma *et al.*, 2009).

The neotropical sandfly, *L. longipalpis* orient to odors of hexanal and 2-methyl-2-butanol with hexanal in bioassay, while electrophysiology indicated that R(+)-α-pinene, R(+)-β-pinene, S(−)-α-pinene, S(−)-β-pinene, α-terpinene, benzaldehyde may also be important in eliciting behavioral responses (Dougherty *et al.*, 1995). With respect to the blow fly, *Lucilia* spp. the bacterial infections result in the production of sulfur-containing compounds that are highly attractive to gravid *Lucilia* spp. Activation, long-distance orientation, and landing occur in response to the sulfur-rich volatiles, while oviposition is elicited by ammonia-rich compounds (Ashworth and Wall, 1994). Whereas, using electrophysiology, Cork (1994) identified 25 nonsulfur-containing compounds that elicited responses from *Cochliomyia hominivorax* (Coquerel).

VI. Predator/Prey Released Kairomones

Avoidance of potential oviposition sites in which potential predators or competitors already exist by detecting their presence prior to oviposition is a highly efficient strategy to safeguard the progeny of ovipositing females in aquatic environment. Gravid *Ae. aegypti* females avoid sites where parasitized larvae occur or water in which they have been reared (Lowenberger and Rau, 1994), with the degree of repellency increasing as the intensity of infections increased (Zahiri *et al.*, 1997a). The repellency is not species-specific (Zahiri *et al.*, 1997c) and repellent activity of the water is retained even after boiling, antibiotic treatment, or filtration (Lowenberger and Rau, 1994), suggesting a stable semiochemical. *Aedes taeniorhynchus* (Wiedemann) avoid sites containing fish (Ritchie and Laidlaw-Bell, 1994) and *Culex* spp. avoids sites with *Notonectids* (Chesson, 1984). This may be mediated by chemicals associated with the predator/competitor. In contrast, Torres-Estrada *et al.* (2001)found that *Ae. aegypti* females preferred to lay eggs in water that currently or previously contained the copepod *Mesocyclops longisetus* Thiebaud, possibly in response to the copepod-derived terpenes in the water despite the efficiency of the copepod predator.

Interestingly, Stav *et al.* (2000) reported that while *Culiseta longiareolata* Macquart avoided sites with free swimming *Anax* nymphs and laid fewer egg rafts, they do not appear to perceive a predation risk when the dragonfly nymphs were caged. *C. longiareolata* mosquitoes avoid laying eggs in habitats that harbor nymphs of the dragonfly *Anax imperator* (Leach) (Stav and Blaustein, 1999; Stav *et al.*, 2000), and also the hemipteran backswimmer *Notonecta maculata* Fabricius (Blaustein, 1998). A predator released chemical present in the *Notonecta* water repelled the oviposition by *C. longiareolata* for 8 days (Blaustein *et al.*, 2004). The mosquitoes continued to avoid ovipositing even after removing the predator in the former *Notonecta* pools for two additional days suggesting a predator-released kairomone as the cue used by the mosquitoes to detect the presence of this predator (Blaustein *et al.*, 2005).

In another study, Arav and Blaustein (2006) found that the pool depth did not affect oviposition habitat selection by temporary pool dipterans *C. longiareolata* (Culicidae) and *Chironomus riparius* Meigan (Chironomidae). Further, the oviposition patterns were consistent with larval vulnerability of the two species to predation by *N. maculata*. The mosquito *C. longiareolata* strongly avoided ovipositing in pools containing this predator, whereas *C. riparius*, whose larvae are considerably less vulnerable, did not display oviposition avoidance. Recently, Silberbush and Blaustein (2008) reported predator released oviposition deterrent kairomones act as air borne cues against *C. longiareolata*, as females of this species oviposited significantly more in the central pools surrounded by channels containing control water than in *Notonecta* conditioned water. Similarly, *Cx. tarsalis* and *Cx. quinquefasciatus* were deterred significantly from egg laying by the presence of predatory fish, *Gambusia affinis* (Baird and Girard) exudates in oviposition cups, while *Ae. aegypti* was not deterred by the presence of fish exudates (Van Dam and Walton, 2008). In another study, Walton *et al.* (2009) found that the number of *Cx. tarsalis* egg rafts laid on mesocosms containing caged mosquito fish was reduced by 84% relative to control, whereas *Cx. quinquefasciatus* did not differentiate between small oviposition sites with mosquito fish conditioned water and aged reservoir water.

VII. Oviposition Cues of Blood Feeding Bugs

Two families of Heteropteran bugs are haematophagous and feed on vertebrate blood: the Cimicidae or bedbugs and the Triatominae (family Reduviidae) called kissing bugs or cone-nose bugs. The bedbug species of *Cimex lectularius* Linnaeus and *Cimex hemipterus* Fabricius rest and breed in the cracks and crevices of walls and furniture in human habitations, emerging at night to feed on their sleeping hosts. *C. lectularius* produces volatile alarm and assembly pheromones to which both adults and nymphs respond (Levinson and Bar-Ilan, 1971; Levinson *et al.*, 1974). The alarm pheromone is emitted by the metasternal scent glands and mainly comprises *trans*-oct-2-en-1-al and *trans*-hex-2-en-1-al. Although the assembly pheromone has not solely involved in oviposition, by maintaining aggregations of all stages of bedbugs, facilitate aggregation of eggs and immatures.

Parashar *et al.* (2003) have reported induced aggregation activity of *C. hemipterus* by the excreta extracts using different solvents like hexane, dichloromethane, methanol, and water. The water and methanol extracts of filter papers on which the bedbugs were growing, exhibited increased attractiveness for male, female, and fifth nymphal instars. An evidence for male and juvenile specific contact pheromones of *C. lectularius* having contrasting functions of marking shelters as safe refugia for development and growth (juveniles) or mate encounter (adults), to result in the aggregation behavior of conspecifics has been shown by Siljander *et al.* (2007). Subsequently, in another study Siljander *et al.* (2008) identified 10 compounds (nonanal, decanal, (E)-2-hexenal, (E)-2-octenal, (2E,4E)—octadienal, benzaldehyde, (+) and (−) limonene, sulcatone, benzyl alcohol) to be essential components of the *C. lectularius* airborne aggregation pheromone.

Pfiester *et al.* (2009) studied the effect of population structure and size on aggregation behavior of *C. lectularius* and reported that the nymphs had a high tendency to aggregate. At densities of 10 and 40 adults at a 1:1 sex ratio, there were significantly more lone females than lone males. Females, were found away from aggregations significantly more often than any other life stage, are potentially the dispersal stage of the bed bug. The alarm pheromones of bed bugs, previously hypothesized to be a predator chemical defence, can be used by newly fed males to signal their sex and reduce the risk of homosexual mating (Ryne, 2009). The mounting males consider the alarm signal a major sex identification cue, suggesting that male bed bugs use alarm pheromone communication to avoid homosexual harassment and mounting. Olson *et al.*, (2009) in a study on the off-host aggregation behavior and sensory basis of arrestment by *C. lectularius* found that the aggregation by bed bugs is a result of arrestment mediated by direct, close-range contact between sensilla on the pedicel and stained experimental disks.

A trap designed for the bed bug baited with CO_2 (50–400 mL/min), heat (37.2–42.2 °C) and a chemical lure comprised of 33 μg propionic acid, 0.33 μg butyric acid, 0.33 μg valeric acid, 100 μg octenol, and 100 μg L-lactic acid impregnated into a gel (Anderson *et al.*, 2009) caught significantly more bed bugs than controls in laboratory experiments. In another study, Benoit *et al.* (2009) has shown that the addition of alarm pheromone components (E)-2-hexenal, (E)-2-octenal, and a (E)-2-hexenal: (E)-2-octenal blend improved the effectiveness of two desiccant formulations, diatomaceous earth (DE) and Dri-die (silica gel) by increasing the excited crawling activity of *C. lectularius*, thereby promoting cuticular changes that increase water loss.

Triatomine bugs occur worldwide but are of major medical importance in South and Central America, Brazil where they feed on humans and transmit *Trypanosoma cruzi*, the causative agent of Chagas disease. Rather like bedbugs, these vectors inhabit the cracks and crevices in walls, the thatched roofs of human or animal dwellings and some species will also inhabit trees and animal burrows and nests. Schilman *et al.* (1996) reported egg laying by the haematophagous bug *Rhodnius prolixus* Stal was maximal on the fresh feathers and minimal on the cardboard in laboratory experiments.

Triatoma infestans Klug exit shelters to actively defecate at the entry point thus marking the site for other bugs that prefer marked refuges (Lorenzo and Lazzari, 1996). Bug feces contain an aggregation or assembly pheromone (Cruz-Lopez *et al.*, 1993; Lorenzo and Lazzari, 1996; Schofield and Patterson, 1977) possibly ammonia (Taneja and Guerin, 1997) which appears to act interspecifically (Lorenzo Figueiras and Lazzari, 1998a). Another assembly odor is deposited by walking insects (Lorenzo Figueiras and Lazzari, 1998b). Oviposition occurs within these assemblies, where all stages rest when not host seeking. In choice experiments, shelters with feces either inside or outside, were significantly preferred by bugs (Lorenzo and Lazzari, 1998). Adults and larvae of *T. infestans* spend daylight hours assembled in shaded places. And the recently fed insects do not aggregate around feces, but show a significant assembling response from the eighth hour after feeding. Freshly deposited feces evoked rejection, but not assembling. Three hours after deposition, the feces became attractive and that persisted for about 10 days (Figueiras and Lazzari, 2000).

Larvae of *Panstrongylus megistus* Burmeister significantly aggregated on papers impregnated with their own excrement and on papers marked with cuticular substances deposited on surfaces on which these insects had walked (Pires *et al.*, 2002). In the same study, *T. infestans* bugs also aggregated on papers impregnated by feces or by cuticular substances of *P. megistus*, and *P. megistus* aggregated on papers contaminated by feces or by cuticular substances of *T. infestans*. The response of *P. megistus* to its cuticular substances was significantly stronger than that to its feces.

Reisenman *et al.* (2000) reported that the haematophagous bug *T. infestans* displayed various aggregation behavior using both visual and olfactory cues, where feces constituted a major attractant source. In the absence of feces, bugs always assembled in dark places. The bugs' response changed depending on the specific combination of spectral light and feces discriminating between lights of different spectral quality through an achromatic mechanism. Whereas, the choice experiments with *Triatoma pseudomaculata* Correa & Espinola, revealed that the insects aggregated significantly around papers impregnated with dry feces. In addition, the bugs also showed a significant aggregation response to papers impregnated with compounds derived from their cuticle that were deposited by contact on the substrate (Vitta *et al.*, 2002). Futher, it has been shown that fecal spots were deposited in a larger density inside the shelter than in the remaining area available for the bugs. *Triatoma brasiliensis* Neiva larvae were significantly attracted towards their own feces (Vitta *et al.*, 2007), and also to those of *T. pseudomaculata*. In contrast to other Triatomine species, footprints did not promote attraction in *T. brasiliensis*. Regarding mating and sexual behavior of these bugs Crespo and Manrique (2007) reported that metasternal glands of the female are involved in the sexual behavior of *T. infestans*, while Brindley's glands have no effect on mating behavior. Copulation and aggregation behavior of males likely result from the eventual release of volatiles from the female's metasternal glands. Further, a lack of endogenous control and the relevance of light cycles (L/D, L/L, and D/D) as a synchronization signal (Minoli *et al.*, 2007) for exhibiting a cyclic aggregation by *T. infestans* during scotophase and photophase has been observed in these bugs.

VIII. Oviposition Cues of Veterinary Insects

Olfactory cues mediating the oviposition response of insects of veterinary importance are diverse in nature (see McCall, 2002). The oviposition substrates selected by many blood feeding females of stable flies, mainly comprise decomposing vegetal matter in which bacterial degradation of the medium results in the production of volatile compounds, such as carboxylic acids, short chain aliphatic alcohols, phenols, indoles, sulfides, terpenes, and carbon dioxide.

Some plants, mainly belonging to Araceae, are known to mimic dung odor to attract pollinators, including many Diptera associated with the ecological recycling of dung and carrion (Kite, 1995; Skubatz *et al.*, 1996). Henceforth, a complex blend of terpenes, carboxylic acids, aliphatic alcohols, aldehydes, ketones, phenols, indoles, and sulfur containing compounds may serve to lure *Stomoxys* spp. searching for dung and dung like substrates on which to oviposit. Robacker and Bartelt (1997) quantified the chemical components of the head space of *C. freundii* cultures and determined that filtrates were composed mainly of ammonia. Romero *et al.* (2006) reported the role of certain bacteria in the oviposition behavior and larval development of stable flies. Jeanbourquin and Guerin (2007) tested horse and cow dung as substrates for oviposition by the stable fly, *Stomoxys calcitrans* (Linnaeus), in laboratory cages and reported that the odor alone from either horse or cow dung was sufficient to attract flies for oviposition. However, in dual choice assays flies preferred the odor of horse dung over cow dung. They identified some predominant chemostimulant compounds in both substrates such as butanoic acid, oct-1-en-3-ol, decanal, octan-3-one, *p*-cresol, skatole, *β*-caryophyllene, and dimethyl trisulphide.

IX. Synthesis of Oviposition Pheromones

Relatively large number of literatures has been published till date from the discovery of *Culex* oviposition attractant pheromone Erythro-6-acetoxy-5-hexadecanolide by Laurence and Pickett (1982). The laboratory synthesis of identified oviposition pheromones increased the potential use of such pheromone molecules for surveillance of specific vector insects. Laboratory synthesis of (5R,6S)-6-acetoxy-5-hexadecanolide, the *Culex* oviposition pheromone (CuOP) has improved a lot in recent years compared to earlier described protocols by various workers using different reaction procedures, from different precursors of various sources. Jefford *et al.* (1986) synthesized CuOP by the stereocontrolled addition of *n*-decylmetallic reagents to acrolein dimer. While Ko and Eliel (1986) adopted asymmetric synthesis of CuOP by Grignard addition of 5-pentenyl-magnesium bromide, Mitsunobu inversion for one of the erythro (5R,6S) isomers and oxidation-hydride reduction for the other isomer with an overall yield of 30–42%.

Synthesis of CuOP by Sharpless epoxidation method was adopted by Dawson *et al.* (1989), whereas Wang *et al.* (1990) synthesized CuOP from 1,2-cyclohexanediol, using kinetic resolution of cyclic alcohol by a modified Sharpless asymmetric epoxidation reagent. Recently, Singh and Guiry (2009) reported stereoselective synthesis of (−)-(5R,6S)-erythro-6-acetoxy-5-hexadecanolide, in seven steps with 28% overall yield by using Sharpless asymmetric epoxidation and $ZrCl_4$-catalyzed cyclic acetal formation as the key steps. However, Dawson *et al.* (1990) suggested a simple 3-step synthesis of CuOP by aldol condensation between 1-trimethylsilyloxycyclopent-1-ene and undecanal, followed by Baeyer-Villiger ring expansion and acetylation. Similarly, Zhang *et al.* (1994) used the mixture of erythro- and threo-isomers of the lactone, synthesized by the aldol condensation from cyclopentanone and undecanol, producing 2-(1-hydroxyl undecyl-1-) cyclopentanone, then by the Baeyer-Villiger reaction and acetylation to produce the oviposition pheromone.

Couladouros and Mihou (1999) synthesized CuOP in eight steps via a carbonate ester, utilizing novel lactonization with inversion of stereochemistry in a straightforward way using the reaction sequence comprising reduction, Wittig–Schlosser coupling, Sharpless asymmetric dihydroxylation, oxidation, and lactonization. Whereas, proline catalyzed asymmetric aldol reactions has been used for synthesis of CuOP by Sun *et al.* (2005) and Ikishima *et al.* (2006) using synthons of straight-chain aliphatic aldehydes and aldehydes bearing a 1,3-dithiane moiety at the beta-position.

Various precursors have been used to synthesize CuOP. For example, Ichimoto *et al.* (1988) synthesized CuOP from 2-doxy-D-ribose via a highly stereocontrolled route, Gallos *et al.* (2000) used D-ribose for CuOP synthesis and (R)-2,3-Cyclo-hexylidene glyceraldehydes was used by Dhotare *et al.* (2005), while Prasad and Anbarasan (2007) synthesized CuOP from the chiral pool compound, L-(+)-tartaric acid. The synthetic sequence includes the elaboration of an alpha-benzyloxy aldehyde derived from tartaric acid with ring closing metathesis as the key step. Recently, Quinn *et al.* (2009) reported a total synthesis of CuOP in six steps, with a 37% overall yield from (2R,3S)-1,2-expoxy-4-penten-3-ol in which a size-selective ring closing/cross metathesis reaction lead to lactone formation and alkyl chain extension in a one-pot process.

Interestingly, Ramaswamy and Oehlschlager (1991) synthesized oviposition pheromone of *Culex* through chemico-microbial synthesis from a common chiral precursor derived from baker's yeast reduction. While, Olagbemiro *et al.* (1999) used the oil extracted from the seeds of the summer cypress plant, *Kochia scoparia* (Chenopodiaceae) as the source for CuOP synthesis.

The process for preparation of *n*-heneicosane an oviposition attractant pheromone of *Ae. aegypti* has been reported by Ganesan *et al.* (2009). The process comprises (a) reacting 2,4-alkaneanedione with 1-bromoocta decane in absolute ethanol in the presence of 18-crown-6 as catalyst to produce 2-heneicosanone; and (b) reducing the 2-heneicosanone using hydrazine hydrate and potassium hydroxide in ethylene glycol to obtain *n*-heneicosane.

X. Evaluation of Oviposition Pheromones

The oviposition pheromones identified from various haematophagous insects have been evaluated for bioactivity in laboratory and field conditions. Bioactivity of pheromone alone and in combined form with other chemicals, infusions, and breeding water had been extensively investigated and reported. The CuOP erythro-6-acetoxy-5-hexadecanolide, and polluted water increased oviposition by *Culex* spp. and when combined the effect was additive. The oviposition behavior is reflected by the antennal sensitivity to these compounds (Blackwell *et al.*, 1993; Mordue *et al.*, 1992). Michaelakis *et al.* (2005) synthesized the oviposition pheromone of *Cx. quinquefasciatus* in a racemic form and tested the synthetic racemic pheromone (SRP) in the laboratory for its bioactivity on *Cx. pipiens* biotype *molestus*. It was found that the best bioactivity was achieved at 1 μg per cage. Further, the combination of the synthetic pheromone with the control agent temephos showed both an acceptable oviposition activity and sufficient larvicidal effect (Michaelakis *et al.*, 2007). Also, the use of an aged infusion combined with aged pheromone (microencapsulated) along with three common plants in Greece as a potential oviposition medium: *Oxalis pes-carpae*, *Jasminum polyanthum*, and *Avena barbata* revealed 80% oviposition attractancy (Michaelakis *et al.*, 2009), in addition, the combination of the synthetic pheromone with the *O. pes-carpae* infusion revealed a synergistic effect.

A. Flight behavior to pheromones

Pile *et al.* (1991) studied the odor-mediated upwind flight of *Cx. quinquefasciatus* mosquitoes to a synthetic pheromone, erythro-6-acetoxy-5-hexadecanolide, and reported that the females had a higher rate of turning, had a lower flight-speed when landing, and stayed longer at oviposition sites containing pheromone than at a comparable site without pheromone. In the laboratory test, Lampman and Novak (1996) showed that *Ae. albopictus* is attracted to sod infusion and females readily oviposit on substrates in contact with the infusion. Females of *Ae. albopictus*, *Ae. triseriatus*, and *Culex* species were collected from gravid traps placed along the edge of woods at distances ranging from 100 to 200 m from the tyre site. Similarly, Seenivasagan *et al.* (2009) in a flight orientation assay using Y-tube olfactometer observed that the gravid *Ae. aegypti* female mosquitoes were attracted to the odor plume of heneicosane at 10^{-6} and 10^{-5} g dose, while the higher dose of 10^{-3} g plume enforced repellency. In response to oviposition substrates in multiple choice conditions, larger number of eggs were deposited in 10 mg/L solutions, indicating that 10 ppm was most attractive compared to lower and higher concentrations. Recently, Lazzari (2009) reviewed the orientational aspects of haematophagous insect to vertebrate host odors for blood feeding and subsequent oviposition.

B. Additive/synergistic effect of pheromones/ semiochemicals

Oviposition responses of haematophagous insects elicited by their respective pheromones either additively or synergistically with other sources have been documented by several authors. Mordue *et al.* (1992) reported that the attraction of gravid *Cx. quinquefasciatus* to the oviposition pheromone, erythro-6-acetoxy-5-hexadecanolide in combination with polluted water produced additive effect in oviposition. Similarly, an additive effect resulted when 0.05 μg oviposition pheromone was combined with the polluted water dilution series (Blackwell *et al.*, 1993). In another study, the oviposition responses gravid *Cx. quinquefasciatus* to blends of a fixed amount of the pheromone with variable doses of 3-methylindole were additive rather than synergistic (Millar *et al.*, 1994). Whereas, Dougherty *et al.* (1993) showed that the combined extract of rabbit food and oviposition pheromone had a synergistic effect on sandfly egg-laying, greatly increasing the number of eggs laid and resulting in a highly targeted response. However, there was a strong additive interaction in the behavior of *L. longipalpis* (Dougherty and Hamilton, 1997) when dodecanoic acid was tested along with hexanal and 2-methyl-2-butanol. Synergistic effects of the combination of plant-derived *Culex* spp. oviposition pheromone and skatole in laboratory as well as under field conditions has been reported by Olagbemiro *et al.* (2004); in the same study synthetic oviposition pheromone (SOP) and skatole combinations showed additive effects for *Cx. quinquefasciatus*. Braks *et al.* (2007) observed synergistic effects between the oviposition pheromone at 3 μg and the hay infusion in semifield experiments with gravid *Cx. quinquefasciatus* females. The combination of the microencapsulated SOP (Michaelakis *et al.*, 2009) with the *O. pes-carpae* infusion revealed a synergistic effect only for the first day for the West Nile virus vector *Culex pipiens* Linnaeus.

C. Formulations of oviposition pheromones

Culex oviposition pheromone loaded onto an effervescent tablet (Otieno *et al.*, 1988) has been found to attract female *Cx. quinquefasciatus* mosquitoes. Metal carboxylate glasses were used by Blair *et al.* (1994) for the controlled release of the bioactive molecules of *Cx. quinquefasciatus* oviposition pheromone. The glasses degrade in a humid environment, releasing the volatile pheromone in a controlled fashion. Dimethyl disulfide, indole, 4-methylphenol, 3-methylindole, and trimethylamine loaded into controlled-release packets induced oviposition by *Ae. albopictus* in field and laboratory experiments (Trexler *et al.*, 2003); however, they exhibited no oviposition preference for any of the baited traps to the adjacent traps containing only water. Another formulation of microencapsulated pheromone (Michaelakis *et al.*, 2009) from aged infusion of *Oxalis pes-carpae*, *Jasminum polyanthum*, and *Avena barbata* as an oviposition medium has been used for the control of *Cx. pipiens*.

D. Field trials

Otieno *et al.* (1988) in a field trial of the synthetic oviposition attractant pheromone 6-acetoxy-5-hexadecanolide in a formulation of 20 mg containing 5 mg of the active (−)-(5R,6S)-isomer in an effervescent tablet observed a high, positive overall response by gravid females of *Cx. quinquefasciatus* with the activity of the pheromone persisting at the breeding site for 4 days after application and significantly more females (82%) ovipositing around the pheromone source compared to a control. The addition of the insect growth regulator pyriproxyfen to the formulation did not affect the activity of the pheromone and caused 100% mortality of the larvae by the pupal stage. Beehler and Defoliart (1990) evaluated fish oil emulsion and water of high optical density as oviposition attractants for *Ae. triseriatus*, in ovitraps in the field and reported that the water containing vegetable dye increased oviposition up to 4-fold over control traps. Laboratory bioassays with fish oil emulsion at both 1% and 5% confirmed the field results.

Ritchie and Long (2003) conducted field trials near Cairns, Queensland, Australia, and reported no significant difference in the number of eggs of *Ae. aegypti* or *Ochlerotatus notoscriptus* (Skuse) laid in ovitraps with or without a methoprene pellet. Similarly a comparison was made by Ritchie *et al.* (2003) on the efficacy of a standard ovitrap and an ovitrap featuring an internal wall covered by a polybutylene adhesive in field studies. Significantly higher numbers of *Ae. aegypti* were collected by traps set outside rather than inside premises.

Burkett *et al.* (2004) made a comparison between commercial mosquito trap and gravid trap oviposition media in field trials and found that significant differences in numbers collected among traps were noted for several species, including *Aedes vexans* (Meigen), *Ae. albopictus*, *Cx. quinquefasciatus*, *Culex restuans* Theobald, and *Culex salinarius* Coquillett. Olagbemiro *et al.* (2004) studied laboratory and field responses of the mosquito, *Cx. quinquefasciatus*, to plant-derived *Culex* spp. oviposition pheromone and the oviposition cue skatole and found that plant derived pheromone (PDP) and SOP were equally attractive. Jackson *et al.* (2005) conducted field studies in southwestern Virginia to determine the ovipositional preferences of *Cx. restuans* and *Cx. pipiens* by using ovitraps and gravid traps baited with four different infusions (manure, hay, grass, and rabbit chow) and observed significant differences among infusions on most sample dates for both species where the hay and grass infusions collected the majority of the egg rafts compared to manure infusion.

Braks *et al.* (2007) in semifield experiments found that the mean number of egg rafts laid by *Cx. quinquefasciatus* in response to a single egg raft in an oviposition jar filled with hay infusion was significantly greater than all other treatments. When the oviposition pheromone dose was increased from 1 to 10 rafts or when 3.0 μg SOP was dispensed on a floating receptacle, synergistic effects were observed between the oviposition pheromone and the hay infusion. Whereas, Barbosa *et al.* (2007) developed and evaluated a ovitrap (BR-OVT) based on physical and chemical stimuli for attracting gravid *Cx. quinquefasciatus* females under laboratory and field conditions and reported a significant preference of gravid females for sites containing conspecific egg rafts, as a response to the natural oviposition pheromone, as well as for sites treated with the SOP.

XI. Oviposition Traps and Baits for Monitoring and Control

Menace of hamatophagous insects had earlier been managed using traps of various design and nature. With respect to the exploitation of oviposition behavior, ovitraps employing different substrates, color, organic infusions, natural and SOPs, oviposition attraction chemicals identified from natural breeding habitat as well as the combinations of above sources have been used to monitor the population dynamics of blood feeding diptera. Literatures on the design and use of such traps with potential for attraction of target insect is large in numbers for mosquitoes compared to other blood feeding insects. The progress made in this subject is listed hereunder.

Reuben *et al.* (1977) designed a new paddle for the black jar ovitrap for surveillance of *Ae. aegypti* and reported the seasonal changes in egg-laying activity of *Aedes* species in Sonepat, India (Reuben *et al.*, 1978). The tree species and trunk diameter significantly affected the distribution, occurrence, and ovitrap site preference of tree hole mosquitoes: *Ae. triseriatus* and *Aedes hendersoni* Cockerell Eggs of *Ae. hendersoni* were found more frequently associated with trees of border and sunny habitat, while *Ae. triseriatus* eggs were more frequently found in association with trees of mesic habitat. Oviposition of *Ae. hendersoni* occurred more often at trees with smaller diameter at breast height than did *Ae. triseriatus* (Ballard *et al.*, 1987). The egg aggregation of the tree hole mosquito *Ae. triseriatus* has been associated with a non-random dispersion pattern (Kitron *et al.*, 1989) of oviposition events indicating more eggs were laid in traps from which eggs were removed.

Lang (1990) reported that *Ae. triseriatus* females preferred horizontally open ovitraps regardless of whether they are depositing eggs which hatch shortly after deposition or whether the eggs diapause because of shortened late summer/early fall photoperiods. The ovitraps exposed outdoors during wet and dry seasons revealed that 86.4% eggs were laid during the wet season (Chadee *et al.*, 1995) in which most eggs (>80%) were laid on hardboad paddle confirming the superiority of the paddle as a device for monitoring oviposition activity.

Infusion traps had been predominantly used for the monitoring of mosquito populations at various locations. These ogranic infusions derived through fermentation, prolonged submergence in water and release certain chemical substances into the breeding water in a habitat, that attract the gravid female mosquito for oviposition. Reiter *et al.* (1991) reported that an ovitrap containing hay infusion and a second ovitrap adjacent to it containing a 10% dilution of the infusion in tap water together yielded eight times more *Ae. aegypti* eggs than single CDC ovitraps containing tap water. In a field study by Chadee *et al.* (1993), significantly more eggs were collected from 25% and 50% hay infusions than tap water controls.

The ether extract of the aqueous infusion from a fermented Bermuda grass infusion contained phenol, 4-methylphenol, 4-ethylphenol, indole, and 3-methylindole fractionated by liquid chromatography was stimulatory to gravid *Cx. quinquefasciatus* (Millar *et al.*, 1992). Bermuda grass infusion fermented for periods of 0–63 days was stimulatory to gravid *Cx. quinquefasciatus*, while only 5–25-day-old infusion was stimulatory to *Cx. tarsalis* (Isoe *et al.*, 1995). Standard-aged infusion (7d old) was as effective or better than infusion of any other age for *Cx. tarsalis*, whereas *Cx. quinquefasciatus* exhibited a distinct preference for 2–4-week old infusion. Lampman and Novak (1996) studied the oviposition preferences of *Cx. pipiens* and *Cx. restuans* for infusion-baited traps and reported that the percentage of egg rafts from *Cx. restuans* was greater in sod and grass infusions than in rabbit chow infusions, whereas *Cx. pipiens* showed a slight preference for rabbit chow infusions over sod and grass infusions.

The organic infusions created by fermenting white oak leaves in water received largest proportion of eggs laid (76.8%) by *Ae. albopictus* in a 60% concentration of 7-d old infusion. In contrast, *Ae. triseriatus* exhibited variable oviposition responses but generally deposited the largest number of eggs in only a few concentrations of older age infusions (Trexler *et al.*, 1998). In laboratory bioassays, Du and Millar (1999b) demonstrated that fermented infusions of dried bulrushes (*Schoenoplectus acutus*) strongly attracted and stimulated oviposition by gravid female *Cx. quinquefasciatus* and *Cx. tarsalis*. Further, they observed that the gravid mosquitoes are attracted to oviposition sites by blends of compounds rather than by individual chemicals, and that the concentration of compounds in the odor is a critical factor in determining whether responses are positive or negative. In another study, using EAG and oviposition responses of *Cx. quinquefasciatus* and *Cx. tarsalis* (Diptera: Culicidae) to chemicals in odors from Bermuda grass infusions, Du and Millar (1999a) identified nine compounds using GC-EAD (phenol, *p*-cresol, 4-ethylphenol, indole, 3-methylindole, nonanal, 2-undecanone, 2-tridecanone, naphthalene) from odor extracts that elicited significant antennal responses from antennae of gravid females of *Cx. quinquefasciatus* and *Cx. tarsalis*.

A modified ovitrap (Lenhart *et al.*, 2005) consisted of a dark blue 300 mL plastic cup lined inside with a layer of an inexpensive, cream-colored, low thread count cotton fabric, covering from the rim of the cup to about 3/4 of the way down and held in place with a single paper clip has been developed and found efficient in detecting oviposition by *Ae. aegypti* mosquitoes. While, Allan *et al.* (2005) collected significantly more *Cx. quinquefasciatus* and *Cx. nigripalpus* in traps baited with cow manure infusion (highest) compared to alfalfa hay infusion (lowest) in field in Florida under laboratory and field conditions at 1% and 10% dilutions in two-choice bioassays. The fermentation age of the grass infusion affects the oviposition response of mosquitoes. Santana *et al.* (2006) found that anaerobically fermented grass infusions were more attractive than either aerobically fermented or sterilized infusions of *Panicum maximum* (Jacq.) evincing that 15 or 20 day anaerobic fermentation made of fresh, fully mature leaves of *P. maximum* is the optimum infusion for ovitrap-based surveillance of *Aedes* mosquitoes. In another study to compare the attractancy of Bermuda-hay infusion to infusions of emergent aquatic vegetation (Burkett-Cadena and Mullen, 2007) for collecting female mosquitoes in the field in east-central Alabama, the females of *Cx. quinquefasciatus* and *Cx. restuans* but not the *Ae. albopictus* showed selectivity in choosing an oviposition site.

A. Traps deploying microbial volatiles

The role of volatiles produced by the microorganism in a habitat proved effective in attracting the blood feeding insects for oviposition, thus it has been exploited for the design of oviposition traps against certain mosquito species. Wallace (1996) designed a field trap for oviposition by *Ae. taeniorhynchus*. The trap consisted of a 50 × 60-cm piece of contaminated 100% cotton bath towel, saturated with 85% tap water, a container, and a cover of dried plant parts placed over the contaminated toweling by populations of bacteria and fungi which attracted the females for initiation of egg deposition. Similarly, the trials conducted in the field showed that mud pots treated with aqueous infusion of a wood inhabiting fungus (*Polyporus* spp.) at 4 ppm placed in both indoor and outdoor locations received significantly more *Ae. aegypti* eggs than the control (Sivagnaname *et al.*, 2001). The treated pots placed in paddy fields attracted significantly more gravid *Anopheles subpictus* Grassi for oviposition than untreated pots. In contrast, the number of egg rafts of *Cx. quinquefasciatus* laid in fungal infusion treated pots was significantly less than in the control ones owing to strong natural olfactory factors associated with the breeding habitat. Lorenzo *et al.* (1998) captured *T. infestans* under natural climatic conditions using yeast-baited traps, also Pimenta *et al.* (2007) used the yeast, *Saccharomyces cerevisiae* as baits for *Triatoma dimidiata* Latreille and *Triatoma pallidipennis* Stal.

B. Sticky and lethal ovitraps

Addition of an adhesive or an insecticide/insect growth regulator to a potential oviposition trap demonstrated its ability, not only to monitor the prevalence of a haematophagous insect but also to lure and kill the target insect. Insecticides with quick knockdown efficacy has been used by

Zeichner and Perich (1999) in lethal ovitraps with a heavy-weight velour paper strips pretreated with insecticide solutions as an alternative to the wooden paddle normally provided as a substrate for mosquito oviposition. Kay *et al.* (2000) deviced a sticky entry–exit trap for sampling gravid, mosquitoes seeking oviposition sites in subterranean habitats such as wells and service manholes and used successfully against *Aedes tremulus* (Theobald) and *Ae. aegypti*. Bifenthrin-treated lethal ovitrap against *Ae. aegypti*, although less acceptable for oviposition caused 92% mortality in the visiting females. A sticky ovitrap collected both *Ae. aegypti* and *Aedes polynesiensis* (Marks) in greatest numbers baited with water or grass infusions rather than leaf infusions (Russell and Ritchie, 2004). The bifenthrin content of strips, that is 0.1 mg/cm^2 or 7 mg/strip remained effective for 4 week of field exposure (Williams *et al.*, 2007). A biodegradable lethal ovitrap (BLO) dyed black developed by Ritchie *et al.* (2008) against *Ae. aegypti* received more egg deposition. In another study, Zhang and Lei (2008) evaluated sticky ovitraps for the surveillance of *Ae. albopictus* in the field, in Wuhan, China and reported that the female *Ae. albopictus* showed no oviposition preference for infusions made from the leaves of the camphorwood tree, box, green bristle grass, Bermuda grass, lotus magnolia, or bamboo. In terms of the attractancy of the sticky ovitraps to female *Ae. albopictus* in the field, the red color of the ovitraps appeared to contribute more than a Bermuda-grass infusion.

XII. Concluding Remarks

The eventual goal of pheromone research focusing on oviposition behavior of haematophagous insects would be a fundamental understanding of olfactory communication systems from molecular phenomena to the ecosystem level, and its practical application in various ways. Current major understandings of the olfactory communication system also need to be expanded from an individual level to more complex systems. Contact chemoreception mechanism also gained importance in recent years, as the largely semivolatile or relatively nonvolatile chemical substances mediate oviposition by a female insect on a treated substrate. Several groups working in the field of managing blood feeding insects in the last decade have made worthy contributions by isolation and identification of pheromone molecules which mediates oviposition behavior of target insects. Extensive work had been accomplished in exploiting such lead molecules of pheromones and parapheromones in ovitraps under laboratory and field conditions. Improvements made in the usage of various types of infusions along with pheromone molecules, synthetic oviposition attractants to influence the gravid females proved efficient in monitoring and surveillance of target insect. Luring the target insect to a trap with an attractant and killing them with an insecticide in a lethal ovitrap helped to reduce the menace of blood feeding insects in endemic areas. Although, the literature available on haematophagous insects is biased to some extent, location specific effort should be undertaken to study the oviposition behavior of blood feeding insects. Modern extraction techniques, such as head space-solid phase microextraction, liquid phase microextraction, and gas chromatography–mass spectrometry could still be efficiently used for the isolation and identification of newer semiochemicals and pheromone molecules and designing cost effective, newer synthetic protocols for maximum recovery of intended pheromone compound is preferred. Research on trapping technologies for the target insects need to be expanded to minimize the vector population and disease transmission. Understanding on the oviposition ecology of haematophagous insects would guide us to device newer strategies which could be combined with the existing methods of integrated vector management.

ACKNOWLEDGEMENTS

The authors wish to thank Professor Gerald Litwack for his invitation to contribute this chapter. The encouragement and help received from the Head of the Department, for writing the chapter is sincerely acknowledged. We thank all the members of our laboratory for their cordial guidance during the course of writing this review. We sincerely thank all those authors, who provided reprints of their literature on request for reference and citation in this work.

REFERENCES

Achee, N. L., Grieco, J. P., Andre, R. G., Roberts, D. R., and Rejmankova, E. (2006). Experimental evaluation of overhanging bamboo in *Anopheles darlingi* larval habitat selection in Belize, Central America. *J. Vector Ecol.* **31,** 145–151.

Ahmadi, A., and McClelland, G. A. H. (1983). Oviposition attractants of the western treehole mosquito, *Aedes sierrensis*. *Mosq. News.* **43,** 343–345.

Allan, S. A., and Kline, D. L. (1998). Larval rearing water and preexisting eggs influence oviposition by *Aedes aegypti* and *Ae. albopictus* (Diptera: Culicidae). *J. Med. Entomol.* **35,** 943–947.

Allan, S. A., Bernier, U. R., and Kline, D. L. (2005). Evaluation of oviposition substrates and organic infusions on collection of *Culex* in Florida. *J. Am. Mosq. Control Assoc.* **21,** 268–273.

Alves, J. C. M., Hamilton, J. G. C., and Brazil, R. P. (2003). Oviposition response of *Lutzomyia renei* (Martins, Falcao & Silva) (Diptera:Psychodidae) to extracts of conspecific eggs in laboratory bioassays. *Entomotropica.* **18,** 121–126.

Anderson, J. F., Ferrandino, F. J., McKnight, S., Nolen, J., and Miller, J. (2009). A carbon dioxide, heat and chemical lure trap for the bed bug, *Cimex lectularius*. *Med. Vet. Entomol.* **23,** 99–105.

Arav, D., and Blaustein, L. (2006). Effects of pool depth and risk of predation on oviposition habitat selection by temporary pool dipterans. *J. Med. Entomol.* **43,** 493–497.

Ashworth, J. R., and Wall, R. (1994). Responses of sheep blowflies *Lucila sericata* and *L. cuprina* to odour and the development of semiochemicals baits. *Med. Vet. Entomol.* **8,** 303–309.

Ballard, E. M., Waller, J. H., and Knapp, F. W. (1987). Occurrence and ovitrap site preference of tree hole mosquitoes: *Aedes triseriatus* and *Aedes hendersoni* in eastern Kentucky. *J. Am. Mosq. Control Assoc.* **3,** 42–44.

Barbosa, R. M. R., Souto, A., Eiras, A. E., and Regis, L. (2007). Laboratory and field evaluation of an oviposition trap for *Culex quinquefasciatus* (Diptera: Culicidae). *Mem. Inst. Oswaldo Cruz.* **102,** 523–529.

Beehler, J. W., and Defoliart, G. R. (1990). A field evaluation of two suggested *Aedes triseriatus* oviposition attractants. *J. Am. Mosq. Control Assoc.* **6,** 721–723.

Beehler, J. W., Millar, J. G., and Mulla, M. S. (1993). Synergism between chemical attractants and visual cues influencing oviposition of the mosquito, *Culex quinquefasciatus* (Diptera: Culicidae). *J. Chem. Ecol.* **20,** 281–291.

Beehler, J. W., Millar, J. G., and Mulla, M. S. (1994). Protein hydrolysates and associated bacterial contaminants as oviposition attractants for the mosquito *Culex quinquefasciatus*. *Med. Vet. Entomol.* **8,** 381–385.

Benoit, J. B., Phillips, S. A., Croxall, T. J., Christensen, B. S., Yoder, J. A., and Denlinger, D. L. (2009). Addition of alarm pheromone components improves the effectiveness of desiccant dusts against *Cimex lectularius*. *J. Med. Entomol.* **46,** 572–579.

Bentley, M. D., and Day, J. F. (1989). Chemical ecology and behavioral aspects of mosquito oviposition. *Annu. Rev. Entomol.* **34,** 401–421.

Bentley, M. D., Mcdaniel, I. N., Lee, H. P., Stiehl, B., and Yatagai, M.,. (1976). Studies of *Aedes triseriatus* oviposition attractants produced by larvae of *Aedes triseriatus* and *Aedes atropalpus* (Diptera: Culicidae). *J. Med. Entomol.* **13,** 112–115.

Bentley, M. D., Mcdaniel, I. N., Yatagai, M., Lee, H. P., and Maynard, R. (1979). *p*-Cresol: An oviposition attractant of *Aedes triseriatus*. *Environ. Entomol.* **8**, 206–209.

Bentley, M. D., Mcdaniel, I. N., and Davis, E. E. (1982). Studies of 4-methylcyclohexanol: An *Aedes triseriatus* (Diptera: Culicidae) oviposition attractant. *J. Med. Entomol.* **19,** 589–592.

Benzon, G. L., Apperson, C. S., and Clay, W. (1988). Factors affecting oviposition site preference by *Toxorhynchites splendens* in the laboratory. *J. Am. Mosq. Control Assoc.* **4,** 20–22.

Birkett, M. A., Agelopoulos, N., Jensen, K. M. V., Jespersen, J. B., Pickett, J. A., Prijs, H. J., Thomas, G., Trapman, J. J., Wadhams, L. J., and Woodcock, C. M. (2004). The role of semiochemicals in mediating host location and selection by nuisance and disease transmitting cattle flies. *Med. Vet. Entomol.* **18,** 313–322.

Blackwell, A., and Johnson, S. N. (2000). Electrophysiological investigation of larval water and potential oviposition chemo-attractants for *Anopheles gambiae s.s. Ann. Trop. Med. Parasitol.* **94,** 389–398.

Blackwell, A., Mordue, A. J., Hansson, B. S., Wadhams, L. J., and Pickett, J. A. (1993). A behavioural and electrophysiological study of oviposition cues for *Culex quinquefasciatus*. *Physiol. Entomol.* **18,** 343–348.

Blair, J. A., Mordue-Luntz, A. J., Duffy, J. A., and Wardell, J. L. (1994). Use of metal carboxylate glasses in the controlled release of bioactive molecules: *Culex quinquefasciatus* oviposition pheromone. *J. Control. Release.* **31,** 145–149.

Blaustein, L. (1998). Influence of predatory backswimmer, *Notonecta maculata*, on invertebrate community structure. *Ecol. Entomol.* **23,** 246–252.

Blaustein, L., Kiflawi, M., Eitam, A., Mangel, M., and Cohen, J. E. (2004). Oviposition habitat selection in response to risk of predation in temporary pools: Mode of detection and consistency across experimental venue. *Oecologia.* **138,** 300–305.

Blaustein, L., Blaustein, J., and Chase, J. (2005). Chemical detection of the predator *Notonecta irrorata* by ovipositing *Culex* mosquitoes. *J. Vector Ecol.* **30,** 299–301.

Braks, M. A., Leal, W. S., and Cardé, R. T. (2007). Oviposition responses of gravid female *Culex quinquefasciatus* to egg rafts and low doses of oviposition pheromone under semi-field conditions. *J. Chem. Ecol.* **33,** 567–578.
Bruno, D. W., and Laurence, B. R. (1979). The influence of the apical droplet of *Culex* egg rafts on ovposition of *Culex pipiens fatigans* (Diptera: Culicidae). *J. Med. Entomol.* **6,** 300–305.
Burkett, D. A., Kelly, R., Porter, C. H., and Wirtz, R. A. (2004). Commercial mosquito trap and gravid trap oviposition media evaluation, Atlanta, Georgia. *J. Am. Mosq. Control Assoc.* **20,** 233–238.
Burkett-Cadena, N. D., and Mullen, G. R. (2007). Field comparison of Bermuda-hay infusion to infusions of emergent aquatic vegetation for collecting female mosquitoes. *J. Am. Mosq. Control Assoc.* **23,** 117–123.
Cabrera, M., and Jaffe, K. (2007). An aggregation pheromone modulates lekking behavior in the vector mosquito *Aedes aegypti* (Diptera: Culicidae). *J. Am. Mosq. Control Assoc.* **23,** 1–10.
Chadee, D. D., Lakhan, A., Ramdath, W. R., and Persad, R. C. (1993). Oviposition response of *Aedes aegypti* mosquitoes to different concentrations of hay infusion in Trinidad, West Indies. *J. Am. Mosq. Control Assoc.* **9,** 346–348.
Chadee, D. D., Corbet, P. S., and Talbot, H. (1995). Proportions of eggs laid by *Aedes aegypti* on different substrates within an ovitrap in Trinidad, West Indies. *Med. Vet. Entomol.* **9,** 66–70.
Chesson, J. (1984). Effect of *Notonectids* (Hemiptera: Notonectidae) on mosquitoes (Diptera: Culicidae): Predation or selective oviposition. *Environ. Entomol.* **13,** 531–538.
Clements, A. N. (1999). The Biology of Mosquitoes. CABI, Wallingford.
Collins, L. E., and Blackwell, A. (1998). Electroantennogram studies of potential oviposition attractants for *Toxorhynchites moctezuma* and *T. amboinensis* mosquitoes. *Physiol. Entomol.* **23,** 214–219.
Collins, L. E., and Blackwell, A. (2002). Olfactory cues for oviposition behavior in *Toxorhynchites moctezuma* and *Toxorhynchites amboinensis* (Diptera: Culicidae). *J. Med. Entomol.* **39,** 121–126.
Cork, A. (1994). Identification of electrophysiologically-active compounds for New world screwworm, *Cochliomyia hominivorax* in larval wound fluid. *Med. Vet. Entomol.* **8,** 151–159.
Couladouros, E. A., and Mihou, A. P. (1999). A general synthetic route towards gamma- and delta-lactones. Total asymmetric synthesis of (−)-muricatacin and the mosquito oviposition pheromone (5R,6S)-6-acetoxy-hexadecanolide. *Tetrahedron Lett.* **40,** 4861–4862.
Crespo, J. G., and Manrique, G. (2007). Mating behavior of the hematophagous bug *Triatoma infestans:* Role of Brindley's and metasternal glands. *J. Insect Physiol.* **53,** 708–714.
Cruz-Lopez, L., Malo, E. A., and Rojas, J. C. (1993). Aggregation pheromone in five species of *Triatominae* (Hemiptera: Reduviidae). *Mem. Inst. Oswaldo Cruz.* **88,** 535–539.
Cruz-López, L., Malo, E. A., Rojas, J. C., and Morgan, E. D. (2001). Chemical ecology of triatomine bugs: Vectors of Chagas disease. *Med. Vet. Entomol.* **15,** 351–357.
Dawson, G. W., Laurence, B. R., Pickett, J. A., Pile, M. M., and Wadhams, L. J. (1989). A note on the mosquito oviposition pheromone. *Pestic. Sci.* **27,** 277–280.
Dawson, G. W., Mudd, A., Pickett, J. A., Pile, M. M., and Wadhams, L. J. (1990). Convenient synthesis of mosquito oviposition pheromone and a highly fluorinated analog retaining biological activity. *J. Chem. Ecol.* **16,** 1779–1789.
Dhileepan, K. (1997). Physical factors and chemical cues in the oviposition behavior of arboviral vectors *Culex annulirostris* and *Culex molestus* (Diptera: Culicidae). *Environ. Entomol.* **26,** 318–326.

Dhotare, B., Goswami, D., and Chattopadhyay, A. (2005). (R)-2,3-Cyclohexylideneglyceraldehyde, a novel template for stereoselective preparation of functionalized δ-lactones. *Tetrahedron Lett.* **46,** 6219–6221.

Dougherty, M., and Hamilton, G. (1997). Dodecanoic acid is the oviposition pheromone of *Lutzomyia longipalpis. J. Chem. Ecol.* **23,** 2657–2671.

Dougherty, M. J., Ward, R. D., and Hamilton, G. (1992). Evidence for the accessory glands as the site of the oviposition attractant and/or stimulant of *Lutzomyia longipalpis* (Diptera: Psychodidae). *J. Chem. Ecol.* **18,** 1165–1175.

Dougherty, M. J., Hamilton, J. G. C., and Ward, R. D. (1993). Semiochemical mediation of oviposition by the phlebotomine sandfly *Lutzomyia longipalpis. Med. Vet. Entomol.* **7,** 219–224.

Dougherty, M. J., Hamilton, J. G. C., and Ward, R. D. (1994). Isolation of oviposition pheromone from the eggs of the sandfly *Lutzomyia longipalpis. Med. Vet. Entomol.* **8,** 119–124.

Dougherty, M. J., Guerin, P. M., and Ward, R. D. (1995) Identification of oviposition attractants pheromone for the sandfly *Lutzomyia longipalpis* (Diptera: Psychodidae) in volatiles of faeces from vertebrates. *Physiol. Entomol.* **20,** 23–32.

Du, Y., and Millar, J. G. (1999a). Electroantennogram and oviposition bioassay responses of *Culex quinquefasciatus* and *Culex tarsalis* (Diptera: Culicidae) to chemicals in odors from Bermuda grass infusions. *J. Med. Entomol.* **36,** 158–166.

Du, Y., and Millar, J. G. (1999b). Oviposition responses of gravid *Culex quinquefasciatus* and *Culex tarsalis* to bulrush (*Schoenoplectus acutus*) infusions. *J. Am. Mosq. Control Assoc.* **15,** 500–509.

El Naiem, D. A., and Ward, R. D. (1990). An oviposition pheromone on the eggs of sandflies [*Lutzomyia longipalpis*] (Diptera: Psychodidae). *Trans. R. Soc. Trop. Med. Hyg.* **84,** 456–457.

El Naiem, D. A., and Ward, R. D. (1991). Response of the sandfly *Lutzomyia longipalpis* to an oviposition pheromone associated with conspecific eggs. *Med. Vet. Entomol.* **5,** 87–91.

El Naiem, D. A., Ward, R. D., and Rees, H. H. (1991). Chemical factors controlling oviposition of *Lutzomyia longipalpis* (Diptera: Psychodidae). *Parasitologia.* **33**(Suppl), 217–224.

Figueiras, A. N. L., and Lazzari, C. R. (2000). Temporal change of the aggregation response in *Triatoma infestans. Mem. Inst. Oswaldo Cruz.* **95,** 889–892.

Gallos, J. K., Mihelakis, D. S., Dellios, C. C., and Pozarentzi, M. E. (2000). A new synthesis of (−)-(5R,6S)-6-acetoxy-5-hexadecanolide, the mosquito *Culex pipiens fatigans* oviposition attractant pheromone. *Heterocycles.* **53,** 703.

Ganesan, K., Mendki, M. J., Suryanarayana, M. V. S., Prakash, S., and Malhotra, R. C. (2006). Studies of *Aedes aegypti* (Diptera: Culicidae) ovipositional responses to newly identified semiochemicals from conspecific eggs. *Aust. J. Entomol.* **45,** 75–80.

Ganesan, K., Malhotra, R. C., Rao, A. N., Gupta, P. K., Jain, A. K., Prakash, S., and Sekhar, K. (2009). Process for the preparation of n-Heneicosane. US Patent, Defence Research & Development Organisation, New Delhi, India, pp. 4.

Geetha, I., Paily, K. P., Padmanaban, V., and Balaraman, K. (2003). Oviposition response of the mosquito, *Culex quinquefasciatus* to the secondary metabolite(s) of the fungus, *Trichoderma viride. Mem. Inst. Oswaldo Cruz.* **98,** 223–226.

George, N., Ramiah, K. D., Sujatha, C. H., Kalyanasundaram, M., and Das, P. K. (1986). Oviposition attractancy of some substituted esters and the pheromone extracted from egg rafts against *Culex quinquefasciatus. Curr. Sci.* **55,** 1205–1207.

Huang, J., Miller, J. R., Chen, S. C., Vulule, J. M., and Walker, E. D. (2006a). *Anopheles gambiae* (Diptera: Culicidae) oviposition in response to agarose media and cultured bacterial volatiles. *J. Med. Entomol.* **43,** 498–504.

Huang, J., Walker, E., Otienoburu, P., Amimo, F., Vulule, J., and Miller, J. (2006b). Laboratory tests of oviposition by the African malaria mosquito, *Anopheles gambiae*, on dark soil as influenced by presence or absence of vegetation. *Malar. J.* **5,** 88.

Ichimoto, I., Yoshizawa, T., Machiya, K., Kirihata, M., and Ueda, H. (1988). An efficient synthesis of mosquito oviposition attractant pheromone, (5R,6S)-(−)-6-acetoxy-5-hexadecanolide. *Chemistry Express.* **3,** 687–690.

Ikishima, H., Sekiguchi, Y., Ichikawa, Y., and Kotsuki, H. (2006). Synthesis of (−)-(5R,6S)-6-acetoxyhexadecanolide based on L-proline-catalyzed asymmetric aldol reactions. *Tetrahedron.* **62,** 311–316.

Isoe, J., Beehler, J. W., Millar, J. G., and Mulla, M. S. (1995). Oviposition responses of *Culex tarsalis* and *Culex quinquefasciatus* to aged Bermuda grass infusions. *J. Am. Mosq. Control Assoc.* **11,** 39–44.

Jackson, B. T., Paulson, S. L., Youngman, R. R., Scheffel, S. L., and Hawkins, B. (2005). Oviposition preferences of *Culex restuans* and *Culex pipiens* (Diptera: Culicidae) for selected infusions in oviposition traps and gravid traps. *J. Am. Mosq. Control Assoc.* **21,** 360–365.

Jeanbourquin, P., and Guerin, P. M. (2007). Chemostimuli implicated in selection of oviposition substrates by the stable fly *Stomoxys calcitrans. Med. Vet. Entomol.* **21,** 209–216.

Jefford, C. W., Jaggi, D., and Boukouvalas, J. (1986). A short, stereodivergent synthesis of the racemic erythro and threo diastereomers of 6-acetoxy-5-hexadecanolide, a mosquito oviposition attractant pheromone. *Tetrahedron Lett.* **27,** 4011–4014.

Jordan, S., and Hubbard, S. F. (1991). Influence of vegetation on the spatial distribution of *Toxorhynchites moctezuma* ovipositions in the field. *J. Am. Mosq. Control Assoc.* **7,** 126–128.

Kabeh, J. D. (2007). Influence of semiochemicals on group behaviors and application in insect pest and vector management. *Int. J. Agric. Biol.* **9,** 937–940.

Kalpage, K. S. P., and Brust, R. A. (1973). Oviposition attractant produced by immature *Aedes atropalpus. Environ. Entomol.* **2,** 729–730.

Kay, B. H., Sutton, K. A., and Russell, B. M. (2000). A sticky entry–exit trap for sampling mosquitoes in subterranean habitats. *J. Am. Mosq. Control Assoc.* **16,** 262–265.

Kite, G. C. (1995). The floral odor of *Arum maculatum. Biochem. Syst. Ecol.* **23,** 343–354.

Kitron, U. D., Webb, D. W., and Novak, R. J. (1989). Oviposition behavior of *Aedes triseriatus* (Diptera: Culicidae): Prevalence, intensity, and aggregation of eggs in oviposition traps. *J. Med. Entomol.* **26,** 462–467.

Kline, D. L. (2007). Semiochemicals, traps/targets and mass trapping technology for mosquito management. *Am. Mosq. Control Assoc. Bull.* **23,** 241–251.

Ko, K. Y., and Eliel, E. L. (1986). Asymmetric synthesis of (5R,6S)-6-acetoxy-5-hexadecanolide, the major component of the oviposition attractant pheromone of the mosquito *Culex pipiens fatigans*, and two of its stereoisomers. *J. Org. Chem.* **51,** 5353–5362.

Kramer, W. L., and Mulla, M. S. (1979). Oviposition attractants and repellents of mosquitoes: oviposition responses of *Culex* Mosquitoes to organic infusions. *Environ. Entomol.* **8,** 1111–1117.

Lampman, R. L., and Novak, R. J. (1996). Oviposition preferences of *Culex pipiens* and *Culex restuans* for infusion-baited traps. *J. Am. Mosq. Control Assoc.* **12,** 23–32.

Lang, J. T. (1990). Ovipositional response of *Aedes triseriatus* females to horizontally and vertically open ovitraps in Southern Illinois. *J. Am. Mosq. Control Assoc.* **6,** 530–531.

Laurence, B. R., and Pickett, J. A. (1982). *Erythro*-6-acetoxy-5-hexadecanolide, the major component of a mosquito oviposition attractant pheromone. *J. Chem. Soc. Chem. Commun.* 59–60.

Laurence, B. R., and Pickett, J. A. (1985). An oviposition pheromone in *Culex quinquefasciatus* Say (Diptera: Culicidae). *Bull. Ent. Res.* **75,** 283–290.

Lazzari, C. R. (2009). Orientation towards hosts in haematophagous insects: An integrative perspective. *In* "Advances in Insect Physiology," (S. J. Simpson and J. Casas, Eds.), Vol. 37, pp. 1–58. Academic Press, New York.

Lenhart, A. E., Walle, M., Cedillo, H., and Kroeger, A. (2005). Building a better ovitrap for detecting *Aedes aegypti* oviposition. *Acta Trop.* **96,** 56–59.

Leonard, D. E., and Saini, R. K. (1993). Semiochemicals from anal exudate of larvae of tsetse flies *Glossina morsitans morsitans* Westwood and *G. morsitans centralis* Machado attract gravid flies. *J. Chem. Ecol.* **19,** 2039–2046.

Levinson, H. Z., and Bar-Ilan, A. R. (1971). Assembling and alerting scents produced by the bedbug *Cimex lectularius* L. *Experientia.* **27,** 102–103.

Levinson, H. Z., Levinson, A. R., Muller, B., and Steinbrecht, R. A. (1974). Structure of sensilla, olfactory perception and behavior of the bedbug *Cimex lectularius* in response to its alarm pheromone. *J. Insect Physiol.* **20,** 1231–1248.

Linley, J. R. (1989). Laboratory tests of the effects of *p*-cresol and 4-methylcyclohexanol on oviposition by three species of *Toxorhynchites* mosquitoes. *Med. Vet. Entomol.* **3,** 347–352.

Logan, J. G., and Birkett, M. A. (2007). Semiochemicals for biting fly control: Their identification and exploitation. *Pest Manag. Sci.* **63,** 647–657.

Lorenzo Figueiras, A. N., and Lazzari, C. R. (1998a). Aggregation behaviour and interspecific responses in three species of *Triatominae*. *Mem. Inst. Oswaldo Cruz.* **93,** 133–137.

Lorenzo Figueiras, A. N., and Lazzari, C. R. (1998b). Aggregation in the haematophagous bug *Triatoma infestans*: A novel assembling factor. *Physiol. Entomol.* **23,** 33–37.

Lorenzo, M. G., and Lazzari, C. R. (1996). The spatial pattern of defaecation in *Triatoma infestans* and the role of faeces as a chemical mark of the refuge. *J. Insect Physiol.* **42,** 903–907.

Lorenzo, M. G., and Lazzari, C. R. (1998). Activity pattern in relation to refuge exploitation and feeding in *Triatoma infestans* (Hemiptera: Reduviidae). *Acta Trop.* **70,** 163–170.

Lorenzo, M. G., Reisenman, C. E., and Lazzari, C. R. (1998). *Triatoma infestans* can be captured under natural climatic conditions using yeast-baited traps. *Acta Trop.* **70,** 277–284.

Lowenberger, C. A., and Rau, M. E. (1994). Selective oviposition by *Aedes aegypti* (Diptera: Culicidae) in response to a larval parasite, *Plagiorchis elegans* (Trematoda: Plagiochiidae). *Environ. Entomol.* **23,** 1269–1276.

Maire, A. (1985). Effect of axenic larvae on the oviposition site selection by *Aedes atropalpus*. *J. Am. Mosq. Control Assoc.* **1,** 320–323.

McCall, P. J. (1995a). The latest in the *Simulium damnosum* oviposition aggregation pheromone story. *Br. Simuliid Group Bull.* **6,** 7–9.

McCall, P. J. (1995b). Oviposition aggregation pheromone in the *Simulium damnosum* complex. *Med. Vet. Entomol.* **9,** 101–108.

McCall, P. J. (2002). Chemoecology of oviposition in insects of medical and veterinary importance. *In* "Chemoecology of Insect Eggs an Egg Deposition," (M. Hilker and T. Meiners, Eds.), pp. 265–289. Blackwell, Berlin.

McCall, P. J., and Cameron, M. M. (1995). Oviposition pheromones in insect vectors. *Parasitol. Today.* **11,** 352–355.

McCall, P. J., Trees, A. J., Walsh, J. F., and Molyneux, D. H. (1994). Aggregated oviposition in the *Simulium damnosum* complex is mediated by eggs in a laboratory bioassay. *Med. Vet. Entomol.* **8,** 76–80.

McCall, P. J., Heath, R. R., Dueben, B. D., and Wilson, M. D. (1997). Oviposition pheromone in the *Simulium damnosum* complex: Biological activity of chemical fractions from gravid ovaries. *Physiol. Entomol.* **22,** 224–230.

McCrae, A. W. (1984). Oviposition by African malaria vector mosquitoes. II. Effects of site tone, water type and conspecific immatures on target selection by freshwater *Anopheles gambiae* Giles, sensu lato. *Ann. Trop. Med. Parasitol.* **78,** 307–318.

McIver, S. B. (1982). Sensilla of mosquitoes (Diptera: Culicidae). *J. Med. Entomol.* **19,** 489–535.

Mendki, M. J., Ganesan, K., Prakash, S., Suryanarayana, M. V. S., Malhotra, R. C., Rao, K. M., and Vaidyanathaswamy, R. (2000). Heneicosane: An oviposition-attractant pheromone of larval origin in *Aedes aegypti* mosquito. *Curr. Sci.* **78,** 1295–1296.

Michaelakis, A., Mihou, A. P., Couladouros, E. A., Zounos, A. K., and Koliopoulos, G. (2005). Oviposition responses of *Culex pipiens* to a synthetic racemic *Culex quinquefasciatus* oviposition aggregation pheromone. *J. Agric. Food Chem.* **53,** 5225–5229.
Michaelakis, A., Mihou, A. P., Koliopoulos, G., and Couladouros, E. A. (2007). Attract-and-kill strategy. Laboratory studies on hatched larvae of *Culex pipiens*. *Pest Manag. Sci.* **63,** 954–959.
Michaelakis, A., Mihou, A. P., Koliopoulos, G., and Couladouros, E. A. (2009). Influence of the microencapsulated pheromone from aged infusion as an oviposition medium of the West Nile virus vector *Culex pipiens*. *Parasitol. Res.* **104,** 1005–1009.
Millar, J. G., Chaney, J. D., and Mulla, M. S. (1992). Identification of oviposition attractants for *Culex quinquefasciatus* from fermented Bermuda grass infusions. *J. Am. Mosq. Control Assoc.* **8,** 11–17.
Millar, J. G., Chaney, J. D., Beehler, J. W., and Mulla, M. S. (1994). Interaction of the *Culex quinquefasciatus* egg raft pheromone with a natural chemical associated with oviposition sites. *J. Am. Mosq. Control Assoc.* **10,** 374–379.
Minoli, S. A., Baraballe, S., and Figueiras, A. N. L. (2007). Daily rhythm of aggregation in the haematophagous bug *Triatoma infestans* (Heteroptera: Reduviidae). *Mem. Inst. Oswaldo Cruz.* **102,** 449–454.
Mordue (Luntz), A. J. (2003). Arthropod semiochemicals: Mosquitoes, midges and sealice. *Biochem. Soc. Trans.* **31,** 128–133.
Mordue (Luntz), A. J., and Mordue, B. (2003). Biting midge chemical ecology. *Biologist.* **50,** 159–162.
Mordue, A. J., Blackwell, A., Hansson, B. S., Wadhams, L. J., and Pickett, J. A. (1992). Behavioural and electrophysiological evaluation of oviposition attractants for *Culex quinquefasciatus* Say (Diptera: Culicidae). *Experientia.* **48,** 1109–1111.
Nash, T. A. M., Trewern, M. A., and Moloo, S. K. (1976). Observations on the free larval stage of *Glossina morsitans morsitans* Westw. (Diptera; Glossinidae). *Bull. Ent. Res.* **71,** 81–96.
Navarro, D. M. A. F., Oliveira, P. E. S. D., Potting, R. P. J., Brito, A. C., and Fital, S. J. F. (2003). The potential attractant or repellent effects of different water types on oviposition in *Aedes aegypti* L. (Diptera: Culicidae). *J. Appl. Entomol.* **127,** 46–50.
Navarro-Silva, M. A., Marques, F. A., and Jonny, E. D. L. (2009). Review of semiochemicals that mediate the oviposition of mosquitoes: A possible sustainable tool for controlling and monitoring of Culicidae. *Rev. Bras. Entomol.* **53,** 1–6.
Olagbemiro, T. O., Birkett, M. A., Mordue, A. J., and Pickett, J. A. (1999). Production of (5R,6S)-6-acetoxy-5-hexadecanolide, the mosquito oviposition pheromone, from the seed oil of the summer cypress plant, *Kochia scoparia* (Chenopodiaceae). *J. Agric. Food Chem.* **47,** 3411–3415.
Olagbemiro, T. O., Birkett, M. A., Mordue Luntz, A. J., and Pickett, J. A. (2004). Laboratory and field responses of the mosquito, *Culex quinquefasciatus*, to plant-derived *Culex* spp. oviposition pheromone and the oviposition cue skatole. *J. Chem. Ecol.* **30,** 965–976.
Olson, J. F., Moon, R. D., and Kells, S. A. (2009). Off-host aggregation behavior and sensory basis of arrestment by *Cimex lectularius* (Heteroptera: Cimicidae). *J. Insect Physiol.* **55,** 580–587.
O'Malley, S. L., Hubbard, S. F., and Chadee, D. D. (1989). Oviposition habitat preferences of *Toxorhynchites moctezuma* mosquitoes in four types of tropical forest in Trinidad. *Med. Vet. Entomol.* **3,** 247–252.
Osgood, C. E. (1971). An oviposition pheromone associated with the egg rafts of *Culex tarsalis*. *J. Econ. Entomol.* **64,** 1038–1041.
Otieno, W. A., Onyango, T. O., Pile, M. M., Laurence, B. R., Dawson, G. W., Wadhams, L. J., and Pickett, J. A. (1988). A field trial of the synthetic oviposition pheromone with *Culex quinquefasciatus* Say (Diptera: Culicidae) in Kenya. *Bull. Ent. Res.* **78,** 463–478.

Parashar, B. D., Ganesan, K., Sukumaran, D., Rao, Y. V. S., Veer, V., and Prakash, S. (2003). Aggregation activity induced by the excreta extracts in *Cimex hemipterus* (Hemiptera: Cimicidae). *Entomon.* **28,** 215–222.

Perry, A. S., and Fay, W. (1967). Correlation of chemical constitution and physical properties of fatty acid esters with oviposition response of *Aedes aegypti*. *Mosq. News* **27,** 175–182.

Pfiester, M., Koehler, P. G., and Pereira, R. M. (2009). Effect of population structure and size on aggregation behavior of *Cimex lectularius* (Hemiptera: Cimicidae). *J. Med. Entomol.* **46,** 1015.

Pickett, J. A., Wadhams, L. J., and Woodcock, C. M. (1998). Mate and host location by insect model systems for exploiting olfactory interactions. *Biochemist.* **20,** 8–13.

Pile, M. M., Simmonds, M. S. J., and Blaney, W. M. (1991). Odour-mediated upwind flight of *Culex quinquefasciatus* mosquitoes elicited by a synthetic attractant. *Physiol. Entomol.* **16,** 77–85.

Pimenta, F. E., Diotaiuti, L., Lima, A. C. L., and Lorenzo, M. G. (2007). Evaluation of cultures of *Saccharomyces cerevisiae* as baits for *Triatoma dimidiata* and *Triatoma pallidipennis*. *Mem. Inst. Oswaldo Cruz.* **102,** 229–231.

Pires, H. H. R., Lorenzo, M. G., Diotaiuti, L., Lazzari, C. R., and Figueiras, A. N. L. (2002). Aggregation behaviour in *Panstrongylus megistus* and *Triatoma infestans*: Inter and intraspecific responses. *Acta Trop.* **81,** 47–52.

Ponnusamy, L., Xu, N., Nojima, S., Wesson, D. M., Schal, C., and Apperson, C. S. (2008). Identification of bacteria and bacteria-associated chemical cues that mediate oviposition site preferences by *Aedes aegypti*. *Proc. Natl. Acad. Sci. USA.* **105,** 9262–9267.

Poonam, S., Paily, K. P., and Balaraman, K. (2002). Oviposition attractancy of bacterial culture filtrates response of *Culex quinquefasciatus*. *Mem. Inst. Oswaldo Cruz.* **97,** 359–362.

Prasad, K. R., and Anbarasan, P. (2007). Stereoselective synthesis of (−)-6-acetoxy hexadecanolide: A mosquito oviposition attractant pheromone. *Tetrahedron Asym.* **18,** 2479–2483.

Quinn, K. J., Curto, J. M., McGrath, K. P., and Biddick, N. A. (2009). Facile synthesis of (−)-6-acetoxy-5-hexadecanolide by size-selective ring-closing/cross metathesis. *Tetrahedron Lett.* **50,** 7121–7123.

Ramaswamy, S., and Oehlschlager, A. C. (1991). Chemico-microbial syntheses of Japanese beetle and mosquito oviposition pheromones. *Tetrahedron.* **47,** 1145.

Reisenman, C. E., Figueiras, A. N. L., Giurfa, M., and Lazzari, C. R. (2000). Interaction of visual and olfactory cues in the aggregation behaviour of the haematophagous bug *Triatoma infestans*. *J. Comp. Physiol. A Sens. Neural. Behav. Physiol.* **186,** 961–968.

Reiter, P., Amador, M. A., and Colon, N. (1991). Enhancement of the CDC ovitrap with hay infusions for daily monitoring of *Aedes aegypti* populations. *J. Am. Mosq. Control Assoc.* **7,** 52–55.

Rejmankova, E., Roberts, D. R., Manguin, S., Pope, K. O., Komarek, J., and Post, R. A. (1996). *Anopheles albimanus* (Diptera: Culicidae) and cyanobacteria: An example of larval habitat selection. *Environ. Entomol.* **25,** 1058–1067.

Rejmankova, E., Higashi, R., Grieco, J., Achee, N., and Roberts, D. (2005). Volatile substances from larval habitats mediate species-specific oviposition in *Anopheles* mosquitoes. *J. Med. Entomol.* **42,** 95–103.

Renou, M., and Guerrero, A. (2000). Insect parapheromones in olfaction research and semiochemical based pest control strategies. *Annu. Rev. Entomol.* **48,** 605–639.

Reuben, R., Panicker, K. N., Dass, P. K., Kasmi, S. J., and Suguna, S. G. (1977). A new paddle for the black jar ovitrap for surveillance of *Aedes aegypti*. *Indian J. Med. Res.* **65**(Suppl.), 115–119.

Reuben, R., Das, P. K., Kazmi, S. J., and Brooks, G. D. (1978). Seasonal changes in egg-laying activity of *Aedes* species in Sonepat by the use of black jar ovitraps. *Indian J. Med. Res.* **67,** 763–766.

Ritchie, S. A., and Laidlaw-Bell, C. (1994). Do fish repel oviposition by *Aedes taeniorhynchus*? *J. Am. Mosq. Control Assoc.* **10,** 380–384.

Ritchie, S. A., and Long, S. (2003). Does S-methoprene affect oviposition by *Aedes aegypti* in an ovitrap? *J. Am. Mosq. Control Assoc.* **19,** 170–171.

Ritchie, S. A., Long, S., Hart, A., Webb, C. E., and Russell, R. C. (2003). An adulticidal sticky ovitrap for sampling container-breeding mosquitoes. *J. Am. Mosq. Control Assoc.* **19,** 235–242.

Ritchie, S. A., Long, S. A., McCaffrey, N., Key, C., Lonergan, G., and Williams, C. R. (2008). A biodegradable lethal ovitrap for control of container-breeding *Aedes*. *J. Am. Mosq. Control Assoc.* **24,** 47–53.

Robacker, D. C., and Bartelt, R. J. (1997). Chemical attractive to Mexican fruit fly from *Klebsiella pneumoniae* and *Citrobacter freundii* cultures sampled by solid-phase microextraction. *J. Chem. Ecol.* **23,** 2897–2915.

Romero, A., Broce, A., and Zurek, L. (2006). Role of bacteria in the oviposition behaviour and larval development of stable flies. *Med. Vet. Entomol.* **20,** 115–121.

Russell, R. C., and Ritchie, S. A. (2004). Surveillance and behavioral investigations of *Aedes aegypti* and *Aedes polynesiensis* in Moorea, French Polynesia, using a sticky ovitrap. *J. Am. Mosq. Control Assoc.* **20,** 370–375.

Ryne, C. (2009). Homosexual interactions in bed bugs: Alarm pheromones as male recognition signals. *Anim. Behav.* **78,** 1471–1475.

Saini, R. K., Hassanali, A., Andoke, J., Ahuya, P., and Ouma, W. P. (1996). Identification of the major components of larviposition pheromone from larvae of tsetse flies *Glossina morsitans morsitans* Westwood and *G.morsitans centralis* Machado. *J. Chem. Ecol.* **22,** 1211–1220.

Santana, A. L., Roque, R. A., and Eiras, A. E. (2006). Characteristics of grass infusions as oviposition attractants to *Aedes* (Stegomyia) (Diptera: Culicidae). *J. Med. Entomol.* **43,** 214–220.

Schilman, P. E., Núñez, J., and Lazzari, C. R. (1996). Attributes of oviposition substrates affect fecundity in *Rhodnius prolixus*. *J. Insect Physiol.* **42,** 837–841.

Schofield, C. J., and Patterson, J. W. (1977). Assembly pheromone of *Triatoma infestans* and *Rhodnius prolixus* nymphs (Hemiptera: Reduviidae). *J. Med. Entomol.* **13,** 727–734.

Seenivasagan, T., Sharma, K. R., Sekhar, K., Ganesan, K., Prakash, S., and Vijayaraghavan, R. (2009). Electroantennogram, flight orientation, and oviposition responses of *Aedes aegypti* to the oviposition pheromone n-heneicosane. *Parasitol. Res.* **104,** 827–833.

Sharma, K. R., Seenivasagan, T., Rao, A. N., Ganesan, K., Agarwal, O. P., Malhotra, R. C., and Prakash, S. (2008). Oviposition responses of *Aedes aegypti* and *Aedes albopictus* to certain fatty acid esters. *Parasitol. Res.* **103,** 1065–1073.

Sharma, K. R., Seenivasagan, T., Rao, A. N., Ganesan, K., Agrawal, O. P., and Prakash, S. (2009). Mediation of oviposition responses in the malaria mosquito *Anopheles stephensi* Liston by certain fatty acid esters. *Parasitol. Res.* **104,** 281–286.

Silberbush, A., and Blaustein, L. (2008). Oviposition habitat selection by a mosquito in response to a predator: Are predator-released kairomones air-borne cues? *J. Vector Ecol.* **33,** 208–211.

Siljander, E., Penman, D., Harlan, H., and Gries, G. (2007). Evidence for male and juvenile specific contact pheromones of the common bed bug *Cimex lectularius*. *Entomol. Exp. Appl.* **125,** 215–219.

Siljander, E., Gries, R., Khaskin, G., and Gries, G. (2008). Identification of the air borne aggregation pheromone of the common bed bug, *Cimex lectularius*. *J. Chem. Ecol.* **34,** 708–718.

Singh, S., and Guiry, P. J. (2009). A facile synthesis of both enantiomers of 6-acetoxy-5-hexadecanolide, a major component of mosquito oviposition attractant pheromones. *Eur. J. Org. Chem.* **12,** 1896–1901.

Sivagnaname, N., Amalraj, D. D., Kalyanasundaram, M., and Das, P. K. (2001). Oviposition attractancy of an infusion from a wood inhabiting fungus for vector mosquitoes. *Indian J. Med. Res.* **114,** 18–24.

Skubatz, H., Kunkel, D. D., Howald, W. N., *et al.* (1996). The *Sauromatum guttatum* appendix as an osmophore: Excretory pathways, composition of volatiles and attractiveness to insects. *New Phytol.* **134,** 631–640.

Srinivasan, R., Radjame, K., Panicker, K. N., and Dhanda, V. (1995). Response of gravid *Phlebotomus papatasi* females to an oviposition attractant/stimulant associated with conspecific eggs. *Indian J. Exp. Biol.* **33,** 757–760.

Starratt, A. N., and Osgood, C. E. (1972). An oviposition pheromone of the mosquito *Culex tarsalis*: Diglyceride composition of the active fraction. *Biochim. Biophys. Acta (BBA)/ Lipids Lipid Metab.* **280,** 187–193.

Starratt, A. N., and Osgood, C. E. (1973). 1,3-Diglycerides from eggs of *Culex pipiens quinquefasciatus* and *Culex pipiens pipiens*. *Comp. Biochem. Physiol. B Biochem. Mol. Biol.* **46,** 857–859.

Stav, G., and Blaustein, L. M. J. (1999). Experimental evidence for predation risk sensitive oviposition by a mosquito, *Culiseta longiareolata*. *Ecol. Entomol.* **24,** 202–207.

Stav, G., Blaustein, L., and Margalit, Y. (2000). Influence of nymphal Anax imperator (Odonata: Aeshnidae) on oviposition by the mosquito *Culiseta longiareolata* (Diptera: Culicidae) and community structure in temporary pools. *J. Vector Ecol.* **25,** 190–202.

Sumba, L. A., Ogbunugafor, C. B., Deng, A. L., and Hassanali, A. (2008). Regulation of oviposition in *Anopheles gambiae* s.s.: Role of inter and intra-specific signals. *J. Chem. Ecol.* **34,** 1430–1436.

Sun, B., Peng, L. Z., Chen, X. S., Li, Y. L., Li, Y., and Yamasaki, K. (2005). Synthesis of (−)—(5R,6S)-6-acetoxyhexadecan-5-olide by L-proline-catalyzed asymmetric aldol reactions. *Tetrahedron Asym.* **16,** 1305–1307.

Taneja, J., and Guerin, P. M. (1997). Ammonia attracts the haematophagous bug *Triatoma infestans*: Behavioral and neurophysiological data on nymphs. *J Comp. Physiol. A* **181,** 21–34.

Torres-Estrada, J. L., Rodríguez, M. H., Cruz-López, L., and Arredondo-Jimenez, J. I. (2001). Selective oviposition by *Aedes aegypti* (Diptera: culicidae) in response to *Mesocyclops longisetus* (Copepoda: Cyclopoidea) under laboratory and field conditions. *J. Med. Entomol.* **38,** 188–192.

Torres-Estrada, J. L., Meza-Alvarez, R. A., Cruz-López, L., Rodríguez, M. H., and Arredondo-Jiménez, J. I. (2007). Attraction of gravid *Anopheles pseudopunctipennis* females to oviposition substrates by *Spirogyra majuscula* (Zygnematales: Zygnmataceae) algae under laboratory conditions. *J. Am. Mosq. Control Assoc.* **23,** 18–23.

Trexler, J. D., Apperson, C. S., and Schal, C. (1998). Laboratory and field evaluations of oviposition responses of *Aedes albopictus* and *Aedes triseriatus* (Diptera: Culicidae) to oak leaf infusions. *J. Med. Entomol.* **35,** 967–976.

Trexler, J. D., Apperson, C. S., Gemeno, C., Perich, M. J., Carlson, D., and Schal, C. (2003). Field and laboratory evaluations of potential oviposition attractants for *Aedes albopictus* (Diptera: Culicidae). *J. Am. Mosq. Control Assoc.* **19,** 228–234.

Van Dam, A. R., and Walton, W. E. (2008). The effect of predatory fish exudates on the ovipositional behaviour of three mosquito species: *Culex quinquefasciatus, Aedes aegypti* and *Culex tarsalis*. *Med. Vet. Entomol.* **22,** 399–404.

Vitta, A. C. R., Figueiras, A. N., Lazzari, C. R., Diotaiuti, L., and Lorenzo, M. G. (2002). Aggregation mediated by faeces and footprints in *Triatoma pseudomaculata* (Heteroptera: Reduviidae), a Chagas disease vector. *Mem. Inst. Oswaldo Cruz.* **97,** 865–867.

Vitta, A. C. R., Mota, T. R. P., Diotaiuti, L., and Lorenzo, M. G. (2007). The use of aggregation signals by *Triatoma brasiliensis* (Heteroptera: Reduviidae). *Acta Trop.* **101,** 147–152.

Wallace, F. L. (1996). Construction of a field trap for initiating an ovipositional response in *Aedes taeniorhynchus*. *J. Am. Mosq. Control Assoc.* **12,** 491–493.

Walton, W. E., Van Dam, A. R., and Popko, D. A. (2009). Ovipositional responses of two *Culex* (Diptera: Culicidae) species to Larvivorous fish. *J. Med. Entomol.* **46,** 1338–1343.

Wang, Z. M., Qian, X. H., and Zhou, W. S. (1990). Stereoselective synthesis of (−)-(5R,6S)-6-acetoxy-5-hexadecanolide, the mosquito oviposition attractant pheromone. *Tetrahedron.* **46,** 1191–1198.

Williams, C. R., Ritchie, S. A., Long, S. A., Dennison, N., and Russell, R. C. (2007). Impact of a bifenthrin-treated lethal ovitrap on *Aedes aegypti* oviposition and mortality in north Queensland, Australia. *J. Med. Entomol.* **44,** 256–262.

Wilson, M. D., Osei-Atweneboana, M. Y., Boakye, D. A., and McCall, P. J. (2000). Improved survival and oviposition of *Simulium damnosum* (Diptera: Simuliidae) in the laboratory. *Bull. Ent. Res.* **90,** 285–289.

Zahiri, N., and Rau, M. E. (1998). Oviposition attraction and repellency of *Aedes aegypti* (Diptera: Culicidae) to waters from conspecific larvae subjected to crowding, confinement, starvation, or infection. *J. Med. Entomol.* **35,** 782–787.

Zahiri, N., Rau, M. E., and Davis, D. J. (1997a). Oviposition responses of *Aedes aegypti* and *Ae.atropalpus* (Diptera: Culicidae) females to waters from conspecific and heterospecific normal larve and from larvae infected with *Plagiorchis elegans* (Trematoda: Plagiorchiidae). *J. Med. Entomol.* **34,** 565–568.

Zahiri, N., Rau, M. E., and Lewis, D. J. (1997b). Starved larvae of *Aedes aegypti* (Diptera: Culicidae) render waters unattractive to ovipositing conspecific females. *Environ. Entomol.* **26,** 1087–1090.

Zahiri, N., Rau, M. E., Lewis, D. J., and Khanizadeh, S. (1997c). Intensity and site of *Plagiorchis elegans* (Trematoda: Plagiorchiidae) infections in *Aedes aegypti* (Diptera; Culicidae)Larvae affect the attractiveness of their waters to ovipositing conspecific females. *Environ. Entomol.* **26,** 920–923.

Zeichner, B. C., and Perich, M. J. (1999). Laboratory testing of a lethal ovitrap for *Aedes aegypti*. *Med. Vet. Entomol.* **13,** 234–238.

Zhang, L. Y., and Lei, C. L. (2008). Evaluation of sticky ovitraps for the surveillance of *Aedes* (Stegomyia) *albopictus* (Skuse) and the screening of oviposition attractants from organic infusions. *Ann. Trop. Med. Parasitol.* **102,** 399–407.

Zhang, J., Liu, X., Kong, J., Zhang, Z., and Bai, Y. (1994). Synthesis and species specific attractancy of an oviposition attractant pheromone of *Culex pipiens quinquefasciatus*. *Acta Parasitol. Med. Entomol. Sin.* **1,** 45–50.

Index

P

Q

R

S

Kolibri 360 GmbH
Ferdinand-Jühlke-Straße 7
99095 Erfurt, Deutschland
produktsicherheit@kolibri360.de